HESI

Comprehensive Review for the

NCLEX-PN®
EXAMINATION

Edition 4

Editors

Sandra Upchurch, PhD, RN

Traci Henry, MSN, RN

Rosemary Pine, PhD, RN, BC, CDE

Amy Rickles, MA

Tina Cuellar, PhD, RN, P/MHCNS-BC

ELSEVIER

3251 Riverport Lane
St. Louis, Missouri 63043

HESI COMPREHENSIVE REVIEW FOR THE NCLEX-PN®
EXAMINATION, FOURTH EDITION   ISBN: 978-1-4557-5106-8
Copyright © 2015, 2012, 2008 by Elsevier Inc.

Notices

Knowledge and best practice in this field are constantly changing. As new research and experience broaden our understanding, changes in research methods, professional practices, or medical treatment may become necessary.

Practitioners and researchers must always rely on their own experience and knowledge in evaluating and using any information, methods, compounds, or experiments described herein. In using such information or methods they should be mindful of their own safety and the safety of others, including parties for whom they have a professional responsibility.

With respect to any drug or pharmaceutical products identified, readers are advised to check the most current information provided (i) on procedures featured or (ii) by the manufacturer of each product to be administered, to verify the recommended dose or formula, the method and duration of administration, and contraindications. It is the responsibility of practitioners, relying on their own experience and knowledge of their patients, to make diagnoses, to determine dosages and the best treatment for each individual patient, and to take all appropriate safety precautions.

To the fullest extent of the law, neither the Publisher nor the authors, contributors, or editors, assume any liability for any injury and/or damage to persons or property as a matter of products liability, negligence or otherwise, or from any use or operation of any methods, products, instructions, or ideas contained in the material herein.

NANDA International Nursing Diagnoses: Definitions and Classifications 2012-2014; Herdman T.H. (ED); copyright © 2012, 1994-2012 NANDA International; Published by John Wiley & Sons, Limited.

NCLEX®, NCLEX-RN®, and NCLEX-PN® are Registered Trademarks of the National Council of State Boards of Nursing, Inc.

Library of Congress Cataloging-in-Publication Data

HESI comprehensive review for the NCLEX-PN examination/editors, Sandra Upchurch, Traci Henry, Rosemary Pine, Amy Rickles. – Edition 4.
      p. ; cm.
  Comprehensive review for the NCLEX-PN examination
  Includes bibliographical references and index.
  ISBN 978-1-4557-5106-8 (pbk. : alk. paper)
  I. Upchurch, Sandra L., editor of compilation. II. Henry, Traci, editor of compilation. III. Pine, Rosemary, editor of compilation. IV. Rickles, Amy, editor of compilation. V. HESI (Firm), issuing body. VI. Title: Comprehensive review for the NCLEX-PN examination.
  [DNLM: 1. Nursing, Practical–Examination Questions. 2. Nursing, Practical–Outlines. 3. Nursing Care–Examination Questions. 4. Nursing Care–Outlines. 5. Nursing Process–Examination Questions. 6. Nursing Process–Outlines. WY 18.2]
  RT62
  610.7306'93076--dc23   2013032249

Executive Content Strategist: Kristin Geen
Associate Content Development Specialist: Laura Goodrich
Publishing Services Manager: Deborah L. Vogel
Project Manager: John W. Gabbert
Design Direction: Brian Salisbury

Printed in China

Last digit is the print number: 9 8 7 6 5 4 3 2 1

CONTRIBUTING AUTHORS

Joanna E. Cain, BSN, BA, RN
President & Founder
Auctorial Pursuits, Inc.
Austin, Texas

REVIEWERS

Linda Ann Aubrey, MSN, CMSRN, CNE
Retention and Recruitment Instructor for Nursing Department
Delaware Technical Community College – Owens Campus
Georgetown, Delaware

Kristen Bagby, RN, MSN, CNL
Saint Peters, Missouri

Carol Deresz Barrera, MSN, RNC-OB
Clinical Assistant Professor
University of Texas Health Science Center at San Antonio School of Nursing
San Antonio, Texas

Terry Bichsel, RN, BSN
Practical Nursing Coordinator
Moberly Area Community College
Moberly, Missouri

Barbara Callahan, RN, NCC, MEd
ADN Program Faculty
Lenoir Community College
Kinston, North Carolina

Judy Carlyle, MNSc, RN
ARNEC Faculty/Clinical Liaison
Cossatot Community College, University of Arkansas
Nashville, Arkansas

Kim Clevenger, EdD, MSN, RN, BC
Associate Professor of Nursing
BSN & RN-BSN Program Coordinator
Morehead State University
Grayson, Kentucky

Linda Crawford, RN, MSN
Lead Instructor for PN to ADN Courses
Trident Technical College
Charleston, South Carolina

Mattie Davis, DNP, RN
Nursing Instructor
JF Drake State College
Huntsville, Alabama

Kathy A. Dillard, RN
Instructor
School Nurse, K-12th grades
Bossier Parish School System
Dealing, Louisiana

Mary L. Dowell, PhD, RN, BC
Assistant Professor
San Antonio College
San Antonio, Texas

Laura R. Durbin, BSN, RN, CHPN
Assistant Professor
West Kentucky Community and Technical College
Paducah, Kentucky

Gretchen N. Ezaki, RN, MSN
Nursing Instructor
Fresno City College
Fresno, California

Abimbola Farinde, PharmD.,MS
Clinical Pharmacist Specialist
Clear Lake Regional Medical Center
Webster, Texas

Margie L. Francisco, EdD(c), MSN, RN
Nursing Professor
Illinois Valley Community College
Oglesby, Illinois

Crystal Gillihan, MHA, BSN, RN
ARNEC Director
Arkansas Rural Nursing Education Consortium
Mountain View, Arkansas

Susan Golden, MSN, RN
Interim Dean of Health
Eastern New Mexico University-Roswell
Roswell, New Mexico

Jennifer Heck, MS, RNC-NIC, CNE
Instructor
East Central University
Ada, Oklahoma

Judith M. Hochberger, PhD, MS, RN
Assistant Professor of Nursing
Roseman University of Health Sciences Henderson, Nevada

Tiffany Jakubowski, RN
Adjunct Faculty
Front Range Community College
Longmont, Colorado

Christina D. Keller, RN, MSN-Educator
Instructor
Radford University Clinical Simulation Center
Fairlawn, Virginia

Hana Malik, RN, MSN, FNP-BC
Academic Director
Illinois College of Nursing
Lombard, Illinois

Janet H. McClintock, RN, MSN, LPC, MS
Coordinator of Clinical Education
Rogers Memorial Hospital
West Allis, Wisconsin

Jane V. McCloskey, RN, MSN
Faculty
Carolinas College of Health Sciences
Charlotte, North Carolina

Linda C. Nance, EdD, RN-BC, MSN, FNP
Professor of Nursing Curriculum
    Development Facilitator
Scottsdale Community College
Scottsdale, Arizona

Jennifer Ponto, RN, BSN
Faculty, Vocational Nursing
    Program
South Plains College
Levelland, Texas

Margaret R. Rateau, PhD, RN, CNE
Associate Professor of Nursing
Kent State University-Columbiana
    at East Liverpool
Liverpool, Ohio

Susan D. Rymer, RN, MSN
Assistant Professor of Nursing
Bellin College
Green Bay, Wisconson

Russlyn A. St. John, RN, MSN
Professor, Practical Nursing
St. Charles Community College
Cottleville, Missouri

Lisa Tardo-Green, MSN, RN
ADN Faculty/Simulation & Skills
    Lab Coordinator
Cabarrus College of Health
    Sciences
Concord, North Carolina

Anne Van Landingham, RN, BSN, MSN
Nursing Instructor Practical
    Nursing Program
Orlando Tech
Casselberry, Florida

Laura C. Williams, MSN, CNS, ONC, CCNS
Orthopedic Clinical Nurse
    Specialist
Orlando Regional Medical Center
Orlando, Florida

Donna Wilsker, MSN, RN
Assistant Professor
Lamar University
Beaumont, Texas

The editors and publisher would also like to acknowledge the following individuals for their contributions to the previous editions of this book:

Mary Anderson, RN, MSN, CNS
Elizabeth Arnold, RN, MSN, CNS
Sara Bishop, PhD, RNC
Mary Ann Boyd, PhD, DNS, APRN, BC
Mary Cassem, RN, MS
Daria M. Close, RN, MSN
Carol L. Collins, RN, MS
Nancy Cox, RN, CCRN
Pat Crotwell, RN, MSN
Debra Danforth, RN, MS, ARNP
Deborah Davenport, RN, MSN, CCRN
Judith Driscoll, RN, MEd, MSN
Karen F. Duncan, RN, MS
Laurie K. Erford, RN, MSN
Jean Flick, RN, MS
Judy Hammond, PhD, RNC
Patricia Handley, MSN, RN
Mary M. Hinds, PhD, RN, CNS
Judy R. Hyland, MS, RN
Florence Jemes, RN, MSN, CS

Jean Joublanc, MSN, RN, CS
Barbara Kearney, PhD, RN
Robin Lockhart, PhD(c), RN
Mary Lou Martin, RN, MSN, CPNP
Jane Mathis, RNC, MSN, CCE
Kathleen Mikilitus, MPA, RN, CNA
Susan Morrison, PhD, RN
Lee Nelson, MSN, RN
Susan Nelson, MSN, RN
Ainslie Nibert, PhD, RN
Leslie Pafford, MSN, RN, FNP
Lorene Payne, MSN, RN
Cynthia K. Peterson, RN, MSN
Phyllis L. Rowe, MSN, RN, ANP
Judy Siefert, MSN, RN
Sylvia Stone, MSN, RN, CNS
Betty Tracy, RN, MN
Cheryle Whitney, MSN, RN, BC
Mary Yoho, PhD, RN

PREFACE

Welcome to *HESI Comprehensive Review for the NCLEX-PN® Examination* with online study exams by HESI.

Congratulations! This outstanding review manual with the companion Evolve site is designed to prepare nursing students for what is very likely the most important examination they will ever take, the NCLEX-PN Licensing Examination. As a graduate of a PN Nursing program, the student has the basic knowledge required to pass tests and perform safely and successfully in the clinical area. *HESI Comprehensive Review for the NCLEX-PN Examination* with companion Evolve site allows the nursing student to prepare for the NCLEX-PN licensure exam in a structured way.

- Organize basic nursing knowledge previously learned.
- Review content learned during basic nursing curriculum.
- Identify weaknesses in content knowledge, so study efforts can be focused appropriately.
- Develop test-taking skills so application of safe nursing practice from knowledge can be demonstrated.
- Reduce anxiety level by increasing ability to correctly answer NCLEX-type questions.
- Boost test-taking confidence by being well prepared and knowing what to expect.

Organization

Chapter 1, *Introduction to the NCLEX-PN® Examination,* gives an overview of the NCLEX-PN Licensing Exam history and test plan for the examination. A review of the nursing process (updated with the latest NANDA-approved nursing diagnoses), client needs, and prioritizing nursing care is also presented.

Chapter 2, *Leadership and Management,* reviews the legal aspects of nursing, leadership, and management, along with disaster nursing.

Chapter 3, *Advanced Clinical Concepts,* presents nursing assessment (data collection), analysis (nursing diagnosis), planning, and intervention at the practical nurse level. Respiratory failure, shock, disseminated intravascular coagulation (DIC), resuscitation, fluid and electrolyte balance, acid-base balance, ECG, perioperative care, HIV, pain, and death and grief are reviewed.

Chapters 4 through 8, *Medical-Surgical Nursing, Pediatric Nursing, Maternity Nursing, Psychiatric Nursing,* and ***Gerontologic Nursing,*** are presented in traditional clinical areas.

Each clinical area is divided into physiologic components, but essential knowledge about basic anatomy, medications, nutrition, communication, client and family education, acute and chronic care, leadership and management, and clinical decision-making are integrated throughout the different components.

Open-ended style questions appear at the end of each chapter, which encourage the student to think in depth about the content presented throughout the individual chapter. When a variety of learning mechanisms are used, students have the opportunity to comprehensively prepare for the NCLEX. These strategies include:

- Reading the review book.
- Discussing content with others.
- Answering open-ended questions.
- Practicing with study exams that simulate the licensure examination.

These learning experiences are all different ways that students should use to prepare for the NCLEX. The purpose of the open-ended questions appearing at the end of the chapter is not a focused practice session on managing NCLEX-style multiple-choice questions, but instead this learning approach allows for more in-depth thinking about the particular topics in the chapter. Practice with multiple-choice style questions alone cannot provide the depth of critical thinking and analysis possible with the short–answer-style questions at the end of the chapter. Additionally, the open-ended questions provide a summary experience that helps students focus on the main topics that were covered in the chapter. Teachers use open–ended-style questions to stimulate the critical-thinking process, and *HESI Comprehensive Review for the NCELX-PN Examination* facilitates the critical-thinking process by posing the same type of questions the teacher might ask.

When students need to practice multiple-choice style questions, the Study Exams offer extensive opportunities for practice and skill-building to improve their test-taking abilities. The Study Exams contain seven content-specific exams (Medical-Surgical Nursing, Pharmacology, Pediatrics, Fundamentals, Maternity, Psychiatric-Mental Health Nursing, and Gerontology) and two comprehensive exams patterned after categories on the NCLEX. The Study Exams can be accessed as many times as necessary, and no questions are repeated. For instance, the Medical Surgical exam does not contain questions that are on the Pediatrics exam. The purpose of providing these exams is to allow practice and exposure to the critical-thinking–style questions that students will encounter on the NCLEX-PN. However, the Study Exams should not be used to predict performance on the NCLEX. Only the HESI Exit Exam—a secure, computerized exam that simulates the NCLEX test plan and has evidenced-based results from numerous research studies indicating a high level of accuracy in predicting NCLEX success—is offered as a true predictor of NCLEX performance. Students are allowed unlimited practice on each Study Exam so that they can have the opportunity to review all of the rationales for the questions.

Here is a plan for student to use with the companion Evolve site:

- Trial 1: Take the PN Practice Exam without studying for it to see your areas of strengths and weaknesses.
- Trial 2: After going over the content that relates to the practice questions on a particular practice test (for instance, Pediatrics, Medical-Surgical, Maternity, etc.), review that section of the manual and take the test again to determine whether you have been able to improve your scores.
- Trial 3: Purposely miss every question on the exam so that you can view rationales for every question.
- Trial 4: Take the exam again under timed conditions at the pace that you would have to progress in order to complete the NCLEX in the time allowed (approximately 1 minute per question). Find out whether being placed under timing constraints affects your performance.
- Trial 5: Put the exam away for a while, and continue review and remediation with other textbook resources, results of any secure exams that you are taking at your school, etc. Take the practice exams again following this study period to see whether your performance improves after in-depth study and following a few weeks' break from these questions.

Trial 5 represents a good activity in preparation for the HESI Exit Exam presented in your final semester of the program, especially if you have not used the Evolve question site for several weeks. Repeated exposure to the questions, however, will make them less useful over time because students tend to memorize the answers. For this reason, these tests are useful only for practice and are not a prediction of NCLEX-PN success. The tendency to memorize the questions after viewing them multiple times falsely elevates the student's scores on the study exams.

Additional assistance for students to study for the NCLEX-PN Licensing Examination can be obtained from a variety of products in the Elsevier family. Many nursing schools have also adopted the following resources:

- HESI Examinations—A comprehensive set of examinations designed to prepare nursing students for the NCLEX exam. They enable customized remediation from Mosby and Saunders textbooks that saves time for faculty and students. Each student is given an individualized report detailing exam results and is allowed to view questions and rationales for items that were answered incorrectly. The electronic remediation, a complimentary feature of the HESI specialty and exit exams, can be obtained on the subject matter in which the student did not answer a question correctly.
- HESI-PN Practice Test—A test that provides an introduction to real-world client situations with critical thinking questions. These questions cover nursing care for clients with a wide range of physiologic and psychosocial alterations and a related coordination of client care, pharmacology, and nursing concepts.
- HESI Complete PN Case Study Collection—Prepares students to manage complex patient conditions and make sound clinical judgments. These online case studies cover a broad range of physiologic and psychosocial alterations, in addition to related coordination of care, pharmacology, and therapeutic concepts.
- HESI Live Review—A Live Review Course presented by an expert faculty member who has received training by the Manager of Review Courses for Elsevier Review and Testing. Students are presented with a workbook and practice NCLEX-style questions that are used during the course.
- eBooks—Online versions of the all Mosby and Saunders textbooks used in the student's Nursing Curriculum. Search across titles, highlight, make notes, and more—all on your PC.
- Elsevier Simulations—Using virtual clinical cases, standardized simulation scenarios, and electronic documentation software, Elsevier Simulations allow students to practice and apply skills in a controlled, monitored environment.
- Evolve Courses—Created by experts using instructional design principles, this interactive content engages students with reading, animation, video, audio, interactive exercises, and assessments.

CONTENTS

INTRODUCTION TO TESTING AND THE NCLEX-PN® EXAMINATION

The NCLEX-PN Licensing Exam

A. The main purpose of a licensing exam such as the NCLEX-PN is to protect the public.
B. The NCLEX-PN:
   1. Developed by the National Council of State Boards of Nursing.
   2. Administered by the State Board of Nursing.
   3. Designed to test the candidate's capability for safe and effective nursing practice by measuring current, entry-level practical nursing behavior.

Job Analysis Studies

A. *"Essential"* knowledge on the NCLEX-PN test is determined by practice analysis studies.
B. Practical nurses (PNs or vocational nurses [VNs]) submit statements about the frequency of nursing activities and the related impact on client safety.

> **HESI Hint** • The 2012 LPN/VN Practice Analysis: Linking the NCLEX-PN Examination to Practice (Vol. 58) determines how frequently new practical nurses perform more than 150 different types of nursing care activities. From the analysis, the 2014 NCLEX-PN Test Plan (Effective April 1st, 2014) identifies four major client needs categories, and two of those categories are further divided into a total of six subcategories and five fundamental nursing processes. They provide a basis for establishing a minimum level of knowledge and skills for PNs to use with a diverse patient population, in any setting, and within the laws and rules of each state (Table 1-1, *Client Needs*, and Table 1-2, *Practical/Vocational Nursing Processes*).

> **HESI Hint** • For more information on the NCLEX-PN Test Plan and content related to each category go to *www.ncsbn.org*.

The Nursing Process and Nursing Diagnoses

A. PN role in the nursing process: Practical nurses use the nursing process to critically think and problem solve (see Table 1-2).
B. Practical nurses assist the health care team to gather and organize data and recognize client needs and problems regardless of the client's developmental stage or the health care setting. They also assist the RN in formulating nursing diagnoses and developing plans of care.
C. The National Conference of the North American Nursing Diagnosis Association (NANDA) guides nurses in the selection of nursing interventions for the purpose of achieving specific outcomes; outcomes and interventions are associated with specific diagnoses (Table 1-3, *Components of a Nursing Diagnosis*, and Box 1-1, *NANDA-Approved Nursing Diagnoses*).

> **HESI Hint** • A nursing diagnosis is not a medical diagnosis because a nursing diagnosis:
> Is subject to nursing management.
> May/may not come from a medical diagnosis.
> Is formulated and written by nurses.
> Is implemented from nursing orders (care plan and nursing interventions).

Prioritizing Nursing Care on NCLEX-PN

A. Many NCLEX-PN test items are designed to test your ability to set priorities.
B. Some examples include:
   1. Identify the MOST IMPORTANT client needs.
   2. Identify the MOST IMPORTANT nursing intervention.
   3. Which nursing action should be done FIRST?
   4. Which client should be cared for FIRST?

Exam Item Formats

A. Several different item types (alternate item formats) are presented on the NCLEX-PN examination.

TABLE 1-1 **Client Needs**

Category of Client Needs	% of NCLEX-PN Test	Practical Nursing Actions	Category of Client Needs	% of NCLEX-PN Test	Practical Nursing Actions
Safe and Effective Care Environment • Coordinated Care • Safety and Infection Control	16%-22% 10%-16%	**Coordinated Care** • Advance Directive • Advocacy • Client Care Assignments • Collaboration with Interdisciplinary Team • Concepts of Management and Supervision • Confidentiality/Information Security • Continuity of Care • Establishing Priorities • Ethical Practice • Informed Consent • Information Technology • Legal Responsibility • Performance Improvement (Quality Improvement) • Referral Process • Resource Management **Safety and Infection Control** • Accident/Error/Injury Prevention • Emergency Response Plan • Ergonomic Principles • Handling Hazardous and Infectious Materials • Home Safety • Reporting of Incident/Event/Irregular Occurrence/Variance • Least Restrictive Restraints and Safety Devices • Safe Use of Equipment • Security Plan • Standard Precautions/Transmission-Based Precautions/Surgical Asepsis	Psychosocial Integrity	8%-14%	• Abuse and Neglect • Behavioral Management • Chemical and other dependencies • Coping Mechanisms • Crisis Interventions • Cultural Awareness • End-of-life Concepts • Grief and Loss • Mental Health Concepts • Religious and Spiritual Influences on Health • Sensory/Perceptual Alterations • Stress Management • Support Systems • Therapeutic Communication • Therapeutic Environment
Health Promotion and Maintenance	7%-13%	• Aging Process • Ante/Intra/Postpartum and New-born Care • Data Collection Techniques • Developmental Stages and Transitions • Health Promotion/Disease Prevention • High Risk Behaviors • Lifestyle Choices • Self-care	Physiologic Integrity • Basic Care and Comfort • Pharmacologic Therapies • Reduction of Risk Potential • Physiologic Adaptation	7%-13% 11%-17% 10%-16% 7%-13%	**Basic Care and Comfort** • Assistive Devices • Elimination • Mobility/Immobility • Nonpharmacological Comfort Interventions • Nutrition and Oral Hydration • Personal Hygiene • Rest and Sleep **Pharmacological Therapies** • Adverse Effects/Contraindications/Side Effects/Interactions • Dosage Calculations • Expected Actions/Outcomes • Medication Administration • Pharmacological Pain Management **Reduction of Risk Potential** • Changes/Abnormalities in Vital Signs • Diagnostic Tests • Laboratory Values • Potential for Alterations in Body Systems • Potential for Complications of Diagnostic Tests/Treatments/Procedures • Potential for Complications from Surgical Procedures and Health Alterations • Therapeutic Procedures **Physiological Adaption** • Alterations in Body Systems • Basic Pathophysiology • Fluid and Electrolyte Imbalances • Medical Emergencies • Unexpected Responses to Therapies

Based on the results of the *2014 LPN/VN Practice Analysis: Linking the NCLEX-PN Examination to Practice (Vol. 58).* The percentages indicate the amount of questions written for each client need category in the *2011 NCLEX-PN Test Plan.*
Adapted from National Council of State Boards of Nursing, Inc. NCLEX-PN Examination: Test Plan for the National Council Licensure Examination for Licensure Practical/Vocational Nurses, 2011, Chicago, IL. *www.ncsbn.org.*

1. The majority of the questions are multiple-choice items with four choices (answers) from which to choose one correct answer.
2. Multiple-response items require the candidate to select one or more responses from five to seven choices. The item instructs the candidate to choose *all* that apply.
3. Fill-in-the-blank questions require the candidate to calculate the answer and type in the numbers.
4. Hot-spot items require the candidate to identify an area on a picture or graph and click on the area.
5. Chart/exhibit format presents a chart or exhibit that the candidate needs to read to be able to answer the problem.
6. Ordered response items require a candidate to rank order or move options to provide the correct order of actions or events.

BOX 1-1   *NANDA-Approved Nursing Diagnoses—cont'd*

F—cont'd
Interrupted **Family** Processes
Readiness for Enhanced **Family** Processes
Fatigue
Fear
Ineffective Infant **Feeding** Pattern
Readiness for Enhanced **Fluid** Balance
Risk for Imbalanced **Fluid** Volume
Deficient **Fluid** Volume
Excess **Fluid** Volume
Risk for Deficient **Fluid** Volume

G
Impaired **Gas** Exchange
Risk for Dysfunctional **Gastrointestinal** Motility
Dysfunctional **Gastrointestinal** Motility
Risk for Ineffective **Gastrointestinal** Perfusion
Grieving
Complicated **Grieving**
Risk for Complicated **Grieving**
Risk for Disproportionate **Growth**
Delayed **Growth** and Development

H
Deficient Community **Health**
Risk-Prone **Health** Behavior
Ineffective **Health** Maintenance
Impaired **Home** Maintenance
Readiness for Enhanced **Hope**
Hopelessness
Risk for Compromised **Human** Dignity
Hyperthermia
Hypothermia

I
Readiness for Enhanced **Immunization** Status
Ineffective **Impulse** Control
Functional Urinary **Incontinence**
Overflow Urinary **Incontinence**
Reflex Urinary **Incontinence**
Stress Urinary **Incontinence**
Urge Urinary **Incontinence**
Risk for Urge Urinary **Incontinence**
Bowel **Incontinence**
Risk for **Infection**
Risk for **Injury**
Insomnia
Decreased **Intracranial** Adaptive Capacity

J
Neonatal **Jaundice**
Risk for Neonatal **Jaundice**

K
Deficient **Knowledge**
Readiness for Enhanced **Knowledge**

L
Latex Allergy Response

Risk for **Latex** Allergy Response
Sedentary **Lifestyle**
Risk for Impaired **Liver** Function
Risk for **Loneliness**

M
Risk for Disturbed **Maternal-Fetal** Dyad
Impaired **Memory**
Impaired Bed **Mobility**
Impaired Physical **Mobility**
Impaired Wheelchair **Mobility**
Moral Distress

N
Nausea
Unilateral **Neglect**
Noncompliance
Readiness for Enhanced **Nutrition**
Imbalanced **Nutrition**: Less Than Body Requirements
Imbalanced **Nutrition**: More Than Body Requirements

O
Impaired **Oral** Mucous Membrane

P
Acute **Pain**
Chronic **Pain**
Impaired **Parenting**
Readiness for Enhanced **Parenting**
Risk for Impaired **Parenting**
Risk for Perioperative **Positioning** Injury
Risk for **Peripheral** Neurovascular Dysfunction
Disturbed **Personal** Identity
Risk for Disturbed **Personal** Identity
Risk for **Poisoning**
Posttrauma Syndrome
Risk for **Posttrauma** Syndrome
Readiness for Enhanced **Power**
Powerlessness
Risk for **Powerlessness**
Ineffective **Protection**

R
Rape-Trauma Syndrome
Ineffective **Relationship**
Readiness for Enhanced **Relationship**
Risk for Ineffective **Relationship**
Impaired **Religiosity**
Readiness for Enhanced **Religiosity**
Risk for Impaired **Religiosity**
Relocation Stress Syndrome
Risk for **Relocation** Stress Syndrome
Risk for Ineffective **Renal** Perfusion
Impaired Individual **Resilience**
Readiness for Enhanced **Resilience**
Risk for Compromised **Resilience**
Parental **Role** Conflict
Ineffective **Role** Performance

Continued

BOX 1-1 *NANDA-Approved Nursing Diagnoses—cont'd*

S
Bathing **Self-Care** Deficit
Dressing **Self-Care** Deficit
Feeding **Self-Care** Deficit
Toileting **Self-Care** Deficit
Readiness for Enhanced **Self-Care**
Readiness for Enhanced **Self-Concept**
Chronic Low **Self-Esteem**
Situational Low **Self-Esteem**
Risk for Chronic Low **Self-Esteem**
Risk for Situational Low **Self-Esteem**
Ineffective **Self-Health** Management
Readiness for Enhanced **Self-Health** Management
Risk for **Self-Mutilation**
Self-Mutilation
Self-Neglect
Sexual Dysfunction
Ineffective **Sexuality** Pattern
Risk for **Shock**
Impaired **Skin** Integrity
Risk for Impaired **Skin** Integrity
Sleep Deprivation
Readiness for Enhanced **Sleep**
Disturbed **Sleep** Pattern
Impaired **Social** Interaction
Social Isolation
Chronic **Sorrow**
Spiritual Distress
Risk for **Spiritual** Distress
Readiness for Enhanced **Spiritual** Well-Being
Stress Overload
Risk for **Suffocation**

Risk for **Suicide**
Delayed **Surgical** Recovery
Impaired **Swallowing**

T
Ineffective Family **Therapeutic** Regimen Management
Risk for **Thermal** Injury
Ineffective **Thermoregulation**
Impaired **Tissue** Integrity
Ineffective Peripheral **Tissue** Perfusion
Risk for Decreased Cardiac **Tissue** Perfusion
Risk for Ineffective Cerebral **Tissue** Perfusion
Risk for Ineffective Peripheral **Tissue** Perfusion
Impaired **Transfer** Ability
Risk for **Trauma**

U
Impaired **Urinary** Elimination
Readiness for Enhanced **Urinary** Elimination
Urinary Retention

V
Risk for **Vascular** Trauma
Impaired Spontaneous **Ventilation**
Dysfunctional **Ventilatory** Weaning Response
Risk for Other-Directed **Violence**
Risk for Self-Directed **Violence**

W
Impaired **Walking**
Wandering

In order to make safe and effective judgments using NANDA-I nursing diagnoses, it is essential that nurses refer to the definitions and defining characteristics of the diagnoses listed in this work. For more information, see *www.nanda.org*.

B. Pearson VUE is responsible for adapting the NCLEX-PN exam to the CAT format, processing candidate applications, and transmitting test results to its data center for scoring.
C. The NCSBN generates the NCLEX-PN test items.

Understanding CAT

A. NCLEX-PN consists of 85 to 205 multiple-choice or alternative format items.
B. The candidate is presented with a test item.
   1. If the question is answered correctly, a slightly more difficult item follows, and the level of difficulty increases with each item until an item is missed.
   2. If the question is answered incorrectly, a slightly less difficult item follows, and the level of difficulty decreases with each item until the candidate answers an item correctly.
C. The process continues until the candidate has achieved a definite "pass" or "fail" score. A message indicating

that the candidate has completed the exam appears on the screen.
D. The item number the candidate is currently answering appears in the upper right side of the screen.
E. The greatest number of items appearing on your exam is 205.

Taking the Test

A. A test administrator provides each candidate with an erasable note board that may be replaced as needed while testing. A candidate may not bring his or her own note boards, scratch paper, or writing instruments to the exam.
B. You must answer each question before proceeding to the next one. Returning to a question or skipping a question is not allowed during testing. You will not be able to change an answer once you proceed to the next question; this works in your favor.
C. When taking the exam, read carefully and maintain a reasonable pace.

Time Frame and Breaks

A. The candidate receives up to 5 hours to complete the exam. The 5 hours include a tutorial, sample questions, breaks, and completion of the examination.

B. Two programmed optional breaks are given, one after 2 hours of testing and another after 3½ hours of testing. A candidate may take an unscheduled break at any time. All breaks count against testing time.

C. When candidates take a break, they must leave the testing room and will be required to provide a fingerprint before and after the break.

Results and Scoring

A. When the candidate answers the minimum number of items (85) and has performed with 95% certainty above or below the passing standard, the computer test stops and calculates that the candidate has passed or failed.

B. If a candidate has answered the maximum number of items (205) and is not at the end of the 5-hour limit, the candidate's ability estimate is precise. So if the ability estimate is at or above the passing standard, the candidate passes, and if the ability estimate is at or below the passing standard, the candidate fails.

C. If a candidate has run out of time (5-hour limit) and has not answered the maximum number of items (205) but shows a consistent pattern above the passing standard, then the candidate will pass even if he or she has run out of time.

D. A specific passing score is recommended by the NCSBN. All states require the same score to pass, so if you pass in one state, you are eligible to practice nursing in any other state.

> **HESI Hint** • Results are not given at the testing centers. Results are mailed to the candidate by the boards of nursing about 1 month after taking the examination. The testing center staff does not have access to test results. The NCSBN does not want the testing center to be in a position of managing candidates' reactions to scores, nor does it want those waiting to take their exams to be influenced by such reactions.

Item Strategy

A. Every question must be answered to move to the next question, so make your best guess if you are not sure of the answer.

B. One or more choices are likely to be very wrong. Quickly eliminate those choices that do not answer the question.

C. Decide between two choices by:
   1. Rereading the question for qualifiers or other words that specify what the question is asking.
   2. Rereading the choices and deciding what makes them different from one another.
   3. Examining the choice; it may contain correct information but not answer the question.
   4. Using information from Maslow's Hierarchy of Needs (Table 1-4) or Erikson's Stages of Development (Table 1-5) to choose the correct response.

D. Trust your instincts. The first response you have is a gut instinct and is an educated guess. Do not second-guess yourself.

Tips for NCLEX-PN Success

Overall Planning

A. Eat a well-balanced diet and drink plenty of water.

B. Maintain a normal exercise program. This is the perfect activity for a study break.

C. Get plenty of sleep while studying because you will study more efficiently when well rested.

D. Limit your social life for this short period of time before the exam so you have plenty of time to study. This will help you achieve your goal of becoming a nurse.

E. Eliminate alcohol and recreational drugs from your lifestyle because the time involved in their use will waste the time you have to prepare for the test.

F. Avoid negative people and think positively. Stay away from people who have test anxieties or project their problems onto you. Sometimes this person is a fellow classmate, a colleague, or your best friend. They will still be present when the exam is over. Right now you need to take care of yourself; therefore, surround yourself with positive, optimistic people.
   1. Write "I WILL BE SUCCESSFUL!" on a "sticky note" and put it where you will see it every day.
   2. Choose a relaxation and affirmation method that you are comfortable with and that meets your needs.
   3. Repeat to yourself, "I have the knowledge to successfully complete the NCLEX-PN."

Study Skills

Logically, you will study less-familiar topics more than those you have already mastered. When developing a study plan, consider the following:

A. Study plan.
   1. Study every day until you take the exam. Schedule study time on your daily calendar.
   2. Make a list of topics you want to study in order of importance.
   3. Build your confidence by alternating areas of strength with areas that need further review.

B. Vary learning techniques: study alone, in a group, or study content or sample NCLEX-PN questions.

C. Organize the material in each topic. Increasing the time you work with the material will increase your

TABLE 1-4 Maslow's Hierarchy of Needs

Need	Definition	Nursing Implications
Physiologic	Biologic needs for food, shelter, water, sleep, oxygen, sexual expression	The priority biologic need is breathing—that is, an open airway. Review Table 1-1 *Client Needs*, the activities associated with physiologic integrity. If you were asked to identify the *most important* action, you would identify needs associated with physiologic integrity—for example, providing an open airway—as the *most important* nursing action.
Safety	Avoiding harm; attaining security, order, and physical safety	Review Table 1-1 *Client Needs*, the activities associated with Safe and Effective Care Environment. Ensuring that the client's environment is SAFE is a priority—for example, teaching an older client to remove throw rugs that pose a safety hazard when ambulating would have a greater priority than teaching him/her how to use a walker—*first* priority is *SAFETY*, then coping skills, unless coping is a safety issue (e.g., self-harm).
Love and Belonging	Giving and receiving affection; companionship; and identification with a group	Although these needs are important, (described in Table 1-1 *Client Needs*, activities associated with Psychosocial Integrity) they are less important than physiologic or safety needs. For example, it is more important for a client to have an open airway and a safe environment for ambulating than it is to assist him/her to become part of a support group. However, assisting the client in becoming a part of a support group would have higher priority than assisting him/her in developing self-esteem. The sense of belonging would come *first*, and such a sense might help in developing self-esteem.
Esteem and Recognition	Self-esteem and respect of others; success in work; prestige	
Self-Actualization	Fulfillment of unique potential	It is important to understand the last two needs in Maslow's Hierarchy. They could deal with Client Needs associated with Health Promotion and Maintenance such as continued growth and development and self-care, as well as those associated with Psychosocial Integrity. However, you will probably not be asked to prioritize needs at this level. Remember, it is the goal of the Council to ensure SAFE nursing practice, and such practice does not usually deal with the client's self-actualization or aesthetic needs.
Aesthetic	Search for beauty and spiritual goals	

knowledge base and confidence. Use organizational methods such as:
1. Write your own fill-in-the-blank tests.
2. Prepare flash cards.
3. Rewrite material in your own words.
4. Make charts and tables of the material.
5. Label or explain pictures.
D. Rewrite test questions in your own words, with special emphasis on understanding the rationale.
E. Identify areas for further review and seek clarification for complete understanding.
F. Develop test-taking skills to demonstrate your knowledge. This is very important because these skills help increase your ability to:
1. Determine what each question is asking.
2. Eliminate test responses or answers that are obviously incorrect.
3. Identify the best response or prioritize.
G. Know what to expect. Remember: "Knowledge is power" when you know what to expect. In addition, your confidence will soar and your anxiety will decrease.
H. Read the NCLEX-PN Candidate Bulletin.

Test-Day Preparation

A. **Test-Day Checklist:** Gather all necessary materials the night before the exam and put them in a large envelope.

1. Admission ticket
2. Directions to the testing center
3. Identification
4. Money for lunch
5. Glasses or contact lenses
B. **Approved Items:** Candidates are allowed to bring only identification forms into the testing room. The following items are not allowed: watches, candy, chewing gum, food, drinks, purses, wallets, pens, pencils, beepers, cellular phones, Post-it® notes, study materials or aids, or calculators.
C. **Allow Plenty of Traveling Time:** Plan to arrive 30 minutes early. Allow for traffic jams and time for parking. Arriving early will give you a chance to get settled before beginning the test.
D. **Dress Comfortably:** Dress in loose layers so you can adjust your clothing to the temperature of the testing room.
E. **Do Not Discuss the Exam:** Avoid discussing the exam during breaks and while waiting to take the exam.
F. **Avoid Distraction:** If the typing noise of other test takers is a problem, ask the test administrator for earplugs, which are available at each center.

TABLE 1-5 Stages of Development

Stage	Features	Developmental Task
Infant		
0-3 Months	• Posterior fontanel closes • Makes noise when spoken to • Holds head up when prone	• Trust vs. Mistrust: can learn to trust environment, depending on the response to crying, nurturing, and feeding
3-6 Months	• Birth weight doubles, teeth emerge • Sits up, rolls over, makes sounds • Puts objects in mouth	
6-9 Months	• Fears separation from mother • Combines syllables • Transfers objects, crawls	
9-12 Months	• Birth weight triples; anterior fontanel closes by 18 months • Words emerge • Stands alone; begins to walk	
Toddler (1-3 Years)	• Importance of rituals, training, and instruction • Temper tantrums, parallel play • Partial to total toilet training	• Autonomy vs. Shame and Doubt: reassurance and self-respect are obtained through learning, exploring, and independence
Preschool (3-6 Years)	• Conscience develops; learns the rules • Transitions from fantasy to reality; has feelings; fears intrusions into body • Teeth completely emerge; leg and foot growth rapid; tie shoes at 6 years	• Initiative vs. Guilt: performance of activities to gain approval
School-Age (6-12 Years)	• Begin to discard parental standards; competence and perseverance; able to classify; seek sense of accomplishment • Lose baby teeth; develop speed and strength	• Industry vs. Inferiority: working through competition to completion and tangible results
Preadolescent (10-12 Years)	• Variability in growth and maturation • Strong desire to conform	• Preparation for Adolescence
Adolescent (12-18 Years)	• Rational sense of self; actualizes abilities; moral judgment • Confused; indecisive; antisocial • Rapid growth; bone growth completed; secondary sexual features develop	• Identity vs. Inferiority (or Role Confusion): establish independence with ideals and goals, understand and enact adulthood
Young Adult (18-35 Years)	• Leave home; commit to personal relationships and career • Develop a lifestyle; increase responsibility • Physical growth complete; chronic disease is uncommon	• Intimacy vs. Isolation: seek close, personal relationships to develop productivity and contentment
Middle Adult (36-65 Years)	• Desire to accomplish unfilled goals • Examine the past; assess current life; plan for future; and realize mortality • Chronic disease emerges; life subtly changes	• Generativity vs. Stagnation: pursues self-fulfillment for sense of accomplishment
Older Adult	• Desire to find satisfaction with life • Assure housing and relationships • Adjust to losses; manage illness; prepare for death	• Ego Integrity vs. Despair: adjust to aging with self-worth; reflect on life with satisfaction

2

LEADERSHIP AND MANAGEMENT

Legal Aspects of Nursing

Laws Governing Nursing

A. Nurse Practice Acts provide the laws that control the practice of nursing in each state. Under the law, the practice of nursing is restricted to licensed professionals. All states have nursing practice acts, and these laws contain state standards for nursing care.

B. Nurse Practice Acts govern the practical nurse's (PN) responsibility in assigning, supervising, and accepting assignments and making assignments.
   1. Assignments should be commensurate with the nursing personnel's educational preparation, experience, and knowledge.
   2. The PN should supervise care provided by nursing personnel delegated by a registered nurse (RN) or assigned PN. Some states do not authorize PNs to delegate nursing care.
   3. Sterile or invasive procedures should be assigned to and/or supervised by RNs.

Organization of Laws

A. Laws are divided into two large groups: criminal (public) law and civil (private) law. Criminal laws are crimes against the country, state, or local government (Table 2-1, *Organization of Law*). Constitutional, administrative, and criminal are the three types of criminal law. Civil law is separated into two large groups: contract and tort law. Tort law is further divided into intentional and unintentional torts.

Crime

A. Nurses remain bound by all criminal laws, although court cases involving nurses generally involve tort laws. Crimes occur when criminal statutes are violated. These acts are crimes against the state (government), they usually include intent, and they are punishable by the state.

B. A crime is committed when:
   1. The act is contrary to a criminal law or statute.
   2. An act is not performed when a legal obligation exists to perform the act—for example, refusing to assist in childbirth if the refusal results in injury to the child.
   3. Two or more persons agree to commit a crime—that is, criminal conspiracy.
   4. One person is aware a crime is being committed and helps another person in committing the crime. Both participants are equally guilty.
   5. A law is ignored—for example, a nurse observes another nurse removing narcotics from the unit and ignores the observation. Using this concept as a defense is usually ineffective.
   6. Assault is unjustified and not in self-defense. To be justified, only enough force can be used to maintain self-protection.
   7. When child abuse is not reported. It is a nurse's legal responsibility to report suspected child abuse. In some states, reporting elder abuse and domestic violence also is mandated.

Torts

Description: an act involving injury or damage to another, other than a breach of contract, that results in civil liability (i.e., the victim can sue) instead of criminal liability (see Crime). Victims (the plaintiffs) can sue in civil courts (Table 2-2, *Comparison of Nursing Negligence and Malpractice*).

Unintentional Torts

Negligence and Malpractice
A. **Negligence:** performing an act that a reasonable and prudent person would not perform under similar conditions. Negligence includes:
   1. Lack of skill
   2. Errors
   3. Professional misconduct
   4. Failure to act

TABLE 2-1 Organization of Law

Courts	Types of Law	Description	Example
Criminal (public)	Constitutional	• Constitutional and amendments • Government operation	• Right to free speech • Right to vote
	Administrative	• Creates government and official agencies	• Control of nursing through boards of nursing • Nurse Practice Act
	Criminal	• Misdemeanors and felonies	• Theft • Partner abuse
Civil (private)	Contract	• Legally binding agreement between two or more individuals or groups	• Hospital hires an agency nurse • Buying/selling a car
	Tort	• Unintentional • Negligence • Malpractice	• Heat application extending beyond time limit imposed by hospital policy • Amputating the wrong limb
		• Intentional • Assault • Battery • Defamation • False imprisonment • Fraud • Invasion of privacy	• Threatening to withhold pain medication • Performing CPR on a client with a DNR order • Intentionally making damaging verbal or written statements about a client's physician • Unauthorized use of restraints • Providing false documents on an employment application • Releasing test results to the parents of an emancipated minor

CPR, Cardiopulmonary resuscitation; DNR, do not resuscitate.

TABLE 2-2 Comparison of Nursing Negligence and Malpractice

Nursing Negligence	Nursing Malpractice
Leaving a heating pad on a client's skin without damage against institutional policy	Burning a client's skin as a result of leaving a heating pad on against institutional policy
Failing to assess a restrained client as required in institutional policy	Failing to assess a restrained client as required by institutional policy, resulting in a head injury occurring when the client tries to climb out of bed
Failing to notice the warning signs of a myocardial infarction (MI)	Failing to notice the warning signs of an MI, resulting in an acute MI
Forgetting to administer antianginal medication	Forgetting to administer antianginal medication, resulting in an acute MI

B. **Malpractice:** equates to professional negligence. The plaintiff must prove all four of the following elements to prove malpractice:
   1. **Duty:** obligation to maintain a nursing standard—that is, what a reasonable and prudent nurse would do. Nurses are expected to anticipate foreseeable risk. For example, if water is on the floor, the nurse is responsible for anticipating the risk to the client.
   2. **Breach of Duty:** failure to maintain the nursing standard. A reasonable and prudent nurse in the same situation would not have performed this act or performed it in this manner. This is a failure to perform according to the established standard of conduct in providing nursing care.
   3. **Injury/Damages:** a failure to meet the standard of practice caused mental or physical injury or damage to the plaintiff.
   4. **Proximate Cause:** the breach of duty caused the harm, and the nurse's action or lack of action caused harm to the plaintiff. A connection exists between conduct and the resulting injury, referred to as *proximate cause* or *remoteness of damage*.

Intentional Torts
Assault and Battery
A. **Assault:** mental or physical threat to touch without permission—for example, forcing (without touching) a client to take a medication or treatment.
B. **Battery:** touching without permission, with or without the intent to do harm—for example, hitting or striking a client. If a mentally competent adult is forced to have a treatment that he/she has refused, battery occurs.

Invasion of Privacy. Definition: Intrusion into another's body or into confidential information. This includes encroachment or trespassing on another's body and/or personality.

A. **False Imprisonment:** detaining a competent person against his/her will—for example, confinement or use of restraints and protective devices without the client's consent, referred to as confinement without authorization.

B. **Exposure of a Person:** after death, the client has a right to be unobserved, excluded from unwarranted operations, and protected from unauthorized touching of the body.

C. **Defamation:** revealing privileged information.
   1. **Libel:** written statement that may cause harm to a person's reputation.
   2. **Slander:** verbal statement that may cause harm to a person's reputation. This includes divulgence of privileged information or communication—for example, from charts, conversations, or observations.

D. **Fraud:** willful and purposeful misrepresentation resulting in loss or harm to another.

Legal Issues in Practical Nursing

A. **Incident Reports:** Incident reports, or occurrence reports, are an essential part of reducing mistakes and errors, preparing the administration for possible liability claims and the need to investigate events or processes. The reports serve as internal institutional documentation of the event and not as protection for negligence, malpractice, or criminal acts. Incident reports are not a part of the legal record of client care.

B. **Institutional Policies and Procedures:** These rules govern nursing practice and guide nursing actions in a particular institution. They are not laws, but courts generally rule as though they were laws. Institutions can be held liable for poorly formulated or implemented policies.

C. **Client Identification:** This information is used to meet safety goals.
   1. Two client identifiers must be used when taking blood samples or administering medications.
   2. The client room number may *not* be used as an identifier.

Consent

A. Nurses are responsible for obtaining consent forms and ensuring that completed consent forms are on the chart prior to a procedure. Nurses are not responsible for obtaining informed consent (i.e., explaining the procedure to the client). *Informed consent* is consent obtained after the risks and benefits of having or not having the procedure (or treatment) to be performed are explained by the person performing the procedure.

B. The law does not require written consent to perform all medical treatment.
   1. Treatment can be performed if the client has been fully informed about the procedure.
   2. Treatment can be performed if the client voluntarily consents to the procedure.
   3. If informed consent cannot be obtained and immediate treatment is required to save "life or limb," emergency laws, such as the *Good Samaritan Act,* can be applied.

C. **Verbal consent** requires documentation in the client's medical record to:
   1. Describe in detail how and why verbal consent was obtained.
   2. Identify and record the signatures of two witnesses to the consent who are not directly related to the treatment or procedure.

D. **Written consent** requires that the person giving consent, usually the client, be:
   1. Alert, coherent, and an otherwise competent adult.
   2. Parent or legal guardian. Person in "loco parentis" (person standing in for a parent with parental rights, duties, and responsibilities) for a minor or incompetent adult; this also may be called *power of attorney.*

> **HESI Hint** • A minor client 14 years of age and older must agree to treatment, along with his/her legally responsible parent or guardian. Competent, emancipated minors can consent to treatment without the consent of a parent or guardian. The definition of an emancipated minor may vary from state to state.

E. **Surgical consent,** or surgical permit, is obtained before any surgical procedure, however minor the procedure is. The health care provider, the hospital, and the hospital staff are protected against claims of unauthorized procedures. To serve as a legal document, the consent must be:
   1. Written
   2. Obtained voluntarily
   3. Explained to the client and parent or guardian by the person performing the procedure, including in the cases of:
      a. Possible complications and disfigurements
      b. Removal of any organs or body parts
   4. Witnessed
   5. Signed by a competent adult, emancipated minor, or competent parent or guardian

> **HESI Hint** • The Good Samaritan Act protects health care practitioners against malpractice claims for emergency care provided in "good faith" (e.g., a nurse gives aid at the scene to an automobile accident victim). Health care personnel are required to deliver care in a reasonable and prudent manner.

Nursing Practice and the Law

Psychiatric Nursing

A. **Civil Procedures:** methods used to protect the rights of psychiatric clients.
B. **Voluntary Admission:** client admits himself/herself to an institution for treatment and retains civil rights. Client can withdraw from such treatment at any time.
C. **Involuntary Admission:** someone other than the client applies for admission to an institution.
   1. Requires certification by a health care provider and/or a police officer that the person is a danger to self and/or others (depending on the state, one or two health care provider certifications are required).
   2. Individuals have the right to a legal hearing within a certain number of hours or days.
   3. Most states limit commitment to 90 days.
   4. Extended commitment is usually no longer than 1 year.
D. **Emergency Admission:** any adult may apply for emergency detention of another. However, medical or judicial approval is required to detain anyone longer than 24 hours.
   1. Persons held against their will can file a habeas corpus to try to get the court to hear their case and release them.
   2. The court determines the sanity and alleged unlawful restraint of a person.
E. Legal and civil rights of hospitalized clients:
   1. Right to wear their own clothes, keep personal items, and keep a reasonable amount of cash for small purchases.
   2. Right to have individual storage space for their own use.
   3. Right to see visitors daily.
   4. Right to have reasonable access to a telephone and the opportunity to have private conversations by telephone.
   5. Right to receive and send mail (unopened).
   6. Right to refuse shock treatments and/or lobotomy.
F. **Competency Hearing:** legal hearing that is held to determine a person's capability to make responsible decisions about self, dependents, or property.
G. Persons declared incompetent have the legal status of a minor—that is, they cannot:
   1. Vote.
   2. Make contracts or wills.
   3. Drive a car.
   4. Sue or be sued.
   5. Hold a professional license.
H. A guardian is appointed by the court for the incompetent person. Declaring a person incompetent can be initiated by the state or the family.
I. **Determination of Competency**
   1. **Insanity:** a legal term meaning the accused is not criminally responsible for the unlawful act committed because he/she is mentally ill.

   2. **Inability to Stand Trial:** the person accused of committing a crime is not mentally capable of standing trial. He/she:
      a. Cannot understand the charge against him/her.
      b. Must be sent to a psychiatric unit until legally determined competent for trial.
      c. Once the person is mentally fit, he/she must stand trial and serve any sentence, if convicted.

Prescriptions and the Health Care Provider

A. The nurse is required to obtain a health care provider prescription (order) to carry out medical procedures.
B. Although verbal phone prescriptions should be avoided, the nurse should follow the agency's policy and procedures. Failure to follow such rules could be considered *negligence.* The Joint Commission (TJC) requires that organizations implement a process for taking verbal or telephone orders that includes a "read-back" of critical values and prescriptions. The employee receiving the prescription should write the verbal order/critical value on the chart or record it in the computer and then read back the order/value to the health care provider.
C. If a nurse questions a health care provider's prescription because he/she believes it is *wrong* (e.g., the wrong dosage for a medication was prescribed), the nurse should do the following:
   1. Inform the health care provider.
   2. Record that the health care provider was informed and record the health care provider's response to such information.
   3. Inform the nursing supervisor.
   4. Refuse to carry out the prescription.
D. If the nurse believes that a health care provider's prescription was made with *poor judgment* (e.g., the nurse believes the client does not need as many tranquilizers as the health care provider prescribed, the client is difficult to arouse or has slurred speech), the nurse should:
   1. Record that the health care provider was notified and that the prescription was questioned.
   2. Notify the nursing supervisor.
   3. Carry out the prescription if the patient's safety is not jeopardized because a nurse's nursing judgment cannot be substituted for a health care provider's medical judgment.
E. If a nurse is asked to perform a task for which he/she has not been prepared educationally (e.g., obtain a urine specimen from a premature infant by needle aspiration of the bladder) or has not had the necessary experience (e.g., a nurse who has never worked in labor and delivery is asked to perform a vaginal exam and determine cervical dilation), the nurse should do the following:
   1. Inform the health care provider that he/she does not have the education or experience necessary to carry out the prescription.
   2. Refuse to carry out the prescription.

3. Arrange to have an RN supervisor or nurse who is prepared by education and/or experience to carry out the procedure.

> **HESI Hint** • If the nurse carries out a health care provider's prescription for which he/she is not prepared and does not inform the health care provider of his/her lack of preparation, the nurse is solely liable for any damages.
>
> If the nurse informs the health care provider of his/her lack of preparation in carrying out a prescription and carries out the prescription anyway, the nurse and the health care provider are liable for any damages.

F. The nurse cannot, without a health care provider's prescription, alter the amount of drug given to the client. For example, if a health care provider has prescribed pain medication in a certain amount and the client's pain is not, in the nurse's judgment, severe enough to warrant the dosage prescribed, the nurse *cannot* reduce the amount without first checking with the health care provider. Remember, nursing judgment cannot be substituted for medical judgment (unless patient safety is compromised, based on an assessment that the patient is overly sedated [e.g., decreased respirations, falling]).

Restraints

A. Clients may be restrained only under the following circumstances:
   1. In an emergency
   2. For a limited time
   3. For the limited purpose of protecting the client from injury or harm or for the safety of others
B. Nursing responsibilities with regard to restraints:
   1. The nurse must notify the health care provider immediately that the client has been restrained and obtain an order to continue the use of restraints.
   2. The nurse should document the rationale for restraining the client.
C. When restraining a client, the nurse should do the following:
   1. Use the least restrictive restraints, physical or chemical, after exhausting all reasonable alternatives.
   2. Apply the restraints in accordance with facility policy.
   3. Check frequently to see that the restraints do not impair circulation or cause pressure sores or other injuries.
   4. Allow for nutrition, hydration, and stimulation at frequent intervals.
   5. Remove restraints as soon as possible.
   6. Document the need for application, monitoring, and removal of restraints.

> **HESI Hint** • Restraints of any kind may constitute false imprisonment.
>
> Freedom from unlawful restraint is a basic human right and is protected by law.

Health Insurance Portability and Accountability Act of 1996

A. Congress passed the Health Insurance Portability and Accountability Act of 1996 (HIPAA) to create a national client record privacy standard.
B. **Who and What Is Covered?** HIPAA privacy rules pertain to health care providers, health plans, and health clearinghouses and their business partners that engage in computer-to-computer transmission of health care claims, payment and remittance, benefit information, and/or health plan eligibility information, and who disclose personal health information that specifically identifies an individual and is transmitted electronically, in writing, or verbally.
C. Client privacy rights are of key importance. Clients must provide written approval for the disclosure of any of their health information for almost any purpose. Health care providers must offer specific information to clients that explains how their personal health information will be used. Clients must have access to their medical records, and they can receive copies of these and request that changes be made if they identify inaccuracies.
D. Health care providers who do not comply with HIPAA regulations and/or make unauthorized disclosures risk civil and criminal liability.
E. For further information, the U.S. Department of Health and Human Services, Health Information Privacy website contains frequently asked questions about HIPAA at http://www.hhs.gov/ocr/privacy/hipaa/understanding/summary/index.html.

Safe Practice

A. **Assess, Monitor, and Observe:** PN practice requires the necessary skills and knowledge to properly assess (collect data) and monitor, including implementation. Notify the nursing supervisor and/or health care provider, or seek help when appropriate, and evaluate nursing care until the client is stable.
B. **Plan Care:** Maintain and update a written plan for nursing care based on the client's current status.
C. **Implement Nursing Care:** Provide nursing care according to the plan, advocate for the client, intervene to prevent harm, and follow up as necessary.
D. **Implement Specific Nursing Actions:** Respond to the client, reinforce educational information provided to the client, and adequately supervise nursing care provided by others.
E. **Evaluate Nursing Care—Observe, Monitor, Communicate, and Document:** Nurses must know the client's baseline and

current status to observe and appreciate significant changes in the client's condition. Report and document changes, and provide appropriate follow-up care.

F. **Maintain Adequate Documentation:** The client's medical record must be accurate, current, and complete.

Although verbal testimony is considered, courts clearly prefer written documentation.

G. **Work within the Scope of Your Practice:** Perform only those nursing activities outlined in your job description and within your agency policies and procedures.

Review of Legal Aspects of Nursing

1. How does a PN decide whether he/she can perform a procedure?
2. Negligence is measured by how "reasonable" an action is. How does a PN decide whether an action is "reasonable"?
3. What four elements are necessary to prove malpractice?
4. List and define the types of intentional tort cases heard by a civil court.
5. What determines competency? List five activities a person who is declared incompetent cannot do.
6. Under what conditions can a client be involuntarily admitted to a psychiatric facility?
7. Name three legal requirements of a surgical permit.
8. When can a procedure be performed without written consent?
9. What role does a PN have in obtaining consent? Informed consent?
10. What law protects a PN who renders first aid in an emergency? What protection does the law provide in an emergency?
11. What action should a PN take when a prescription or medical order is inappropriate?
12. Describe the nursing care of a restrained client.
13. Describe six client rights guaranteed under HIPAA regulations that PNs must apply to their practice.

Answers to Review

1. Has the PN received sufficient education, training, and experience? Refer to job description, policies, and procedures of the health care facility; be consistent with the state's Nurse Practice Act.
2. Is the action something that a rational, responsible, and prudent nurse would do in a similar situation?
3. *Duty:* nurse was responsible for delivering care; *breach of duty:* failure to perform according to established standards; *causation:* failure to follow the standard resulted in client injury or damage; and *damages:* client suffers a physical, mental, or financial loss.
4. *Assault:* threats or acts that cause fear; *battery:* unauthorized physical contact; *defamation:* using false information to harm another's reputation; *false imprisonment:* unauthorized interference with someone's personal freedom; *fraud:* providing false information with the potential to cause harm; and *invasion of privacy:* failure to protect bodily and confidential property.
5. A person's ability to make responsible decisions; client must be alert, coherent, emancipated, or have a parent or legal guardian. A person declared incompetent cannot vote, make contracts or wills, drive a car, sue or be sued, or hold a professional license.
6. Client is declared a threat to self or others as certified by a licensed health care provider (one or two required). Client must receive a legal hearing shortly after admission; confinement is usually limited to 90 days and may possibly be extended to a 1-year commitment.
7. Must be written, voluntary, informed, witnessed, and signed by a competent adult, emancipated minor, or parent or legal guardian.
8. When the client is fully informed, the client voluntarily agrees to the procedure, verbal consent is obtained, and is necessary to save "life or limb."
9. A PN is responsible for making sure the consent form is signed and in the client's chart. Nurses do not obtain informed consent; that is obtained by the person performing the procedure.
10. The Good Samaritan Law. The person rendering aid is not held liable for civil acts for emergency care rendered "in good faith." The care delivered must be reasonable and prudent.
11. The PN should inform the health care provider, record that the health care provider was informed, and record the health care provider's response to such information. The PN should inform the nursing supervisor and decline to perform the order.
12. Apply restraints according to the manufacturer's instructions and institutional policy; check restraints regularly and frequently; prevent injury from the restraint; record all monitoring; remove restraints as soon as possible; and demonstrate and record repeated efforts to avoid restraint use.

13. Client must give written consent before health care providers can use or disclose personal health information; health care providers must give clients notice about provider responsibilities regarding client confidentiality; clients must have access to their medical records; providers who restrict access must explain why and must offer clients a description of the complaint process; clients have the right to request that changes be made in their medical records to correct inaccuracies; health care providers must follow specific tracking procedures or any disclosures made that ensure accountability for maintenance of client confidentiality; and clients have the right to request that health care providers restrict use and disclosure of their personal health information, although the provider may decline to do so.

Leadership and Management

A. Leaders have specific goals and are able to enlist others to support the goals.
B. Leadership is the process a leader uses to achieve goals. It includes excellent communication skills and the ability to influence others.
C. Managers work to accomplish the goals of an organization, usually the employer.
D. Nurse-managers organize the staff and resources to provide safe, effective client care according to the standards and goals of the institution. Nurse-managers have authority, are responsible to the institution, and support the institutional goals and standards.

Qualities of Effective Leaders

A. **Supportive:** Create a positive environment with open-minded, fair, and consistent behavior; handle conflict.
B. **Assertive:** Make their thoughts, needs, and desires clearly known to others without personal or malicious attacks.
C. **Sensitive and Objective:** Use listening skills and consider other individuals' positions carefully while being able to act based on comprehensive facts.
D. **Responsible:** Are dependable and answerable for personal and group actions.
E. **Facultative:** Provide the necessary motivation, resources, time, and encouragement to meet goals.

> **HESI Hint** • Look for NCLEX-PN questions that demonstrate assertive communication skills.

Effective Leadership Skills

A. **Communication:** Clearly define goals and expectations; provide information and consistent verbal and nonverbal messages.
B. **Organization:** Effectively use human, material, and financial resources to promote goals.
C. **Delegation:** Transfer responsibility and authority for the completion of delegated tasks to another person, but retain responsibility for the task. Delegation must be within the policies and procedures of an institution. In some states it is not legal for the PN to delegate

under his/her state Nurse Practice Act. The PN may assign and supervise tasks to unlicensed assistive personnel (UAP) (Table 2-3, *Role Comparison PN-RN*).
D. **Supervision**
   1. Provide guidance and direction; include instruction, expected outcome, time frame, limits, and understanding of assignment.
   2. Evaluate care: frequently check personnel, communication, and status of task.
   3. Perform follow-up; communicate evaluation findings to appropriate personnel, and teach and guide as needed.
E. **Critical Thinking:** Problem-solve for solutions to problems, using the nursing process and skills such as collaboration, reasoning, and time management (see Table 1-2, *Practical/Vocational Nursing Processes*, p. 3).
F. **Team Building:** Foster positive team environment with motivation and coaching; handle change and conflict.

> **HESI Hint** • **FIVE RIGHTS OF DELEGATION**
> Tasks appropriately delegated will answer "Yes" to the following questions. Is it the:
>   1. Right task? Can it be delegated by an RN or a PN?
>   2. Right situation? Consider the setting and available resources, and the appropriateness of the delegated task.
>   3. Right person? Has it been delegated by the proper person and to the proper person? Refer to the job description.
>   4. Right communication? Provide expectations, complete instructions, and well-defined limits. Ensure understanding by the delegate.
>   5. Right supervision? Has the delegatee received the proper guidance, evaluation, and follow-up?

Qualities of Effective Nurse-Managers

A. A nurse-manager acts to achieve safe, effective care within the goals of an institution by being:
   1. **Clinically proficient:** maintains and practices current nursing skills.
   2. **Educationally focused:** identifies need and provides necessary training and knowledge for safe clinical performance and professional growth.

TABLE 2-3 Role Comparison PN-RN

PN	RN
• Data collection • Focused assessment • Participate in planning nursing care needs • Participate in modifying nursing care plan • Implement care within scope of practice rather than legal, ethical, and educational parameters • Implement teaching plan for common health problems and well-defined learning needs • Provide direct basic care to assigned multiple clients in structured settings • Assist in evaluation of client's responses and outcomes to therapeutic interventions • Use a problem-solving approach as the basis for decision making in practice	• Perform initial assessment • Perform comprehensive assessments • Determine nursing diagnoses • Formulate nursing care plan • Implement nursing care • Develop and implement teaching plans rather than promotion, maintenance, and restoration of health • Provide for care of multiple clients either through direct care or assignment and/or delegation of care to other members of the health care team • Evaluate client's responses and outcomes to therapeutic interventions • Use critical thinking approach to analyze clinical data and current literature as a basis for decision making in nursing practice • Evaluate impact of care • Make independent decisions • Communicate and consult with other health care team members
Coordinator of Care-PN	**Coordinator of Care-RN**
• Assign specific tasks, activities, and functions • Maintain appropriate supervision of licensed and unlicensed personnel in compliance with current state Board of Nursing rules in structured health settings for clients with predictable health care needs in accordance with designated job descriptions and/or job duties	• Make assignments to licensed staff (PNs, RNs) • Delegate to unlicensed staff in compliance with current Board of Nurse Examiners (BNE) rules in both structured and unstructured health settings for clients with predictable as well as unpredictable health needs

3. **Resourceful:** identifies and uses available supplies, tools, and personnel (see Table 2-3).

HESI Hint • The nurse-manager needs to analyze all the desired outcomes involved when assigning:

  Rooms: a client with an infection should not be assigned to share a room with a surgical or immunocompromised client.

  Nursing assignments: a nurse's client care management should be based on the nurse's abilities, the individual client's needs, and the needs of the entire group of assigned clients.

B. **Managing Change:** Change may cause anxiety; unwanted change leads to resistance. An effective nurse-manager uses problem-solving skills to identify factors that contribute to resistance. Critical thinking and communication skills assist the nurse-manager in overcoming the resistance.
C. **Facilitate Change**
   1. Seek input of nurses and staff.
   2. Show respect.
   3. Value opinions.
   4. Build trust.
   5. Provide information.

Roles of the Practical/Vocational Nurse

A. **Provider of Care**
   1. Assist in determining health status and health needs of the client based on interpretation of health-related data and preventive health practices in collaboration with clients (individual), their families, and other members of the multidisciplinary health care team.
   2. Assist in the formulation of goals/outcomes and a plan of care in collaboration with the client (individual), their families, and interdisciplinary health care team members.
   3. Implement plan of care within legal and ethical parameters, including scope of education, in collaboration with the client (individual) and interdisciplinary health care team to assist client in meeting health care needs.
   4. Implement or reinforce teaching plan for client with common health problems and well-defined learning needs.

5. Assist in the evaluation of the client's responses and outcomes to therapeutic interventions.
6. Provide direct basic care to assigned multiple clients in structured settings.
7. Use the problem-solving approach as the basis for decision making in practice.

B. **Coordinator of Care**
1. Assist in the coordination of human and material resources for the provision of care for assigned clients.
2. Collaborate with clients and the interdisciplinary health care team to provide direct care to assigned clients.
3. Participate in the identification of client needs for referral to resources that facilitate continuity of care.
4. Participate in activities that support the organizational framework of structured health care settings.

C. **Member of a Profession**
1. Demonstrate accountability for own nursing practice.
2. Participate as an advocate in activities that focus on improving the health care of clients (individual).
3. Demonstrate behaviors that promote the development and practice of vocational nursing.

Legal Aspects of Management

A. Nurses are usually responsible for the acts of people they supervise unless that person acts outside of nursing standards. State laws control this aspect of delegation.
B. **Key Points**
1. The most common source of nursing standards is the policies and procedures manual.
2. State law requires nurses to follow nursing standards.
3. Inform and update staff about policies and procedures.
4. Be familiar with nursing staff job descriptions before delegation or assignment.
5. Provide adequate supervision and correct inadequate performance.

Management of Care

A. **Delegation**
1. Delegation is the process by which responsibility and authority are transferred to another individual.
2. Responsibility is the obligation to complete a task.
3. Authority is the right to act or command the actions of others.
4. Accountability is the ability and willingness to assume responsibility for actions and related consequences.

BOX 2-1 Delegation Do's and Don'ts

Do's
• Always use the 5 Rights of Delegation
• Provide adequate supervision of delegated tasks:
  • Guidance and direction
  • Evaluation and monitoring
  • Follow-up
• Understand the qualifications of each delegatee:
  • Appropriate education
  • Training
  • Experience
  • Skills
  • Demonstrated and documented competence
Don'ts
• Delegate tasks that require *nursing* judgment:
  • Assessment
  • Diagnosis
  • Planning
  • Evaluation
• Delegate invasive or sterile procedures

5. The authority and responsibility for delegation come from the state Nurse Practice Act. However, delegation is also based on professional practice standards, institutional policies, and ethical codes for PNs. The authority and responsibility for the completion of the delegated task are transferred to another nurse, but the nurse remains responsible for proper delegation (Box 2-1, *Delegation Do's and Don'ts*).

HESI Hint • When delegating, the nurse delegating must understand the qualifications of the person receiving the task or assignment.

B. **Critical Thinking**
1. The ability to maintain a safe, effective care environment depends on a nurse's ability to think critically. Critical thinking is the basis for clinical judgment, clinical decision making, and is:
   a. Driven by goals.
   b. Directed toward an outcome.
   c. Focused on the needs of the client.
   d. Based on the nursing process and available resources.
   e. Developed with logical reasoning, facts, and nursing standards.
   f. Reevaluated for improvement.
2. Critical thinking checklist
   a. Assessment: What are the needs or problems?
   b. Analysis: What is the priority?
   c. Plan:
      (1) What goals and outcomes need to be accomplished?

(2) What are the available resources?
   (a) Nursing staff
   (b) Interdisciplinary team members
   (c) Time
   (d) Equipment and supplies
   (e) Space
d. Implement:
   (1) Communicate clear expectations.
   (2) Complete documentation.
e. Evaluate:
   (1) Were the outcomes achieved?
   (2) Is the care safe and effective?

C. Prioritizing ranks items in order. The order will vary depending on the situation, the client, and so on. To determine a priority, ask yourself:
1. Which client is the most critically ill?
2. Which client should be cared for first? Second?
3. Which client is most likely to have a significant change in condition?
4. Which client requires an assessment by an RN?
5. Which intervention is most effective? Which should the PN perform next?
6. Which diagnosis is most appropriate? Most important?
7. Are Maslow's Hierarchy of Needs or Erikson's developmental stages applicable?

> **HESI Hint** • NCLEX-PN questions may require you to determine the priority.

D. Collaboration requires health care teams to:
1. Share common goals, commitment, and accountability.
2. Communicate clearly and openly.
3. Respect the expertise of team members.
E. Critical pathways are predetermined care plans for high-volume, high-risk clients and are integrated into individualized care plans; they do not replace individual care plans. They are developed:
1. By an interdisciplinary team.
2. For diagnoses and care that can be standardized.
3. To guide and track client progress.
F. Case management coordinates client care by an interdisciplinary team. Case managers use critical pathways to organize care and help to effectively use resources.
G. Quality assurance, also known as (CQI/TQM), is an organized approach to improving the achievement of outcomes and the quality of client care. Quality is a measure of how well institutional standards are implemented and results in positive outcomes.

Review of Leadership and Management

1. Which aspect of supervision is the PN performing?
   a. Checks on the staff after making assignments.
   b. Carefully explains details of an assignment.
   c. Suggests an improvement in technique to a UAP after completing a task.
2. What is the difference between supervision and delegation?
3. What are the five rights of delegation?
4. Which of these tasks can be delegated to a UAP?
   a. Insert a Foley catheter.
   b. Measure and record urine output from a Foley catheter.
   c. Teach a client how to perform self-care for a urinary catheter.
   d. Assess for symptoms of a urinary tract infection (UTI).
5. What systematic problem-solving method in nursing is used for critical thinking?
6. How does a nurse prioritize?
7. For what kind of client are critical pathways developed?

Answers to Review

1. Aspect:
   a. Evaluates care.
   b. Provides guidance and direction.
   c. Provides follow-up.
2. Transferring the responsibility of a task or assignment occurs only with delegation.
3. Right task, right person, right situation, right communication, and right supervision.

4. Task:
   a. Should not be delegated because it is a sterile procedure.
   b. Can be delegated because it is an intervention that is part of the implementation phase of the nursing process.
   c. Requires nursing knowledge and skills and thus cannot be delegated.
   d. Must be performed by a nurse and cannot be delegated.
5. Nursing process.
6. Prioritize by ranking the items according to a criterion such as "first," "next," or "most important."
7. High volume—a large number of clients receive this care—and high risk—have a high potential to experience a change in condition.

Disaster Nursing

A. The role of the nurse takes place at all three levels of disaster management:
   1. Disaster preparedness
   2. Disaster response
   3. Disaster recovery
B. To achieve effective disaster management:
   1. Organization is the key.
   2. All personnel must be trained.
   3. All personnel must know their role.

Levels of Prevention in Disaster Management

A. **Primary Prevention**
   1. Participate in development of disaster plan.
   2. Train rescue workers in triage/basic first aid.
   3. Educate personnel for shelter management.
   4. Educate the public on disaster plan and personal preparation for disaster.
B. **Secondary Prevention**
   1. Triage
   2. Treatment of injuries
   3. Treatment of other conditions, mental health
   4. Shelter supervision
C. **Tertiary Prevention**
   1. Follow-up care for injuries
   2. Follow-up care for psychologic problems
   3. Recovery assistance
   4. Prevention of future disasters and their consequences

Triage

A. French word meaning "to sort or categorize."
B. Goal—maximize the number of survivors by sorting the injured according to treatable and untreatable victims (Table 2-4, *Triage Color Code System*).
C. **Primary Criteria Used**
   1. Potential for survival
   2. Availability of resources

Nursing Interventions and Roles in Triage

A. Assist with triage duties using a systemic approach such as the START method (Figure 2-1, *Simple Triage and Rapid Treatment (START) Method for Triage*).
B. **Treatment of Injuries**
   1. Render first aid for injuries.
   2. Provide additional treatment as needed in definitive care areas.
C. **Treatment of Other Conditions, Mental Health**
   1. Observe for health needs other than injury.
   2. Refer for medical treatment as required.
   3. Provide treatment for other conditions based on medically approved protocols.

Shelter Supervision

A. Coordinate activities of shelter workers.
B. Oversee records of victims admitted and discharged from shelter.
C. Promote effective interpersonal and group interactions of victims in shelter.
D. Promote independence and involvement of victims housed in the shelter.

TABLE 2-4 Triage Color Code System

	Red	Yellow	Green	Black
Urgency	Most urgent—first priority	Urgent—second priority	Third priority	Dying or dead
Injury type	Life-threatening injuries	Injuries with systemic effects and complications	Minimal injuries with no systemic complications	Catastrophic injuries
May delay treatment?	NO	30 to 60 minutes	Several hours	No hope for survival—no treatment

Bioterrorism

A. Learn symptoms of illnesses that are associated with exposure to likely biologic and/or chemical agents.

B. Could appear days to weeks after exposure.

C. Nurses and other health care providers would be the first responders as victims seek medical evaluation as symptoms manifest. "First responders" are critical in identification of an outbreak, determination of cause of outbreak, identification of risk factors, and implementation of measures to control and minimize the outbreak.

D. **Possible Agents** (Table 2-5, *Biologic Agents, Chemical Agents, and Radiation*)

   1. **Biologic Agents**
      a. Anthrax
      b. Pneumonic plague
      c. Botulism
      d. Smallpox
      e. Inhalation tularemia
      f. Viral hemorrhagic fever
   2. **Chemical Agents**
      a. Biotoxin agents: ricin
      b. Nerve agents: sarin
   3. Radiation

> **HESI Hint** • It is important to remember that in disaster/bioterrorism management, the nurse must consider both the individual and the community.

Nursing Assessment (Data Collection)

A. Community disaster risk assessment

B. Measures to mitigate disaster effect

C. Exposure symptom identification

Analysis (Nursing Diagnoses)

A. Deficient knowledge related to . . .

B. Risk for poisoning related to . . .

C. Risk for trauma related to . . .

D. Risk for suffocation related to . . .

E. Fear related to . . .

F. Ineffective community coping related to . . .

G. Posttrauma syndrome related to . . .

Nursing Plans and Interventions

A. Participate in development of disaster plan.

B. Reinforce the education of the public on disaster plan and personal preparation for disaster.

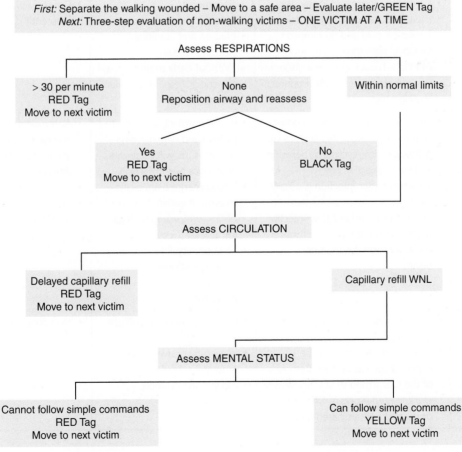

First: Separate the walking wounded – Move to a safe area – Evaluate later/GREEN Tag
Next: Three-step evaluation of non-walking victims – ONE VICTIM AT A TIME

Assess RESPIRATIONS

> 30 per minute RED Tag Move to next victim

None Reposition airway and reassess

Within normal limits

Yes RED Tag Move to next victim

No BLACK Tag

Assess CIRCULATION

Delayed capillary refill RED Tag Move to next victim

Capillary refill WNL

Assess MENTAL STATUS

Cannot follow simple commands RED Tag Move to next victim

Can follow simple commands YELLOW Tag Move to next victim

FIGURE 2-1 Simple Triage and Rapid Treatment (START) method for triage.

TABLE 2-5 Biologic Agents, Chemical Agents, and Radiation

Biologic Agents		
	Anthrax	**Pneumonic Plague**	**Botulism**
Agent	*Bacillus anthracis* • A bacterium that forms spores • Three types: • Cutaneous • Inhalation • Digestive	*Yersinia pestis* • A bacterium found in rodents and their fleas	*Clostridium botulinum* • A toxin made by a bacterium
Transmission	• Inhalation of powder form • Inhalation of spores from infected animal products (such as wool) • Handling of infected animals • Eating undercooked meat from infected animals • Cannot be spread from person to person	• Aerosol release into the environment • Respiratory droplets from an infected person (6-foot range) • Untreated bubonic plague sequelae	• Foodborne botulism occurs when a person ingests pre-formed toxin • Wound botulism occurs when wounds are infected with *C. botulinum* that secretes the toxin • Cannot be spread person to person
Incubation Period	• Within 7 days (all types) • Inhalation incubation period extends to 42 days	• 1 to 6 days	• Few hours to a few days • Foodborne: most commonly 12 to 36 hours, but range is 6 hours to 2 weeks
Signs and Symptoms	• Cutaneous: sores that develop into painless blisters, then ulcers with black centers • GI: nausea, anorexia, bloody diarrhea, fever, severe stomach pain • Inhalation: cold and flu symptoms, including sore throat, mild fever, muscle aches, cough, chest discomfort, shortness of breath, tiredness, muscle aches	• Fever • Weakness • Rapidly developing pneumonia • Bloody or watery sputum • Nausea and vomiting • Abdominal pain • Without early treatment, will see shock, respiratory failure, and rapid death	• Double and/or blurred vision • Drooping eyelids • Slurred speech • Difficulty swallowing • Descending muscle weakness
Treatment	• Prevention after exposure consists of the use of antibiotics such as ciprofloxacin, doxycycline, or penicillin and vaccination • Treatment after infection is usually a 60-day course of antibiotics • Success of treatment after infection depends on the type of anthrax and how soon the treatment begins	• If close contact with infected person and within 7 days of exposure, will treat with antibiotics prophylactically • Recommended antibiotic treatment within 24 hours of first symptom and treat for at least 7 days • Oral: tetracyclines, fluoroquinolones • IV: streptomycin or gentamicin	• Antitoxin to reduce severity of disease (most effective when administered early in course of disease) • Supportive care • May require mechanical ventilation
Miscellaneous	• Vaccine available, but not to the general public • Given to those who may be exposed, such as certain members of the U.S. armed forces, laboratory workers, and workers who enter or reenter contaminated areas	• Easily destroyed by sunlight and drying • In air can survive up to 1 hour • No vaccine available	• No vaccine available

TABLE 2-5 Biologic Agents, Chemical Agents, and Radiation—cont'd

	Smallpox	Inhalation Tularemia	Viral Hemorrhagic Fever
Agent	*Variola virus* • An *Orthopoxvirus*	*Francisella tularensis* • A highly infectious bacterium	• Five families of viruses (examples: Ebola, Lassa, dengue, yellow, Marburg) • RNA viruses enveloped in a lipid coating
Transmission	• Aerosol released into the environment • Contact with infected person (direct and prolonged face-to-face) • Bodily fluids • Contaminated objects • Air in enclosed settings (rare)	• Insect (usually tick and deer-fly) bites • Handling sick or dead infected animals • Contaminated food or water • Inhalation of airborne bacterium • Cannot be spread person to person	• From viral reservoirs such as rodents and arthropods or an animal host; some hosts remain unknown • May be transmitted person to person via close contact or bodily fluids • Objects contaminated with bodily fluids
Incubation Period	• 7 to 17 days	• Most commonly 3 to 5 days, but may range from 1 to 14 days	• 2 to 21 days (varies by virus)
Signs and Symptoms	• High fever • Head and body aches • Vomiting • Rash that progresses to raised bumps and pus-filled blisters that crust and scab, then fall off in about 3 weeks, leaving a pitted scar	• Skin ulcers • Swollen and painful lymph glands • Sore throat • Mouth sores • Diarrhea • Pneumonia • If inhaled: abrupt onset of fever and chills, headache, muscle aches, joint pain, dry cough, and progressive weakness • Those who develop pneumonia may exhibit chest pain, difficulty breathing, bloody sputum, and respiratory failure	• Varies by individual virus, but common symptoms exist • Marked fever • Exhaustion • Muscle aches • Loss of strength • As disease worsens, more severe symptoms emerge • Bleeding under skin, in internal organs, or from body orifices (mouth, eyes, ears) • Shock • CNS malfunction • Seizures • Coma • Renal failure
Treatment	• No proven treatment • Supportive therapy • Antibiotic treatment for secondary infections • Research being done with antivirals	• Antibiotics for 10 to 14 days • Oral: tetracyclines, fluoroquinolones • IM or IV: streptomycin, gentamicin	• Supportive therapy • Generally no established cure • May use ribavirin with Lassa fever
Miscellaneous	• A fragile virus—aerosolized die within 24 hours, even quicker if in sunlight • Vaccine available	• Can remain alive in water and soil for 2 weeks • No vaccine available	• Need a reservoir to survive: humans are not the natural reservoir, but once infected by the host can transmit to one another; although these viruses were once geographically restricted to where the host lived, the increasing incidence of international travel brings outbreaks to places where the viruses have never been seen before • No vaccines available except for Argentine and yellow fevers

Continued

TABLE 2-5 Biologic Agents, Chemical Agents, and Radiation—cont'd

	Chemical Agents and Radiation		
	Ricin	**Sarin**	**Radiation**
Agent	• Poison made from waste left over from processing castor beans • Forms include powder, mist, pellet • Dissolved in water or weak acid	• Human-made chemical • Similar to, but far more potent than, organophosphate pesticides • Clear, odorless, and tasteless liquid that can evaporate to a gas and spread into the environment	• A form of energy, both man-made and natural
Transmission	• Deliberate act of poisoning by inhalation or injection (need minuscule amount [500 mcg] to kill) • Deliberate act of contamination of food and water supply (requires greater amount to kill) • Cannot be spread person to person through casual contact	• Agent in air: exposed through skin, eyes, inhalation • Ingested in water or food • Clothing can release sarin for approximately 30 minutes after contact	• External exposure comes from the sun or from man-made sources such as x-rays, nuclear bombs, or nuclear disasters (such as Chernobyl) • Small quantities in air, water, food cause internal exposure
Incubation Period	• Inhalation: within 8 hours • Ingestion: less than 6 hours	• Vapor: a few seconds • Liquid: a few minutes to 18 hours	• Exposure is cumulative—low-dose exposure effects may not be seen for several years • A high dose received in a matter of minutes results in acute radiation syndrome (ARS)
Signs and Symptoms	• Inhalation: respiratory distress, fever, nausea, tightness in chest, heavy sweating, pulmonary edema, decreased B/P, respiratory failure, death • Ingestion: vomiting and diarrhea that becomes bloody, severe dehydration, decreased B/P, hallucinations, seizures, hematuria; within several days liver, spleen, and kidney failure will occur • Skin and eyes: redness and pain	• Runny nose • Watery eyes • Pinpoint pupils • Eye pain and blurred vision • Drooling • Excessive sweating • Respiratory symptoms • Diarrhea • Altered LOC • Nausea and vomiting • Headache • Decreased or increased B/P • In large doses: loss of consciousness, convulsions, paralysis, respiratory failure, death	• ARS: nausea, vomiting, diarrhea, then bone marrow depletion, weight loss, loss of appetite, flu symptoms, infection, and bleeding • Mild effects include skin reddening • May lead to cancers (low dose or those surviving ARS)
Treatment	• Supportive care	• Remove from body as soon as possible • Supportive care • Antidote available: most effective if given as soon as possible after exposure	• Dependent on dose and type of radiation • Supportive care

Continued

TABLE 2-5 Biologic Agents, Chemical Agents, and Radiation—cont'd

	Chemical Agents and Radiation		
	Ricin	**Sarin**	**Radiation**
Miscellaneous	• Stable agent: not affected by very hot or very cold temperatures • Death usually occurs in about 36 to 72 hours • If survives for 3 to 5 days, victim will usually recover • No vaccine available	• A heavy vapor, this agent sinks to low-lying areas • Mildly or moderately exposed people usually recover completely • Severely exposed people usually do not survive • May experience neurologic problems lasting 1 to 2 weeks post exposure	• Survival dependent on dose • Full recovery may take a few weeks to a few years

For further information, see *www.bt.cdc.gov/index.asp.*
CNS, Central nervous system; *GI,* gastrointestinal; *IM,* intramuscular; *IV,* intravenous; *LOC,* level of consciousness; *B/P,* blood pressure.

Nursing Plans and Interventions (continued)

C. Assist in training rescue workers in triage/basic first aid.
D. Reinforce the education of personnel for shelter management.
E. Assist with triage.
F. Treat injuries and illness.
G. Treat other conditions, mental health.
H. Supervise shelter.
I. Perform follow-up care for injuries.
J. Perform follow-up care for psychologic problems.
K. Assist in recovery.
L. Prevent future disasters and their consequences.

Review of Disaster Nursing

1. List the three levels of disaster management.
2. List examples of the three levels of prevention in disaster management.
3. Define *triage.*
4. Identify three bioterrorism agents.

Answers to Review

1. Disaster preparedness, disaster response, disaster recovery.
2. *Primary:* assist with development of plan, training/education plan, train/educate personnel and public; *secondary:* triage, treatment shelter supervision; *tertiary:* follow-up, recovery assistance, prevention of future disasters.
3. To sort or categorize.
4. Anthrax, pneumonic plague, botulism, smallpox, inhalation tularemia, viral hemorrhagic fever, ricin, sarin, radiation.

3

ADVANCED CLINICAL CONCEPTS

Respiratory Failure

Acute Respiratory Distress Syndrome

Description: The exchange of oxygen for carbon dioxide in the lungs is inadequate for oxygen consumption and carbon dioxide production within the body's cells.

A. This is sometimes referred to as adult respiratory distress syndrome (ARDS). ARDS is characterized by:
  1. Hypoxemia: P_{O_2} below 60 mm Hg.
  2. Hypoventilation: P_{CO_2} above 45 mm Hg.

> **HESI Hint** • ARDS is an unexpected, catastrophic pulmonary complication occurring in a person with no previous pulmonary problems. Clients are critically ill and are managed in an intensive care setting. The mortality rate is high.

B. During acute failure, the arterial pH falls below 7.35, indicating acidosis.

> **HESI Hint** • In ARDS, a common laboratory finding is a lowered P_{O_2}; however, these clients are not very responsive to high concentrations of oxygen.

C. Common causes of respiratory failure include:
  1. Exacerbation of chronic obstructive pulmonary disease (COPD)
  2. Pneumonia
  3. Tuberculosis
  4. Contusion
  5. Aspiration
  6. Inhaled toxins
  7. Emboli
  8. Drug overdose
  9. Fluid overload
  10. Disseminated intravascular coagulation (DIC)
  11. Shock

Nursing Assessment (Data Collection)

A. Dyspnea, tachypnea, crackles (or rales)
B. Intercostal retractions, nasal flaring
C. Cyanosis
D. Hypoxemia: P_{O_2} less than 60 mm Hg with F_{IO_2} (fraction of inspired oxygen) greater than 60%
E. Diffuse pulmonary infiltrates seen on chest x-ray films as "white-out" appearance
F. Verbalized anxiety; restlessness
G. Change in level of consciousness

Analysis (Nursing Diagnoses)

A. Impaired gas exchange related to . . .
B. Ineffective airway clearance related to . . .
C. Ineffective breathing pattern related to . . .
D. Decreased cardiac output related to . . .

Nursing Plans and Interventions

A. Monitor client on a ventilator.
B. Provide care for either an oral airway or a tracheostomy.

> **HESI Hint** • Suction only when secretions are present (see Table 4-3, *Nursing Skills: Respiratory Client*, p. 68).

C. Monitor breath sounds for pneumothorax (diminished or absent breath sounds), especially when positive end expiratory pressure (PEEP) is used to keep small airways open.
D. Monitor respiratory effort—rate, depth, use of accessory muscles, and so on.
E. Provide emotional support to decrease anxiety and allow ventilator to "work" the lungs.
F. Monitor client hemodynamically with essential vital signs and cardiac monitor.
G. Monitor arterial blood gases (ABGs) routinely.
H. Monitor vital organ status: central nervous system, level of consciousness, renal system output, and myocardium (apical pulse, blood pressure).
I. Monitor metabolic status through routine lab work (Table 3-1, *Arterial Blood Gases*).
J. Sedate per prescription to decrease anxiety and decrease O_2 use.

TABLE 3-1 Arterial Blood Gases

Blood Gases	Normal Values
pH	7.35 to 7.45
Po_2	80 to 100 mm Hg
Pco_2	35 to 45 mm Hg
HCO_3 (mEq/L)	21 to 28 mEq/L
Anion gap (mEq/L)	10 to 18

Respiratory Failure in Children

Description: Common causes of respiratory failure in children include:
A. Congenital heart disease
B. Respiratory distress syndrome
C. Infection, sepsis
D. Neuromuscular diseases
E. Trauma and burns
F. Aspiration
G. Fluid overload or dehydration
H. Anesthesia and narcotic overdose

Nursing Assessment (Data Collection)
A. Child who looks "bad"
B. Very slow or very rapid respiratory tachypnea rate, dyspnea, gasping
C. Tachycardia
D. Cyanosis, pallor, or mottled color (connotes deterioration of systemic perfusion)
E. Irritability and, later, lethargy (connotes a deteriorating level of consciousness)
F. Retractions, nasal flaring, poor air movement
G. Grunting
H. Hypoxemia, hypercapnia, respiratory acidosis
I. Laboratory data: values should be evaluated, keeping in mind the percent of oxygen the child receives

> **HESI Hint** A child in severe distress should be on 100% O_2.

Review of Respiratory Failure

1. What Po_2 value indicates hypoxemia? *PCO ↓ 60*
2. What blood value indicates hypoventilation? *↑ 45*
3. Identify the condition that exists when the Po_2 is less than 60 mm Hg and Fio_2 is greater than 60%.
4. List three symptoms of respiratory failure in the adult. *dyspnea, tachy*
5. List four common causes of respiratory failure in children. *infection / trauma*
6. What percentage of O_2 should a child in severe respiratory distress receive? *100*

Answers to Review

1. Below 60 mm Hg.
2. Pco_2 above 45 mm Hg.
3. Hypoxemia.
4. Dyspnea/tachypnea, intercostal retractions, cyanosis.
5. Congenital heart disease, infection or sepsis, respiratory distress syndrome, aspiration, fluid overload, or dehydration.
6. 100%.

Shock

Description: Widespread, serious reduction of tissue perfusion (lack of O_2 and nutrients) that, if prolonged, leads to generalized impairment of cellular functioning
A. Arterial pressure is the driving force of blood flow through all the organs.
   1. It is dependent on cardiac output to perfuse the body.
   2. It is dependent on peripheral vasomotor tone to return blood and other fluids to the heart.
   3. It is dependent on the amount of circulating blood.
   4. Marked reduction in either cardiac output or peripheral vasomotor tone, without a compensatory elevation in the other, results in system hypotension.
   5. Those at risk for development of shock include:
      a. Very young and very old clients
      b. Post–myocardial infarction (MI) clients
      c. Clients with severe dysrhythmia
      d. Clients with adrenocortical dysfunction
      e. Persons with a history of recent hemorrhage or blood loss
      f. Clients with burns
      g. Clients with massive or overwhelming infection

> **HESI Hint** • Early signs of shock are agitation and restlessness resulting from cerebral hypoxia.

B. Types of shock
   1. Hypovolemic—related to external or internal blood or fluid loss (the most common cause of shock; Table 3-2).
   2. Cardiogenic—related to ischemia or impairment in tissue perfusion resulting from MI, serious arrhythmia, or heart failure. All of these cause decreased cardiac output.

3. Distributive (anaphylactic, neurogenic, and septic)—results from excessive vasodilation and the impaired distribution of blood flow.
   a. Anaphylatic—related to allergens (anaphylaxis), can be acute and life threatening with respiratory distress related to bronchial constriction leading to airway obstruction; vascular collapse may follow.
   b. Neurogenic—related to injury to the descending sympathetic pathways in the spinal cord. This results from loss of vasomotor tone and sympathetic innervation to the heart.

TABLE 3-2 Stages of Hypovolemic Shock

Stage	Signs and Symptoms	Clinical Description
Stage I		
• Initial stage • Blood loss of less than 10% • Compensatory mechanisms triggered	• Apprehension and restlessness (first signs of shock) • Increased heart rate • Cool, pale skin • Fatigue	• Arteriolar constriction • Increased production of antidiuretic hormone (ADH) • Arterial pressure is maintained • Cardiac output usually normal (for healthy individuals) • Selective reduction in blood flow to skin and muscle beds
Stage II		
• Compensatory stage • Blood volume reduced by 15% to 25% • Decompensation begins	• Flattened neck veins and delayed venous filling time • Increased pulse and respirations • Pallor, diaphoresis, and cool skin • Decreased urinary output • Sunken, soft eyeballs • Confusion	• Marked reduction in cardiac output • Arterial pressure decline (despite compensatory arteriolar vasoconstriction) • Massive adrenergic compensatory response resulting in tachycardia, tachypnea, cutaneous vasoconstriction, and oliguria • Decreased cerebral perfusion
Stage III		
• Progressive stage	• Edema • Increased blood viscosity • Excessively low BP • Dysrhythmia, ischemia, and myocardial infarction (MI) • Weak, thready, or absent peripheral pulses	• Rapid circulatory deterioration • Decreased cardiac output • Decreased tissue perfusion • Reduced blood volume
Stage IV		
• Irreversible stage	• Profound hypotension, unresponsive to vasopressor drugs • Severe hypoxemia, unresponsive to O₂ administration • Anuria, renal shutdown • Heart rate slows, BP falls, with consequent cardiac and respiratory arrest	• Cell destruction so severe that death is inevitable • Multiple organ system failure • It is the nurse's responsibility to recognize the signs and symptoms of shock early in the course of the disease process to prevent the devastating clinical course that the progression of shock can take.

> **HESI Hint** • Severe shock leads to widespread cellular injury and impairs the integrity of the capillary membranes. Fluid and osmotic proteins seep into the extravascular spaces, further reducing cardiac output. A vicious cycle of decreased perfusion to *all* cellular level activities ensues. All organs are damaged, and if perfusion problems persist, the damage can be permanent.

c. Septic—related to endotoxins released by bacteria, which cause vascular pooling, diminished venous return, and reduced cardiac output.
4. Obstructive—physical obstruction related to tamponade, emboli, or compartment syndrome and that impedes the filling or outflow of blood, resulting in reduced cardiac output.

> **HESI Hint** • If cardiogenic shock exists with the presence of pulmonary edema (i.e., from pump failure), position client to REDUCE venous return (HIGH-FOWLER with legs down) so as to decrease venous return further to the left ventricle.

Medical Treatment for Shock

A. Correct decreased tissue perfusion and restore cardiac output.
   1. **Oxygenation and Ventilation**
      a. Optimize oxygen delivery and reduce demand on heart.
      b. Increase arterial oxygen saturation with supplemental oxygenation and mechanical ventilation.
      c. Space activities that decrease oxygen consumption.
   2. **Fluid Resuscitation**
      a. Cause of shock dictates the type of treatment. Rapid infusion of volume-expanding fluids is the cornerstone of treatment for hypovolemic shock and anaphylactic shock.
      b. Whole blood, plasma, plasma substitutes (colloid fluids) may be used.
      c. Isotonic, electrolyte intravenous solutions such as Ringer's lactate solution and normal saline may also be used.
      d. If shock is cardiogenic in nature, the infusion of volume-expanding fluids may result in pulmonary edema.
   3. **Drug Therapy**
      a. Restoration of cardiac function should take priority. Drug selection is based on the effect of the shock on preload, afterload, or contractility.
         i. Drugs that increase preload (i.e., blood products, crystalloids) or decrease preload (i.e., morphine, nitrates, diuretics)
         ii. Drugs that increase afterload (i.e., vasopressors, dopamine) or decrease afterload (i.e., nitroprusside, ACE-I, ARB)
         iii. Drugs that decrease contractility (i.e., beta blockers, calcium channel blockers) or that increase contractility (i.e., digoxin [Lanoxin], dobutamine)
   4. **Monitoring**
      a. Central venous pulmonary artery catheters are inserted in the operating room (OR) and intensive care unit (ICU) to monitor shock.
      b. Serial measurements of central venous pressure (CVP), urinary output, heart rate, and the clinical and mental state of the client are taken every 5 to 15 minutes.
      c. Following immediate attention to improvement of perfusion, attention is directed toward treating the underlying cause of the condition.
      d. Administration of drugs is usually withheld until circulating volume has been restored.

Nursing Assessment (Data Collection)

A. Vital signs:
   1. Tachycardia (pulse more than 100 bpm)
   2. Tachypnea (respirations more than 24/minute)
   3. Blood pressure decreased (systolic less than 80 mm Hg)
B. Mental status exam:
   1. Early shock: restless, hyperalert
   2. Late shock: decreased alertness, lethargy, coma
C. Skin changes:
   1. Cool, clammy (warm skin in vasogenic and early septic shock)
   2. Diaphoresis
   3. Pale
D. Fluid status (acute renal tubular necrosis can happen quickly in shock):
   1. Urine output decreases or an imbalance between intake and output occurs.
   2. Abnormal CVP (less than 4 cm of H_2O).
   3. Urine specific gravity more than 1.02 (indicates hypovolemia).

Analysis (Nursing Diagnoses)

A. Deficit fluid volume related to . . .
B. Decreased cardiac output related to . . .
C. Anxiety related to . . .
D. Ineffective peripheral tissue perfusion related to…

Nursing Plans and Interventions

A. Monitor arterial pressure by understanding the concepts related to arterial pressure (Table 3-3, *Arterial Pressure*).
B. Monitor blood pressure (BP), pulse, respirations, and dysrhythmias every 15 minutes or more often, depending on stability of client.
C. Monitor urine output every hour to maintain *at least* 30 mL/hour (Foley catheter placement necessary).
D. Notify health care provider if urine output drops below 30 mL/hr (reflects decreased renal perfusion and may result in acute renal failure).
E. Fluids are administered as prescribed by provider to improve preload: blood, colloids, or electrolyte solutions until designated CVP is reached. (In shock situations, the health care provider often orders fluids to elevate CVP 16 to 19 cm of H_2O as compensation for decreased cardiac output; Table 3-4, *Administration*

TABLE 3-3 Arterial Pressure

Concept	Definition
Mean Arterial Pressure (MAP)	• Level of pressure in the central arterial bed measured indirectly by blood pressure measurement • MAP = cardiac output × total peripheral resistance = systolic blood pressure + 2 (diastolic blood pressure)/3 • In adults, usually approaches 100 mm Hg • MAP ≥60 for renal perfusion • Can be measured directly through arterial catheter insertion
Cardiac Output	• Volume of blood ejected by the left ventricle per unit of time • Stroke volume (amount of blood ejected per beat) × heart rate
Peripheral Resistance	• Resistance to blood flow offered by the vessels in the peripheral vascular bed
Central Venous Pressure	• Pressure within the right atrium; normal CVP/RAP ranges from 2 to 6 mm Hg

of Blood Products.) For fluid administration, PNs must work in accordance with agency policies and their state Scope of Practice.

F. Remember client's bed position is dependent on cause of shock.

G. Do not administer medications intramuscularly or subcutaneously until perfusion improves in muscles and subcutaneous tissue.

H. Keep client warm (increase heat in room or put warm blankets on client, but not *too* hot).

I. Keep side rails up during all procedures. (Clients in shock experience mental confusion and may easily be injured by falls and may require physical/medical restraint for safety.)

J. Assist in the procurement of blood for lab work as prescribed: complete blood count (CBC), electrolytes, blood urea nitrogen (BUN), creatinine (renal damage), lactate (sepsis), and blood gases (oxygenation).

K. When vasopressors/adrenergic stimulants such as epinephrine (Bronkaid), dopamine, dobutamine (Dobutrex), norepinephrine (Levophed), or isoproterenol (Isuprel) are administered:
1. Monitor BP (hemodynamic status) every 5 to 15 minutes. Arterial line placement is necessary with long-term vasopressors for continuous BP monitoring.
2. Watch intravenous site carefully for extravasation and tissue damage.
3. Ask health care provider for target mean systolic blood pressure (usually 80 to 90 mm Hg or mean arterial pressure [MAP] of 60 or more).

L. Provide family support:
1. Notify appropriate support persons for waiting family during crisis—that is, call spiritual advisor, other family members, or anyone the family thinks will be supportive.
2. At intervals, notify family of actions/progress or lack of progress in realistic terms.
3. Collaborate with health care provider before notifying family of medical interventions.

M. Glucose levels should be maintained at 140 and 180 mg/dL.

Disseminated Intravascular Coagulation

Description: Disseminated intravascular coagulation (DIC) is a coagulation disorder with paradoxic thrombosis and hemorrhage.

A. DIC is an acute complication of conditions such as hypotension and septicemia, suspected when there is bloody oozing from two or more unexpected sites. DIC can also be a complication of pregnancy.

B. The first phase involves abnormal clotting in the microcirculation, which uses up clotting factors and results in an inability to form clots, and hemorrhage occurs.

C. The diagnosis is based on laboratory findings:
1. Prothrombin time (PT): prolonged
2. Partial thromboplastin time (PTT): prolonged
3. Fibrinogen: decreased
4. Platelet count: decreased
5. Fibrin degradation (split) products (FDP): increased

Nursing Assessment (Data Collection)

A. Petechiae, purpura, hematomas
B. Oozing from IV sites, drains, gums, and wounds
C. Gastrointestinal (GI) and genitourinary (GU) bleeding
D. Hemoptysis
E. Mental status change
F. Hypotension, tachycardia
G. Pain

Analysis (Nursing Diagnoses)

A. Risk for injury related to . . .
B. Ineffective tissue perfusion altered (specify type) related to . . .

Nursing Plans and Interventions

A. Monitor client for bleeding.
B. Monitor vital signs frequently.
C. Monitor PT/INR.
D. Monitor intake and output.
E. Protect client from injury and bleeding.

TABLE 3-4 **Administration of Blood Products**

Component therapy has replaced the use of whole blood, which now accounts for less than 10% of all transfusions.

Blood Products

Description	Special Considerations	Indications for Use
Packed red blood cells (RBCs)	Less danger of fluid overload	Acute blood loss
Frozen RBCs: prepared from RBCs using glycerol for protection and then frozen	Must be used within 24 hours of thawing	Auto transfusion: infrequently used because filters remove most of white blood cells
Platelets: pooled—300 mL One unit contains single donor—200 mL	Bag should be agitated periodically	Bleeding caused by thrombocytopenia
Fresh-frozen plasma (FFP): liquid portion of whole blood is separated from cells and frozen	The use of FFP is being replaced by albumin plasma expanders	Bleeding caused by deficiency in clotting factors
Albumin: prepared from plasma and is available in 5% and 20% solutions	Albumin 25 g/100 mL is osmotically equal to 500 mL of plasma	Hypovolemic shock, hypoalbuminemia
Cryoprecipitates and commercial concentrates: prepared from fresh-frozen plasma with 10 to 20 mL/bag	Used in treating hemophilia	Replacement of clotting factors, especially factor VIII and fibrinogen

Transfusion Reactions

Reactions/Complications	Assessment	Nursing Interventions
Acute hemolytic	Chills, fever, low back pain, flushing, tachycardia, hypotension progressing to acute renal failure, shock, and cardiac arrest	*Stop transfusion* Change tubing, then continue saline IV Treat for shock if present Draw blood samples for serologic testing Monitor hourly urine output Give diuretics as prescribed
Febrile nonhemolytic (most common)	Sudden chills and fever, headaches, flushing, anxiety, and muscle pain	Give antipyretics as prescribed
Mild allergic	Flushing, itching, urticaria (hives)	Give antihistamine as directed
Anaphylactic and severe allergic	Anxiety, urticaria, wheezing, progressive cyanosis leading to shock and possible cardiac arrest	Stop transfusion Initiate CPR
Circulatory overload	Cough, dyspnea, pulmonary congestion, headache, hypertension	Place client in upright position with feet in dependent position and administer diuretics, oxygen, morphine; slow IV rate
Sepsis	Rapid onset of chills, high fever, vomiting, marked hypotension, or shock	Ensure a patent airway, obtain blood for culture, administer prescribed antibiotics, take vital signs every 5 minutes until stable

Continued

TABLE 3-4 Administration of Blood Products—cont'd

Nursing Skills

- Obtain venous access, use central venous catheter or 19-gauge needle.
- Use only blood administration tubing to infuse blood products.
- Run blood products with saline solutions only. Dextrose solutions and Ringer's lactate solution will induce RBC hemolysis.
- Run infusion at prescribed rate and remain with client for the first 15 to 30 minutes of infusion.
- The blood should be administered as soon as it is brought to the patient.
- Check vital signs frequently before, during, and immediately following infusion; note any increase in temperature.
- Follow agency policy regarding specific timetable for blood infusion.
- Check and double-check the product before infusing to see that it is the:
- Correct product, as prescribed; double-check with a second licensed person.
- Correct blood type and Rh factor, matched with the client

HESI Hint • Administration of blood and blood products is not permitted by the Scope of Practice for PNs in many states. Knowing the Scope of Practice in your state is essential.

1. Provide gentle oral care with mouth swabs.
2. Minimize needle sticks, and use smallest-gauge needle possible.
3. Turn frequently to eliminate pressure points.
4. Minimize number of BPs taken by cuff.
5. Use gentle suction to prevent trauma to mucosa.
6. Apply pressure to any oozing site.
F. Monitor heparin IV during the first phase to inhibit coagulation.
G. Provide emotional support to decrease anxiety.

Review of Shock and DIC

1. Define shock.
2. What is the most common cause of shock?
3. What causes septic shock?
4. What is the goal of treatment for hypovolemic shock?
5. What intervention is used to restore cardiac output when hypovolemic shock exists?
6. It is important to differentiate between hypovolemic and cardiogenic shock. How might the nurse determine the existence of cardiogenic shock?
7. If a client is in cardiogenic shock, what might result from administration of volume-expanding fluids? What intervention can the nurse expect to perform in the event of such an occurrence?
8. List five assessment findings found in most shock victims.
9. What is the established minimum renal output per hour?
10. List four measurable criteria that are the major expected outcomes of a shock crisis.
11. Define DIC.
12. What is the effect of DIC on the following laboratory tests: PT, PTT, platelets?
13. What drug is used in the treatment of DIC?
14. Name four nursing interventions to prevent injury in clients with DIC.

Answers to Review

1. Widespread, serious reduction of tissue perfusion, which leads to generalized impairment of cellular function.
2. Hypovolemia.
3. Release of endotoxins from bacteria that act on nerves in vascular space in periphery, causing vascular pooling, reduced venous return, and decreased cardiac output, resulting in poor systemic perfusion.
4. Quick restoration of cardiac output and tissue perfusion.
5. Rapid infusion of volume-expanding fluids.
6. History of MI with left ventricular failure or possible cardiomyopathy, with symptoms of pulmonary edema.
7. Pulmonary edema; administer cardiotonic drugs such as digitalis preparations.

8. Tachycardia; tachypnea; hypotension; cool, clammy skin; decrease in urinary output.
9. 30 mL/hr.
10. BP mean of 80 to 90 mm Hg; Po_2 more than 50 mm Hg; CVP above 6 cm of H_2O; urine output at least 30 mL/hr.
11. A coagulation disorder in which there is paradoxic thrombosis and hemorrhage.
12. Prothrombin time—prolonged; partial thromboplastin time—prolonged; platelets—decreased.
13. Heparin.
14. Gently provide oral care with mouth swabs. Minimize needle sticks and use the smallest-gauge needle possible when injections are necessary. Eliminate pressure by turning the client frequently. Minimize the number of BPs taken by cuff. Use gentle suction to prevent trauma to mucosa. Apply pressure to any oozing site.

Resuscitation

Cardiopulmonary Arrest

A. Usually caused by myocardial infarction (MI): necrosis of the heart muscle caused by inadequate blood supply to heart.
B. MIs usually occur at rest or with moderate activity, contrary to the belief that they occur with strenuous activity.
C. Symptoms immediately preceding MI:
   1. Chest pain/discomfort either at rest or with ordinary activity.
   2. Change in previously stable anginal pain—that is, an increase in frequency or severity or rest angina occurring for the first time.
   3. Chest pain in a client with known coronary heart disease that is unrelieved by rest and/or nitroglycerin.

> **HESI Hint** • NCLEX-PN questions on cardiopulmonary resuscitation (CPR) often deal with prioritization of actions.
> **Question:** What actions are required for each of the following situations?
> A 24-year-old motorcycle accident victim with a ruptured artery of the leg. The client is pulseless and apneic.
> A 36-year-old first-time pregnant woman who arrests during labor.
> A 17-year-old with no pulse or respirations who is trapped in an overturned car that is starting to catch fire.
> A 40-year-old businessman who arrests 2 days after a cervical laminectomy.

D. O_2 is necessary for survival; all other injuries are secondary—except for removal of any source of imminent danger, such as a fire.
E. Chest pain of myocardial ischemia:
   1. Usually described as crushing, pressing, constricting, oppressive, or heavy.
   2. Tends to increase in intensity over a few minutes.
   3. May be substernal or more diffused.
   4. May radiate to one or both shoulders and arms, or to neck, jaw, or back.
   5. Atypical symptoms occur with women and patients diagnosed with diabetes. For example, women experience unexpected shortness of breath, breaking out in a cold sweat, or sudden fatigue, nausea, or lightheadedness.
F. Occasions for cardiopulmonary resuscitation are often *unwitnessed* cardiac arrests.

> **HESI Hint** • **WHEN TO SEEK EMERGENCY MEDICAL SERVICE**
> The American Heart Association recommends that those with known angina pectoris activate an emergency medical system (EMS) if chest pain does not go away immediately with rest, if it is not relieved in 5 minutes after taking nitroglycerin, or if additional symptoms such as nausea and sweating are also present with the chest pain.
> A person with previously unrecognized coronary disease experiencing chest pain persisting for 2 minutes or longer should seek emergency medical treatment.

Management of Cardiac Arrest

> **HESI Hint** • It is important for the nurse to stay current with the American Heart Association's (AHA) guidelines for basic life support (BLS) by being certified every 2 years, as required. See the American Heart Association website for *2010 CPR Guidelines* and to locate a CPR class: www.heart.org/HEARTORG/.
> Major components of BLS consist of immediate recognition of cardiac arrest and activation of the emergency response system, CPR with emphasis on chest compression, and rapid defibrillation if indicated. The AHA *2010 Guidelines for Cardiopulmonary Resuscitation (CPR) and Emergency Cardiovascular Care (ECC)* have changed focus for the BLS steps.
> One change is that CPR for the trained layperson is a hands-only CPR (chest compressions–only CPR). The focus is on early, high-quality chest compressions.

A change for the health care provider includes chest compressions before rescue breaths—that is, a change from the well-known "A-B-C" (Airway, Breathing, and Chest Compressions) to "C-A-B" (Chest Compressions, Airway, and Breathing) for adults and children (steps for newborns remain "A-B-C"). Chest compressions are described by the phrase "push hard and push fast." The phrase reflects an increased emphasis on high-quality chest compressions and a deemphasis on pulse checks. High-quality chest compressions mean the chest in adults is compressed at a rate of 100 compressions per minute at a depth of at least 2 inches (5 cm).

In-Hospital Cardiac Arrest

A. Determine responsiveness of client:
 1. If no response occurs, call a "code," or cardiac arrest, in order to initiate response of cardiac arrest team. Obtain AED or emergency crash cart with defibrillator.
 2. Position client on cardiac board or put bed in CPR position. If pulse is not identified within 10 seconds, begin chest compressions.
 3. Initiate chest compressions—30 compressions with both hands over the lower half of the sternum at a rate of 100 compressions per minute with a depth of 2 inches (5 cm).
 4. After 30 compressions, ventilate by mask or bag over 1 second per breath for 2 breaths.
B. Team leader arrives and assesses client, directs team members, and obtains history and precipitating events to arrest.
 1. Without interrupting CPR, apply cardiac portable monitor "quick-look" paddles or AED to determine whether defibrillation is necessary or whether asystole has occurred.
 2. Follow hospital policies and procedures to convert client to a normal sinus rhythm.
 3. Resume CPR, beginning with compressions, immediately after defibrillations.

Pediatric Resuscitation

For newborn resuscitation, see *Maternity Nursing*, p. 284.
1. If no response occurs, call a "code," or cardiac arrest, in order to initiate response of cardiac arrest team. Obtain AED or emergency crash cart with defibrillator.
2. Check for pulse:
 a. Infant younger than 1 year old: brachial pulse
 b. Children 1 year to puberty: carotid or femoral
3. Begin compressions within 10 seconds:
 a. Infant compressions cover at least one third of the anterior/posterior diameter of the chest at 1½-inch depth in most infants.
 b. Children compressions cover at least one third of the anterior/posterior diameter of the chest at 2-inch depth in most children.
 c. Do 30 compressions to 2 breaths with one rescuer; 15 compressions to 1 breath with 2 rescuers.
4. Deliver each breath over 1 second (avoid excess ventilation [gastric inflation]).
5. Minimize interruption in chest compression.
6. Allow full chest recoil.

HESI Hint • One primary action for the practical nurse is to record the activities (CPR, drug administration, intubation, IV insertion, etc.) that occur during the resuscitation.

HESI Hint • The compression to ventilation ratio for a lone rescuer is 30:2, and for a two-rescuer situation, it is 15:1. Ventilations should be delivered with minimal interruptions in chest compressions. If the client has an endotracheal tube in place, the cycles of compressions and ventilations are no longer delivered. Instead, the compressing rescuer should deliver at least 100 compressions per minute without pausing for ventilation. The ventilation rescuer delivers 8 to 10 breaths per minute, being careful to avoid excessive ventilation.

Management of Foreign Body Airway Obstruction

Adults and Children 1 Year and Older

A. If unable to ventilate the person during CPR, suspect a foreign body in the airway.
B. Signs of foreign body airway obstruction (FBAO) that require rescuer intervention include silent cough, inability to speak or breathe, or cyanosis. The victim typically clutches the neck.
C. Ask "Are you choking?" If patient nods without talking, then intervention is required.
B. If person is conscious, stand behind person, grasp around waist with clenched fist (halfway between navel and xiphoid), and exert palmar thrust inward at epigastrium (Heimlich maneuver) in rapid sequence.
C. Chest thrust should be used in obese or pregnant patients.
D. Continue until object is expelled or person falls to ground unconscious; then activate EMS and begin CPR.
E. Use a finger sweep only if the object is seen obstructing the airway.

Infants and Children

A. For a child, perform subdiaphragmatic abdominal thrusts (Heimlich maneuver) until the object is expelled or the victim becomes unresponsive. For an infant, deliver repeated cycles of five back blows (slaps) followed by five chest compressions until the object is expelled or the victim becomes unresponsive. Abdominal thrusts are not recommended for infants because they may damage the infant's relatively large and unprotected liver.

Open a conscious child's mouth and attempt to clear obstruction manually if the object can be seen (*no* blind sweeps; they may push the foreign object farther down the throat).

B. For a child, perform subdiaphragmatic abdominal thrusts (Heimlich maneuver) in rapid sequence until the obstruction is relieved.

C. If the infant is able to cry, cough, or breathe, do *not* interfere.

D. If the infant is conscious and *cannot* cry, cough, or breathe:
   1. Place infant facedown, head lower than trunk, with legs straddling your arm and chest supported by your upturned hand.
   2. Give five firm blows to back with heel of hand (compresses rib cage between two hands).
   3. Position face upward and give five chest thrusts as you would for cardiac massage.
   4. Repeat until the object is expelled or the infant becomes unresponsive.

E. If unresponsive, begin CPR.

Review of Resuscitation

1. What are the priorities when a client with sudden cardiac arrest is found?
2. Define *myocardial infarction*.
3. What criteria should alert a client with known angina who takes nitroglycerin tablets sublingually to call the EMS?
4. Name two changes from the 2005 AHA BLS guidelines to the present 2010 guidelines.
5. True or False: When feeling for the presence of a carotid pulse, no more than 5 seconds should be used.
6. During one-rescuer CPR, what is the ratio of compressions to ventilations for an adult who has no pulse?
7. A client in cardiac arrest is noted on the bedside monitor to be in pulseless ventricular tachycardia. What is the first action that should be taken?
8. How would the nurse assess the adequacy of compressions during CPR? How would the nurse assess for adequacy of ventilations during CPR?
9. If a person is choking, when should the rescuer intervene?
10. One should never make blind sweeps into the mouth of a choking child or infant. Why?

Answers to Review

1. Immediate activation of the emergency response system and the start of chest compressions.
2. Necrosis of the heart muscle because of poor perfusion of the heart.
3. Unrelieved chest pain after rest, 5 minutes after taking nitroglycerin, or if accompanied by other symptoms such as nausea or sweating.
4. Increased focus on high-quality, immediate chest compressions and a deemphasis on pulse checks.
5. False: palpate for at least but no more than 10 seconds, recognizing that dysrhythmias or bradycardia could be occurring.
6. 30 compressions and two breaths.
7. Defibrillation.
8. Check for a carotid or femoral pulse. Watch for chest excursion and auscultate bilaterally for breath sounds.
9. When the person points to his/her throat and can no longer cough, talk, or make sounds.
10. Because the object might be pushed farther down into the throat.

Fluid and Electrolyte Balance

Homeostasis

Description: The process of maintaining a relative state of equilibrium.

A. Homeostasis occurs in relation to maintenance of the composition of fluids.

B. Fluid composition is maintained by changes in osmolarity (Table 3-5, *Fluid Volume*).

> **HESI Hint** • Changes in osmolarity cause shifts in fluid. The osmolarity of the extracellular fluid (ECF) is almost entirely caused by sodium. The osmolarity of intracellular fluid (ICF) is related to many particles, with potassium being the primary electrolyte. The pressures in the ECF and ICF are almost identical. If either ECF or ICF changes in concentration, fluid shifts from the area of lesser concentration to the area of greater concentration.

TABLE 3-5 Fluid Volume

Variable	Deficit	Excess
Description	• Occurs when the body loses water and electrolytes isotonically—that is, in the same proportion as in the normal body fluid • Serum electrolyte levels remain normal • Dehydration: state in which the body loses water and serum sodium levels increase	• Occurs when the body retains water and electrolytes isotonically • Water intoxication: state in which the body retains water and serum sodium levels decrease
Causes	• Vomiting • Diarrhea • GI suctioning • Sweating • Inadequate fluid intake • Massive edema, as with initial stage of major burns • Ascites • Elderly—forgetting to drink	• Heart failure (HF) • Renal failure • Cirrhosis, liver failure • Excessive ingestion of table salt • Overhydration with sodium-containing fluid • Poorly controlled IV therapy, especially in young and old clients
Symptoms	• Weight loss (1 liter of fluid weight loss or gain is approximately equal to 2.2 pounds or 1 kilogram) • Decreased skin turgor • Oliguria, concentrated urine • Dry and sticky mucous membranes • Postural hypotension or weak, rapid pulse	• Peripheral edema • Increased bounding pulse • Elevated BP • Distended neck and hand veins • Dyspnea; moist crackles heard when lungs auscultated • Attention loss, confusion, aphasia • Altered level of consciousness
Lab Findings	• Elevated BUN and creatinine • Increased serum osmolality • Elevated Hgb and Hct	• Decreased BUN • Decreased Hgb and Hct • Decreased serum osmolality • Decreased urine osmolality and specific gravity
Treatment and Nursing Care	• Strict I&O • Replace fluids isotonically, preferably orally • *WATER IS A HYPOTONIC FLUID* • If intravenous hydration is needed, isotonic fluids are used	• Diuretics • Fluid restriction with total divided among three 8-hour periods • Strict I&O • Sodium-restricted diet • Weigh daily • Monitor K^+ serum

HESI Hint · Fluid Volume Deficit: Dehydration

Elevated BUN: The BUN measures the amount of urea nitrogen in the blood. Urea is formed in the liver as the end product of protein metabolism. The BUN is directly related to the metabolic function of the liver and the excretory function of the kidneys.

Creatinine, as with BUN, is excreted entirely by the kidneys and is therefore directly proportional to renal excretory function. However, unlike BUN, the creatinine level is affected very little by dehydration, malnutrition, or hepatic function. The daily production of creatinine depends on muscle mass, which fluctuates very little. Therefore, it is a better test of renal function than is the BUN. Creatinine is generally used in conjunction with the BUN test, and they normally are in a 1:20 ratio.

Serum osmolality measures the concentration of particles in a solution. It refers to the fact that the same amount of solute is present, but the amount of solvent (fluid) is decreased. Therefore, the blood can be considered "more concentrated."

Urine osmolality and specific gravity increase.

BP, Blood pressure; *BUN,* blood urea nitrogen; *GI,* gastrointestinal; *Hct,* hematocrit; *Hgb,* hemoglobin; *I&O,* intake and output.

> **HESI Hint** • Dextrose 10% is a hyperosmolar solution and should be administered IV.
> Normal saline is an isotonic solution and is used for irrigations, such as bladder irrigations or IV flush lines with intermittent IV medication.
> Use only isotonic (neutral) solutions in irrigations, infusions, and so on, unless the specific aim is to shift fluid to intracellular or extracellular spaces.

Role in Electrolyte Balance

A. **Kidney**
1. Selectively maintain and excrete body fluids.
2. Selectively retain needed substances and excrete unneeded substances—that is, electrolytes.
3. Regulate pH by excreting or maintaining hydrogen ions and bicarbonate.
4. Excrete metabolic wastes and toxic substances.
B. **Lungs**
1. Rid the body of approximately 300 mL of fluid per day and play a role in acid-base balance.
2. Regulate carbon dioxide concentration.
C. **Heart:** Pumps with sufficient force to perfuse the kidneys, necessary for their functioning.
D. **Adrenal Glands:** Secrete aldosterone, which causes sodium retention (which causes water retention) and potassium excretion.
E. **Parathyroid Glands:** Regulate calcium and phosphorus balance.
F. **Pituitary Gland:** Secretes antidiuretic hormone (ADH), which causes the body to retain water.

Electrolyte Imbalance

Nursing Assessment (Data Collection). See Table 3-6, *Electrolyte Imbalances.*

Nursing Plans and Interventions
See Table 3-7, *Types of IV Solutions.*

> **HESI Hint** • Potassium imbalances are potentially life threatening; they must be corrected immediately. A low magnesium often accompanies a low potassium, especially with the use of diuretics.

> **HESI Hint**
> **Aldosterone:** Na retaining (K-excreting hormone)
> **Antidiuretic hormone (ADH):** Water-retaining hormone
> Where Na^+ goes, water flows.

Intravenous (IV) Therapy

Description: IV solutions are used to supply electrolytes, nutrients, and water (see Table 3-7). Even though the PN may not administer IV solutions and medications, it is important for the PN to apply the following information to assist the RN and other health care providers to monitor the client receiving intravenous therapy.

Administration of IV Therapy
A. The purpose and duration of the IV therapy determine the type of equipment, such as IV tubing, and the size of the needle that should be used—for example, administration of blood requires an 18-gauge needle or larger.
B. Gloves *must* be worn during venipuncture and when discontinuing an IV.
C. Assess the IV site frequently (minimum of every 2 hours). It is the nurse's legal responsibility to observe the client, report any reactions, and take measures necessary to prevent complications.
D. Intermittent IV therapy may be given through a saline lock; regular flushing maintains patency.
E. IV tubing and dressing should be changed according to hospital policy.
F. When the IV is discontinued, apply pressure to the site for 1 to 3 minutes after the needle is removed (longer for clients on anticoagulants, the elderly, or those with prolonged PT/PTT).

Complications Associated with IV Administration
A. Infections such as septicemia:
1. Aseptic and antiseptic technique should be used when starting an IV and caring for an IV site.
2. Inspect all fluids and containers before use to be sure they have not been opened, otherwise contaminated, or expired.
3. Change administration sets per agency policy.
4. Primary IV solution bags should not hang for more than 24 hours.
5. Do not irrigate blocked cannulas.
B. A pulmonary embolism occurs when a substance or clot is propelled by venous circulation to the right side of the heart and subsequently into the pulmonary artery.
1. Special blood tubing with a clot filter is used when infusing blood or blood products.
2. Lower-extremity veins should be avoided for cannulation.
3. Do not irrigate plugged cannulas.
4. Subsequent IVs should not be started lower on the extremity.
C. An air embolism can be fatal if the pulmonary capillaries are blocked.
1. Watch for empty IV fluid containers.

TABLE 3-6 **Electrolyte Imbalances**

Abnormalities and Common Causes	Signs and Symptoms	Treatment
Hyponatremia (↓Na)		
• Diuretics • GI fluid loss • Hypotonic tube feeding • D₅W or hypotonic IV fluids • Diaphoresis	• Anorexia, nausea, and vomiting • Weakness • Lethargy • Confusion • Muscle cramps, twitching • Seizures • Na below 135 mEq/L	• Restrict fluids (safer) • If IV saline solutions prescribed, the solution should be administered very slowly; use isotonic saline if fluid restriction is not effective
Hypernatremia (↑Na)		
• Water deprivation • Hypertonic tube feeding • Diabetes insipidus • Heatstroke • Hyperventilation • Watery diarrhea • Renal failure • Cushing syndrome	• Thirst • Hyperpyrexia • Sticky mucous membranes • Dry mouth • Hallucinations • Lethargy • Irritability • Seizures • Na above 145 mEq/L	• Restrict sodium in the diet • Beware of "hidden" sodium in foods and medications • Increase water intake
Hypokalemia (↓K)		
• Diuretics • Diarrhea • Vomiting • Gastric suction • Steroid administration • Hyperaldosteronism • Amphotericin B • Bulimia • Cushing syndrome	• Fatigue • Anorexia • Nausea, vomiting • Muscle weakness • Decreased GI motility • Dysrhythmias • Paresthesia • Flat T waves on ECG • K⁺ less than 3.5 mEq/L	• Potassium supplements can be given both orally or IV • Oral forms of potassium are unpleasant tasting and are irritating to the GI tract (Do not give on empty stomach; dilute) • Potassium IV should *never* be given as a bolus • Assess renal status—that is, urinary • Encourage foods high in potassium, such as bananas, oranges, cantaloupe, avocadoes, spinach, potatoes
Hyperkalemia (↑K)		
• Hemolyzed serum sample produces pseudohyperkalemia • Oliguria • Acidosis • Renal failure • Addison disease • Multiple blood transfusions	• Muscle weakness • Bradycardia • Dysrhythmias • Flaccid paralysis • Intestinal colic • Tall T waves on ECG • K⁺ above 5 mEq/L	• Do not give parenteral potassium • 50% glucose with regular insulin can be given to reduce the potassium level • Kayexalate can also be used to reduce serum potassium • Monitor ECG • Calcium gluconate is given to protect the heart • IV loop diuretics may be prescribed • Renal dialysis may be required
Hypocalcemia (↓Ca)		
• Renal failure • Hypoparathyroidism • Malabsorption • Pancreatitis • Alkalosis	• Diarrhea • Numbness • Tingling of extremities • Convulsions • Positive Trousseau sign • Chvostek sign • Calcium (Ca) below 8.5 mEq/L • At risk for tetany	• Administer calcium supplements orally 30 minutes before meals • IV calcium should be given slowly and can cause tissue necrosis • Increase calcium intake, such as dairy products, greens

TABLE 3-6 Electrolyte Imbalances—cont'd

Abnormalities and Common Causes	Signs and Symptoms	Treatment
Hypercalcemia (↑Ca)		
• Hyperparathyroidism • Malignant bone disease • Prolonged immobilization • Excess calcium supplementation • Diuretic phase of acute renal failure	• Muscle weakness • Constipation • Anorexia • Nausea, vomiting • Polyuria • Polydipsia • Neurosis • Dysrhythmias • Ca above 10.5 mEq/L	• Eliminate parenteral calcium • Administer agents to reduce calcium such as calcitonin • Avoid calcium-based antacids • Loop diuretics may be used • Renal dialysis may be required
Hypomagnesemia (↓Mg)		
• Alcoholism • Malabsorption • Diabetic ketoacidosis • Prolonged gastric suction • Diuretics	• Anorexia, distention • Neuromuscular irritability • Depression • Disorientation • Mg below 1.5 mEq/L	• Magnesium sulfate IV should be given • Encourage foods high in magnesium, such as meats, nuts, legumes, fish, and vegetables
Hypermagnesemia (↑Mg)		
• Renal failure • Adrenal insufficiency • Excess replacement	• Flushing • Hypotension • Drowsiness, lethargy • Hypoactive reflexes • Depressed respirations • Bradycardia • Mg above 2.5 mEq/L	• Avoid magnesium-based antacids and laxatives • Restrict dietary intake of foods high in magnesium
Hypophosphatemia (↓pH)		
• Refeeding after starvation • Alcohol withdrawal • Diabetic ketoacidosis • Respiratory alkalosis	• Paresthesias • Muscle weakness • Muscle pain • Mental changes • Cardiomyopathy • Respiratory failure • pH below 2 mEq/L	• Correct underlying cause • Administer oral replacement of phosphates with vitamin D
Hyperphosphatemia (↑pH)		
• Renal failure • Excess intake of phosphorus	• Short term: tetany symptoms • Long term: phosphorus precipitation in nonosseous sites • pH above 4.5 mEq/L	• Administer aluminum hydroxide with meals to bind phosphorus • Dialysis may be required if renal failure is underlying cause

D. A circulatory overload is especially hazardous for clients with impaired renal or cardiac functioning.
  1. The infusion rate should be maintained at the prescribed rate.
  2. Observe for signs of circulatory overload: weight gain; edema; pulmonary edema, which is characterized by dyspnea, cough, sweating, and frothy pinkish sputum; decreased SaO_2; puffy eyelids; and ascites.

E. Phlebitis can occur because of mechanical, chemical, and/or septic causes.
  1. Cannulation sites should not be over a joint.
  2. Cannulas should be well anchored to prevent motion, thereby reducing the risk of entry of microorganisms into the puncture wound.
  3. The cannula size should be smaller than the vein.
  4. Use aseptic and antiseptic technique.

TABLE 3-7 Types of IV Solutions

Isotonic	Hypotonic	Hypertonic

• Have an osmolality close to the ECF
• Do not cause red blood cells to swell or shrink
• Indicated for intravascular dehydration
• Isotonic solutions:
  →Normal saline (0.9% NS)
  →Lactated Ringer's (LR)
  →5% Dextrose in water (D_5W)
• (D_5W is on the low end of isotonic—some sources classified as hypotonic)
• Used to treat intravascular dehydration (not enough fluid in vascular system)
• Common type of dehydration
• Examples: dehydration caused by running, labor, fever, and so on
	• Have an osmolality lower than the ECF
	• Causes fluid to move from ECF to ICF
	• Indicated for cellular dehydration
	• Used in the management of the client who is both volume-depleted and hyperosmolar (e.g., in cases of hypernatremia or hyperglycemia).
	• Hypotonic solutions:
	  →0.5% Normal saline (HNS or 0.45% NS)
	  →2.5% Dextrose in 0.45% saline ($D_{25}0.45\%$ NS)
	• Used to treat intracellular dehydration (cells have too many osmoles, need to drive fluid into the cells)
	• Not a common occurrence
	• Examples: dehydration caused by prolonged dehydration (may also see in clients who are on TPN for prolonged periods)
		• Have an osmolality higher than the ECF
		• Indicated for intravascular dehydration with interstitial or cellular overhydration
		• Use with extreme caution
		• High concentrations of dextrose are given for caloric replacement such as intravenous hyperalimentation into a central vein for rapid dilution
		• Hypertonic saline solutions are available but used only when serum osmolality is dangerously low
		• Hypertonic solutions:
		  →5% Dextrose in lactated Ringer's (D_5 LR)
		  →5% Dextrose in 0.45% saline (D_5 ½ NS)
		  →5% Dextrose in 0.9% saline (D_5 NS)
		  →10% dextrose in water (D10W)
		• Used to treat intravascular dehydration with cellular or interstitial overhydration
		• Examples: dehydration resulting from surgery; blood loss causes intravascular dehydration, but the edematous tissue caused by manipulation during surgery can pull fluid into the area, causing interstitial overhydration
		• May also see with ascites and third spacing

Flow Rate Calculation

- Several formulas exist for calculating intravenous flow rates.
- Infusion pumps are used when measurement of exact flow is necessary.
- Using the following steps for IV calculation will ensure proper calculation:
  1. mL/hr: rate for IV infusion on a pump
  2. gtts/min: rate for IV infusions by gravity

HESI Hint • Check the IV tubing container to determine the drip factor because drip factors vary. The most common drip factors are 10, 12, 15, 20, and 60 drops per milliliter. A microdrip is 60 drops per milliliter.

ECF, Extracellular fluid; *ICF,* intracellular fluid.

5. Remove the cannula within 72 hours or immediately if one of the following occurs:
   a. Erythema
   b. Induration
   c. Tenderness when palpating the vein
   d. Leaking at insertion site

HESI Hint • Intravenous administration is limited by law for the licensed practical nurse (LPN) in many states. The practical nurse needs to be aware of the Scope of Practice in his or her state and the agency's policies.

Acid-Base Balance

Description: An acid-base balance must be maintained in the body because cells and enzymatic processes do not function well beyond the normal range and can result in alkalosis or acidosis.

A. Maintaining the acid-base balance is imperative and involves three systems:
   1. A chemical buffer system
   2. The kidneys
   3. The lungs
B. Acid-base balance is determined by the hydrogen ion concentration in body fluids.

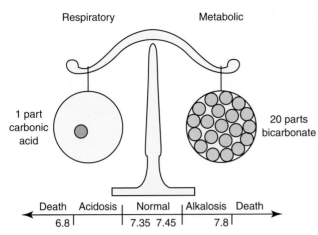

Respiratory   Metabolic

1 part carbonic acid

20 parts bicarbonate

Death Acidosis   Normal   Alkalosis Death
6.8   7.35 7.45   7.8

FIGURE 3-1 Relationship of sodium bicarbonate to carbonic acid. (From Potter PA, Perry AG: *Fundamentals of nursing*, ed 7, St. Louis, 2009, Mosby.)

TABLE 3-8 Arterial Blood Gas Comparisons

Acid-Base Conditions	pH	P_{CO_2} (mm Hg)	HCO_3 (mEq/L)
Normal	7.35 to 7.45	35 to 45	21 to 28
Respiratory acidosis	↓	↑	Normal
Respiratory alkalosis	↑	↓	Normal
Metabolic acidosis	↓	Normal	↓
Metabolic alkalosis	↑	Normal	↑

1. Normal range is 7.35 to 7.45 expressed as the pH (Figure 3-1, *Relationship of Sodium Bicarbonate to Carbonic Acid*).
2. pH less than 7.35 indicates acidosis.
3. pH greater than 7.45 indicates alkalosis.
4. Measurement is by arterial blood gases (ABG) (Table 3-8, *Arterial Blood Gas Comparisons*).

Chemical Buffer System

A. Chemical buffers act quickly to prevent major changes in body fluid pH by removing or releasing hydrogen ions.
B. The main chemical buffer is the bicarbonate-carbonic acid (HCO_3-H_2CO_3) system.
   1. Normally there are 20 parts of bicarbonate to 1 part carbonic acid. If the 20:1 ratio is altered, the pH is changed (ratio is important, not absolute values).
   2. Carbonic acid (H_2CO_3) is formed when carbon dioxide (CO_2) combines with water (H_2O).
   3. Excess CO_2 in the body alters the ratio and creates an imbalance. Other buffer systems:
      a. Phosphate
      b. Protein
      c. Hemoglobin

Lungs

A. Control CO_2 content through respirations (is actually carbonic acid content).
B. Control, to a small extent, water balance ($CO_2 + H_2O = H_2CO_3$).
C. Release excess CO_2 by increasing respiratory rate.
D. Retain CO_2 by decreasing respiratory rate.

Kidneys

A. Regulate bicarbonate levels by retaining or reabsorbing bicarbonate as needed.
B. Provide a very slow, but important, compensatory mechanism (can require hours or days).
C. Cannot help with compensation when metabolic acidosis is created by renal failure.

Determining Acid-Base Disorders

A. In uncompensated acid-base disturbances, it is easy to determine when a disorder exists. Draw arrows to indicate whether the pH, P_{CO_2}, or HCO_3 are increased (↑), decreased (↓), or within normal limits (WNL).
B. When pH is increased (↑), alkalosis is present; when pH is decreased (↓), acidosis is present.
C. In respiratory disorders, the HCO_3 is normal, and the arrows for pH and P_{CO_2} are in opposite directions.

HESI Hint
Hyperventilation: Associated with an increase in pH or a decrease in P_{CO_2} (CO_2 is lost).
Hypoventilation: Associated with a decrease in pH or an increase in P_{CO_2} (CO_2 is retained).

D. In metabolic disorders, the P_{CO_2} is normal, and the arrows for pH and HCO_3 are in the same direction or equal (Table 3-9, *Analysis of Arterial Blood Gases*).
E. The body will begin to compensate in acid-base disorders to bring the pH back within the normal range of 7.35 to 7.45.
F. Example: For a client with a pH of 7.29 (↑), a P_{CO_2} of 50 (↓), and an HCO_3 of 26:
   1. Determine the pH: acidosis.
   2. Determine the P_{CO_2}: respiratory.
   3. Determine HCO_3: not metabolic.
   4. Respiratory acidosis is the disorder (Table 3-10, *Potential Etiologies of Acid-Base Conditions*).

HESI Hint • The acronym **ROME** can help you remember: **R**espiratory, **O**pposite (pH and P_{CO_2}); **M**etabolic arrows; **E**qual (pH and HCO_3).

HESI Hint • Learn either acidosis or alkalosis for the respiratory and the metabolic types. Then the opposite type will have the opposite problem with all laboratory findings.

Review of Fluid and Electrolyte Balance

1. List four common causes of fluid volume deficit.
2. List four common causes of fluid volume overload.
3. Identify two examples of isotonic IV fluids.
4. List three systems that maintain acid-base balance.
5. Cite the normal ABG levels for the following:
   A. pH
   B. P_{CO_2}
   C. HCO_3

Answers to Review

1. GI causes: vomiting, diarrhea, GI suctioning; decrease in fluid intake; increase in fluid output, such as sweating; massive edema, ascites.
2. Heart failure (HF); renal failure; cirrhosis; excess ingestion of table salt or overhydration with sodium-containing fluids.
3. Ringer's lactate; normal saline.
4. Lungs; kidneys; chemical buffers.
5. Normal levels:
   A. 7.35 to 7.45 pH
   B. 35 to 45 mm Hg P_{CO_2}
   C. 21 to 28 mEq/L HCO_3

TABLE 3-9 Analysis of Arterial Blood Gases

Component	Description	Values
pH	• Measures hydrogen ion (H^+) concentration • ↑ in ions (acidosis) reflects in pH • ↓ in ions (alkalosis) reflects in pH	• 7.35 to 7.45 • <7.35 • >7.45
P_{CO_2}	• Partial pressure of CO_2 in arteries • Respiratory component of acid-base regulation • Hypoventilation (respiratory acidosis) • Hyperventilation (respiratory alkalosis)	• 35 to 45 mm Hg • >45 mm Hg • <35 mm Hg
HCO_3	• Measures serum bicarbonate • May reflect primary metabolic disorder or compensatory mechanism to respiratory acidosis • Metabolic acidosis • Metabolic alkalosis	• Normal 21 to 28 mEq/L • <21 mEq/L • >28 mEq/L

Electrocardiogram

Description: An electrocardiogram (ECG or EKG) is a noninvasive visual representation of the electrical activity of the heart reflected by changes in the electrical potential at the skin surface. Abnormalities are related to conduction, rate, rhythm, chamber enlargement, myocardial ischemia, myocardial infarction, and electrolyte imbalance. The 12-lead EKG assesses different views of the heart.

> **HESI Hint** • **REVIEW THE ORDER OF BLOOD FLOW THROUGH THE HEART**
> Unoxygenated blood flows from the superior and inferior vena cava into the right atrium, and then to the right ventricle. It flows out of the heart through the pulmonary artery, to the lungs for oxygenation. The pulmonary vein delivers oxygenated blood back to the left atrium, and then to the left ventricle (largest, strongest chamber) and out the aorta.
> Review the three structures that control the one-way flow of blood through the heart:
> **Valves**
> A. Atrioventricular valves
>   1. Tricuspid (right side)
>   2. Mitral (left side)
> B. Semilunar valves
>   1. Pulmonic (in pulmonary artery)
>   2. Aortic (in aorta)
> **Chordae tendineae**
> **Papillary muscles**

TABLE 3-10 Potential Etiologies of Acid-Base Conditions

Condition	Primary Etiology	Contributing Etiology
Respiratory acidosis	• Hypoventilation	• COPD (primary etiology) • Pulmonary disease • Drugs • Obesity • Mechanical asphyxia • Sleep apnea
Metabolic acidosis	• Addition of large amounts of fixed acids to body fluids	• Lactic acidosis (circulatory failure) • Ketoacidosis (diabetes, starvation) • Phosphates and sulfates (renal disease) • Acid ingestion (salicylates) • *Secondary to respiratory alkalosis* • Adrenal insufficiency
Respiratory alkalosis	• Hyperventilation	• Overventilation on a ventilator • Response to acidosis • Bacteremia • Thyrotoxicosis • Fever • Hepatic failure • Response to hypoxia • Hysteria
Metabolic alkalosis	• Retention of base or removal of acid from body fluids	• Excessive gastric drainage • Vomiting • Potassium depletion (diuretic therapy) • Burns • Excessive $NaHCO_3$ administration

COPD, Chronic obstructive pulmonary disease.

A. The visual representation of an ECG can be recorded as a tracing on a strip of graph paper or can be seen on an oscilloscope.

B. The following conditions can interfere with normal heart functioning:
   1. Disturbances of rate or rhythm
   2. Disorders of conductivity
   3. Enlarged heart chambers
   4. Presence of myocardial infarction
   5. Fluid and electrolyte imbalances

C. Each ECG should include identifying information:
   1. Client's name and identification number
   2. Location, time, and date of recording
   3. Client's age, gender, and cardiac and noncardiac medications currently being taken
   4. Height, weight, and BP
   5. Clinical diagnosis and current clinical status
   6. Any unusual position of the client during the recording
   7. If present, thoracic deformities, respiratory distress, or muscle tremor

D. Standard ECG is the 12-lead EKG.

E. Bedside monitoring through telemetry is more commonly seen in the clinical setting.
   1. Telemetry uses three or five leads transmitted to an oscilloscope.
   2. Graphic information is printed either upon request or at any time the set parameters are transcended.

F. A portable continuous monitor (Holter monitor) can be placed on the client to provide a magnetic tape recording. While wearing a Holter monitor, the client is instructed to keep a diary concerning the following:
   1. Activity
   2. Medications
   3. Chest pains

G. The ECG graph paper consists of small and large squares (Figure 3-2, *Composition of ECG Paper*).
   1. The small squares represent 0.04 seconds each, with five of these small squares combining to form one large square.
   2. Each large square represents 0.20 seconds (0.04 seconds × 5). Five large squares represent 1 second. Calculation of heart rate using the 6-second rule (Box 3-1, *Methods for Estimating Heart Rate Using an Electrocardiogram Tracing*):
      a. The easiest means of calculating the heart rate.
      b. Cannot be used when the heart rate is irregular.
      c. Large squares equal one 6-second time interval.
      d. Count the number of RR intervals in the 30 large squares, and multiply by 10 to determine the heart rate for 1 minute (the R is the high peak on the strip) (Figure 3-3, *The Cardiac Conduction System*).

Analysis (Nursing Diagnoses)

Dysrhythmia

A. Activity intolerance related to . . .
B. Ineffective health maintenance related to . . .
C. Ineffective tissue perfusion related to . . .
D. Death anxiety related to . . .
E. Decreased cardiac output related to . . .

Composition of the ECG

A. P wave: atrial systole.
   1. Represents depolarization of the atrial muscle.
   2. Should be rounded without peaking or notching.
B. QRS complex: ventricular systole.
   1. Represents depolarization of the ventricular muscle.
   2. Normally follows the P wave.

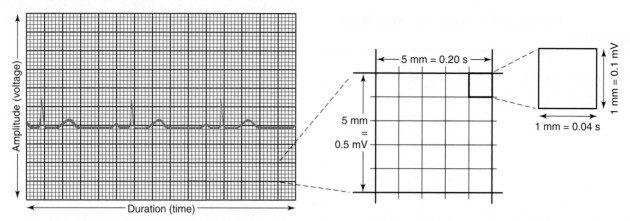

FIGURE 3-2 Composition of ECG Paper. Electrocardiograph waveforms are measured in amplitude (voltage) and duration (time.) (From Ignatavicius DD, Workman ML: *Medical-surgical nursing: patient-centered collaborative care*, ed 7, St. Louis, 2012, Saunders.)

BOX 3-1 *Methods for Estimating Heart Rate Using an Electrocardiogram Tracing*

1. Measure the interval between consecutive QRS complexes, determine the number of small squares, and divide 1500 by that number. This method is used only when the heart rhythm is regular.
2. Measure the interval between consecutive QRS complexes, determine the number of large squares, and divide 300 by that number. This method is used only when the heart rhythm is regular.
3. Determine the number of RR intervals within 6 seconds and multiply by 10. The ECG paper is conveniently marked at the top with slashes that represent 3-second intervals. This method can be used when the rhythm is irregular. If the rhythm is extremely irregular, an interval of 30 to 60 seconds should be used.

4. Count the number of big blocks between the same point in any two successive QRS complexes (usually R wave to R wave) and divide by 300 because there are 300 big blocks in 1 minute. It is easiest to use a QRS that falls on a dark line. If little blocks are left over when counting big blocks, count each little block as 0.2, add this to the number of big blocks, and then divide by 300.
5. The memory method relies on memorization of the following sequence: 300, 150, 100, 75, 60, 50, 43, 37, 33, 30. Find a QRS complex that falls on the dark line representing 0.2 second or a big block, and count backward to the next QRS complex. Each dark line is a memorized number. This is the method most widely used in hospitals for calculating heart rates for regular rhythms.

Calculation of heart rate. In this example, the heart rate using the big block method is 300 ÷ 4 big blocks (between QRS complexes), or 75 bpm. The memory method is also demonstrated with a heart rate of 75 bpm. (From Ignatavicius DD, Workman ML: *Medical-surgical nursing: critical thinking for collaborative care*, ed 5, Philadelphia, 2006, Saunders.)

Adapted from Monahan, FD, et al: *Phipps' medical-surgical nursing: health and illness perspectives*, ed 8, St. Louis, 2007, Mosby; and Ignatavicius DD, Workman ML: *Medical-surgical nursing: patient-centered collaborative care*, ed 6, St. Louis, 2010, Saunders.

---

3. QRS interval measured from the beginning of the QRS to the end of the QRS (normally less than 0.11 seconds).
4. T wave: ventricular diastole.
   a. Represents repolarization of the ventricular muscle.
   b. Follows the QRS complex.
   c. Usually slightly rounded without peaking or notching.

HESI Hint • Because the T wave represents repolarization of the ventricle, this is a critical time in the heartbeat. This action represents a resting and regrouping stage so that the next heartbeat can occur. If defibrillation occurs during this phase, the heart can be thrust into a life-threatening dysrhythmia.

C. ST segment:
   1. Represents early ventricular repolarization.
   2. Measured from the end of the S wave to the beginning of the T wave.
D. PR interval:
   1. Represents the time required for the impulse to travel through the atria (SA node), through the AV node, to the Purkinje fibers in the ventricles.
   2. Measured from beginning of the P wave to the beginning of the QRS complex.
   3. Represents AV nodal function (normal 0.12-0.20 seconds).
E. U wave:
   1. Not always present.
   2. Most prominent in the presence of hypokalemia.
F. QT interval:
   1. Represents the time required to completely depolarize and repolarize the ventricles.

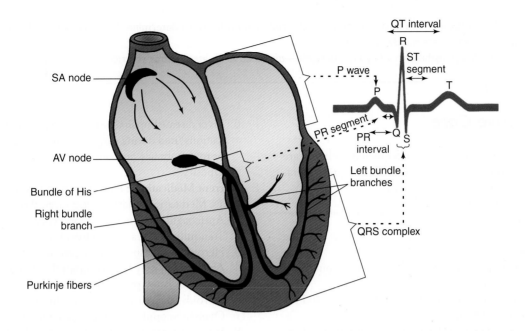

FIGURE 3-3 The cardiac conduction system. (From Ignatavicius DD, Workman ML: *Medical-surgical nursing: patient-centered collaborative care*, ed 7, St. Louis, 2012, Saunders.)

  2. Measured from the beginning of the QRS complex to the end of the T wave.
G. RR interval:
  1. Reflects the regularity of the heart rhythm.
  2. Measured from one QRS to the next QRS.

> **HESI Hint** • Observe the client for tolerance of the current rhythm. This information is the most important data the nurse can collect on the client with a dysrhythmia.

> **HESI Hint** • NCLEX-PN questions are likely to relate to early recognition of abnormalities and associated nursing actions.
> *Remember* to monitor the client as well as the machine! If the ECG monitor shows a severe dysrhythmia, but the client is sitting up quietly watching television without any sign of distress, assess to determine whether the leads are attached properly.

Review of Electrocardiogram

1. Identify the waveforms found in a normal ECG.
2. In an ECG reading, which wave represents depolarization of the atrium?
3. In an ECG reading, what complex represents depolarization of the ventricle?
4. What does the PR interval represent?
5. If the U wave is most prominent, what condition might the nurse suspect?
6. Describe the calculation of the heart rate using an ECG rhythm strip.
7. What is the most important assessment data for the nurse to obtain on a client with a dysrhythmia?
8. What are the possible lethal dysrhythmias?

Answers to Review

1. P wave, QRS complex, T wave, ST segment, PR interval.
2. Represented by the P wave.
3. QRS complex.
4. The time required for the impulse to travel from the atria through the AV node.

5. Hypokalemia.
6. Count the number of RR intervals in the 30 large squares and multiply by 10 to determine the heart rate for 1 minute.
7. Ability of the client to tolerate the dysrhythmia.
8. Any atrial or ventricle dysrhythmia that becomes unstable—that is, atrial fib, atrial flutter, ventricle fib, ventricle flutter, 3° AV block.

Perioperative Care

Description: The perioperative period includes client care before surgery (preoperative), during surgery (intraoperative), and after surgery (postoperative).

A. The nurse's role is to:
1. Provide an overview of the experience.
2. Provide continuity of care using the nursing process.
3. Reduce anxiety—for example, anxiety about postoperative pain.
4. Promote an uncomplicated perioperative period for the client and family.

B. Surgery is performed under aseptic conditions, in a hospital or alternate hospital setting (ambulatory surgical center or health care provider's office).

C. Client safety is a serious concern during the perioperative period. Steps should be implemented to ensure safety. An implementation plan for the reduction and elimination of preventable surgical complications, known as the Surgical Care Improvement Project (SCIP) core measures, is mandatory for patient safety.

Surgical Risk Factors

A. **Age:** The very young and very old are greater surgical risks than children and adults.

B. **Nutrition:** Obesity and malnutrition increase surgical risk.

C. **Fluid and Electrolyte Status:** Dehydration and hypovolemia increase surgical risk because of imbalances in calcium, magnesium, potassium, and phosphorus.

D. **General Health:** Any infection or pathology increases surgical risk.
1. Cardiac conditions: angina, MIs, hypertension, heart failure (well-controlled cardiac problems pose little risk).
2. Blood coagulation disorders can lead to severe bleeding, hemorrhage, and shock.
3. Upper respiratory tract infections (surgery is usually delayed when the client has an upper respiratory infection) and chronic obstructive pulmonary disease are exacerbated by general anesthesia and adversely affect pulmonary function.
4. Renal disease, such as a renal insufficiency, impairs fluid and electrolyte regulation.
5. Diabetes mellitus predisposes clients to wound infection and delayed healing.

6. Liver disease impairs the liver's ability to detoxify medications used during surgery, to produce prothrombin, or to metabolize nutrients for wound healing.
7. Obesity.

E. **Current Medications:** Prescription and over-the-counter drugs. Medications that increase surgical risk include:
1. Anticoagulants (increase blood coagulation time).
2. Tranquilizers (may cause hypotension).
3. Heroin (decreases central nervous system response).
4. Antibiotics (may be incompatible with anesthetics).
5. Diuretics (may precipitate electrolyte imbalance).
6. Steroids (decreased wound healing).
7. Over-the-counter natural supplements.
8. Vitamin E (may increase the risk of bleeding when used with warfarin or other herbal medications such as ginkgo, ginger, and garlic).

Preoperative Care

Description: Care provided from the time the client/family makes the decision to have surgery until the client is taken to the operative suite.

Data to Obtain When Taking a Preoperative Nursing History

A. Age
B. Allergies to medications, foods (shellfish), and topical antiseptics (especially iodine)
C. Current medications; prescriptions, over-the-counter drugs, and herbal preparations
D. History of medical and surgical problems
E. Previous surgical experiences
F. Previous experience with anesthesia
G. Tobacco, alcohol, and drug abuse
H. Understanding of surgical procedure
I. Coping resources
J. Cultural and ethnic factors that may influence surgery or postoperative care
K. Latex allergy

Key Components of Preoperative Teaching Plans

A. Regulations concerning valuables, jewelry, dentures, glasses, hearing aids
B. Food and fluid restrictions, such as nothing given orally (NPO) after midnight, per prescription by health care provider; clear liquids may be given up to 6 hours prior surgery for the no-risk client per prescription by the health care provider.

C. Invasive procedures such as urinary catheters, IVs, nasogastric (NG) tubes, enemas, douches
D. Preoperative medications
E. Operating room, transportation, skin preparation, postanesthesia
F. Postoperative procedures:
   1. Respiratory care such as ventilator, incentive spirometer, deep breathing, splinting
   2. Activity such as range of motion (ROM) exercises, leg exercises, early ambulation, turning
   3. Pain control such as IM medications, PCA (patient-controlled analgesia)
   4. Dietary restrictions
   5. Intensive care unit or postanesthesia care unit orientation (recovery room)

Preoperative Checklist Information

A. "Informed consent," surgical consent, signed and witnessed consent for treatment per hospital policy; signature must be obtained before administration of any narcotics or other medications affecting client cognition. Consents are valid for 45 days.
B. Site is marked by the person performing surgery. Before the incision is initiated, all team members confirm identity, procedure, site of surgery, and consents.
C. Accurate height and weight charted.
D. History and physical completed (by health care provider) in chart.
E. Chest x-ray film, ECG, urinalysis.
F. Hemoglobin (Hgb), hematocrit (Hct), electrolytes, glucose, and type/cross-match for blood.
G. Old medical records.
H. Identification band on client, including allergies.
I. Addressograph information.
J. Contact lenses, glasses, dentures, partial plates, wigs, jewelry, artificial eye, prostheses, makeup, nail polish removed.
K. Client voided or catheterized.
L. Client in hospital gown.
M. Vital signs: BP, temperature, pulse, respirations.
N. Premedication given: type and time.
O. Skin preparation (if prescribed by health care provider/physician):
   1. Wash with soap and water.
   2. Scrub or shower with povidone/iodine or another antibacterial solution per prescription.
   3. Do not remove hair unless it will interfere with the operation, and remove it using only electric clippers if possible.
P. Signature of nurse certifying completion.

> **HESI Hint** • Marking the operative site is required for procedures involving right/left distinctions, multiple structures (fingers, toes), or levels (spinal procedures). Site marking should be done with the involvement of the client.

Intraoperative Care

Description: From the time the client is received in the operative suite until admission to the recovery room, an operating room nurse is in charge of care.
A. Maintain quiet during induction.
B. Maintain safety:
   1. Conduct client identification: right client, right procedure, right anatomic site.
   2. Ensure that sponge, needle, and instrument counts are accurate.
   3. Position during procedure to prevent injury.
   4. Apply grounding device to client if electrocautery is to be used.
   5. Strictly adhere to asepsis during *all* intraoperative procedures.
   6. Ensure adequate, functioning suction setup(s).
   7. Responsible for correct labeling, handling, and deposition of any and all specimens.
C. Monitor physical status:
   1. If excessive blood loss occurs, calculate effect on client.
   2. Report changes in pulse, temperature, respirations, blood pressure to surgeon in conjunction with anesthesiologist/certified registered nurse anesthetist (CRNA).
D. Provide psychologic support:
   1. Provide emotional support to client/family immediately before, during, and after surgery.
   2. Arrange with physician to provide information to the family if surgery is prolonged or complications or unexpected findings occur.
   3. Communicate emotional state of client to other health care team members.

Postoperative Care

Description: From admission to recovery room until client is recovered.
A. Initially the client goes to the recovery room or postanesthesia care unit or to the ICU.
B. O$_2$ applied/continued.
C. On arrival, the nurse will check the vital signs (BP, pulse, respirations, temperature, and pain—the fifth vital sign), level of consciousness, skin color and condition, dressing location and condition, intravenous fluids, drainage tubes, position, and oxygen saturation levels.
D. When stabilized and prescribed by the health care provider, the client is then transferred to the general nursing unit or the intensive care unit.
E. Immediate postoperative nursing care should include:
   1. Monitor for signs of shock and hemorrhage: hypotension; narrow pulse pressure; rapid, weak pulse; cold, moist skin; increased capillary filling time (Table 3-11, *Common Postoperative Complications*).

TABLE 3-11 Common Postoperative Complications

Postoperative Complication	Occurrence	Interventions for Preventions
Urinary retention	8 to 12 hours postoperatively	• Monitor hydration status and encourage oral intake if allowed • Monitor for first void after surgery • Offer bedpan or assist to commode • Catheterize as needed per prescription
Pulmonary problems • Atelectasis • Pneumonia • Embolus	1 to 2 days postoperatively	• Assist client to turn, cough, deep breathe every 2 hours • Keep client hydrated • Early ambulation • Early incentive spirometer (per hospital protocol)
Wound-healing problems	5 to 6 days postoperatively	• Splint incision when client coughs • Monitor for signs of infection, malnutrition, dehydration • High-protein diet • Maintain dressing per prescription • Keep wound clean and dry
Urinary tract infections	5 to 8 days postoperatively	• Oral fluid intake • Emptying of bladder every 4 to 6 hours • Monitor intake and output • Avoid catheterizations if possible
Thrombophlebitis	6 to 14 days postoperatively	• Leg exercises every 2 hours while in bed • Early ambulation • Apply antiembolus (TED) stockings or sequential hose as prescribed; remove TEDs every 8 hours and reapply • Apply alternating compression devices • Avoid pressure that may obstruct venous flow; do not raise knee gatch on bed, do not place pillows beneath knees, avoid crossing legs at knees • Low-dose heparin may be used prophylactically
Decreased gastrointestinal peristalsis • Constipation • Paralytic ileus	2 to 4 days postoperatively	• NG tubing to decompress GI tract • Client to limit use of narcotic analgesics that decrease peristalsis • Encourage early ambulation • Encourage oral fluid intake if allowed

HESI Hint • Wound dehiscence is separation of the wound edges and is more likely to occur with vertical incisions. It usually occurs after the early postoperative period, when the client's own granulation tissue is "taking over" the wound, after absorption of the sutures has begun. Evisceration of the wound is protrusion of intestinal contents (in an abdominal wound) and is more likely in clients who are older, diabetic, obese, or malnourished and have prolonged paralytic ileus.

2. Monitor surgical sites frequently to determine possible presence of bleeding.
3. Position on side (if not contraindicated) to prevent aspiration, and allow client to cough out airway; side rails should be up at all times.
4. Provide warmth with heated blanket.
5. Manage nausea/vomiting with antiemetic drugs and NG suctioning.
6. Manage pain with analgesics.
7. Check with anesthesiologist about intraoperative medications before administering pain medications.
8. Determine intraoperative irrigations/instillations with drains to help evaluate amount of drainage on dressing and/or in drainage collection devices.

HESI Hint • NCLEX-PN items will focus on the nurse's role in terms of the entire perioperative process.
Sample: A 43-year-old mother of two teenage daughters enters the hospital to have her gallbladder removed in a same-day surgery using a scope instead of an incision. What nursing needs will dominate each phase of her short hospital stay?
Preparation phase: Reinforce education about postoperative care, NPO, assist with meeting family needs.
Operative phase: Assessment, management of the operative suite.
Postanesthesia phase: Pain management, postanesthesia precautions.
Postoperative phase: Prevent and assess for complications, pain management, dietary restrictions, activity.

Review of Perioperative Care

1. List five variables that increase surgical risk.
2. Why is a client with liver disease at increased risk for operative complications?
3. Preoperative teaching should include demonstration and explanation of expected postoperative client activities. What activities should be included?
4. What items should the nurse assist the client in removing before surgery?
5. How and why is the client positioned in the immediate postoperative period?
6. List three nursing actions to prevent postoperative wound dehiscence/evisceration.
7. Identify three nursing interventions to prevent postoperative urinary tract infections.
8. Identify nursing/medical interventions to prevent postoperative paralytic ileus.
9. List four nursing interventions to prevent postoperative thrombophlebitis.
10. During the intraoperative period, what activities should the operating room nurse do to ensure safety during surgery?

Answers to Review

1. Age: very young and very old; obesity and malnutrition; preoperative dehydration/hypovolemia; preoperative infection; use of anticoagulants preoperative (aspirin).
2. Impairs ability to detoxify medications used during surgery. Impairs ability to produce prothrombin to reduce hemorrhage.
3. Respiratory activities: coughing and breathing, use of spirometer. Exercises: range of motion exercises, leg exercises, turning. Pain management: medications, splinting. Dietary restrictions: NPO to progressive diet. Dressings and drains. Orientation to recovery room environment.
4. Contact lenses, glasses, dentures, partial plates, wigs, jewelry, prostheses, makeup, and nail polish.
5. Usually on the side or with head to side so as to prevent aspiration of any emesis.
6. Splint incision when coughing, encourage coughing/deep breathing in *early* postoperative period when sutures are *strong*. Monitor for signs of infection, malnutrition, and dehydration. Encourage high-protein diet.
7. Avoid postoperative catheterization. Increase oral fluid intake. Empty bladder q4 to 6 hours, early ambulation.
8. Early ambulation. Limit use of narcotic analgesics. NG tube decompression.
9. Perform in-bed leg exercises. Early ambulation. Apply antiembolus stockings. Avoid positions/pressure that obstruct venous flow.
10. Ascertain correct sponge, needle, and instrument count. Position client to avoid injury. Apply ground during electrocautery use. Strict use of surgical asepsis.

HIV Infection

Description: Infection with human immunodeficiency virus (HIV).

A. HIV is caused by a retrovirus, which is attracted to CD4 T-cells, lymphocytes, macrophages, and cells of the central nervous system.

B. The virus enters the cell and begins to replicate. Some event, such as cofactors (herpes simplex and cytomegalovirus [CMV]) can stimulate this replication.

C. The destruction of the CD4 T-cell causes depletion in the number of CD4 T-cells and a loss of the body's ability to fight infection. Individuals with fewer than 200 CD4 T-cells are at risk for opportunistic infections. (The normal CD4 T-cell count is 600 to 1200.)

D. Initially, the individual often suffers an acute infection, which is quite similar to mononucleosis (Table 3-12, *Stages of HIV*).

E. Initial symptoms usually occur within 3 weeks of initial exposure to HIV, after which the person becomes asymptomatic. Persons infected with HIV can transmit the virus to others any time after infection has occurred, whether they are symptomatic or asymptomatic.

F. Current Centers for Disease Control (CDC) definition of AIDS (end-stage infection) includes persons with specific, serious, opportunistic infections such as *Pneumocystis carinii* pneumonia (PCP), disseminated cytomegalovirus, or Kaposi sarcoma.

G. Risk groups include the following:
   1. Homosexual or bisexual males.
   2. IV drug abusers or those who have had tattoos or acupuncture.
   3. Heterosexual partner of a risk group member.
   4. Recipients of blood products prior to blood product screening—for example, those with hemophilia who were diagnosed and treated before 1985.

TABLE 3-12 Stages of HIV

Stage	Description/Symptoms
Primary Infection (Acute HIV Infection or Acute HIV Syndrome)	
CD4 T-cell counts of at least 800 cells/mm³	• Flu-like symptoms, fever, malaise • Mononucleosis-like illness, lymphadenopathy, fever, malaise, rash • Symptoms usually occur within 3 weeks of initial exposure to HIV, after which the person becomes asymptomatic
HIV Asymptomatic (CDC Category A)	
CD4 T-cell counts more than 500 cells/mm³	• No clinical problems • Characterized by continuous viral replication • Can last for many years, 10 years or longer
HIV Symptomatic (CDC Category B)	
CD4 T-cell counts between 200 and 499 cells/mm³	• Persistent generalized lymphadenopathy • Persistent fever • Weight loss, diarrhea • Peripheral neuropathy • Herpes zoster • Candidiasis • Cervical dysplasia • Hairy leukoplakia, oral
AIDS (CDC Category C)	
CD4 T-cell counts less than 200 cells/mm³	• Occurs when a variety of bacteria, parasites, or viruses overwhelm the body's immune system • Once classified as category C, the client remains classified as category C; this provides eligibility for entitlements such as health benefits, housing, food stamps, and so on (if certain financial requirements exist)

5. Those taking medications such as steroids or other agents that cause immunosuppression.
6. Infants born to infected mothers.
7. Breastfeeding infants of infected mothers.

Nursing Assessment (Data Collection)

A. Laboratory testing:
   1. Positive ELISA (enzyme-linked immunosorbent assay)—can have false positive.
   2. Confirmation by the Western Blot test, which uses electrophoreses and evaluates virus-specific bands.
   3. Polymerase chain reaction test (PCR) may be used to differentiate between HIV infection in the neonate and antibodies neonates receive from the mother.
   4. Seroconversion to positive on these tests occurs usually within 6 weeks to 3 months, but may take as long as 12 months.
   5. Before seroconversion to antibody-positive status, P24 antigen assay will be positive. (This test detects the core antigen of the virus.)

B. Symptoms:
   1. Extreme fatigue
   2. Loss of appetite and unexplained weight loss of more than 10 pounds in 2 months
   3. Swollen glands
   4. Leg weakness or pain
   5. Unexplained fever for more than a week
   6. Night sweats
   7. Unexplained diarrhea
   8. Dry cough; may represent *Pneumocystis carinii* pneumonia (PCP)
   9. White spots in the mouth and throat, may represent candidiasis
   10. Painful blisters, may represent shingles
   11. Painless, purple-blue lesions on the skin
   12. Confusion, disorientation
   13. In women, recurrent vaginal infections that are resistant to treatment

C. Opportunistic infections (Table 3-13, *Opportunistic Infections*).

> **HESI Hint** • HIV clients with tuberculosis require respiratory isolation. Tuberculosis is the only real risk to nonpregnant caregivers that is not related to a break in standard precautions (i.e., needle sticks, etc.).

Analysis (Nursing Diagnoses)

A. Risk for infection related to . . .
B. Imbalanced nutrition: less than body requirements related to . . .
C. Disturbed body image related to . . .
D. Social isolation related to . . .
E. Fatigue related to . . .
F. Risk for complicated grieving related to . . .

Nursing Plans and Interventions

A. Monitor respiratory functioning frequently.
B. Avoid known sources of infection.
C. Use strict asepsis for all invasive procedures.
D. Obtain vital signs frequently.
E. Plan activities to allow rest periods.
F. Elevate head of bed.
G. Coordinate a referral to the nutritionist.

TABLE 3-13 Opportunistic Infections

Pneumocystis Carinii Pneumonia (PCP)	Kaposi Sarcoma	Cryptosporidiosis	Candidiasis of Oral Cavity and Esophagus
• Fever • Dry cough • Dyspnea at rest • Chills	• Purple-blue lesions on skin, often arms and legs • Invasion of gastrointestinal tract, lymphatic system, lungs, and brain	• Severe, watery diarrhea (may be 30 to 40 stools per day) • Abdominal cramps • Nausea • Electrolyte imbalance • Malaise	• Thick, white exudate in the mouth • Unusual taste to food • Retrosternal burning • Oral ulcers
Cryptococcal Meningitis	**Cytomegalovirus (CMV) Retinitis**	**CMV Colitis**	**Disseminated CMV**
• Headache • Changes in level of consciousness • Nausea, vomiting • Stiff neck • Blurred vision	• Most common CMV infection in persons with AIDS • Impaired vision in one or both eyes • Can lead to blindness	• Diarrhea • Malabsorption of nutrients • Weight loss	• Malaise • Fever • Pancytopenia • Weight loss • Positive cultures from blood, urine, or throat
Perirectal Mucocutaneous Herpes Simplex Viral Infections	**Lymphomas of Central Nervous System (CNS)**	**Tuberculosis (TB)**	**HIV Encephalopathy**
• Severe pain • Bleeding, rectal discharge • Ulceration in the rectal area	• Change in mental status • Apathy • Psychomotor slowing • Seizures	• Pulmonary and extrapulmonary • Lymphatic and hematogenous TB are common; negative skin testing does not rule out TB • TB skin test is positive if induration of 5 mm or more if client is immunosuppressed	• Memory loss and impaired concentration • Apathy • Depression • Psychomotor slowing (most prominent symptom) • Incontinence • CAT scan findings: diffuse atrophy and ventricular enlargement

H. Offer small, frequent feedings.

I. Weigh daily.

J. Encourage client to avoid fatty foods.

K. Monitor for skin breakdown, offer good skin care.

L. Use safety precautions for clients with neurologic symptoms or loss of vision.

M. Orient client who is confused.

N. Provide emotional support for grieving client who is losing relationships and skills.

O. Provide emotional support for significant others: family, family of choice, lovers, friends.

P. Monitor the client's status while receiving IV fluids for hydration, as prescribed.

Q. Monitor the client while receiving total parenteral nutrition (TPN), as prescribed.

R. Administer agents that treat specific, opportunistic infections and medications for HIV (Table 3-14, *HIV Drugs*).

S. Assist with pain management; administer prescribed narcotics or analgesics.

T. Collaborate with RN to develop and implement client/family teaching about ways to avoid infection (i.e., stay away from enclosed crowded areas, avoid changing cat litter, avoid gardening, clean toothbrush daily in dishwasher, etc.).

HESI Hint • STANDARD PRECAUTIONS

Wash hands, even if gloves have been worn to give care.

Wear exam gloves for touching blood or body fluids or any nonintact body surface.

Wear gowns during any procedure that might generate splashes (changing clients with diarrhea).

Use masks and eye protection during activity that might disperse droplets (suctioning).

Do not recap needles; dispose of in puncture-resistant containers.

Use mouthpiece for resuscitation efforts.

For additional information, see *www.CDC.gov*.

HESI Hint • Caregivers who are pregnant may choose not to care for a client with cytomegalovirus (CMV).

TABLE 3-14 HIV Drugs

Drugs	Indications	Adverse Reactions	Nursing Implications
NRT (nucleoTide) Inhibitors • Tenofovir (Viread)	HIV infection classifications used in various combinations to reduce viral load and slow development of resistance	• Headache • Renal insufficiency • Fever, rash, N/V, abdominal cramps	• Monitor for lactic acidosis
Non-NRT Inhibitors • Efavirenz (Sustiva) • Delavirdine (Rescriptor) • Nevirapine (Viramune) • Etravirine (Intelence		• CNS changes • Nausea • Rash • Triglycerides • Hepatotoxicity	• Many drug–drug interactions • Monitor liver function tests • Reduces contraceptive effects • Do not confuse Viramune with Viracept
Protease Inhibitors • Indinavir (Crixivan) • Amprenavir (Agenerase) • Saquinavir (Invirase) • Ritonavir (Norvir, Kaletra) • Nelfinavir (Viracept) • Lopinavir + ritonavir (Kaletra) • Fosamprenavir (Lexiva) • Atazanavir (Reyataz)		• Depression • Ketoacidosis • Seizures • Angioedema • Stevens-Johnson syndrome	• Many drug–drug interactions • High-fat, high-protein foods reduce absorption • Give most of these with food • Reduces contraceptive effects • Do not confuse ritonavir (Norvir) with trade name zidovudine (Retrovir)
Combination Products • Lamivudine + zidovudine (Combivir) • Zidovudine + lamivudine + abacavir (Trizivir) • Emtricitabine + tenofovir (Truvada) • Tenofovir + emtricitabine + efavirenz (Atripla)		• Monitor for side effects associated with the individual drugs	• Note implications of the individual drugs in the combination product
CCR5 Inhibitors • Maraviroc (Selzentry)		• Hepatotoxicity • Cough, fever, rash, hypotension • Increased risk of infection	• Use cautiously in patients with underlying liver, renal, and cardiac disease
Fusion Inhibitors • Enfuvirtide (Fuzeon)		• Infection risk and lipodystrophy if injection site is not rotated	• Monitor skin reactions at injection site
Antiprotozoals • Atovaquone (Mepron) • Trimethoprim/sulfamethoxazole (Bactrim) • Pentamidine isethionate (Pentam 300)	Mepron used for PCP in those unable to tolerate trimethoprim/sulfamethoxazole prophylaxis Prophylaxis for PCP Treatment of PCP	• CNS disturbances • Agranulocytosis • Phlebitis if IV • Renal calculi with Bactrim • Leukopenia • ECG abnormalities	• Enhances effects of oral hypoglycemics • Increases thrombocytopenia risk if given with thiazide diuretics • Check for allergy to sulfonamide • IV or aerosol; not oral • Use careful precautions against potential spread of TB

TABLE 3-14 HIV Drugs—cont'd

Drugs	Indications	Adverse Reactions	Nursing Implications
Antivirals • Acyclovir sodium (Zovirax) • Valcyclovir (Valtrex) • Famciclovir (Famvir) • Ganciclovir (Cytovene) • Valganciclovir (Valcyte)	Herpes simplex CMV retinitis	• Granulocytopenia • Thrombocytopenia	• Give with or without food • Many incompatibilities: IV, PO, topical • Monitor liver function tests
Antifungals • Ampherotericin B (Fungizone) • Caspofungin (Cancidas) • Fluconazole (Diflucan) • Flucytosine (Ancobon) • Anidulafungin (Eraxis) • Posaconazole (Noxafil) • Itraconazole (Sporanox) • Micafungin (Mycamine) • Voriconazole (Vfend)	IV: Cryptococcal meningitis PO: Oral candidiasis	• Nephrotoxicity • Hypotension • Hypokalemia • Febrile reaction • Muscle cramps • Circulatory problems	• Many drug–drug interactions • Vesicant: monitor IV site closely; premedicate with antipyretic; give slowly • Swish as long as possible before swallowing PO form

Note: Client should have regular blood counts to track CD4 levels and viral load.

Pediatric HIV Infection

Description: Infection with HIV in infants and children.
A. Sources of infection for pediatric clients:
1. Perinatal transmission: 30% to 50% of children born to HIV-positive mothers will be infected unless the mother is treated with zidovudine during pregnancy and neonate is treated after birth; then rate decreases to 4% to 8%.
2. HIV-infected blood products
3. Breast milk
4. Sexual abuse
B. Although maternal antibodies may be present at birth in some children, the antibody tests convert to negative before 18 months of age.

Nursing Assessment (Data Collection)

A. Risk groups:
1. Infants born to mothers who are HIV positive
2. Hemophiliacs
3. Infants/children who have received blood transfusions
B. Symptoms:
1. Failure to thrive
2. Lymphadenopathy
3. Organomegaly
4. Neuropathy
5. Cardiomyopathy
6. Chronic recurrent infections, such as thrush
7. Unexplained fevers

HESI Hint • Pediatric HIV is often evidenced by lymphoid interstitial pneumonitis, pulmonary lymphoid hyperplasia, and opportunistic infection.

HESI Hint • The focus of NCLX-PN questions is likely to be assessment of early signs of the disease and management of complications associated with HIV.

Analysis (Nursing Diagnoses)

All diagnoses for adults may be experienced by children depending on the age of the child.
A. Interrupted family processes related to . . .
B. Delayed growth development related to . . .

Nursing Plans and Interventions

A. Avoid exposure to persons with infections, especially chickenpox.
B. Administer NO live virus vaccines.
C. Collaborate with RN to develop/implement client/family teaching plan:
1. Family to use gloves when diapering the child if child has diarrhea.
2. Family to clean any soiled surfaces (wearing gloves) with 1:10 bleach to water solution.
3. Family to identify signs of opportunistic infections.

D. Monitor growth parameters.
E. Administer gammaglobulin as prescribed, usually each month.
F. Support use of social services.

G. Support child attending school as much as child is able.
H. Refer back to the care plan for adult HIV client.
I. Assist in community and school education programs.

Review of HIV Infection

1. Identify the way HIV is transmitted.
2. Vertical transmission (from mother to fetus) occurs how often if the mother is not treated during pregnancy?
3. Describe universal precautions.
4. What does the CD4 T-cell count describe?
5. Why does the CD4 T-cell count drop in those with HIV infections?
6. Describe the ways a pediatric client might acquire HIV infection.

Answers to Review

1. Transmitted through blood and body fluids—for example, unprotected sexual contact with an infected person, sharing needles among drug-abusing persons, infected blood products (rare), maternal to fetus transmission through maternal placental circulation, breaks in universal precautions (needle sticks or similar occurrences).
2. Vertical transmission occurs 30% to 50% of the time.
3. Protection from blood and body fluids is the goal of standard precautions. Standard precautions: initiate barrier protection between caregiver and client through hand washing, use of gloves, use of gown and mask, eye protection as indicated, depending on activity of care and the likelihood of exposure. Prevent needle sticks by not recapping needles.
4. CD4 T-cell count describes the number of infection-fighting lymphocytes the person has.
5. CD4 T-cell count drops because the virus destroys CD4 T-cells as it invades them and replicates.
6. Through infected blood products, sexual abuse, and/or breast milk.

Pain

Description: An individual's subjective experience, including perception and response to an uncomfortable stimulus. Only the individual experiencing pain can know its characteristics. The pain is accepted as described by the client.
A. Client's pain often goes unrecognized and untreated.
   1. Health care professionals may poorly identify, assess, and manage pain.
   2. Health care professionals often cling to biases, including fear of addiction.
   3. Neonates have a fully developed and functioning pain perception mechanism.
B. Pain is classified as acute or chronic. Other types include intractable and referred.
   1. Acute pain
      a. Acute pain warns that something is wrong and usually is sudden and localized.
         (1) Chest pain may indicate myocardial hypoxia or other related thoracic structures—that is, broken ribs, intercostal muscles, or pulmonary or pleural origin.
         (2) Abdominal pain may reflect pathology from underlying structures—that is, gallbladder, hepatic, gastric, or renal problems.
      b. Signs of acute pain:
         (1) Increased heart rate and cardiac output
         (2) Increased blood pressure
         (3) Pupillary dilation
         (4) Palmar sweating
         (5) Hyperventilation
         (6) Hypermotility
         (7) Escape behavior
         (8) Anxiety state
   2. Chronic pain
      a. Chronic pain is insidious and may persist for months.
      b. Signs of chronic pain:
         (1) Sleep disturbances
         (2) Irritability
         (3) Appetite disturbances
         (4) Constipation
         (5) Psychomotor retardation
         (6) Pain intolerance
         (7) Social withdrawal
         (8) Mental depression
   3. Intractable pain includes persistent and intense pain caused by invasive, degenerative, or neurologic conditions—that is, cancer, arthritis, phantom limb, nerve entrapment, or neuralgias.

4. Referred pain is perceived at a site remote from its source.
   a. Deep structures may share the same dermatomes as superficial areas—that is, MI pain referred down medial aspect of left arm.
   b. Other referred pain may not share innervations along the same dermatome—that is, angina pain referred to the jaw.
C. An individual's response to pain is influenced by a variety of changing and interacting factors.
   1. Anxiety, fear, psychosocial stressors, fatigue, boredom, distraction
   2. Chemical and biochemical factors—that is, alcohol, drugs, biofeedback
   3. Culture and religion
   4. Emotional meaning and lifestyle impact
   5. History of pain: childhood experiences may impact adult perception and reaction to pain
   6. Intensity related to pathology
   7. Mental health—that is, depression, psychosis
D. Theories of pain
   1. *Gate control theory:* It is thought that stimulation of large, fast-conducting sensory fibers oppose input from small pain fibers, thus blocking pain perception.
   2. *Endorphin/enkephalin theory:* Endorphins and enkephalins are naturally occurring neurotransmitters that bind with opiate receptors in the central nervous system (CNS) and modulate pain.
E. Pain management modalities
   1. Analgesics and adjuvant medications
   2. Neurosurgical procedures—that is, nerve blocks, nerve resection (sympathectomy)
   3. Transcutaneous electrical nerve stimulation (TENS)
   4. Acupuncture, acupressure
   5. Massage, heat, cold applications
   6. Biofeedback
   7. Behavior modification
   8. Distraction, relaxation, guided imagery
   9. Hypnosis

Nursing Assessment (Data Collection)

A. Location: localized, radiating, or referred.
B. Intensity: ask client to rate pain.
   1. Before and after intervention.
   2. Use scale such as 0 to 10, with 0 being no pain.
   3. Use picture scale for children and cognitively impaired clients.
C. Comfort: often clients can describe what relieves pain better than describing the pain itself.
D. Quality: sharp, dull, aching, soreness, and so on.
E. Chronology: ask the client.
   1. When did pain start?
   2. What time of day does pain occur?
   3. How often does pain appear?
   4. How long does pain last?
   5. Is pain constant or intermittent?
   6. Has the intensity changed?
F. Subjective experience: ask the client.
   1. What decreases or aggravates pain?
   2. What other symptoms are associated with pain?
   3. What interventions provide relief?
   4. What limitations does the pain inflict?
G. Objective experience:
   1. Observe client's facial expressions to help judge client's level of pain.
   2. Observe cues—that is, groaning, moaning, crying, and requests for pain medication.
   3. Sleep deprivation can lead to sleepiness, fatigue, negative mood, disorientation, a decrease in growth hormone secretion, and lower pain threshold.

> **HESI Hint** • A subject assessment of pain can be collected by asking the client to rate his or her pain on a scale from 0 to 10, where 0 = no pain and 10 = the worst pain possible.

Analysis (Nursing Diagnoses)

A. Acute or chronic pain related to . . .
B. Ineffective coping related to . . .
C. Disturbed sleep pattern related to . . .
D. Activity intolerance related to . . .
E. Self-care deficit (specify) related to . . .

Nursing Plans and Interventions for Pain Management

A. Pharmacologic interventions (Table 3-15, *Routes of Administration for Analgesics*)
   1. Nonnarcotics, nonsteroidal anti-inflammatory drugs (NSAIDs) (see Table 4-27, *Nonsteroidal Antiinflammatory Drugs [NSAIDs]*, p. 125).
      a. Act by a peripheral mechanism at level of damaged tissue by inhibiting prostaglandin and other chemical mediator syntheses involved in pain.
      b. Antipyretic activity by action on the hypothalamic heat-regulating center to reduce fever.
      c. Examples: salicylates—aspirin (Bayer); non-salicylates—acetaminophen (Tylenol), ibuprofen (Motrin)
   2. Narcotic mixed agonists/antagonists
      a. Act as narcotics (agonists) that antagonize the "pure" agonists (counteract narcotic effects).
      b. Administration after client has been receiving narcotics may cause withdrawal symptoms.
      c. Side effects include drowsiness, occasional nausea, and psychomimetic effects such as hallucinations and euphoria.
      d. Examples: butorphanol (Stadol), nalbuphine (Nubain)

TABLE 3-15 Routes of Administration for Analgesics

Route	Administration
Oral	• Preferred method of administration • Drug levels usually peak at 1 to 2 hours
Intramuscular	• Acceptable method of managing acute, short-term pain • Onset 30 minutes, peak effect 1 to 3 hours, duration of action 4 hours
Rectal	• Useful with clients who are nauseated and unable to take analgesics by mouth • Useful for home care and with elderly clients as an alternative to oral and IV administration; reduced effectiveness with constipation
IV bolus (IV push)*	• Provides the most rapid onset (5 minutes), but with the shortest duration (1 hour) • Useful with acute pain, such as a client in labor
Patient-controlled analgesia (PCA)*	• Ideal method of pain control in that the client is able to prevent pain by administering to himself/herself smaller doses of the narcotic (usually morphine) as soon as the first sign of discomfort arises • Usually administered IV • A predetermined dose and a set lockout interval (5 to 20 minutes) is prescribed by physician, and pump is calibrated to deliver the specified dose for bolus, basal, and whenever client "hits the button" • Pump can deliver a bolus amount as a loading dose, a basal rate, intermittent doses, or a combination of any of the above • Lockout mechanism prevents overdosage • Pump can record number of times the client uses the pump and the cumulative dose delivered • Danger of respiratory depression • Teach family members at bedside to not push PCA if client is sleeping
Continuous subcutaneous narcotic infusion (CSI)	• Useful with clients who cannot take anything by mouth and who require prolonged administration of parenteral narcotics • Provides a constant level of analgesia by continuous infusion of a narcotic • Site should be inspected q8 hrs and changed at least every 7 days • Risk for respiratory depression
Continuous epidural analgesia (management of this route of administration is not within the scope of the PN)	• Catheter threaded into epidural space with continuous infusion of fentanyl citrate, morphine, or other narcotic analgesics • Risk of respiratory depression
Transdermal patches	• Applied to skin (self-adhesive or with overlay to secure patch) • Also used to deliver hormonal therapy, nitroglycerin, and nicotine • Sites for application and frequency of application are specific to each medication • Document removal of old patch as well as site and application date/time of new patch

*Depending on the state where you practice, administration of intravenous medications may not be within the PN's Scope of Practice. Monitoring the client's response to the medication should be done by the PN.

3. Narcotics
   a. Act as opioids, binding with specific opiate receptors throughout the CNS to reduce pain perception.
   b. Side effects include nausea and vomiting, constipation, respiratory depression, and CNS depression.
   c. Examples: hydromorphone (Dilaudid), morphine sulfate (Table 3-16, *Onset of Commonly Administered Narcotics*)

HESI Hint • For narcotic-induced respiratory depression, naloxone (Narcan) 0.1 mg to 0.4 mg IV can be given every 2 to 3 minutes as needed, until 1 mg is achieved.

TABLE 3-16 Onset of Commonly Administrated Narcotics*

Medication	Mode	Onset	Comments
Codeine	Oral	30 to 45 minutes	• Do *not* administer discolored injection solutions • May also be prescribed as an antitussive or antidiarrheal
	IM or subcut	10 to 30 minutes	
Hydromorphone (Dilaudid)	Oral	30 minutes	• Fast-acting, potent narcotic • More likely to cause appetite loss than other narcotics
	IM	15 minutes	
	IV	10 to 15 minutes	
Morphine sulfate	Oral	60 to 90 minutes	• Drug of choice in relieving pain associated with myocardial infarction • May cause transient decrease in blood pressure • Drug of choice for use with chronic cancer pain
	IM	10 to 30 minutes	
	IV	10 minutes	
Fentanyl citrate (Duragesic)	IM IV Intradermal Intrabuccal Intrathecal	7 to 15 minutes Within 5 minutes Within 12 hours 5 to 15 minutes Immediate	• Synthetic narcotic, morphine sulfate-like • Acts more quickly; shorter duration

*Although IV medication administration may not be within your Scope of Practice, the IV mode is included for your information.

B. Adjuvant to analgesics.
  1. Given in combination with an analgesic to potentiate or enhance the analgesic's effectiveness.
  2. Helpful in controlling discomforts associated with pain such as nausea, anxiety, and depression—for example, promethazine (Phenergan).

HESI Hint • USE NONINVASIVE METHODS FOR PAIN MANAGEMENT WHEN POSSIBLE
Relaxation exercises
Distraction
Imagery
Biofeedback
Interpersonal skills
Physical care: altering positions, touch, hot and cold applications (as ordered by HCP)

Nursing Assessment of Pain Relief Techniques

A. Pain (Table 3-17, *Pain Relief Techniques*)
B. Response to pharmacologic intervention: tolerance to pharmacologic interventions may occur—that is, the client physiologically requires increasingly larger doses to provide the same effect.
  1. First sign of tolerance is a decreased duration of drug effectiveness.
  2. Increased dosages can be a result of increased pain rather than tolerance—for example, clients with advanced cancer.

TABLE 3-17 Pain Relief Techniques

Noninvasive: Cutaneous Stimulation that Is Useful Alone or in Combination with Other Pain-Management Techniques

• Heat and cold applications decrease pain and muscle spasm.
• Transcutaneous electrical nerve stimulation (TENS) provides continuous mild electrical current to the skin via electrodes.
• Massage provides a simple, inexpensive, and effective method of pain relief.
• Distraction diverts client's attention from the pain; useful during short periods of pain or during painful procedures such as IV venipunctures.
• Relaxation can be used as a distraction and to facilitate sedation or sleep; rarely decrease pain sensation.
• Biofeedback techniques: control of autonomic responses (tachycardia, muscle tension) to pain through electrical feedback.
• Positioning, guided imagery meditation.

Invasive: Any Procedure Used to Relieve Pain that Invades the Body

• Nerve blocks: injection of anesthetic into or near a nerve to decrease pain pathways—for example, "deadening" area for dental work, regional anesthesia used in obstetrics.
• Neurosurgical procedures: surgical or chemical (alcohol) interruption of nerve pathways; commonly used in clients with cancer who have severe pain.
• Acupuncture: insertion of needles at various points into the body to relieve pain.

HESI Hint • Narcotic analgesics are preferred for pain relief because they bind to the various opiate receptor sites in the central nervous system (CNS). Morphine is often the preferred narcotic. (*Remember*, it causes respiratory depression.)

Narcotic antagonists block the attachment of narcotics to the receptors, such as naloxone (Narcan). Once Narcan has been given, additional narcotics cannot be given until the Narcan effects have passed.

Review of Pain

1. What modalities are associated with the gate control pain theory?
2. What modalities are thought to increase the production of endogenous opiates?
3. What six factors should the nurse include when assessing the pain experience?
4. What mechanism is involved in the reduction of pain through the administration of nonsteroidal anti-inflammatory medications?
5. If narcotic agonist/antagonist drugs are administered to a client already taking narcotic drugs, what may be the result?
6. List four side effects of narcotic medications.
7. What is the antidote for narcotic-induced respiratory depression?
8. What is the first sign of tolerance to pain analgesics?
9. Which route of administration for pain medications has the quickest onset and the shortest duration?
10. List the six modalities that are considered noninvasive, nonpharmacologic pain relief measures.

Answers to Review

1. Massage, heat and cold, acupuncture, TENS
2. Acupuncture, administration of placebos, TENS
3. Location, intensity, comfort measures, quality, chronology, and subjective view of pain
4. NSAIDs act by a peripheral mechanism at the level of damaged tissue by inhibiting prostaglandin synthesis and other chemical mediators involved in pain transmission.
5. Initiation of withdrawal symptoms
6. Nausea/vomiting, constipation, CNS depression, respiratory depression
7. Naloxone (Narcan)
8. Decreased duration of drug effectiveness
9. Intravenous push or bolus
10. Heat and cold applications, TENS, massage, distraction, relaxation techniques, biofeedback techniques

Death and Grief

Description: Death is the last developmental task for an individual. It completes the life cycle. Grief is the process an individual goes through to deal with loss.

Nursing Assessment (Data Collection)

A. Types of death:
   1. Natural/expected
   2. Sudden/unexpected
   3. Suicide
B. Stages of preparing for death or dying as described by Dr. Kübler-Ross:
   1. Denial
      a. Coping style used to protect self/ego.
      b. May be noncompliant, refusing to seek treatment, ignoring symptoms.
      c. Client changes the subject when speaking about illness.
      d. Client might state, "Not me. It must be a mistake."
   2. Anger
      a. Often directed at family and/or health care team members.
      b. "Why me?"; "It's not fair."
   3. Bargaining
      a. Usually makes a deal with God to prolong life.
      b. Usually does not share this with anyone. It is a very private experience.
   4. Depression
      a. Results from the losses experienced because of health status and hospitalization.

      b. Anticipation of the loss of life.
   5. Acceptance
      a. Accepts the inevitable.
      b. May begin to emotionally separate.

> **HESI Hint** • Although this is the normal progression of grief stages, it is not unusual for a client to go back and forth between stages.

C. Stages of dealing with loss (grief)
   1. Shock, disbelief, rejection, or denial
      a. Anger and crying
      b. Conflicting emotions
      c. Anger toward the deceased
      d. Guilt
      e. Preoccupation with loss
   2. Resolution
      a. Process can take up to 1 year or more
      b. Renewed interest in activities
D. Complicated grief
   1. If grief is unresolved, determine level of dysfunction.
   2. Physical symptoms similar to the deceased.
   3. Clinical depression
   4. Social isolation
   5. Failure to acknowledge loss

Analysis (Nursing Diagnoses)

A. Complicated grief related to . . .
B. Powerlessness related to . . .

> **HESI Hint** • Health care providers may refer clients to hospice during the dying process. The goal of hospice is to provide the highest quality of end-of-life care for dying individuals. The care includes comfort and support for the individual as well as for the family.

Nursing Plans and Interventions

A. Signs and symptoms of dying
   1. Progressive loss of appetite
      a. Result in dehydration and decreased cerebral function
      b. Interventions for decreased oral intake
        (1) Provide small amounts of light food and supplements (forcing food causes nausea, vomiting, or distention).
        (2) Avoid IVs and forcing fluids.
        (3) Moisten lips and mouth.
   2. Withdrawal
      a. Separation begins.
      b. Client uses energy to self-evaluate and prepare emotionally and spiritually.
        (1) Life review should be encouraged.

        (2) Focus on positive and negative remembrances.
        (3) Review accomplishments and impact on others.
      c. Reconciliation with others
        (1) Offer client/family referral to spiritual advisor.
        (2) Discuss cultural expectations with client and family.
      d. Financial concerns and final arrangements may be addressed.
   3. Sleep pattern changes
      a. Usually, more alert in the AM hours of the day.
      b. Progress into comatose state.
      c. Hearing is the last sense to go.
   4. Confusion and disorientation
      a. Client at risk for falls.
      b. Remind client of names.
      c. Client may have dreams or visions of others.
   5. Progressive loss of energy
   6. Decrease in bowel function
      a. Avoid laxatives and enemas.
      b. All orifices relax and expel contents at time of death; therefore, use pads and draw sheets on bed.
   7. Diminished circulation
      a. Fever
        (1) Sponge with cool water.
        (2) Cover lightly.
      b. Sweating
      c. Edema
      d. Decreased urine output
      e. Decubitus
        (1) Change positions frequently, as tolerated.
        (2) Keep bed linen wrinkle free.
        (3) Use moisturizing lotions.
      f. Skin color changes.
        (1) Peripheral circulation diminished.
        (2) Increased circulation to vital organs.
   8. Changes in breathing patterns
      a. Shortness of breath related to increasing weakness
        (1) Elevate head of bed.
        (2) Reposition client on side to facilitate postural drainage.
        (3) Administer O_2 per provider's order.
      b. Dyspnea
        (1) Administer pain medication as prescribed (oral, patches, and suppositories).
        (2) Comfort client and family.
      c. Congestion
        (1) "Death rattle"—accumulation of fluid and mucus in airways because of loss of cough reflex.
        (2) Position head to the side to drain secretions.
        (3) Transdermal scopolamine patch may be ordered.
      d. Cheyne-Stokes respirations
        (1) Periods of apnea lasting 10 to 60 seconds.
        (2) Followed by increasing depth and frequency of respirations.

e. Final breaths: provide support to client and family.
9. Rigor mortis (death rigor)
   a. Muscles begin to stiffen 3 to 4 hours after death.
   b. Peak rigidity occurs at 12 hours.
   c. Gradually dissipates over the next 48 to 60 hours.

> **HESI Hint** • Do not take away the coping style of *denial* when it's being used in a crisis state. It can be a very useful and a needed tool at the initial stage for some individuals. Support, do not challenge, unless it hinders/ blocks treatment—endangering the client.

Review of Death and Grief

1. Identify the five stages of death and dying.
2. A client has been told of a positive breast biopsy report. She asks no questions and leaves the health care provider's office. She is overheard telling her husband, "The doctor didn't find a thing." What coping style is operating at this stage of grief?
3. Your client, an incest survivor, is speaking of her deceased father, the perpetrator. "He was a wonderful man, so good and kind. Everyone thought so." What would be the most useful intervention at this time?
4. Your client feels responsible for his sister's death because he took her to the hospital where she died. "If I hadn't taken her there, they couldn't have killed her." It has been 1 month since her death. Is this response indicative of a normal or complicated grief reaction?
5. Mrs. Green lost her husband 3 years ago. She has not disturbed any of his belongings and continues to set a place at the table for him nightly. Is this response indicative of a normal or complicated grief reaction?

Answers to Review

1. Denial, anger, bargaining, depression, acceptance
2. Denial
3. Gently point out both the positive and negative aspects of her relationship with her father. Try to minimize the idealization of the deceased.
4. This is a normal expression of anger and guilt that occurs. Try to minimize the rumination of these thoughts.
5. This is a dysfunctional grief reaction. Mrs. Green has never moved out of the denial stage of her grief work.

MEDICAL-SURGICAL NURSING

Respiratory System

Pneumonia

Description: Pneumonia is an inflammation of the lower respiratory tract.

A. Pneumonia is commonly caused by infectious agents.
B. Organisms that cause pneumonia reach the lungs by three methods:
1. Aspiration
2. Inhalation
3. Hematogenous spread
C. Pneumonia is generally classified according to causative agents:
1. Bacterial
2. Viral
3. Fungal (rare)
4. Chemical
D. Pneumonia may be community acquired or nosocomial (hospital/agency acquired).
E. High-risk groups include individuals who are:
1. Debilitated with accumulated lung secretions
2. Cigarette smokers
3. Immobile
4. Immunosuppressed
5. Experiencing a depressed gag reflex and/or cough
6. Sedated
7. Impaired by neuromuscular disorders
8. Nasogastric/orogastric intubation
9. Hospitalized client

Nursing Assessment (Data Collection)

A. Tachypnea: shallow respirations, often with use of accessory muscles
B. Abrupt onset of fever with shaking and chills (not reliable with older adults)
C. Productive cough with pleuritic pain
D. Rapid, bounding pulse
E. In the older adults, symptoms include:
1. Confusion
2. Lethargy/malaise

3. Anorexia
4. Rapid respiratory rate
5. Tachycardia
F. Pain and dullness on percussion over the affected lung area
G. Bronchial breath sounds; crackles
H. Chest x-ray indication of infiltrates with consolidation or pleural effusion
I. Elevated white blood cell count (WBC)
J. Arterial blood gases (ABGs) indicate hypoxemia
K. A drop in oxygen saturation when using a pulse oximetry (should be more than 90%, ideally more than 95%)

> **HESI Hint** • Fever can cause dehydration from excessive fluid loss in diaphoresis. Increased temperature also increases metabolism and the demand for oxygen.

> **HESI Hint** • **HIGH RISK FOR PNEUMONIA**
> Any person who has an altered level of consciousness, has depressed or absent gag and cough reflexes, or is susceptible to aspirating oropharyngeal secretions (including alcoholics, anesthetized individuals, those with brain injury, those in a state of drug overdose, stroke victims, those with asplenia, and those who are immunocompromised) is at high risk.

Analysis (Nursing Diagnoses)

A. Impaired gas exchange related to . . .
B. Ineffective airway clearance related to . . .
C. Activity intolerance related to . . .
D. Risk for deficient fluid volume related to . . .

Nursing Plans and Interventions

A. Examine and report sputum for volume, color, consistency, and clarity.

B. Assist client to cough productively by:
1. Deep breathing every 2 hours (may use incentive spirometer).
2. Using humidity to loosen secretions (may be oxygenated).
3. Suctioning the airway, if necessary.
4. Chest physiotherapy as prescribed.

C. Provide fluids up to 3 liters/day unless contraindicated (helps liquefy lung secretions).

D. Auscultate lung sounds before and after coughing.

E. Monitor rate, depth, and pattern of respirations regularly (normal adult rate is 16 to 20 breaths/min).

F. Monitor ABGs (Po_2 more than 80 mm Hg; Pco_2 less than 45 mm Hg).

G. Monitor O_2 saturation with pulse oximetry (ideally more than 95%).

H. Report skin color.

I. Monitor mental status, restlessness, and irritability.

J. Administer O_2 as prescribed.

K. Monitor temperature regularly.

L. Provide adequate rest periods, including uninterrupted sleep.

M. Administer antibiotics as prescribed (Table 4-1, *Anti-Infectives*).

N. Collaborate with RN to develop a client/family teaching plan about risk factors and include preventive measures.

O. Encourage at-risk groups to get pneumonia and flu immunizations.

P. Promote rest and conserve energy.

TABLE 4-1 Anti-Infectives

Drugs	Indications	Adverse Reactions	Nursing Implications
Penicillins			
• Procaine penicillin G (Wycillin) • Benzathine penicillin (Bicillin L-A) • Penicillin V (Pen-Vee K)	• Anti-infectives • Used primarily for gram-positive infections	• Allergic reactions • Anaphylaxis • Phlebitis at IV site • Diarrhea • GI distress • Superinfection • False positive for glucose using Clinitest	• Use with caution in clients allergic to cephalosporins • Monitor for allergic reactions • Observe all clients for at least 30 minutes after parenteral administration • Oral penicillin G should be taken on an empty stomach • Probenecid decreases renal excretion, thereby resulting in an increased blood level of the drug • Alters contraceptive effectiveness
Semisynthetic			
• Oxacillin sodium • Nafcillin sodium • Cloxacillin sodium • Dicloxacillin sodium	• Anti-infectives • Used primarily for gram-positive infections	• Allergic reactions • Anaphylaxis • Superinfection • *See Penicillins*	• Cannot be used in clients allergic to penicillin • Caution in clients allergic to cephalosporins • Monitor for superinfection (sore mouth, vaginal discharge, diarrhea, cough) • *See Penicillins*
Antipseudomonal Penicillins and Combinations			
• Ampicillin • Ticarcillin + clavulanate (Timentin) • Piperacillin + tazobactam (Zosyn) • Ampicillin + sulbactam (Unasyn)	• Anti-infectives • Broad spectrums	• Similar to penicillin • Ampicillin rash	• Contraindicated in clients allergic to penicillin • *See Penicillins*

TABLE 4-1 Anti-Infectives—cont'd

Drugs	Indications	Adverse Reactions	Nursing Implications
Tetracyclines			
• Tetracycline HCL • Doxycycline hyclate (Vibramycin) • Minocycline (Minocin)	• Anti-infectives	• Hypersensitivity reactions • Photosensitivity	• Decreases the effectiveness of oral contraceptives • Avoid concurrent use of antacids, milk products • Inspect IV site frequently • Monitor for superinfections • Avoid exposure to sunlight during use • Avoid use in pregnant clients and children under 8 years; can cause yellow-brown discoloration of teeth and growth retardation
Aminoglycosides			
• Gentamicin sulfate • Tobramycin sulfate (Nebcin) • Amikacin sulfate Miscellaneous Agents • Vancomycin hydrochloride • Metronidazole (Flagyl)	• Anti-infectives • Used with gram-negative bacteria	• Neuromuscular blockade • Nephrotoxicity • Ototoxicity	• Monitor renal function, BUN, creatinine, and I&O • Monitor for ototoxicity; headache, dizziness, hearing loss, tinnitus • Monitor for superinfection • Monitor vancomycin serum drug concentrations • Red-neck syndrome
Cephalosporins			
First Generation: • Cefazolin (Kefzol) • Cephalexin (Keflex) Second Generation: • Cefaclor (Ceclor) • Cefamandole (Mandol) • Cefuroxime (Ceftin-PO, Zinacef-IV) • Cefoxitin (Mefoxin) • Cefotetan (Cefotan) • Cefprozil (Cefzil) Third Generation: • Cefotaxime (Claforan) • Ceftriaxone (Rocephin) • Ceftazidime (Fortaz) • Cefdinir (Omnicef) • Cefixime (Suprax) • Cefpodoxime (Vantin) • Ceftibuten (Cedax) Fourth Generation • Cefepime (Maxipime)	• Anti-infectives	• Allergic reactions • Thrombophlebitis • GI distress • Superinfection	• Use with caution in clients allergic to penicillin and cephalosporins • *See Penicillins*

Continued

TABLE 4-1 Anti-Infectives—cont'd

Drugs	Indications	Adverse Reactions	Nursing Implications
Carbapenems			
• Imipenem (Primaxin) • Meropenem (Merrem IV) • Ertapenem (Invanz)			
Monobactam			
• Aztreonam (Azactam)	• *Pseudomonas aeruginosa* + many otherwise resistant organisms • Most effective against gram negatives	• Phlebitis • Pseudomembranous colitis • CNS changes • EEG changes • Headache/diplopia • Hypotension	• Monitor renal and hepatic function, especially in older adults • Carefully monitor for diarrhea • Assess motor sensory function and cardiac rhythm
Macrolides			
• Clarithromycin (Biaxin) • Azithromycin (Zithromax) • Erythromycin	• Biaxin (oral): URI, including Strep; as adjunct treatment for *H. pylori* • Zithromax (IV): gram-negative and gram-positive organisms	• Pseudomembranous colitis • Phlebitis—a vesicant • Superinfections • Dizziness • Dyspnea	• Give Biaxin XL with food • Space MAO inhibitors 14 days before start and after end of Biaxin • Report diarrhea, abdominal cramping—all macrolides • Monitor liver, renal labs • Oral Zithromax—give on empty stomach
Fluoroquinolones			
• Ciproflaxin (Cipro) • Levoflaxin (Levaqin) • Moxifloxacin (Avelox)	• All three of the most difficult to treat respiratory infections, UTIs, skin, bone, and joint infections • Has been used as conjunctive treatment for TB and AIDS	• Superinfections • CNS disturbances • Arroyos and cataracts possible with Cipro • Cipro—a vesicant	• Prompt onset • Crosses placenta and in breast milk • Can lower seizure threshold • Monitor liver, renal, and blood counts • Safety for children not known • Many drug–drug interactions
Lincosamides			
• Clindamycin HCl (Cleocin HCl)	• *Pneumocystis carinii* pneumonia (PCP) in AIDS • Soft tissue infections caused by streptococci, staphylococci, and anaerobes • Severe infections resistant to penicillins and cephalosporins • Used in penicillin or erythromycin-sensitive clients	• Agranulocytosis • Pseudomembranous colitis • Superinfections	• Highly toxic drug; use only when absolutely necessary • Periodic liver, renal and blood counts • Report diarrhea immediately

TABLE 4-1 Anti-Infectives—cont'd

Drugs	Indications	Adverse Reactions	Nursing Implications
Streptogramin			
• Quinupristin/dalfopristin (Synercid)	• Life-threatening vancomycin-resistant enterococcus (VRE)	• Arthralgia, myalgia • Severe vesicant • Pseudomembranous colitis • Nausea/vomiting, diarrhea • Rash, pruritus	• Incompatible with any saline solutions or heparin • Functionally related to both macrolides and lincosamides • Monitor total bilirubin • Many drug–drug interactions
Oxazolidinone			
• Linezolid (Ziox)	• Life-threatening vancomycin resistant enterococcus (VRE) and methicillin-resistant *Staphylococcus aureus* (MRSA)	• GI disturbances • Headache • Pancytopenia • Pseudomembranous colitis • Superinfections	• Monitor renal and liver labs, + blood count • May exacerbate hypertension, especially if foods ingested with tyramine • Report diarrhea immediately

HESI Hint • Bronchial breath sounds are heard over areas of density or consolidation. Sound waves are easily transmitted over consolidated tissue.

HESI Hint • **HYDRATION**
Enables liquefaction of mucus trapped in the bronchioles and alveoli, facilitating expectoration. Essential for client experiencing fever. Important because 300 to 400 mL of fluid are lost daily by the lungs through evaporation.

HESI Hint • Irritability and restlessness are early signs of cerebral hypoxia; the client is not getting enough oxygen to the brain.

HESI Hint • **PNEUMONIA PREVENTATIVES**
• **Older adults:** Flu shots; pneumonia immunizations; avoiding sources of infection and indoor pollutants (dust, smoke, and aerosols); no smoking
• **Immunosuppressed and debilitated persons:** Flu shots, pneumonia immunizations, infection avoidance, sensible nutrition, adequate fluid intake, balance of rest and activity
• **Comatose and immobile persons:** Elevation of head of bed to feed and for 1 hour after feeding; frequently turning

Chronic Airflow Limitation

Description: Chronic airflow limitation (CAL) includes chronic bronchitis, pulmonary emphysema, and asthma (Table 4-2, *Chronic Airflow Limitation*).
A. Emphysema and bronchitis termed as chronic obstructive pulmonary disease (COPD) are characterized by bronchospasm and dyspnea. The damage to the lung is not reversible and increases in severity.
B. Asthma, unlike COPD, is an intermittent disease with reversible airflow obstruction.
C. Alveoli beyond the chronic obstruction are overinflated, causing chronic hypoxemia, hypoxia, and hypercapnia (in emphysema).

HESI Hint • Respiratory compensation happens through the lungs most often to correct acid-base imbalances.

Nursing Assessment (Data Collection)
A. Changes in breathing pattern (e.g., an increase in rate with a decrease in depth)
B. Use of accessory breathing muscles (barrel chest)
C. Generalized cyanosis of lips, mucous membranes, face, nail beds ("blue bloater")
D. Cough (dry or productive)
E. Higher CO_2 than average
F. Low O_2, as determined by pulse oximetry
G. Decreased breath sounds
H. Coarse crackles in lung fields, which tend to disappear after coughing; wheezing

TABLE 4-2 Chronic Airflow Limitation

Chronic Bronchitis	Emphysema	Asthma
• Cough with sputum production on a daily basis for a minimum of 3 months per year • Chronic hypoxemia, cor pulmonale • Increase in mucus, cilia production • Increase in bronchial wall thickness (obstructs air flow) • Reduced responsiveness of respiratory center to hypoxemix stimuli	• Reduced gas exchange surface area • Increased air trapping (increased A-P diameter) • Decreased capillary network • Increased work, increased O_2 consumption	• Narrowing or closure of the airway due to a variety of stimulants
Precipitating Factors		
• Higher incidence in smokers	• Cigarette smoking • Environment and/or occupational exposure • Genetic	• Mucosal edema • V/Q abnormalities • Increased work of breathing • Beta-blockers • Respiratory infection • Allergic reaction • Emotional stress • Exercise • Environmental or occupational exposure • Reflux esophagitis
Assessment		
• Generalized cyanosis "Blue Bloaters" • Right-sided heart failure • Distended neck veins • Crackles • Expiratory wheezes	• "Pink Puffers" • Barrel chest • Pursed-lip breathers • Distant, quiet breath sounds • Wheezes • Pulmonary blebs on radiograph	• Dyspnea, wheezing, chest tightness • Monitor precipitating factors • Medication history
Nursing Plans and Interventions		
• Lowest FiO_2 possible to prevent CO_2 retention • Monitor for s/s of fluid overload • Maintain PaO_2 between 55 and 60 • Baseline ABGs • Teach pursed-lip breathing and diaphragmatic breathing • Teach tripod position	• Lowest FiO_2 possible to prevent CO_2 retention • Monitor for s/s of fluid overload • Maintain PaO_2 between 55 and 60 • Baseline ABGs • Teach pursed-lip breathing and diaphragmatic breathing • Teach tripod position	• Administer bronchodilators • Administer fluids and humidification • Reinforce teaching (causes, medication regimen) • ABGs • Ventilatory patterns

I. Dyspnea, orthopnea
J. Poor nutrition, weight loss
K. Activity intolerance
L. Anxiety concerning breathing, manifested by:
   1. Anger
   2. Fear of being alone
   3. Fear of not being able to "catch breath"

Gastric distention becomes a priority in these clients because it elevates the diaphragm and inhibits full lung expansion.

HESI Hint • Productive cough and comfort can be facilitated by semi-Fowler or high Fowler positions, which lessen pressure on the diaphragm from abdominal organs.

HESI Hint • **NORMAL ABG VALUES**

Blood Gas	Adult	Child
Ph	7.35 to 7.45	7.36 to 7.44
Pco_2	35 to 45 mm Hg	Same as adult
Po_2	80 to 100 mm Hg	Same as adult
HCO_3	22 to 26 mEq/L	Same as adult

Continued

HESI Hint • **Pink Puffer:** Barrel chest is indicative of emphysema and is caused by use of accessory muscles to breathe, which causes the person to work harder to breathe, but the amount of O_2 taken in is adequate to oxygenate the tissues.

Blue Bloater: Insufficient oxygenation occurs with chronic bronchitis and leads to generalized cyanosis and often right-sided heart failure (cor pulmonale).

HESI Hint • **HEALTH PROMOTION**

Eating consumes energy needed for breathing. Offer mechanically soft diets that do not require as much chewing and digestion. Assist with feeding if needed.

Prevent secondary infections—avoid crowds, contact with persons who have infectious diseases, and respiratory irritants (tobacco smoke).

Reinforce client teaching to report any change in characteristics of sputum.

Encourage client to hydrate well and to obtain immunizations needed (flu and pneumonia).

Analysis (Nursing Diagnoses)

A. Ineffective airway clearance related to . . .
B. Ineffective breathing pattern related to . . .
C. Impaired gas exchange related to . . .
D. Activity intolerance related to . . .
E. Knowledge deficit related to . . .

HESI Hint • Cells of the body depend on oxygen to carry out their functions. Inadequate arterial oxygenation is manifested by cyanosis and slow capillary refill (more than 3 seconds). A chronic sign is clubbing of the fingernails, and a late sign is clubbing of the fingers.

Nursing Plans and Interventions

A. Collaborate with RN to develop and implement a client teaching plan about sitting upright and bending slightly forward to promote breathing.
  1. In bed—sitting with arms resting on or over the bed table (tripod position)
  2. In chair—leaning forward with elbows resting on knees (tripod position) (Figure 4-1, *Forward-Leaning-Position*)
B. Reinforce the client teaching plan regarding diaphragmatic and pursed-lip breathing.
C. Collaborate with RN to develop and implement a client teaching plan about prolonged expiratory phase to clear trapped air.
D. Administer O_2 at 1 to 2 liters per nasal cannula (Table 4-3, *Nursing Skills: Respiratory Client*).

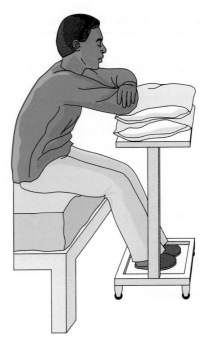

Sitting on the edge of a bed with the arms folded and placed on two or three pillows positioned over a nightstand.

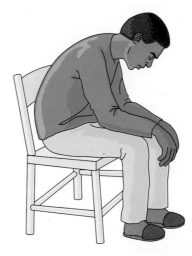

Sitting in a chair with the feet spread shoulder-width apart and leaning forward with the elbows on the knees. Arms and hands are relaxed.

FIGURE 4-1 Forward-Leaning-Position. A, The client sits on the edge of the bed with arms folded on a pillow placed on the elevated bedside table. **B,** Client in three-point position. The client sits in a chair with the feet approximately 1 foot apart and leans forward with elbows on knees. (From Ignatavicius DD, Workman ML: *Medical-surgical nursing: patient-centered collaborative care,* ed 6, St. Louis, 2010, Saunders.)

HESI Hint • Caution must be used in administering O_2 to a COPD client. The stimulus to breathe is hypoxia (hypoxic drive), not the usual hypercapnia, the stimulus to breathe for healthy persons. Therefore, if too much oxygen is given, the client may stop breathing!

TABLE 4-3 Nursing Skills: Respiratory Client

Suctioning (Tracheal)
• Suction when adventitious breath sounds are heard, when secretions are present at endotracheal tube, or when gurgling sounds are noted.
• Use aseptic/sterile technique throughout procedure.
• Wear mask and goggles.
• May liquefy secretions with 3 mL saline instilled before suctioning.
• Advance catheter until resistance is felt.
• Apply suction only when withdrawing catheter (gently rotate catheter when withdrawing).
• Never suction more than 10 to 15 seconds, and only pass the catheter three or fewer times.
• Oxygenate with 100% O_2 for 1 to 2 minutes before and after suctioning to prevent hypoxia.
Maintain Ventilator Setting
• Verify that alarms are on.
• Maintain settings and check often to insure they are specifically set as prescribed by health care provider.
• Verify functioning of ventilator at least every 4 hours.
Oxygen Administration
• Nasal cannula: low oxygen flow for low oxygen concentrations (good for COPD).
• Simple face mask: low flow but effectively delivers high oxygen concentrations; cannot deliver less than 40% O_2.
• Nonrebreather mask: low flow but delivers high oxygen concentrations (60% to 90%).
• Partial rebreather mask: low flow oxygen reservoir bag attached; can deliver high oxygen concentrations.
• Venturi mask: high-flow system; can deliver exact oxygen concentration.
Pulse Oximetry
• Easy measurement of oxygen saturation.
• Should be greater than 90%, ideally above 95%.
• Noninvasive, fastens to finger, toe, or earlobe.
Tracheostomy Care
• Aseptic technique (remove inner cannula only).
• Clean disposable inner cannula with hydrogen peroxide—rinse with sterile saline.
• 4 × 4 gauze dressing is butterfly folded.
Respiratory Isolation Technique
• Mask required for anyone entering room.
• Private room required.
• Client must wear mask if leaving room.
Proper Use of an Inhaler
• Have client exhale completely.
• Only grip (in mouth) if client has a spacer, otherwise keep mouth open to bring in volume of air with misted medication. While inhaling slowly, push down firmly on the inhaler to release the medication.
• Use bronchodilator inhaler before steroid inhaler and rinse mouthpiece after every use.

E. Pace activities to conserve energy.

F. Maintain adequate dietary intake, but do not overfeed.
1. Small, frequent meals
2. Favorite foods
3. Dietary supplements (protein-rich shakes, vitamins)

G. Provide an adequate fluid intake (3 liters/day) unless contraindicated.

H. Collaborate with the RN to develop and implement a client/family teaching plan about relaxation techniques.

I. Reinforce the teaching plan regarding prevention of secondary infections.

J. Collaborate with RN to develop and implement a client/family teaching plan about medication regimen (Table 4-4, *Bronchodilators/Corticosteroids*).

K. Collaborate with RN to develop and implement a client/family teaching plan about proper technique for inhalers.

L. Smoking cessation is imperative.

M. Encourage health promotion activities.

TABLE 4-4 Bronchodilators/Corticosteroids

Drugs	Indications	Adverse Reactions	Nursing Implications
Adrenergics/Sympathomimetics			
• Epinephrine • Isoproterenol HCL (Isuprel) • Albuterol (Proventil) • Isoetharine (Bronkometer) • Terbutaline (Brethine) • Salmeterol (Serevent) • Metaproterenol (inhaled) (Alupent) • Levalbuterol (Xopenex)	• Bronchodilator	• Anxiety • Increased heart rate • Nausea, vomiting • Urinary retention	• Check heart rate • Monitor for urinary retention, especially in men older than 40 • Reinforce teaching in proper use of inhaler • Use bronchodilator inhaler before steroid inhaler • May cause sleep disturbance
Methylxanthines			
• Aminophylline (IV) • Theophylline (oral)	• Bronchodilator	• GI distress • Sleeplessness • Cardiac dysrhythmias • Hyperactivity	• Administer oral forms with food • Avoid foods containing caffeine • Can also be administered intravenously • Check heart rate • Reinforce teaching in proper use of inhaler • Monitor therapeutic range 10 to 20 mg/mL • Crosses placenta
Corticosteroids			
• Prednisone (oral) • Methylprednisolone (Solu-Medrol) (IV) • Beclomethasone dipropionate (inhaled) (Vanceril) • Budesonide (inhaled) (Pulmicort) • Fluticasone (inhaled) (Flovent) • Triamcinolone (inhaled) (Azmacort) • Flunisolide (inhaled) (AeroBid) • Mometasone (inhaled) (Asmanex)	• Anti-inflammatory	• Cardiac dysrhythmias that occur with long-term steroid use	• Reinforce teaching in proper use of inhaler
Anticholinergics			
• Ipratropium (Atrovent) • Tiotropium (Spiriva)	• Bronchodilator • Control of rhinorrhea	• Dry mouth • Blurred vision • Cough	Do not exceed 12 doses in 24 hours (Ipratropium)
Combination Products			
• Fluticasone + albuterol (Advair) • Ipratropium + albuterol (Combivent) • Budesonide + fomoterol (Symbicort)	See individual drugs	See individual drugs	See individual drugs
Phosphodiesterase 4 Inhibitors			
• Roflumilast (Daliresp)	• Reduced lung inflammation in severe COPD	• Insomnia • Weight loss • Depression	• Many drug–drug interactions

HESI Hint • When asked to prioritize nursing actions, use the ABC rule:
- Airway first
- Then breathing
- Then circulation

In CPR circumstances, follow the CAB guidelines.

HESI Hint • *Look and listen!* If breath sounds are clear, but the client is cyanotic and lethargic, adequate oxygenation is not occurring.

HESI Hint • The key to respiratory status is to auscultate breath sounds as well as visualize the client. Breath sounds are better "described," not named (e.g., sounds should be described as "crackles," "wheeze," "high-pitched whistling sound," rather than "rales," "rhonchi," etc., which may not mean the same thing to each clinical professional).

HESI Hint • Watch for NCLEX-PN® questions that deal with oxygen delivery. In adults, O_2 must bubble through some type of water solution so it can be humidified if given at more than 4 L/min or delivered directly to the trachea. If given at 1 to 4 L/min or by mask or nasal prongs, the oropharynx and nasal pharynx provide adequate humidification.

Cancer of the Larynx

Description: Neoplasm occurring in the larynx, most commonly squamous cell in origin.
A. The combined effects of prolonged use of alcohol and/or tobacco are directly related to development.
B. Other contributing factors include the following:
 1. Vocal straining
 2. Chronic laryngitis
 3. Family predisposition
 4. Industrial exposure to carcinogens
 5. Nutritional deficiencies; riboflavin
C. Men are affected eight times more often than women.
D. Diagnosis usually occurs between ages 55 and 70.
E. Earliest sign is hoarseness or a change in vocal quality that lasts more than 2 weeks.
F. Medical management includes radiation therapy, often with adjuvant chemotherapy or surgical removal of the larynx (laryngectomy).

Nursing Assessment (Data Collection)
A. Hoarseness for greater than 2 weeks (early)
B. Color changes in mouth or tongue
C. Later changes include dysphagia, dyspnea, cough, hemoptysis, weight loss, neck pain radiating to the ear, enlarged cervical nodes, and halitosis.

HESI Hint • With cancer of the larynx, the tongue and mouth often appear white, gray, dark brown, or black, and they may appear patchy.

D. Direct laryngoscopy
E. X-ray films of head, neck, and chest
F. CT scan of neck and biopsy
G. MRI

Analysis (Nursing Diagnoses)
For client undergoing a laryngectomy:
A. Anxiety related to . . .
B. Ineffective airway clearance related to . . .
C. Impaired verbal communication related to . . .
D. Knowledge deficit related to . . .

Nursing Plans and Interventions
A. Collaborate with the RN to develop and implement a client/family perioperative teaching plan.
 1. Allow client/family to observe and handle tracheostomy tubes and suctioning equipment.
 2. Explain how and why suctioning will take place after surgery.
 3. Plan for acceptable communication method after surgery. Consider literacy level.
 4. Coordinate referral to speech pathologist.
 5. Discuss the planned rehabilitation program.
B. Provide postoperative care.
 1. Simplify communications.
 2. Use planned alternate communication method.
 3. Keep call bell/light within reach at all times.
 4. Ask client yes/no questions whenever possible.
 5. Invite family member to remain at bedside to provide support.
C. Promote respiratory functioning.
 1. Monitor respiratory rate and characteristics every 1 to 2 hours.
 2. Keep bed in semi-Fowler position at all times.
 3. Keep laryngeal airway humidified at all times.
 4. Auscultate lung sounds every 2 to 4 hours.
 5. Provide tracheostomy care every 2 to 4 hours and as needed.

HESI Hint • Tracheostomy care involves cleaning the inner cannula, suctioning, and applying a clean dressing.

 6. Administer tube feedings as prescribed.
 7. Encourage ambulation as early as possible.
 8. Coordinate referral for speech rehabilitation with artificial larynx and/or to learn esophageal speech.
 9. Humidification of environment.

HESI Hint • Air entering the lungs is humidified along the nasobronchial tree. This natural humidifying pathway is gone for the client who has had a laryngectomy. If the air is not humidified before entering the lungs, secretions tend to thicken and become crusty.

HESI Hint • A laryngectomy tube has a larger lumen and is shorter than the tracheostomy tube. Observe the client for any signs of bleeding or occlusion, which are the greatest immediate postoperative risks (first 24 hours).

HESI Hint • Fear of choking is very real for laryngectomy clients. They cannot cough as before because the glottis is gone. Teach the "glottal stop" technique to remove secretions (take a deep breath, momentarily occlude the tracheostomy tube, cough, and simultaneously remove the finger from the tube).

Pulmonary Tuberculosis

Description: Pulmonary tuberculosis (TB) is a communicable lung disease caused by an infection with the *Mycobacterium tuberculosis* bacteria.
A. Airborne transmission.
B. After initial exposure, the bacteria encapsulate (form Ghon lesion).
C. Bacteria remain dormant until a later time when clinical symptoms appear.

Nursing Assessment (Data Collection)

A. Often asymptomatic.
B. Symptoms include:
   1. Fever with night sweats
   2. Anorexia, weight loss
   3. Malaise, fatigue
   4. Cough, hemoptysis
   5. Dyspnea, pleuritic chest pain with inspiration
   6. Cavitation or calcification as evidenced on chest x-ray film
   7. Positive sputum culture
   8. Repeated upper respiratory infections (URIs)

HESI Hint • **TB SKIN TEST**
A positive TB skin test in a healthy client is exhibited by an induration 10 mm or greater in diameter 48 hours after skin test. Anyone who has received a bacillus Calmette-Guerin vaccine will have a positive skin test and must be evaluated with an initial chest radiograph. A health history with signs and symptoms form may be filled out annually until signs and symptoms arise; then another chest x-ray is required. Chest x-rays are required on new employment; employer may require an x-ray every 5 years.

Analysis (Nursing Diagnoses)

A. Deficit knowledge (specify) related to . . .
B. Risk for infection (of others) related to . . .
C. Imbalanced nutrition: less than body requirements related to . . .
D. Ineffective breathing pattern related to . . .

Nursing Plans and Interventions

A. Collaborate with the RN to develop and implement a client/family teaching plan.
   1. Cough into tissues and dispose of immediately into special bags.
   2. Take all prescribed medications daily for 9 to 12 months.
   3. Hand hygiene using proper technique.
   4. Report symptoms of deteriorating condition, especially hemorrhage.
B. Collect sputum cultures as needed; client may return to work after three negative cultures.
C. Place client in respiratory isolation while hospitalized. All personnel should wear a particulate respirator mask to filter the small tuberculosis organism.
D. Administer antituberculosis medications as prescribed (Table 4-5, *Drug Therapy for Tuberculosis [TB]*).
E. Coordinate referral for client and high-risk persons to local or state health department for testing and prophylactic treatment.
F. Promote adequate nutrition.

Lung Cancer

Description: Neoplasm occurring in the lung.
A. Lung cancer is the leading cause of cancer-related deaths in men and women in the United States.
B. Cigarette smoking is responsible for 80% to 90% of all lung cancers.
C. Exposure to occupational hazards such as asbestos and radioactive dust poses significant risk.
D. Lung cancer tends to appear years after exposure; it is most commonly seen in persons in the fifth or sixth decade of life.

Nursing Assessment (Data Collection)

A. Dry, hacking cough early, with cough turning productive as disease progresses
B. Hoarseness
C. Dyspnea
D. Hemoptysis; rust-colored or purulent sputum
E. Pain in the chest area
F. Diminished breath sounds, occasional wheezing
G. Abnormal chest x-ray
H. Positive sputum for cytology

Analysis (Nursing Diagnoses)

A. Chronic pain related to . . .
B. Ineffective breathing pattern related to . . .

TABLE 4-5 Drug Therapy for Tuberculosis (TB)

Drug	Mechanisms of Action	Side Effects	Comments
First-Line Drugs			
• Isoniazid (INH)	• Interferes with DNA metabolism of tubercle bacillus	• Peripheral neuritis, hepatotoxicity, hypersensitivity (skin rash, arthralgia, fever), optic neuritis, vitamin B_6, neuritis	• Metabolism primarily by liver and excretion by kidneys, pyridoxine (vitamin B_6) administration during high-dose therapy as prophylactic measure • Use as single prophylactic agent for active TB in individuals whose PPD converts to positive • Ability to cross blood-brain barrier
• Rifampin (Rifadin)	• Has broad-spectrum effects • Inhibits RNA polymerase of tubercle bacillus	• Hepatitis, febrile reaction, GI disturbance, peripheral neuropathy, hypersensitivity	• Most common use with isoniazid • Low incidence of side effects • Suppression of effect of birth control pills • Possible orange urine
• Ethambutol (Myambutol)	• Inhibits RNA synthesis and is bacteriostatic for the tubercle bacillus	• Skin rash, GI disturbance, malaise, peripheral neuritis, optic neuritis	• Side effects uncommon and reversible with discontinuation of drug • Most common use as substitute drug when toxicity occurs with isoniazid or rifampin
• Streptomycin	• Inhibits protein synthesis and is bactericidal	• Ototoxicity (eighth cranial nerve), nephrotoxicity, hypersensitivity	• Cautious use in older adults, those with renal disease, and pregnant women • Must be given parenterally
• Pyrazinamide	• Bactericidal effect (exact mechanism is unknown)	• Fever, skin rash, hyperuricemia, jaundice (rare)	• High rate of effectiveness when used with streptomycin or capreomycin
• Rifapentine (Priftin)	• Inhibits DNA-dependent RNA polymerase	• Red discoloration of body fluids and tissues	• Many drug interactions • Always use in conjunction with at least one other antituberculosis drug
Second-Line Drugs			
• Ethionamide (Trecator)	• Inhibits protein synthesis	• GI disturbance, hepatotoxicity, hypersensitivity	• Valuable for treatment of resistant organisms; contraindicated in pregnancy
• Capreomycin (Capastat)	• Inhibits protein synthesis and is bactericidal	• Ototoxicity, nephrotoxicity	• Cautious use in older adults
• Kanamycin (Kantrex) and amikacin	• Interferes with protein synthesis	• Ototoxicity, nephrotoxicity	• Use in selected cases for treatment of resistant strains
• Para-aminosalicylic acid (PAS) • Streptomycin • Levofloxacin (Levaquin) and moxifloxacin (Avelox)	• Interferes with metabolism of tubercle bacillus • Inhibits protein synthesis and is bactericidal • Inhibits DNA gyrase	• GI disturbance (frequent), hypersensitivity, hepatotoxicity • Ototoxicity (eighth cranial nerve), nephrotoxicity, hypersensitivity • Increased risk of tendinitis	• Interferes with absorption of rifampin; infrequent use • Cautious use in older adults, those with renal disease, and pregnant women; must be given parenterally • Many drug–drug interactions

TABLE 4-5 Drug Therapy for Tuberculosis (TB)—cont'd

Drug	Mechanisms of Action	Side Effects	Comments
• Cycloserine (Seromycin)	• Inhibits cell-wall synthesis	• Personality changes, psychosis, rash	• Contraindicated in individuals with a history of psychosis; use in treatment of resistant strains

HESI Hint • Teaching is very important with the TB client. Drug therapy is usually long term (9 months or longer). It is essential that the client take the medications as prescribed for the entire time. Skipping doses or prematurely terminating the drug therapy can result in a public health hazard.

HESI Hint • **TEACHING POINTS**
Rifampin: reduces effectiveness of oral contraceptives; should use other birth control methods during treatment; gives body fluids orange tinge; stains soft contact lenses. Isoniazid (INH): increases Dilantin levels. Ethambutol: vision check before starting therapy and monthly; may have to take 1 to 2 years or longer. The rationale for combination drug therapy is to increase compliance. Resistance develops more slowly if several anti-TB drugs are given instead of just one drug at a time.

C. Impaired gas exchange related to . . .
D. Imbalanced nutrition: less than body requirements related to . . .
E. Anxiety related to . . .

Nursing Plans and Interventions
A. Nursing interventions are similar to those implemented for the client with COPD.
B. Place client in semi-Fowler position.
C. Collaborate with RN to develop and implement a client/family teaching plan for pursed lip breathing to improve gas exchange.
D. Collaborate with RN to develop and implement a client/family teaching plan for relaxation techniques; client often becomes anxious about breathing difficulty.
E. Administer oxygen, as indicated by pulse oximetry or arterial blood gases (ABGs).
F. Take measures to allay anxiety:
   1. Keep client/family informed of impending tests and procedures.
   2. Give client as much control as possible over personal care.
   3. Encourage client/family to verbalize concerns.
G. Decrease pain to manageable level by administering analgesics as needed (within safety range for respiratory difficulty).
H. Surgery
   1. Thoracotomy for clients who have a resectable tumor. Unfortunately, detection is often so late that the tumor is no longer localized and not amenable to resection.
   2. Pneumonectomy—removal of entire lung
      a. Position on back.
      b. Chest tubes not usually used.
      c. Never turn to unoperative side.
   3. Lobectomy and segmental resection
      a. Position on back.

b. Check to ensure tubing is not kinked or obstructed.
c. Chest tubes usually inserted (Figure 4-2, *Chest Tubes*).

HESI Hint • Some tumors are so large that they fill entire lobes of the lung. When removed, large spaces are left. Chest tubes are not usually used with these clients because it is helpful if the mediastinal cavity, where the lung used to be, fills up with fluid. This fluid helps prevent a shift of the remaining chest organs to fill the empty space.

4. Chest tubes
   a. Keep all tubing coiled loosely below chest level, with connections tight and taped.
   b. Keep water seal and suction control chamber at the appropriate water levels.
   c. Monitor the fluid drainage, and mark the time of measurement and the fluid level.
   d. Observe for air bubbling in the water seal chamber and fluctuations (tidaling).
   e. Monitor the client's clinical status.
   f. Check the position of the chest drainage system.
   g. Encourage the client to breathe deeply periodically.
   h. Do not empty collection container. Replace unit when full.
   i. Do not strip or milk chest tubes.
   j. Chest tubes are not clamped routinely. If the drainage system breaks, place the distal end of the chest tubing connection in a sterile water container at a 2-cm level as an emergency water seal.
   k. Maintain dry occlusive dressing.

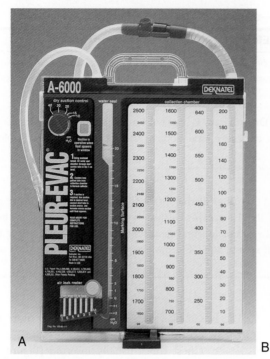

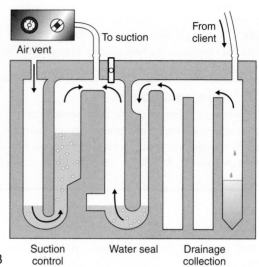

FIGURE 4-2 Chest Tubes. Chest tubes are used to remove or drain blood or air from the intrapleural space, to expand the lung after surgery, or to restore subatmospheric pressure to the thoracic cavity. Many brands of commercial chest drainage systems are available; all are based upon the traditional three-bottle water seal system. **A,** Commonly used disposable chest drainage system. **B,** Diagram of chambers of water-seal chest drainage. From Ignatavicius DD, Workman ML: *Medical-surgical nursing: Patient-centered collaborative care,* ed 7, St. Louis, 2013, Saunders.

HESI Hint • CHEST TUBES

- If the chest tube becomes disconnected, do not clamp! Immediately place the end of the tube in a container of sterile saline or water until a new drainage system can be connected.
- If the chest tube is accidentally removed from the client, the nurse should cover with a dry, sterile dressing. If an air leak is noted, tape the dressing on three sides only; this allows air to escape and prevents the formation of a tension pneumothorax. Notify the health care provider immediately.

HESI Hint • NCLEX-PN CONTENT ON CHEST TUBES

Fluctuations (tidaling) in the fluid will occur if there is no external suction. These fluctuating movements are a good indicator that the system is intact and should move upward with each inspiration and downward with each expiration. If fluctuations cease, check for kinked tubing, accumulation of fluid in the tubing, occlusions, or change in the client's position because expanding lung tissue may be occluding the tube opening. Remember, when external suction is applied, the fluctuations cease. Most hospitals *do not milk* chest tubes as a means of clearing or preventing clots. It is too easy to remove chest tubes. Mediastinal tubes may have orders to be stripped because of location, compared with larger thoracic cavity tubes.

I. Chemotherapy
   1. Nursing care for immunosuppression (see Oncology, p. 149).
   2. Administer antiemetics before administration of chemotherapy as prescribed.
   3. Take precautions for the administration of antineoplastics (see Oncology, p. 149).
J. Radiation therapy
   1. Provide skin care according to health care provider's request.
   2. Reinforce instructions to the client to not wash off the lines drawn by the radiologist.
   3. Reinforce instructions to the client to wear soft, cotton garments only.
   4. Avoid use of powders or creams to radiation site unless specified by radiologist.

HESI Hint • Various pathophysiologic conditions can be related to the nursing diagnosis "ineffective breathing patterns."
1. Inability of air sacs to fill and empty properly (emphysema, cystic fibrosis)
2. Obstruction of the air passages (carcinoma, asthma, chronic bronchitis)
3. Accumulation of fluid in the air sacs (pneumonia)
4. Respiratory muscle fatigue (COPD, pneumonia, degenerative diseases such as multiple sclerosis [MS], myasthenia gravis [MG])

Review of Respiratory System

1. List four common symptoms of pneumonia the nurse might note on physical exam.
2. State four nursing interventions for assisting the client to cough productively.
3. What symptoms of pneumonia might the nurse expect to see in an older client?
4. What should the O₂ flow rate be for the client with COPD?
5. How does the nurse prevent hypoxia during suctioning?
6. During mechanical ventilation, what are three major nursing interventions?
7. When examining a client with emphysema, what physical findings is the nurse likely to see?
8. What is the most common risk factor associated with lung cancer?
9. Describe the preoperative nursing care for a client undergoing a laryngectomy.
10. List five nursing interventions to implement after chest tube insertion.
11. What immediate action should the nurse take when a chest tube becomes disconnected from a bottle or suction apparatus? What should the nurse do if a chest tube is accidentally removed from the client?
12. What instructions should be given to a client after radiation therapy?
13. What precautions are required for clients with TB when placed on respiratory isolation?
14. List four components of teaching for the client with tuberculosis.

Answers to Review

1. Tachypnea, fever with chills, productive cough, bronchial breath sounds.
2. Deep breathing, fluid intake increased to 3 liters/day, use humidity to loosen secretions, suction airway to stimulate coughing.
3. Confusion, lethargy, anorexia, rapid respiratory rate.
4. The flow rate should be 1 to 2 liters per nasal cannula; too much O₂ may eliminate the COPD client's stimulus to breathe. A COPD client has a hypoxic drive to breathe.
5. Deliver 100% oxygen (hyperinflating) before and after each endotracheal suctioning.
6. Monitor client's respiratory status and secure connections, establish a communication mechanism with the client, keep airway clear by coughing/suctioning.
7. Barrel chest, dry or productive cough, decreased breath sounds, dyspnea, crackles in lung fields.
8. Smoking.
9. Involve family/client in manipulation of tracheostomy equipment before surgery, plan acceptable communication method, refer to speech pathologist, discuss rehabilitation program.
10. Maintain a dry occlusive dressing to chest tube site at all times. Keeping all tubing connections tight and taped, monitor client's clinical status. Encourage the client to breathe deeply periodically. Monitor the fluid drainage and mark the time of measurement and of fluid level.
11. Place the end of the tube in a sterile water container at a 2-cm level. Apply an occlusive dressing and notify health care provider *STAT*.
12. Do *not* wash off lines; wear soft cotton garments; avoid use of powders/creams on radiation site.
13. Mask for anyone entering room; private room; client *must* wear mask if leaving room.
14. Cough into tissues and dispose immediately into special bags. Long-term need for daily medication. Good hand washing technique. Report symptoms of deterioration, such as blood in secretions.

Renal System

Acute Renal Failure

Description: Acute renal failure (ARF) is the abrupt deterioration of the renal system; may be a reversible syndrome.

> **HESI Hint** • Normally, kidneys excrete approximately 1 mL of urine per kg of body weight per hour, which is about 1 to 2 liters in a 24-hour period for adults.

A. Acute renal failure occurs when metabolites accumulate in the body and urinary output changes.

TABLE 4-6 Acute Renal Failure

Types	Description	Etiologic Factors
• Prerenal	• Interference with renal perfusion	• Hemorrhage • Hypovolemia • Decreased cardiac output • Decreased renal perfusion
• Intrarenal	• Damage to renal parenchyma	• Prolonged prerenal state • Nephrotoxins • Intratubular obstruction • Infections (glomerulonephritis) • Renal injury • Vascular lesions • Acute pyelonephritis
• Postrenal	• Obstruction in the urinary tract anywhere from the tubules to the urethral meatus	• Calculi • Prostatic hypertrophy • Tumors

B. There are three major types of acute renal failure (Table 4-6, *Acute Renal Failure*).
C. There are three phases of acute renal failure:
   1. Oliguric phase
   2. Diuretic phase
   3. Recovery phase

Nursing Assessment (Data Collection)

A. History of taking nephrotoxic drugs (salicylates, antibiotics, nonsteroidal anti-inflammatory drugs [NSAIDs], angiotensin converting enzyme [ACE] inhibitors, angiotensin receptor blocker [ARB])
B. Alterations in urinary output
C. Edema, weight gain (ask if waistbands have suddenly become too tight)
D. Change in mental status
E. Hematuria
F. Dry mucous membranes
G. Drowsiness, headache (HA), muscle twitching, seizures

HESI Hint • Electrolytes are profoundly affected by kidney problems (a favorite NCLEX-PN topic). There must be a balance between extracellular fluid and intracellular fluid to maintain homeostasis. A change in the number of ions or in the amount of fluid will cause a shift in one direction or the other. Sodium and chloride are the primary extracellular ions. Potassium and phosphate are the primary intracellular ions.

E. Diagnostic findings in the oliguric phase:
   1. Increased blood urea nitrogen (BUN) and creatinine
   2. Increased potassium (hyperkalemia)
   3. Decreased sodium (hyponatremia)
   4. Decreased pH (acidosis)
   5. Fluid overloaded (hypervolemic).
   6. High urine specific gravity greater than 1.02

F. Diagnostic findings in the diuretic phase:
   1. Decreased fluid volume (hypovolemia)
   2. Decreased potassium (hypokalemia)
   3. Further decrease in sodium (hyponatremia)
   4. Low urine specific gravity less than 1.02 g/mL
G. Diagnostic lab work returns to normal range in recovery phase

HESI Hint • In some cases, a person in ARF may not experience the oliguric phase but may progress directly to the diuretic phase, during which the urine output may be as much as 10 liters per day.

Analysis (Nursing Diagnoses)

A. Excess fluid volume related to . . .
B. Deficient fluid volume related to . . .
C. Anxiety related to . . .
D. Imbalanced nutrition: less than body requirements related to . . .

Nursing Plans and Interventions

A. Monitor input and output (I&O) accurately; give only enough fluids in oliguric phase to replace losses—usually 400 to 500 mL/24 hours.
B. Document and report any change in fluid volume status.
C. Monitor lab values for both serum and urine to assess electrolyte status, especially hyperkalemia indicated by serum potassium levels over 7 mEq/L and electrocardiogram (ECG) changes.
D. Identify changes in the level of consciousness.
E. Weigh daily: in oliguric phase gain up to 1 lb/day.
F. Prevent cross infection.
G. Sodium polystryene (Kayexalate) may be prescribed if K+ too high.
H. Provide low-protein, moderate-fat, high-carbohydrate diet.

HESI Hint • Body weight is a good indicator of fluid retention and renal status. Obtain accurate weights on all clients with renal failure—done on the same scale at the same time every day.

HESI Hint • **FLUID VOLUME ALTERATIONS**
Excess fluid symptoms:
• Dyspnea
• Tachycardia
• Jugular vein distention
• Peripheral edema
• Pulmonary edema
Deficient fluid symptoms:
• Decreased urine output
• Reduction in body weight
• Decreased skin turgor
• Dry mucous membranes
• Hypotension
• Tachycardia

HESI Hint • Watch for signs of hyperkalemia: dizziness, weakness, cardiac irregularities, muscle cramps, diarrhea, and nausea.

HESI Hint • Potassium has a critical safe range (3.5 to 5.0 mEq/L) because it affects the heart, and any imbalance must be corrected by medications or dietary modification. Limit high-potassium foods (bananas, avocados, spinach, fish) and salt substitutes, which are high in potassium.

HESI Hint • Clients with renal failure retain sodium. With water retention, the sodium becomes diluted, and serum levels may appear near normal. With excessive water retention, the sodium levels appear decreased (dilution). Limit fluid and sodium intake in ARF clients.

I. Monitor cardiac rate and rhythm (acute cardiac dysrhythmias are usually related to hyperkalemia).
J. Monitor drug levels and interactions.

HESI Hint • During the oliguric phase, minimize protein breakdown and prevent rise in BUN by limiting protein intake. When the BUN and creatinine return to normal, ARF is determined to be resolved.

Chronic Renal Failure–End Stage Renal Disease

Description: Chronic renal failure–end stage renal disease (ESRD) is progressive, irreversible damage to the nephrons and glomeruli, resulting in uremia.
A. Causes of chronic renal failure are multitudinous.
B. As renal function diminishes, dialysis becomes necessary.
C. Transplantation is an alternative to dialysis for some clients.

Nursing Assessment (Data Collection)

A. History of high medication usage
B. Family history of renal disease
C. Increased blood pressure (BP) and/or chronic hypertension
D. Edema, pulmonary edema
E. Neurologic impairment (weakness, drowsiness)
F. Decreasing urinary function:
   1. Hematuria
   2. Proteinuria
   3. Cloudy urine
   4. Oliguric (100 to 400 mL/day)
   5. Anuric (less than 100 mL/day)
G. Jaundice
H. Gastrointestinal (GI) upsets
I. Metallic taste in mouth
J. Ammonia breath
K. Pain, discomfort
L. Peripheral neuropathy
M. Dialysis (Table 4-7, *Renal Dialysis*)
N. Previous kidney transplant
O. Lab information
   1. Azotemia
   2. Increased creatinine and BUN
   3. Decreased calcium
   4. Elevated phosphorus and magnesium
   5. Anemia

HESI Hint • Accumulation of waste products from protein metabolism is the primary cause of uremia. Protein must be restricted in ESRD clients. However, if protein intake is inadequate, a negative nitrogen balance occurs, causing muscle wasting. The glomerular filtration rate (GFR) is most often used as an indicator of level of protein consumption.

HESI Hint • **DIALYSIS COVERED BY MEDICARE**
• All persons in the United States are eligible for Medicare as of their first day of dialysis under special ESRD funding.
• Medicare card will indicate ESRD.
• Transplantation is covered by Medicare procedure; coverage terminates 6 months postoperative if dialysis is no longer required.

TABLE 4-7 Renal Dialysis

Type of Dialysis	Description	Nursing Implications
• Hemodialysis	• Requires venous access (AV shunt, fistula, or graft) • Treatment is 3 to 8 hours in length, 3 times per week • Correction of fluid and electrolyte imbalance is rapid • Potential blood loss • Does not result in protein loss	• Heparinization is required • Requires expensive equipment • Inconvenient for home use • Rapid shifts of fluid and electrolytes can lead to disequilibrium syndrome (an unpleasant sensation and potentially dangerous situation) • Potential for hepatitis B and C • Do NOT take blood pressure or perform venipunctures on the arm with the AV shunt, fistula, or graft • Monitor the access site for thrill and bruit
• Continuous arterio-venous hemofiltration (CAVH)	• Requires vascular access: usually femoral or subclavian catheters • Slow process • Correction of fluid and electrolyte imbalance is slow • Does not cause blood loss • Does not result in protein loss	• Requires heparinization of filter tubing • Filters are costly • Equipment is simple to use • Limited to special care units, NOT for home use • Filter may rupture, causing blood loss

• Peritoneal	• Surgical placement of abdominal catheter is required (Tenckhoff, Gore-Tex, column-disk)
	• Slow process
	• Correction of fluid and electrolyte imbalance is slow
	• Does not cause blood loss
	• Protein is lost in dialysate
		• Heparinization is NOT required
		• Fairly expensive
		• Simple to perform
		• Easy to use at home
		• Dialysate is similar to IV fluid and is prescribed for the individual client's electrolyte needs
		• Potential complications:
		  o Bowel or bladder perforation
		  o Exit site and tunnel infection
		  o Peritonitis

HESI Hint • The major difference between dialysate for hemodialysis and peritoneal dialysis is the amount of glucose. Peritoneal dialysis dialysate is much higher in glucose. For this reason, if the dialysate is left in the peritoneal cavity too long, hyperglycemia may occur.

Analysis (Nursing Diagnoses)

A. Excess fluid volume related to . . .
B. Imbalanced nutrition: less than body requirements related to . . .
C. Decreased cardiac output related to . . .

Nursing Plans and Interventions

A. Monitor serum electrolyte levels.
B. Weigh daily.
C. Strict I&O.
D. Check for jugular vein distention (JVD) and other signs of fluid overload.
E. Monitor edema, pulmonary edema.
F. Provide low-protein, low-sodium, low-potassium, low-phosphate diet.

HESI Hint • Protein intake is restricted until blood chemistry shows the ability to handle protein catabolites: urea, creatinine. Ensure high-calorie intake so protein is spared for its own work; give hard candy, jelly beans, flavored carbohydrate powders.

G. Administer phosphate binders with food because client is unable to excrete phosphates (no magnesium-based antacids). Timing is important.
H. Encourage protein intake of high biologic value (eggs, milk, meat) because the client is on a low-protein diet.
I. Alternate periods of rest with periods of activity.
J. Encourage strict adherence to medication regimen; teach client to obtain health care provider's permission before taking any over-the-counter medications.

TABLE 4-8 Antianemic: Biologic Response Modifier (BRM)

Drug	Indications	Adverse Reactions	Nursing Interventions
• Erythropoietin (Epogen)	• Anemia resulting from decreased production of erythropoietin in end-stage renal disease • Stimulates RBC production, increases Hgb, reticulocyte count, and Hct	• Use with caution in older clients because of increased risk of thrombosis	• Monitor Hct weekly; report levels over 30% to 33% or increases of more than 4 points in less than 2 weeks • Explain that pelvic and limb pain should dissipate after 12 hours • Do not shake vial; shaking may inactivate the glycoprotein • Discard unused contents—does not contain preservatives

HESI Hint • As kidneys fail, medications must often be adjusted. Of particular importance is digoxin toxicity because digitalis preparations are excreted by the kidneys. Signs of toxicity in adults include nausea, vomiting, anorexia, visual disturbances, restlessness, headache, cardiac dysrhythmias, and pulse less than 60 beats per minute.

TABLE 4-9 Postoperative Care: Kidney Surgery

Assessment	Nursing Interventions	Rationale
• Respiratory status	• Auscultate lung sounds to detect "wet" sounds indicating infection • Demonstrate method of splinting incision for comfort when coughing and deep breathing	• Flank incision causes pain with BOTH inspiration and expiration; therefore, client avoids deep breathing and coughing, which can lead to respiratory difficulties, including pneumonia
• Circulatory status	• Check vital signs to detect early signs of bleeding, shock • Monitor skin color and temperature (pallor and cold skin are signs of shock) • Monitor urinary output (will decrease with circulatory collapse) • Monitor surgical site for frank bleeding	• The kidney is very vascular • Bleeding is a constant threat • Circulatory collapse will occur with hemorrhage and can occur very quickly
• Pain relief status	• Administer narcotic analgesics as needed to relieve pain	• Relief of pain will improve the client's cooperation with deep breathing exercises • Relief of pain will improve client's cooperation with early ambulation
• Urinary status	• Check urinary output and drainage from ALL tubes inserted during the surgery • Maintain accurate intake and output	• Mechanical drainage of bladder will be implemented after surgery

K. Observe for complications:
   1. Anemia, administer antianemic drug (Table 4-8, *Antianemic: Biologic Response Modifier [BRM]*)
   2. Renal osteodystrophy (abnormal calcium metabolism causes bone pathology)
   3. Severe, resistant hypertension
   4. Infection
   5. Metabolic acidosis
L. Living-related or cadaver renal transplant (Table 4-9, *Postoperative Care: Kidney Surgery*).
   1. Monitor for rejection.
   2. Monitor for infection.
   3. Reinforce client teaching about meticulously maintaining immunosuppressive drug therapy.

Urinary Tract Infections

Description: Infection or inflammation at any site in the urinary tract. (Kidney = pyelonephritis, urethra = urethritis, bladder = cystitis, prostate = prostatitis.)
A. Normally, the entire urinary tract is sterile.
B. The most common infectious agent is *Escherichia coli*.
C. Persons at highest risk for acquiring urinary tract infection (UTI):
   1. Clients diagnosed with diabetes
   2. Pregnant women
   3. Men with prostatic hypertrophy
   4. Immunosuppressed persons
   5. Catheterized clients

6. Anyone with urinary retention, either short term or long term
7. Older women (bladder prolapse)
8. Sexually active women, who are more vulnerable to UTIs

D. Diagnosis:
1. Clean-catch midstream urine collection for culture to identify specific causative organism (prior to administering anti-infective medications).
2. Intravenous pyelogram (IVP) to determine kidney functioning.
3. Cystogram to determine bladder functioning.
4. Cystoscopy to determine bladder or urethral abnormalities.

Nursing Assessment (Data Collection)

A. Signs of infection including malaise, fever, and chills
B. Urinary frequency, urgency, or dysuria
C. Hematuria
D. Pain at the costovertebral angle
E. Elevated serum WBC (greater than 10,000)
F. Characteristics of urine: cloudy, dark, and foul smelling
G. Bladder spasms
H. Nausea and vomiting

Analysis (Nursing Diagnoses)

A. Pain related to . . .
B. Impaired urinary elimination related to . . .
C. Deficient knowledge (specify) related to . . .

Nursing Plans and Interventions

A. Administer prescribed antibiotics specific to infection agent.
B. Instruct client in the appropriate medication regimen.
C. Encourage fluid intake of 3000 mL fluid/day.
D. Maintain I&O.
E. Administer mild analgesics (acetaminophen or aspirin).
F. Encourage to void every 2 to 3 hours to prevent residual urine from stagnating in bladder.

> **HESI Hint** • The key to resolving UTIs with most antibiotics is to keep the blood level of the antibiotic constant. It is important to tell the client to take the antibiotics around the clock and not to skip doses so a consistent blood level can be maintained for optimal effectiveness.

G. Collaborate with RN and implement a teaching plan.
1. Take entire prescription as directed.
2. Encourage oral fluid intake to 3 liters/day (water, juices). Should not consume citrus juices.
3. Shower rather than bathe as a preventive measure. If bathing is necessary, never take a bubble or oil bath.

4. Women/girls should cleanse from front to back after toileting.
5. Avoid urinary tract irritants: alcohol, sodas, citrus juices, spices.
6. Women should void immediately after intercourse.
7. Void every 2 to 3 hours during the day.
8. Wear cotton undergarments and loose clothing to help decrease perineal moisture.
9. Practice good hand-washing technique.
10. Obtain follow-up care.

Urinary Tract Obstruction

Description: Partial or complete blockage of the flow of urine at any point in the urinary system.
A. Urinary tract obstruction is usually caused by:
1. Foreign body (calculus)
2. Tumor
3. Stricture
4. Functional (e.g., neurogenic bladder)
B. When urinary tract obstruction occurs, urine is retained above the point of obstruction.
1. Hydrostatic pressure builds, causing dilation of the organs above the obstruction.
2. If hydrostatic pressure continues to build, then hydronephrosis develops, which can lead to renal failure.

Nursing Assessment (Data Collection)

A. Pain, usually quite severe, acute.
1. May be colicky
2. Radiating down the thigh and to the genitalia
B. Symptoms of obstruction:
1. Fever, chills
2. Nausea, vomiting, diarrhea
3. Abdominal distention

> **HESI Hint** •
> Location of the pain can help determine location of the stone.
> Flank pain usually means the stone is in the kidney or upper ureter. If it radiates to the abdomen or scrotum, the stone is likely to be in the ureter or bladder.
> Excruciating, spastic-type pain is called *colic*.
> During kidney stone attacks, it is preferable to administer pain medications at regularly scheduled intervals rather than PRN to prevent spasms and optimize comfort.

C. Change in voiding pattern.
1. Dysuria, hematuria
2. Urgency, frequency, hesitancy, nocturia, dribbling
3. Difficulty in starting a stream
4. Incontinence

D. Those with the following conditions are at risk for developing calculi:
   1. Strictures
   2. Prostatic hypertrophy
   3. Neoplasms
   4. Congenital malformations
   5. History of calculi
   6. Family history of calculi

Analysis (Nursing Diagnoses)

A. Pain related to . . .
B. Risk for infection related to . . .
C. Risk for injury related to . . .

Nursing Plans and Interventions

A. Administer narcotic analgesics.
B. Apply moist heat to the painful area unless prescribed otherwise.
C. Encourage high oral fluid intake to help dislodge the stone.
D. Monitor intravenous antibiotics if infection is present.
E. Strain all urine.
F. Send any stones found from straining to the laboratory for analysis.
G. Accurately document I&O.
H. Endourologic procedures.
   1. Cystoscopy
   2. Cystolitholapaxy
   3. Ureteroscopy
   4. Percutaneous nephrolithotomy
I. Lithotripsy
   1. Ultrasonic
   2. Electrohydraulic
   3. Laser
   4. Extracorporeal shock wave
J. Surgical therapy
   1. Nephrolithotomy
   2. Pyelolithotomy
   3. Ureterolithotomy
   4. Cystectomy

> **HESI Hint · PERCUTANEOUS NEPHROSTOMY**
> A needle/catheter is inserted through the skin into the calyx of the kidney. The stone may be dissolved by percutaneous irrigation with the liquid that will dissolve the stone, or ultrasonic sound waves (lithotripsy) can be directed through the needle/catheter to break up the stone that then can be eliminated through the urinary tract.

K. Collaborate with the RN and implement a teaching plan to include the following:
   1. Encourage follow-up care because stones tend to recur.
   2. Maintain a high fluid intake of 3 to 4 liters per day.

   3. Follow prescribed diet (based on composition of stone).
   4. Avoid long periods of supine position.

Benign Prostatic Hyperplasia

(Sometimes called *hypertrophy of the prostate.*)
   Description: Benign prostatic hyperplasia (BPH) is enlargement or hypertrophy of the prostate.
A. BPH tends to occur in men over 40 years of age.
B. Intervention is required when symptoms of obstruction occur.
C. The most common treatment is transurethral resection of the prostate gland (TURP). The prostate is removed by endoscopy (no surgical incision is made), allowing for a shorter hospital stay.

Nursing Assessment (Data Collection)

A. Increased frequency with a decrease in amount of each voiding
B. Nocturia
C. Hesitancy
D. Terminal dribbling
E. Changes in size and force of urinary stream
F. Acute urinary retention
G. Bladder distention
H. Dribbling
I. Hematuria
J. UTIs

Analysis (Nursing Diagnoses)

A. Pain related to . . .
B. Risk for injury related to . . .
C. Infection related to . . .
D. Impaired urinary elimination related to . . .

Nursing Plans and Interventions

A. Assist with preoperative teaching to include information concerning pain from bladder spasms that occur postoperatively.
B. Postoperatively maintain patent urinary drainage system to decrease the spasms.
C. Provide pain relief as prescribed: analgesics, narcotics, and antispasmodics.

> **HESI Hint ·** Bladder spasms frequently occur after TURP. Inform the client that the presence of the oversized balloon on the catheter (30 to 45 mL inflate) will cause a continuous feeling of needing to void. The client should not try to void around the catheter because that can precipitate bladder spasms. Medications to reduce or prevent spasms should be given.

D. Minimize catheter manipulation by taping catheter to abdomen or leg or by using a leg strap.

E. Maintain gentle traction on urinary catheter.
F. Check the urinary drainage system for clots.
G. Irrigate bladder as prescribed (may be continuous or intermittent). If continuous, keep Foley bag emptied to avoid retrograde pressure.

> **HESI Hint** • Instillation of the hypertonic or hypotonic solution into a body cavity will cause a shift in cellular fluid. Use only sterile saline for bladder irrigation after TURP because the irrigation must be isotonic to prevent fluid and electrolyte imbalance.

H. Observe the color and content of urinary output.
1. Normal drainage after prostate surgery is reddish pink clearing to light pink within 24 hours after surgery.
2. Monitor for bright red bleeding with large clots and increased viscosity.
I. Monitor vital signs frequently for indication of circulatory collapse.
J. Monitor hemoglobin (Hgb) and hematocrit (Hct) for pattern of decreasing values that indicates bleeding.
K. After catheter is removed:
1. Monitor amount and number of times client voids.
2. Have the client use urine cups to provide a specimen with each voiding.
3. Observe for hematuria after each voiding (urine should progress to clear yellow color by the fourth day).

4. Inform client that burning on urination and urinary frequency are usually experienced in the first postoperative week.
5. Generally the client is not impotent after surgery, but sterility may occur.
6. Reinforce instructions for client to immediately report any frank bleeding to health care provider.
7. Monitor for signs of urethral stricture: straining, dysuria, weak urinary stream.
8. Administer antispasmodics as prescribed.

> **HESI Hint** • Inform the client before discharge that some bleeding is expected after TURP. Large amounts of blood or frank, bright bleeding should be reported. However, it is normal for the client to pass small amounts of blood during the healing process, as well as small clots. He should rest quietly and continue drinking large amounts of fluid.

L. Encourage client to increase fluid intake to 3000 mL/day.
M. Prepare client for discharge with instructions to:
1. Continue to drink 12 to 14 glasses of water a day.
2. Avoid constipation, straining.
3. Avoid strenuous activity, lifting, intercourse, or engaging in sports during the first 3 to 4 weeks after surgery.
4. Schedule a follow-up appointment.

Review of Renal System

1. Differentiate between acute renal failure and chronic renal failure.
2. During the oliguric phase of renal failure, protein should be severely restricted. What is the rationale for this restriction?
3. Identify two nursing interventions for the client on hemodialysis.
4. What is the highest-priority nursing diagnosis for clients in any type of renal failure?
5. A client in renal failure asks why he is being given antacids. How should the nurse reply?
6. List four essential elements of a teaching plan for clients with frequent urinary tract infections.
7. What are the most important nursing interventions for clients with possible renal calculi?
8. What discharge instructions should be given to a client who has had urinary calculi?
9. Following transurethral resection of the prostate gland (TURP), hematuria should subside by what postoperative day?
10. After the urinary catheter is removed in the TURP client, what are three priority nursing actions to be taken?
11. After kidney surgery, what are the primary assessments the nurse should make?

Answers to Review

1. Acute renal failure: often reversible, abrupt deterioration of kidney function. Chronic renal failure: irreversible, slow deterioration of kidney function characterized by increasing BUN and creatinine. Eventually dialysis is required.
2. Toxic metabolites that accumulate in the blood (urea, creatinine) are derived mainly from protein catabolism.
3. Do not take blood pressure (BP) or perform venipunctures on the arm with the A-V shunt, fistula, or graft. Assess access site for thrill and bruit.
4. Risk for imbalanced fluid volume.

5. Calcium and aluminum antacids bind phosphates and help to keep phosphates from being absorbed into the bloodstream, thereby preventing rising phosphate levels, and must be taken with meals.
6. Fluid intake 3 liters/day; good hand washing; void every 2 to 3 hours during waking hours; take all prescribed medications; wear cotton undergarments.
7. Straining all urine is the most important intervention. Other interventions include accurate intake and output documentation and administering analgesics as needed.
8. Maintain high fluid intake of 3 to 4 liters per day. Follow-up care (stones tend to recur). Follow prescribed diet based on calculi content. Avoid supine position.
9. Fourth day.
10. Continued strict I&O. Continued observations for hematuria. Inform client that burning and frequency may last for a week.
11. Respiratory status (breathing is guarded because of pain); circulatory status (the kidney is very vascular, and excessive bleeding can occur); pain assessment; urinary assessment (most importantly, assessment of urinary output).

Cardiovascular System

> **HESI Hint** • What is the relationship of the kidneys to the cardiovascular system?
> - The kidneys filter about a liter of blood per minute.
> - If cardiac output is decreased, the amount of blood going through the kidneys is decreased; urinary output is decreased. Therefore, a decreased urinary output may be a sign of cardiac problems.
> - When the kidneys produce and excrete 0.5 mL of urine per kg of body weight or average 30 mL/hour output, the blood supply is considered to be minimally adequate to perfuse the vital organs.

Angina

Description: Angina is chest discomfort or pain occurring when myocardial oxygen demands exceed supply. This temporary deficiency of blood flow is called ischemia. Common causes include:
A. Atherosclerotic heart disease
B. Hypertension
C. Coronary artery spasm
D. Hypertrophic cardiomyopathy
E. Any activity that increases the heart's oxygen demand: physical exertion, cold temperatures

Nursing Assessment (Data Collection)
A. Pain:
   1. Mild to severe intensity, described as heavy, squeezing, pressing, burning, choking, aching, and feeling of apprehension
   2. Substernal, radiating to left arm and/or shoulder, jaw, or right shoulder
   3. Transient or prolonged, with gradual or sudden onset; typically short duration
   4. Often precipitated by exercise, exposure to cold, heavy meal, mental tension, sexual intercourse
   5. Relieved by rest and/or nitroglycerin

B. Dyspnea, tachycardia, palpitations
C. Nausea, vomiting
D. Fatigue
E. Diaphoresis, pallor, weakness
F. Syncope
G. Dysrhythmias
H. Diagnostic information:
   1. ECG: generally at client baseline unless taken during anginal attack, when ST depression and T wave inversion may occur.
   2. Exercise stress test shows ST segment depression and hypotension.
   3. Stress echocardiogram: looks for changes in wall motion (indicated in women).
   4. Coronary angiogram: detects coronary artery spasms.
   5. Cardiac catheterization: detects arterial blockage.
I. Risk factors:
   1. Nonmodifiable:
      a. Heredity
      b. Gender: risk greater for male than female until menopause, then equal risk
      c. Ethnic background: African Americans have greater risk
      d. Age
   2. Modifiable:
      a. Hyperlipidemia
      b. Those with serum cholesterol above 300 mg/dL have four times greater risk of developing coronary artery disease (CAD) than those with levels less than 200 mg/dL (desirable level).
      c. Low-density lipoprotein (LDL) "bad" cholesterol. A molecule of LDL is approximately 50% cholesterol by weight (less than 100 mg/dL optimal, less than 130 mg/dL desirable).
      d. High-density lipoprotein (HDL) "good cholesterol." HDL is inversely related to the risk of developing CAD (more than 60 mg/dL is desirable). In fact, HDL may serve to remove cholesterol from tissues.
      e. Hypertension

f. Cigarette smoking
g. Obesity
h. Physical inactivity
i. Diabetes mellitus
j. Stress

Analysis (Nursing Diagnoses)

A. Pain related to . . .
B. Anxiety related to . . .
C. Decreased cardiac output related to . . .

Nursing Plans and Interventions

A. Monitor medications and instruct client in proper administration.
B. Determine factors precipitating pain, and assist client/family in adjusting lifestyle to decrease these factors.

C. Collaborate with RN to develop and implement client/family teaching plan about risk factors, and identify client's own risk factors.
D. During an attack:
   1. Provide immediate rest.
   2. Take vital signs.
   3. Record an ECG.
   4. Administer no more than three nitroglycerin tablets, 5 minutes apart (Table 4-10, *Antianginals*).
   5. Seek emergency treatment if no relief has occurred after taking nitroglycerin.
E. Physical activity:
   1. Avoid isometric activity.
   2. Implement an exercise program.
   3. Sexual activity may be resumed after exercise is tolerated, usually when able to climb two flights of

TABLE 4-10 Antianginals

Drugs	Indications/Actions	Adverse Reactions	Nursing Implications
Nitrates			
• Nitroglycerin (NTG) • Isosorbide dinitrate (Isordil) • Isosorbide mononitrate (Imdur)	• Anginal prophylaxis • Acute attack • Reduces vascular resistance	• Headache • Flushing • Dizziness • Weakness • Hypotension • Nausea	• Monitor relief • Have client rest • Monitor vital signs • Store in original container • Replace NTG tablets every 3 to 5 months
Beta-Blockers			
• Propranolol HCL (Inderal) • Atenolol (Tenormin) • Nadolol (Corgard)	• Anginal prophylaxis • Reduce oxygen demand	• Fatigue • Lethargy • Hallucinations • Impotence • Bradycardia • Hypotension • HF • Wheezing	• Monitor apical heart rate • Watch for a decreased BP • Do not stop abruptly • Clients with HF, bronchitis, asthma, COPD, renal or hepatic insufficiency have increased likelihood of incurring adverse reactions
Calcium Channel Blockers			
• Verapamil (Calan) • Nifedipine HCL (Procardia) • Diltiazem HCL (Cardizem, Norvasc)	• Anginal prophylaxis • Inhibits influx of calcium ions	• Dizziness • Hypotension • Fatigue • Headache • Syncope • Peripheral edema • Hypokalemia • Dysrhythmia • HF	• Clients with HF and older adults have an increased likelihood of incurring adverse reactions • Watch for a decreased BP • Monitor serum potassium • Swallow pills whole • Store at room temperature • Do not stop abruptly • Take 1 hour before meals or 2 hours after meals
Other			
• Ranolazine (Ranexa)	• Anginal prophylaxis • Inhibits influx of sodium ions	• Dysrhythmia • Constipation	• Many drug–drug interactions • Contraindication in all levels of hepatic cirrhosis

stairs without exertion. Nitroglycerin can be taken prophylactically before intercourse.

F. Provide nutritional information concerning modifying fats (saturated) and sodium. Antilipemic medications may be prescribed to lower cholesterol levels (Table 4-11, *Antilipemics*, and Appendix B, *Recommended Daily Requirements and Food Sources*, p. 346).

G. Medical interventions include:
1. Percutaneous transluminal coronary angioplasty (PTCA): a balloon catheter is repeatedly inflated to split or fracture plaque and the arterial wall is stretched, enlarging the diameter of the vessel. A rotoblade is used to pulverize plaque.
2. Arthrectomy: a catheter with a collection chamber is used to remove plaque from a coronary artery by shaving, cutting, or grinding.
3. Coronary artery bypass graft (CABG)
4. Coronary laser therapy
5. Coronary artery stent

Myocardial Infarction (MI)

Description: Myocardial infarction (MI) is the disruption or deficiency of coronary artery blood supply resulting in necrosis (death) of myocardial tissue.

Causes of MI:

A. Thrombus or clotting
B. Shock or hemorrhage

Nursing Assessment (Data Collection)

A. Sudden onset of pain in the lower sternal region (substernal).
1. Severity increases until it becomes nearly unbearable.
2. Heavy and viselike pain often radiates to the shoulders and down the arms and/or to the neck, jaw, and back. Common locations for pain are substernal, retrosternal, or epigastric areas.
3. It differs from angina pain in its sudden onset.
4. Pain is not relieved by rest.

TABLE 4-11   Antilipemics

Drugs	Indications	Adverse Reactions	Nursing Implications
Bile Sequestrants			
• Colestipol HCL (Colestid) • Colesevelam (Welchol) • Cholestyramine (Questran)	• Treat type IIA hyperlipidemia (hypercholesterolemia) when dietary changes fail	• Abdominal pain, nausea and vomiting, distention, flatulence, belching, constipation • Reduced absorption of lipid-soluble vitamins: A, D, E, and K • Alters absorption of other oral medications	• Reinforce teaching plan to mix powder forms with liquid or fruits high in moisture content such as applesauce to prevent accidental inhalation or esophageal distress • Monitor prothrombin times • Report visual changes and rickets • Administer other oral medications 1 hour before or 6 hours after giving bile sequestrants
HNG-CoA Reductase Inhibitors (Statins)			
• Atorvastatin (Lipitor) • Fluvastatin (Lescol) • Pravastatin (Pravachol) • Simvastatin (Zocor) • Lovastatin (Mevacor) • Pitavastatin (Livalo) • Rosuvastatin (Crestor)		• S.E. similar to bile sequestrants • May elevate liver enzymes • Hepatitis and/or pancreatitis • Rhabdomyolysis	• Obtain liver enzymes baseline and monitor q6 months • Monitor creatine phosphokinase (CPK) levels • Review specific drug/food interactions; avoid grapefruit juice • Timing with or without food varies with drug • Reinforce teaching with client to report any muscle tenderness • Monitor dose limits when interacting medications prescribed

Continued

TABLE 4-11 Antilipemics—cont'd

Drugs	Indications	Adverse Reactions	Nursing Implications
Fibric Acid Derivatives			
• Gemfibrozil (Lopid) • Fenofibrate (Tricor) • Fenofibric acid (Trilipix) • Clofibrate (Claripex)	• Used with diet changes to lower both elevated cholesterol and triglycerides	• Abdominal/epigastric pain, diarrhea—most common • Flatulence, nausea and vomiting • Heartburn • Dyspepsia • Gallstones • TriCor: weakness, fatigue, H/A • Myopathy	• Obtain baseline labs: liver function, CBC, and electrolytes and monitor every 3 to 6 months • *Administer:* • Lopid: 30 minutes before breakfast and dinner • TriCor: with meals
Water-Soluble Vitamins			
• Niacin (Niaspan) • Nicotinic acid (Nicobid)	• Large doses decrease lipoprotein and triglyceride synthesis and increase HDL	• Flushing of face/neck • Pruritus • H/A • Orthostatic hypotension • Extended-release form: hepatotoxicity • Hyperglycemia • Hyperuricemia • Upper GI distress	• Give with milk or food to avoid GI irritation • Client to change positions slowly • Reinforce teaching with clients taking extended-release form to report darkened urine, light-colored stools, anorexia, yellowing of eyes or skin, severe stomach pain

> **HESI Hint** • Angina is caused by myocardial ischemia. Which cardiac medications would be appropriate for acute angina?
> Digoxin—*Not appropriate*—Increases the strength and contractility of the heart muscle; the problem in angina is that the muscle is not receiving enough oxygen. Digoxin will not help.
> Nitroglycerin—*Appropriate*—Causes dilation of the coronary arteries, allowing more oxygen to get to the heart muscle.
> Atropine—*Not appropriate*—Increases heart rate by blocking vagal stimulation, which suppresses the heart rate. Does not address the lack of O₂ to the heart muscle.
> Propranolol (Inderal)—*Not appropriate*—For acute angina attack; however, is appropriate for long-term management of stable angina because it acts as a beta-blocker to control vasoconstriction.

5. Pain is not relieved by nitroglycerin.
6. Pain may persist for hours or days.
7. Client may not have pain (silent MI), especially those with diabetic neuropathy.
B. Rapid, irregular, and feeble pulse.
C. Decreased level of consciousness, indicating decreased cerebral perfusion.
D. Left heart shift sometimes occurs post-MI.
E. Cardiac dysrhythmias occur in about 90% of MI clients.
F. Cardiogenic shock or fluid retention.
G. Narrowed pulse pressure—for example, 90/80.
H. Bowel sounds absent or high-pitched, indicating possibility of mesenteric artery thrombosis, which acts as an intestinal obstruction (see Gastrointestinal System, p. 102).
I. Heart failure (HF) indicated by wet lung sounds.
J. ECG changes; occur as early as 2 hours post-MI or as late as 72 hours post-MI (Table 4-12, *Post-MI Cardiac Enzyme Elevations*).
K. Nausea, vomiting, gastric discomfort, indigestion

L. Anxiety, restlessness, feeling of impending doom or death
M. Cool, pale, diaphoretic skin
N. Dizziness, fatigue, syncope
O. Women more commonly experience dyspnea, unusual fatigue, and sleep disturbances

Analysis (Nursing Diagnoses)

A. Ineffective tissue perfusion related to . . .
B. Decreased cardiac output related to . . .
C. Activity intolerance related to . . .
D. Pain related to . . .

> **HESI Hint** • **SIGNS OF CARDIOGENIC SHOCK**
> Hypotension
> Urine output of less than 30 mL/hour
> Tachycardia
> Cool, moist skin
> Decreased level of consciousness

TABLE 4-12 Post-MI Cardiac Enzyme Elevations

Enzyme/Marker	Onset	Peak	Return to Normal
CK-MB (recognized indicator of MI by most clinicians)	4 to 8 hours	12 to 24 hours	48 to 72 hours
Myoglobin	1 to 4 hours (elevate before CK-MB)	12 hours	24 hours
Cardiac troponins	As early as 1 hour post injury	10 to 24 hours	5 to 14 days

Nursing Plans and Interventions

A. Administer and/or monitor medications as prescribed.
1. For pain and to increase O_2 perfusion, intravenous morphine sulfate (acts as a peripheral vasodilator and decreases venous return) is the drug of choice.
2. Other medications often prescribed include (see Table 4-10, *Antianginals*):
   a. Nitrates, such as nitroglycerin
   b. ACE inhibitors
   c. Beta-blockers
   d. Calcium channel blockers (when beta-blockers are contraindicated)
   e. Aspirin
   f. Antiplatelet aggregates
B. Obtain vital signs, including ECG rhythm strip, regularly per agency policy.
C. Administer oxygen at 2 to 5 liters per nasal cannula.
D. Obtain cardiac enzymes as prescribed.
E. Provide a quiet, restful environment.
F. Auscultate breath sounds for rales (indicating pulmonary edema).
G. Monitor the patency of the IV line for administration of emergency medications.
H. Monitor fluid balance.
I. Keep in semi-Fowler position to assist with breathing.
J. Maintain bed rest for 24 hours.
K. Encourage client to gradually resume activity.
L. Encourage verbalization of fears.
M. Provide information about the disease process and cardiac rehabilitation.
N. Medical interventions (see Angina, p. 83).
1. Thrombolytic agents, within 1 to 4 hours of MI
2. Intra-aortic balloon pump (IABP) to improve myocardial perfusion
3. Surgical reperfusion with coronary artery bypass graft

Hypertension

Description: Hypertension is persistent blood pressure levels greater than 140/90.
A. Essential (primary) hypertension has no known cause (idiopathic).
B. Secondary hypertension develops in response to an identifiable mechanism or another disease.

> **HESI Hint** • Blood pressure is created by the difference in the pressure of the blood as it leaves the heart and the resistance it meets flowing out to the tissues. Therefore, any factor that alters cardiac output or peripheral vascular resistance will alter blood pressure. Diet and exercise, smoking cessation, weight control, and stress management can control many factors that influence the resistance blood meets as it flows from the heart.

Nursing Assessment (Data Collection)

A. BP greater than 140/90 or diastolic BP greater than or equal to 90 on three separate occasions:
1. Obtain BP with client lying, sitting, and standing.
2. Compare readings taken lying, sitting, and standing. A difference of more than 10 mm Hg of either systolic or diastolic indicates postural hypotension. Take in both arms.
B. Genetic risk factors (nonmodifiable):
1. Positive family history for hypertension
2. Gender (men have greater risk of being hypertensive at an earlier age than women)
3. Age (increasing risk with increasing age)
4. Ethnicity (African Americans at greater risk than whites)
C. Lifestyle and habits that increase risk of becoming hypertensive (modifiable):
1. Use of alcohol, tobacco, and caffeine
2. Sedentary lifestyle, obesity
3. Socioeconomic level (incidence is greater in lower socioeconomic groups)
4. Nutrition history of high salt and fat intake
5. Use of oral contraceptives or estrogens
6. Stress

> **HESI Hint** • Remember the risk factors for hypertension: heredity, race, age, alcohol abuse, increased salt intake, obesity, and use of oral contraceptives.

D. Associated physical problems:
1. Renal failure
2. Impaired renal function

3. Respiratory problems, especially COPD
4. Cardiac problems, especially valvular disorders
5. Dyslipidemia
6. Diabetes

E. Pharmacologic history:
   1. Steroids (increase BP)
   2. Estrogens (increase BP)
F. Gather data related to headache, edema, nocturia, nosebleeds, vision changes (may be asymptomatic).
G. Assist client to identify level of stress and source of stress (job-related, economic, family).
H. Recognize personality type—that is, determine whether client exhibits "Type A" behavior.

Analysis (Nursing Diagnoses)

A. Deficient knowledge (specify) related to . . .
B. Noncompliance (specify) related to . . .
C. Ineffective tissue perfusion, altered (specify) related to . . .
D. Pain related to . . .

Nursing Plans and Interventions

A. Collaborate with RN and implement a teaching plan to include:
   1. Information about disease process:
      a. Risk factors
      b. Causes
      c. Long-term complications
      d. Lifestyle modifications
      e. Relationship of treatment to prevention of complications
   2. Information about treatment plan:
      a. How to take own blood pressure
      b. Reasons for each medication (Table 4-13, *Diuretics*, and Table 4-14, *Antihypertensives*)
      c. How and when to take each medication
      d. Necessity of consistency with medication regimen
      e. Need for ongoing assessment while taking antihypertensives

TABLE 4-13 Diuretics

Drugs	Indications	Adverse Reactions	Nursing Implications
Thiazides			

• Chlorthalidone (Hygroton)
• Hydrochlorothiazide (Esidrix, Microzide)
• Indapamide (Lozol)
• Metolazone (Zaroxolyn)
	• To decrease fluid volume
	• Inexpensive
	• Effective
	• Useful in severe hypertension
	• Effective orally
	• Enhances other antihypertensives
		• Hypokalemia symptoms include:
		  →Dry mouth
		  →Thirst
		  →Weakness
		  →Drowsiness
		  →Lethargy
		  →Muscle aches
		  →Tachycardia
		• Hyperuricemia
		• Glucose intolerance
		• Hypercholesterolemia
		• Sexual dysfunction
			• Observe for postural hypotension, can be potentiated by:
			  →Alcohol
			  →Barbiturates
			  →Narcotics
			• Caution with:
			  →Renal failure
			  →Gout
			  →Client taking lithium
			• Hypokalemia increases risk of digitalis toxicity
			• Administer potassium supplements

Loop			
• Furosemide (Lasix) • Furosemide (Demadex) • Bumetanide (Bumex)	• Rapid action • Potent for use when thiazides fail • Cause volume depletion	• Hypokalemia • Hyperuricemia • Glucose intolerance • Hypercholesterolemia • Hypertriglyceridemia • Sexual dysfunction • Weakness	• Volume depletion and electrolyte depletion are rapid • All nursing implications cited for Thiazides
Potassium-Sparing			
• Spironolactone (Aldactone) • Amiloride (Midamor) • Triamterene (Dyrenium) • Eplerenone (Inspra)	• Volume depletion without significant potassium loss	• Hyperkalemia • Gynecomastia • Sexual dysfunction	• Watch for hyperkalemia or renal failure in those treated with ACE inhibitors or NSAIDs • Watch for increase in serum lithium levels • Give after meals to decrease GI distress

TABLE 4-13 Diuretics—cont'd

Drugs	Indications	Adverse Reactions	Nursing Implications
Combination Thiazide and Potassium-Sparing			
• HCTZ and triamterene (Maxide) • Hydrochlorothiazide (HCTZ) + amiloride (Moduretic) • HCTZ + spironolactone (Aldactazide)	• Decreases fluid volume while minimizing K+ loss	• Side effects of individual drug offset or minimized by its partner	• Caution client previously on a loop or thiazide alone not to overdo K+ foods now because of K+ sparing component in new drug • Follow scheduling dosage to avoid sleep disruption

TABLE 4-14 Antihypertensives

Drugs	Indications	Adverse Reactions	Nursing Implications
Alpha-Adrenergic Blockers			
• Prazosin HCL (Minipress) • Terazosin (Hytrin) • Phentolamine mesylate (Regitine) • Doxazosin (Cardura)	• Used as peripheral vasodilator that acts directly on the blood vessels • Used in extreme hypertension of pheochromocytoma	• Orthostatic hypotension • Weakness • Palpitations	• Use cautiously in older clients • Occasional vomiting and diarrhea • Warn clients of possible: →Drowsiness →Lack of energy →Weakness
Combined Alpha Beta-Blockers			
• Labetalol (Normodyne) • Carvedilol (Coreg)	• Produces decrease in BP without reflex tachycardia or bradycardia	• HF • Ventricular dysrhythmias • Blood dyscrasias • Bronchospasm • Orthostatic hypotension	• Contraindicated with: →HF →Heart block →COPD
Beta-Blockers			
• Metoprolol tartrate (Lopressor) • Nadolol (Corgard) • Propranolol HCL (Inderal) • Timolol maleate (Blocadren) • Atenolol (Tenormin) • Bisoprolol (Zebeta) • Metoprolol (Lopressor, Toprol)	• Blocks the sympathetic nervous system, especially to the heart • Produces a slower heart rate • Lowers blood pressure • Reduces O2 consumption during myocardial contraction	• Bradycardia • Fatigue • Insomnia • Bizarre dreams • Sexual dysfunction • Hypertriglyceridemia • Decreased HDL • Depression	• Check apical or radial pulse daily • Monitor for GI distress • Do not discontinue abruptly • Watch for shortness of breath; give cautiously with bronchospasm • Do not vary how taken (with or without food) • Do not vary time taken • May mask symptoms of hypoglycemia or may prolong a hypoglycemic reaction
Central-Acting Inhibitors			
• Clonidine (Catapres) • Guanabenz acetate (Wytensin) • Guanfacine (Tenex) • Methyldopa (Aldomet)	• Decrease BP by stimulating central alpha receptors resulting in decreased sympathetic outflow from the brain	• Drowsiness • Dry mouth • Fatigue • Sexual dysfunction	• Watch for rebound hypertension if abruptly discontinued • Caution to make position changes slowly, avoid standing still, or taking hot baths and showers

Continued

TABLE 4-14 Antihypertensives—cont'd

Drugs	Indications	Adverse Reactions	Nursing Implications
Vasodilators			
• Hydralazine HCL (Apresoline) • Minoxidil (Loniten)	• Decrease BP by decreasing peripheral resistance	• Headache • Tachycardia • Fluid retention (HF, pulmonary edema) • Postural hypotension	• Monitor BP, pulse routinely • Observe for peripheral edema • Monitor I&O • Weigh daily
Angiotensin II Receptor Antagonists			
• Losartan (Cozaar) • Valsartan (Diovan) • Irbesartan (Avapro) • Azilsartan (Edarbi) • Candesartan (Atacand) • Eprosartan (Teveten) • Olmesartan (Benicar) • Telmisartan (Micardis)	• Blocks the vasoconstrictor and aldosterone producing effects of angiotensin II at various sites (vascular smooth muscle and adrenal glands)	• Hypotension • Fatigue • Hepatitis • Renal failure • Hyperkalemia (rare)	• Monitor liver enzymes, electrolytes • Monitor for angioedema in those with history of it when on ACE inhibitors previously
Angiotensin-Converting Enzyme (ACE) Inhibitors			
• Captopril (Capoten) • Enalapril maleate (Vasotec) • Lisinopril (Zestril) • Ramipril (Altace) • Benazepril (Lotensin) • Quinapril (Accupril) • Fosinopril (Monopril) • Moexipril (Univasc) • Trandopril (Mavik)	• Decreases BP by suppressing renin–angiotensin-aldosterone system and inhibiting conversion of angiotensin I to angiotensin II • Useful with diabetics	• Proteinuria • Neutropenia • Skin rash • Cough	• Watch for acute renal failure (reversible) • Routine renal function tests • Remain in bed 3 hours after first dose
Calcium Channel Blockers			
• Diltiazem (Cardizem) • Nifedipine (Procardia, Adalat) • Verapamil HCL (Calan, Isoptin) • Nisoldipine (Sular) • Felodipine (Plendil) • Nicardipine (Cardene) • Amlodipine (Norvasc)	• Inhibits calcium ion influx during cardiac depolarization • Decreases SA/AV node conduction	• Headache • Hypotension • Dizziness • Edema • Nausea • Constipation • Tachycardia • HF • Dry cough	• Check BP and pulse routinely • Limit caffeine consumption • Take medications before meals • Avoid grapefruit juice with these drugs as it will increase serum levels, causing hypotension • High-fat meals elevate serum levels

HESI Hint • The number one cause of cerebral vascular accident (CVA) with hypertensive clients is noncompliance with medication regimen. Hypertension is often symptomless, and antihypertensive medications are expensive and have side effects. Studies have shown that the more clients know about their antihypertensive medications, the more likely they are to take them; teaching and reinforcement are important.

f. Monitor serum electrolytes every 90 to 120 days for duration of treatment.
g. Monitor renal functioning (BUN and creatinine) every 90 to 120 days for duration of treatment.
h. Monitor BP and pulse rate, usually weekly.

B. Encourage client to implement nonpharmacologic measures to assist with BP control, such as the following:
1. Stress reduction
2. Weight loss
3. Tobacco cessation
4. Exercise
C. Determine medication side effects experienced by client:
1. Impotence
2. Insomnia
D. Provide nutritional guidance, including a sample meal plan and how to eat at restaurants (low-salt, low-fat/low-cholesterol diet).

Peripheral Vascular Disease

Description: Peripheral vascular disease (PVD) involves circulatory problems that can be due to either arterial or venous pathology.

Nursing Assessment (Data Collection)

A. The signs, symptoms, and treatment of PVD can be opposite, depending on the source of the pathology. Therefore, careful assessment is very important.

B. Predisposing factors:
1. Arterial:
   a. Arteriosclerosis: 95% of all cases are caused by atherosclerosis
   b. Advanced age
2. Venous:
   a. History of deep vein thrombosis (DVT)
   b. Valvular incompetence

C. Associated diseases:
1. Arterial:
   a. Raynaud disease (nonatherosclerotic, triggered by extreme heat or cold, spasms of the arteries)
   b. Buerger disease (occlusive inflammatory disease, strongly associated with smoking)
   c. Diabetes
   d. Acute occlusion (emboli/thrombi)
2. Venous:
   a. Varicose veins
   b. Thrombophlebitis
   c. Venous stasis ulcers

D. Skin:
1. Arterial:
   a. Smooth
   b. Shiny
   c. Loss of hair
   d. Thick nails
   e. Dry, thin skin
2. Venous—brown pigment around ankles

E. Color:
1. Arterial:
   a. Pallor on elevation
   b. Rubor when dependent
2. Venous—cyanotic when dependent

F. Temperature:
1. Arterial—cool
2. Venous—warm

G. Pulses:
1. Arterial—decreased or absent
2. Venous—normal

H. Pain:
1. Arterial:
   a. Sharp
   b. Increase with walking and elevation
   c. Intermittent claudication: CLASSIC presenting symptom, occurs in skeletal muscles during exercise; relieved by rest

   d. Rest pain: occurs when the extremities are horizontal; may be relieved by dependent position; often appears when collateral circulation fails to develop
2. Venous:
   a. Persistent, aching, full feeling, dull sensation
   b. Pain relieved when horizontal (elevate extremities and use elastic stockings)
   c. Nocturnal cramps

I. Ulcers:
1. Arterial:
   a. Very painful
   b. Occur on lateral lower leg, toes, heel
   c. Demarcated edges
   d. Small, but deep
   e. Circular in shape
   f. Necrotic
   g. Not edematous
2. Venous:
   a. Slightly painful
   b. Occur on medial leg, ankle
   c. Uneven edges
   d. Superficial, but large
   e. Marked edema
   f. Highly exudative

Analysis (Nursing Diagnoses)

A. Ineffective tissue perfusion (peripheral) related to . . .
B. Activity intolerance related to . . .
C. Impaired skin integrity related to . . .
D. Risk for infection related to . . .
E. Pain related to . . .

Treatment

A. Noninvasive treatment:
1. Arterial:
   a. Elimination of smoking
   b. Topical antibiotic
   c. Saline dressing
   d. Bed rest/immobilization
   e. Fibrinolytic agents: if clots are the problem—not used for Raynaud or Buerger disease
2. Venous:
   a. Systemic antibiotics
   b. Compression dressing (snug)
   c. Limb elevation
   d. For thrombosis (see Table 4-15, *Anticoagulants*)

B. Surgery:
1. Arterial:
   a. Embolectomy: removal of clot
   b. Endarterectomy: removal of clot and stripping of plaque
   c. Arterial bypass: Teflon/Dacron graft or autograft
   d. Percutaneous transluminal angioplasty (PTA): compression of plaque
   e. Amputation: removal of extremity

TABLE 4-15 Anticoagulants

Drug	Indications	Adverse Reactions	Nursing Implications
• Heparin sodium (Hepalean, Hep-lock)	• Administered parenterally (subcutaneous or IV) as an antagonist to thrombin and to prevent the conversion of fibrinogen to fibrin	• Hemorrhage • Agranulocytosis • Leukopenia • Hepatitis	• Monitor PTT, Hgb, Hct, platelets • Obtain stools for occult blood • Avoid IM injection • Notify anyone performing diagnostic testing of medication • *Antagonist*: protamine sulfate
• Warfarin sodium (Coumadin)	• Blocks the formation of prothrombin from vitamin K	• Hemorrhage • Agranulocytosis • Leukopenia • Hepatitis	• See heparin • Given orally • Monitor PT • Avoid sudden change in intake of foods high in vitamin K • *Antagonist*: vitamin K
Antiplatelet Agent • Ticlopidine (Ticlid) • Dipyridamole (Persantine) • Clopidogrel (Plavix) • Prasugrel (Effient) • Ticagrelor (Brilinta)	• Short-term use after cardiac interventions • Reduce risk of thrombolytic stroke for those intolerant to aspirin • Prevention of thrombolytic disorders	• Neutropenia • Thrombocytopenia • Agranulocytosis • Leukopenia • Hemorrhage • GI irritation, bleeding • Pancytopenia	• Give pc with food to decrease gastric irritation (Ticlid) • Advise not to take antacids within 2 hours of taking ticlopidine • Monitor CBC every 2 weeks for 3 months, and thereafter if signs of infection develop • Monitor for signs of bleeding • Give 1 hour ac (Persantine); (Plavix) no regard for meals
• Low molecular weight heparin enoxaparin (Lovenox) • Tinzaparin (Innohep) • Dalteparin (Fragmin)	• Prevention of thrombolytic formation (deep vein)	• Hemorrhage • GI irritation, bleeding • Thrombocytopenia	• Monitor for signs of bleeding • Given subcutaneously • Monitor CBC • Use soft toothbrush; avoid cuts
Factor Xa inhibitor • Fondaparinux	• Prevention of thrombolytic formation (deep vein)	• Hemorrhage • GI irritation, bleeding	• Monitor for signs of bleeding • Give subcutaneously • Monitor CBC • Use soft toothbrush; avoid cuts

2. Venous:
   a. Vein ligation
   b. Thrombectomy
   c. Debridement

Nursing Plans and Interventions

A. Monitor extremities at designated intervals:
   1. Color
   2. Temperature
   3. Sensation and pulse quality in extremities
B. Schedule activities within client's tolerance level.
C. Encourage rest at the first sign of pain.
D. Encourage keeping extremities elevated (if venous) when sitting, and change position often.
E. Encourage client to avoid crossing legs and to wear nonrestrictive clothing.
F. Encourage client to keep the extremities warm by wearing extra clothing such as socks and slippers. Do not use external heat sources such as electric heating pads.
G. Collaborate with RN to develop and implement a client/family teaching plan about methods to prevent further injury.
   1. Change position frequently.
   2. Wear nonrestrictive clothing.
   3. Avoid crossing legs or keeping legs in a dependent position.
   4. Wear shoes when ambulating.
   5. Obtain proper foot and nail care.

HESI Hint • Decreased blood flow results in diminished sensation in the lower extremities. Any heat source can cause severe burns before the client actually realizes the damage is being done.

H. Discourage cigarette smoking (causes vasoconstriction and spasm of arteries).
I. Provide preoperative and postoperative care if surgery is required.
   1. Preoperative: maintain affected extremity at a level position, if venous, or at a slightly dependent position, if arterial (15 degrees); at room temperature; and protected from trauma.
   2. Postoperative: assess surgical site frequently for hemorrhage.
   3. Anticoagulants may be continued after surgery to prevent thrombosis of affected artery and to diminish development of thrombi at the initiating site.

Abdominal Aortic Aneurysm

Description: An abdominal aortic aneurysm (AAA) is dilation of the abdominal aorta caused by an alteration in the integrity of its wall.
A. Most common cause of AAA is atherosclerosis.
B. Without treatment, rupture and death will occur.
C. AAA is often asymptomatic.
D. Most common symptom is abdominal pain or low back pain with the complaint that the client can feel "heart beating."
E. Those taking antihypertensive drugs are at risk of developing AAA.

HESI Hint • A client is admitted with severe chest pain and states that he feels a terrible, tearing sensation in his chest. He is diagnosed with a dissecting aortic aneurysm. What assessment should the nurse obtain in the first few hours?
• Vital signs every 1 hour
• Neurologic vital signs
• Respiratory status
• Urinary output
• Peripheral pulses

Nursing Assessment (Data Collection)

A. Bruit (swooshing sound heard over a constricted artery when auscultated) heard over abdominal aorta, pulsation in upper abdomen.
B. Abdominal or lower back pain.
C. Abdominal x-ray study will confirm diagnosis if aneurysm is calcified (aortogram, angiogram, abdominal ultrasound).
D. Symptoms of rupture: hypovolemic or cardiogenic shock with sudden, severe abdominal pain.

Analysis (Nursing Diagnoses)

A. Activity intolerance related to . . .
B. Impaired skin integrity related to . . .
C. Anxiety related to . . .
D. Risk for infection related to . . .

Nursing Plans and Interventions

A. Palpate and report findings of all peripheral pulses and vital signs regularly:
   1. Radial
   2. Femoral
   3. Popliteal
   4. Posterior tibial
   5. Dorsalis pedis
B. Observe for signs of occlusion after graft:
   1. Change in pulses
   2. Severe pain
   3. Cool to cold extremities below graft
   4. White or blue extremities
C. Observe renal functioning for signs of kidney damage (artery clamped during surgery may result in kidney damage):
   1. Output of less than 30 mL/hour
   2. Amber urine
   3. Elevated BUN and creatinine (early signs of renal failure)
D. Observe for postoperative ileus:
   1. Nasogastric (NG) tube 1 to 2 days postoperative (may help prevent ileus).
   2. Check bowel sounds every shift.

HESI Hint • **THROMBOPHLEBITIS**
Description: Inflammation of the venous walls with the formation of a clot. (Also known as venous thrombosis, phlebothrombosis, deep vein thrombosis [DVT].)

Nursing Assessment (Data Collection)

A. Calf or groin pain
B. Functional impairment of extremity
C. Edema and warmth in extremity
D. Asymmetry
   1. Inspect legs from groin to feet.
   2. Measure diameter of calf.
E. Tender areas noted on affected extremity with very gentle palpation
F. Occlusion noted with diagnostic testing
   1. Venogram
   2. Doppler ultrasound
   3. Fibrinogen scanning
G. Risk factors:
   1. Prolonged strict bed rest
   2. General surgery
   3. Leg trauma
   4. Previous venous insufficiency
   5. Obesity
   6. Oral contraceptives
   7. Pregnancy
   8. Malignancy

Analysis (Nursing Diagnoses)

A. Pain related to . . .
B. Ineffective tissue perfusion (specify) related to . . .
C. Impaired skin integrity related to . . .

HESI Hint • Heparin prevents conversion of fibrinogen to fibrin and prothrombin to thrombin, thereby inhibiting clot formation. Because the clotting mechanism is prolonged, do not cause tissue trauma, which may lead to bleeding when heparin is given subcutaneously. Do not massage area or aspirate; give in the abdomen between the pelvic bones; 2 inches from umbilicus; rotate sites.

Nursing Plans and Interventions

A. Administer anticoagulant therapy as prescribed (see Table 4-15, *Anticoagulants*).

HESI Hint • Anticoagulants
Heparin
  Antagonist: protamine sulfate
  Lab: partial thromboplastin time (PTT) or activated partial thromboplastin time (APTT) determines efficacy
  Keep 1.5 to 2.5 times normal control
Coumadin
  Antagonist: vitamin K
  Lab: prothrombin time (PT) determines efficacy
  Keep 1.5 to 2.5 times normal control
INR (International Normalized Ratio)
  Desirable therapeutic level usually 2 to 3 (reflects how long it takes a blood sample to clot)

---

1. Observe for side effects, especially bleeding.
2. Collaborate with the RN to develop and implement a client teaching plan regarding the side effects of medications included in treatment regimen.
3. Monitor laboratory data to determine the efficacy of medications included in treatment regimen.
4. Include information on all lab requests that client is receiving anticoagulants.
5. Partial thromboplastin time (PTT) determines efficacy of heparin.
6. Prothrombin time (PT) determines efficacy of warfarin (Coumadin).
7. Maintain pressure on venipuncture sites to minimize hematoma formation.
8. Notify health care provider of any unusual bleeding.
   a. Abnormal vaginal bleeding
   b. Nosebleeds
   c. Melena
   d. Hematuria
   e. Gums
   f. Hemoptysis
9. Advise client to use soft toothbrush and floss with waxed floss.
10. Encourage client to wear medical alert symbol.
11. Encourage client to avoid alcoholic beverages.
12. Advise client to avoid safety razor if taking warfarin (Coumadin).
13. No acetylsalicylic acid (ASA).

B. Use antiembolic stockings. Elevate extremity and/or use shock blocks for foot of bed.
C. Bed rest; strict, if prescribed, means no bathroom privileges! Prevent straining.
D. Monitor for decreasing symptomatology:
   1. Pain
   2. Edema
E. Monitor for pulmonary embolus (chest pain, shortness of breath).
F. Reinforce client teaching that there is increased risk for DVT formation in the future.
G. Dietary precautions if taking warfarin (Coumadin)

Dysrhythmias

Description: Dysrhythmias are a disturbance in the heart rate and/or heart rhythm.

A. Dysrhythmias are caused by a disturbance in the electrical conduction of the heart, *not* by abnormal heart structure.
B. Client is often asymptomatic until cardiac output is altered.
C. Common causes of dysrhythmias:
   1. Drugs—for example, digoxin, quinidine, caffeine, nicotine, alcohol
   2. Acid-base and electrolyte imbalances (potassium, calcium, and magnesium)
   3. Marked thermal changes
   4. Disease and trauma
   5. Stress

Nursing Assessment (Data Collection)

A. Change in pulse rate and/or rhythm:
   1. Tachycardia: fast rates (greater than 100 bpm)
   2. Bradycardia: slow rates (less than 60 bpm)
   3. Irregular rhythm
   4. Pulselessness
B. ECG changes
C. Complaints of:
   1. Palpitations
   2. Syncope
   3. Pain
   4. Dyspnea
D. Diaphoresis
E. Hypotension
F. Electrolyte imbalance

Analysis (Nursing Diagnoses)

A. Ineffective tissue perfusion related to . . .
B. Activity intolerance related to . . .

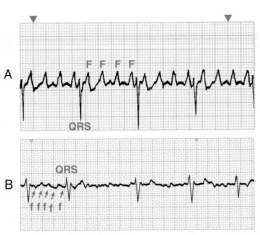

FIGURE 4-3 A, Atrial flutter with a 4:1 conduction (four flutter [F] waves to each QRS complex). **B,** Atrial fibrillation. Note the chaotic fibrillatory (f) waves between the QRS complexes. Note: Recorded from lead V1. (**A,** from Bucher L, Melander S: *Critical care nursing*, Philadelphia, 1999, Saunders; **B,** from Huszar RJ: *Basic dysrhythmias: interpretation and management*, revised ed 3, St. Louis, 2007, Mosby.)

Selected Dysrhythmias

A. Atrial fibrillation (Figure 4-3, A)
   1. Description:
      a. Chaotic activity in the atrioventricular (AV) node
      b. No true P waves visible
      c. Irregular ventricular rhythm
   2. Assessment and treatment:
      a. Anticoagulant therapy is needed due to risk for CVA.
      b. Administer antidysrhythmic drugs.
B. Cardioversion to treat atrial dysrhythmias
C. Atrial flutter (Figure 4-3, B)
   1. Description:
      a. Saw-toothed wave form
      b. Fluttering in chest
      c. Ventricular rhythm stays regular
   2. Assessment and treatment:
      a. May use cardioversion to treat either atrial dysrhythmia.
      b. Administer antidysrhythmic drugs.
      c. Radiofrequency catheter ablation.
D. Ventricular tachycardia (Figure 4-3, C)
   1. Description—wide bizarre QRS
   2. Assessment and treatment:
      a. Assess whether client has a pulse.
      b. Is cardiac output impaired?
      c. Prepare for synchronized cardioversion.
      d. Administer antidysrhythmic drugs.
E. Ventricular fibrillation (Figure 4-3, D)
   1. Description:
      a. Cardiac emergency.
      b. No cardiac output.
   2. Assessment and treatment:
      a. Start CPR.
      b. Defibrillate as quickly as possible.
      c. Administer antidysrhythmic drugs.

Nursing Plans and Interventions

A. Determine medications client is currently taking.
B. Determine serum drug levels, especially digitalis.
C. Determine serum electrolyte levels, especially K^+ and Mg^{++}.
D. Obtain ECG reading upon admission and monitor continuously.

> **HESI Hint** • A Holter monitor offers continuous observation of the client's heart rate. To make assessment of the rhythm strips most meaningful, teach the client to keep a record of:
> • Medication times and doses
> • Chest pain episodes—type and duration
> • Valsalva maneuver (straining at stool, sneezing, coughing)
> • Sexual activity

E. Approach client in a calm, reassuring manner.
F. Monitor client's activity and observe for any symptoms occurring during activity.
G. Ensure proper administration of medications, and monitor for side effects (Table 4-16, *Antidysrhythmics*).
H. Be prepared for emergency measures such as cardioversion or defibrillation.

> **HESI Hint** • Cardioversion is the delivery of synchronized electrical shock to the myocardium.

I. Be prepared for pacemaker insertion.
   1. Temporary pacemaker—used temporarily in emergency situations. Pacing wire is threaded into the right ventricle via the superior vena cava, or an epicardial wire is put in place (through the client's chest incision) during cardiac surgery.
   2. Permanent internal pacemaker with pulse generator implanted in the abdomen or shoulder. May be single or dual chambered. Programmable pacemakers can be reprogrammed by placing a magnetic device over the generator.
   3. Collaborate with RN to develop and implement a client/family teaching plan to:
      a. Report pulse rate lower than the set rate of the pacemaker.
      b. Avoid leaning over an automobile with the engine running.
      c. Stand 4 to 5 feet away from electromagnetic sources, such as operating microwave ovens or radar detectors that are operating.
      d. Avoid MRI diagnostic testing.

TABLE 4-16 Antidysrhythmics

Drugs	Indications	Adverse Reactions	Nursing Implications
Class I (A, B, C)			
• Quinidine • Disopyramide phosphate (Norpace) • Procainamide (Pronestyl) • Moricizine (Ethmozine) • Lidocaine HCL (Xylocaine) • Mexiletine (Mexitil) • Tocainide HCL (Tonocard) • Phenytoin sodium (Dilantin) • Propafenone (Rythmol) • Flecainide acetate (Tambocor)	• Premature beats • Atrial flutter, fibrillation • Contraindicated in heart block • Ventricular dysrhythmias • Unlabeled use: Digitalis-induced dysrhythmias • Ventricular dysrhythmias	• Diarrhea • Hypotension • ECG changes • Cinchonism • Interacts with many common drugs • Hypotension • CNS effects • Seizures • GI distress • Bradycardia • Dizziness • Slurred speech • Ventricular dysrhythmias	• Instruct client to monitor pulse rate and rhythm • Monitor ECG • Monitor for tinnitus and visual disturbances • Lidocaine administered by IV bolus and infusion • Monitor for confusion, drowsiness, slurred speech, seizures with lidocaine • Administer oral drugs with food • May cause digoxin toxicity
Class II			
• Propranolol HCL (Inderal) • Adenosine (Adenocard) • Metoprolol (Lopressor) • Atenolol (Tenormin)	• Supraventricular and ventricular tachydysrhythmias	• Hypotension • Bradycardia • Bronchospasm • Facial flushing	• Monitor vital signs • Contraindicated in asthma, COPD
Class III (Intropics)			
• Amiodarone HCL (Cordarone) • Milrinone (Primacor) • Inamrinone (Inocor) • Sotalol (Betapace) • Dofetilide (Tykosin) • Dronedarone (Multaq) • Ibutilide (Corvert) IV	• Ventricular dysrhythmias	• Dysrhythmias • Hypertension or hypotension • Muscle weakness, tremors • Photophobia	• Amiodarone is now one of the first-choice drugs • Monitor vital signs, ECG • Instruct client taking amiodarone to wear sunglasses and sunscreens when outside
Class IV			
• Verapamil HCL (Isoptin, Calan) • Diltiazem (Cardizem)	• Supraventricular dysrhythmias	• Hypotension • Bradycardia • Constipation	• Monitor BP and pulse • Instruct client to change positions slowly
Miscellaneous Agents			
• Atropine sulfate (Atropisol)	• Bradycardia	• Chest pain • Urinary retention • Dry mouth	• Monitor heart rate and rhythm • Report chest pain • Watch for urinary retention • Avoid use in glaucoma
• Digoxin (Lanoxin) • Digitoxin (Crystodigin)	• Supraventricular dysrhythmias • Atrial fibrillation	• Bradycardia • Dysrhythmias • Anorexia, nausea, vomiting, diarrhea, visual disturbances	• Monitor pulse rate and rhythm • Instruct client to report signs of toxicity • Hypokalemia increases the risk of toxicity • Causes hypercalcemia

TABLE 4-16 Antidysrhythmics—cont'd

Drugs	Indications	Adverse Reactions	Nursing Implications
• Epinephrine (Adrenaline)	• Cardiac arrest	• Tachycardia • Hypertension	• Impaired renal function can cause toxicity—monitor BUN and creatinine • Monitor pulse return in asystole • Monitor vital signs

Additional Drugs That Promote Cardiovascular Perfusion in the Failing Heart

Vasopressors

• Norepinephrine (Levophed)	• Dilates coronary arteries and causes peripheral vasoconstriction for emergency hypotensive states not caused by blood loss, vascular thrombosis, or anesthesia using cyclopropane or halothane	• Can cause SEVERE tissue necrosis, sloughing, and gangrene if infiltrates (blanching along vein pathway = preliminary sign of extravasation)	• Rapidly inactivated by various body enzymes; need to ensure IV patency • Use cautiously in previously hypertensive clients • Check BP every 2 to 5 minutes • Encourage the use of large veins to avoid complications of prolonged vasoconstriction • Pressor effects potentiated by many drugs; check drug–drug interactions • Have phentolamine (Regitine) diluted per protocol for local injection if infiltrates

Cardiotonic/Vasodilator (Human B-Type Natriuretic Peptide: HBNP)

• Nesiritide (Natrecor)	• Treatment of acutely decompensated HF in clients who have dyspnea at rest or with minimal activity • Reduces PCWP and reduces dyspnea	• Hypotension is primary side effect and can be dose limiting • Dysrhythmias • H/A, dizziness, insomnia, tremors, paresthesias • Abdominal pain, nausea, and vomiting	• Many drug–drug interactions • Monitor BP and telemetry • As diuresis occurs, monitor electrolytes, especially K^+ • Watch for overresponse to treatment in older adults

Group IIa-IIIb Inhibitor (Platelet Antiaggregate)

• Eptifibatide (Integrilin) • Tirofiban (Aggrastat) • Abciximab (Reopro)	• Acute coronary syndrome (unstable angina or non-Q waver MI) • Used in combination with heparin, aspirin, and in selected situations, Ticlid and Plavix	• Bleeding, most frequent • Hypotension • Thrombocytopenia • Acute toxicity: decreased muscle tone, dyspnea, loss of righting reflex (unable to maintain balance)	• Check drug–drug interactions before giving other meds • Obtain baseline PT/aPTT, H&H, platelet count and monitor • Dose adjusted by weight for older adults • Same client teaching as with heparin: review activities to avoid • Watch for bleeding • Quickly reversible, so emergency procedures may still be performed shortly after discontinuing infusion

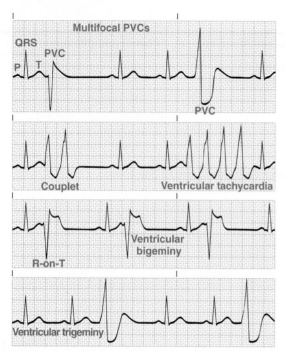

FIGURE 4-4 Various Forms of Premature Ventricular Contractions (PVCs). Note: Recorded from lead II. (From Huszar RJ: *Basic dysrhythmias: interpretation and management*, revised ed 3, St. Louis, 2007, Mosby.)

HESI Hint • Difference in synchronous and asynchronous pacemakers:

- Synchronous or demand pacemaker fires only when the client's heart rate falls below a rate set on the generator.
- Asynchronous or fixed pacemaker fires at a constant rate.

J. Assist in the treatment of premature ventricular contractions (PVCs) as prescribed (tend to be precursors of ventricular tachycardia and ventricular fibrillation) (Figure 4-4, *Premature Ventricular Contractions [PVCs]*).
  1. Occur more often than once in 10 beats.
  2. Occur in groups of 2 and/or 3.
  3. Occur near the T wave.
  4. Take on multiple configurations.

Heart Failure

Description: Heart failure (HF) is the inability of the heart to pump enough blood to meet the tissue's oxygen demands. Primary underlying conditions causing HF include:

A. Ischemic heart disease
B. MI
C. Cardiomyopathy
D. Valvular heart disease
E. Hypertension

Nursing Assessment (Data Collection)

A. Observe for symptoms associated with left-sided or right-sided failure.
  1. Left-sided heart failure—pulmonary edema (left ventricular failure):
    a. Description: results in pulmonary congestion due to the inability of the left ventricle to pump blood to the periphery.
    b. Symptoms:
      (1) Dyspnea
      (2) Orthopnea
      (3) "Wet" lung sounds
      (4) Cough
      (5) Fatigue
      (6) Tachycardia
      (7) Anxiety
      (8) Restlessness
      (9) Confusion
      (10) Paroxysmal nocturnal dypnea
  2. Right-sided heart failure—peripheral edema (right ventricular failure):
    a. Description: results in peripheral congestion due to the inability of the right ventricle to pump blood out to the lungs. Often results from left-sided failure or pulmonary disease.
    b. Symptoms:
      (1) Peripheral edema
      (2) Weight gain
      (3) Distended neck veins
      (4) Anorexia, nausea
      (5) Nocturia
      (6) Weakness
      (7) Hepatomegaly
      (8) Ascites
B. Enlargement of ventricles as indicated by chest x-ray.

HESI Hint • Restricting sodium reduces salt and water retention, thereby reducing vascular volume and preload.

Analysis (Nursing Diagnoses)

A. Decreased cardiac output related to . . .
B. Impaired urinary elimination related to . . .
C. Activity intolerance related to . . .
D. Anxiety related to . . .
E. Ineffective tissue perfusion (specify) related to . . .

Nursing Plans and Interventions

A. Monitor vital signs at least every 4 hours for changes.
B. Monitor apical heart rate with vital signs to detect dysrhythmias, S3 or S4.
C. Assess for hypoxia:
  1. Restlessness
  2. Tachycardia
  3. Angina

TABLE 4-17 Digitalis Preparations

Drugs	Indications	Adverse Reactions	Nursing Implications
• Digitoxin (Crystodigin, Purodigin) • Digoxin (Lanoxin, Lanoxicaps)	• HF • Increases the contractility of cardiac muscle • Slow heart rate and conduction	• Severe: AV block • Headache • Dysrhythmias • Nausea • Vomiting • Blurred vision • Yellow-green halos • Hypotension • Fatigue	• Monitor serum electrolytes; hypokalemia increases risk of digoxin toxicity • Monitor serum digitalis levels if any side effects are present • Check apical pulse before administration; call health care provider if rate is below 60 bpm • Teach client to take radial pulse before administration and call health care provider if below 60 bpm in adults • Therapeutic range: 0.5 to 2 mg
• Digoxin-immune FAB (Digibind)	• Antidote for digitalis toxicity • Binds with digitoxin or digoxin to prevent binding at their site of action	• Decreased cardiac output • Atrial tachydysrhythmias • Use with caution in children and older adults	• Use with 0.22-micron filter • Place client on continuous cardiac monitor • Have resuscitation equipment at bedside before giving first dose

HESI Hint • Digitalis

Side effects of digitalis are increased when the client is hypokalemic. Digitalis has a negative chronotropic effect (i.e., it slows the heart rate). Hold the digitalis if the pulse rate is less than 60 or more than 120 or has markedly changed rhythm. Bradycardia, tachycardia, or dysrhythmias may be signs of digitalis toxicity. These signs include nausea, vomiting, and headache in adults. If withheld, consult with health care provider.

D. Auscultate lungs for indication of pulmonary edema (wet sounds/crackles).
E. Administer oxygen as needed.
F. Elevate head of bed to assist with breathing.
G. Observe for signs of edema:
   1. Weigh daily.
   2. Monitor I&O.
   3. Measure abdominal girth; observe ankles and fingers.
H. Limit sodium intake.
I. Elevate lower extremities while sitting.
J. Obtain apical heart rate before administration of digitalis; withhold medication and call health care provider if rate is below 60 bpm (Table 4-17, *Digitalis Preparations*).
K. Administer diuretics in morning if possible (see Table 4-13, *Diuretics*).
L. Provide periods of rest after periods of activity.

Inflammatory and Infectious Heart Disease

Description: Inflammatory and infectious process involving the endocardium and pericardium.

A. Endocarditis is an inflammatory disease involving the inner surface of the heart, including the valves. Organisms travel through the blood to the heart where vegetations adhere to the valve surface or endocardium. These vegetations can break off and become emboli.

B. Causes of endocarditis:
   1. Rheumatic heart disease
   2. Congenital heart disease
   3. IV drug abuse
   4. Cardiac surgery
   5. Immunosuppression
   6. Dental procedures
   7. Invasive procedures
C. Pericarditis is an inflammation of the outer lining of the heart.
D. Causes of pericarditis:
   1. Post-MI
   2. Trauma
   3. Neoplasm
   4. Connective tissue disease
   5. Following heart surgery
   6. Idiopathic
   7. Infections

Nursing Assessment (Data Collection)

A. Endocarditis:
   1. Fever
   2. Chills, malaise, night sweats, fatigue
   3. Murmurs
   4. Symptoms of heart failure
   5. Atrial embolization

B. Pericarditis:
   1. Pain: sudden, sharp, severe
      a. Substernal, radiating to the back or arm
      b. Aggravated by coughing, inhalation, deep breathing
      c. Relieved by leaning forward
   2. Pericardial friction rub heard best at left lower sternal border
   3. Fever

> **HESI Hint** • Infective endocarditis damage to heart valves occurs with the growth of vegetative lesions on valve leaflets. These lesions pose a risk of embolization; erosion/perforation of the valve leaflets; or abscesses within adjacent myocardial tissue. Valvular stenosis or regurgitation (insufficiency), most commonly of the mitral valve, can occur depending on the type of damage inflicted by the lesions, leading to symptoms of left- or right-sided heart failure (see Valvular Heart Disease, right, and Heart Failure).

> **HESI Hint** • ACUTE AND SUBACUTE INFECTIVE ENDOCARDITIS
> The two types of infective endocarditis are acute, which often affects individuals with previously normal hearts and healthy valves and carries a high mortality rate, and subacute, which typically affects individuals with preexisting conditions, such as rheumatic heart disease, mitral valve prolapse, or immunosuppression. Intravenous drug abusers are at risk for both acute and subacute bacterial endocarditis. When this population develops subacute infective endocarditis, the valves on the right side of the heart (tricuspid and pulmonic) are typically affected because of the introduction of common pathogens that colonize on the skin (*Staphylococcus epidermis* or *Candida*) into the venous system.

> **HESI Hint** • PERICARDITIS
> The presence of a friction rub is an indication of pericarditis (inflammation of the lining of the heart). ST segment elevation and T wave inversion are also signs of pericarditis.

Analysis (Nursing Diagnoses)
A. Decreased cardiac output related to . . .
B. Risk for injury (emboli) related to . . .

Nursing Plans and Interventions
A. Endocarditis
   1. Monitor hemodynamic status (vital signs, level of consciousness, urinary output).
   2. IV antibiotics are usually prescribed for 4 to 6 weeks. Clients may be instructed in IV therapy for home

health care. The American Heart Association no longer recommends the administration of antibiotics before dental or genitourinary procedures except for clients who are at the highest risk of adverse outcomes from infective (bacterial) endocarditis. See www.americanheart.org/.
   3. Collaborate with RN to develop and implement a client/family teaching plan about anticoagulant therapy if prescribed.
   4. Encourage client to maintain good hygiene.
   5. Reinforce client instructions to inform dentist or other health care providers of history.
B. Pericarditis
   1. Provide rest and maintain position of comfort.
   2. Administer analgesics and anti-inflammatory drugs.

Valvular Heart Disease

Description: Heart valves are unable to fully open (stenosis) or fully close (insufficiency or regurgitation).
A. Valve dysfunction most commonly occurs on the left side of the heart, with the mitral valve most frequently involved, followed by the aortic valve.

> **HESI Hint** • With mitral valve stenosis, blood is regurgitated back into the left atrium from the left ventricle. In the early period, there may be no symptoms, but as the disease progresses, the client will exhibit excessive fatigue, dyspnea on exertion, orthopnea, dry cough, hemoptysis, or pulmonary edema. There will be a rumbling apical diastolic murmur, and atrial fibrillation is common.

B. Common causes of valvular disease:
   1. Rheumatic fever
   2. Congenital heart diseases
   3. Syphilis
   4. Endocarditis
   5. Hypertension
C. Prevention of rheumatic heart disease would reduce the incidence of valvular heart disease.

Nursing Assessment (Data Collection)
A. Fatigue
B. Dyspnea, orthopnea
C. Hemoptysis and pulmonary edema
D. Murmurs
E. Irregular cardiac rhythm
F. Angina

Analysis (Nursing Diagnoses)
A. Decreased cardiac output related to . . .
B. Impaired gas exchange related to . . .
C. Activity intolerance related to . . .

Nursing Plans and Interventions

A. See Heart Failure, p. 98.

B. Monitor client for changes in the ECG pattern.

C. Collaborate with RN to develop and implement a teaching plan to help client/family determine the necessity for prophylactic antibiotic therapy before any invasive procedure (e.g., dental procedures).

D. Prepare the client for surgical repair or replacement of heart valves.

E. Reinforce instruction for client who will be receiving valve replacement of the need for lifelong anticoagulant therapy to prevent thrombus formation. Tissue (biologic) valves and autografts do not require lifelong anticoagulant therapy.

Review of Cardiovascular System

1. How do clients experiencing angina describe that pain?
2. Develop a teaching plan for the client taking nitroglycerin.
3. List the parameters of blood pressure for diagnosing hypertension.
4. Differentiate between essential and secondary hypertension.
5. Develop a teaching plan for the client taking antihypertensive medications.
6. Describe intermittent claudication.
7. Describe the nurse's discharge instructions to a client with venous peripheral vascular disease.
8. What is often the underlying cause of abdominal aortic aneurysm?
9. What lab values should be monitored daily for the client with thrombophlebitis who is undergoing anticoagulant therapy?
10. When do PVCs (premature ventricular contractions) present a grave danger?
11. Differentiate between the symptoms of left-sided cardiac failure and right-sided cardiac failure.
12. List three symptoms of digitalis toxicity.
13. What condition increases the likelihood of digitalis toxicity occurring?
14. What lifestyle changes can the client who is at risk for hypertension initiate to reduce the likelihood of becoming hypertensive?
15. What immediate actions should the nurse implement when a client is having a myocardial infarction?
16. What symptoms should the nurse expect to find in the client with hypokalemia?
17. Bradycardia is defined as a heart rate below _____ bpm. Tachycardia is defined as a heart rate above _____ bpm.
18. What precautions should clients with valve disease who have the highest risk for adverse outcomes from infective (bacterial) endocarditis take before invasive procedures or dental work?

Answers to Review

1. Described as squeezing, heavy, burning, radiates to left arm or shoulder, transient, or prolonged.
2. Take at first sign of anginal pain. Take no more than three, 5 minutes apart. Call for emergency attention if no relief in 10 minutes.
3. More than 140/90.
4. Essential has no known cause, while secondary hypertension develops in response to an identifiable mechanism.
5. Explain how and when to take medication, reason for medication, necessity of compliance, need for follow-up visits while on medication, need for certain lab tests, vital sign parameters while initiating therapy.
6. Pain related to peripheral vascular disease occurring with exercise and disappearing with rest.
7. Keep extremities elevated when sitting, rest at first sign of pain, keep extremities warm (but do *not* use heating pad), change position often, avoid crossing legs, wear unrestrictive clothing.
8. Atherosclerosis.
9. PTT, PT, Hgb, Hct, and platelets.
10. When they begin to occur more often than once in 10 beats, occur in 2s or 3s, land near the T wave, or take on multiple configurations.
11. Left-sided failure results in pulmonary congestion due to backup of circulation in the left ventricle. Right-sided failure results in peripheral congestion due to backup of circulation in the right ventricle.
12. Dysrhythmias, headache, nausea, and vomiting.
13. When the client is hypokalemic (which is more common when diuretics and digitalis preparations are given together).
14. Cease cigarette smoking if applicable, control weight, exercise regularly, and maintain a low-fat/low-cholesterol diet.

15. Place the client on immediate strict bed rest to lower oxygen demands of heart, administer oxygen by nasal cannula at 2 to 5 L/min, take measures to alleviate pain and anxiety (administer PRN pain medications and antianxiety medications).
16. Dry mouth and thirst, drowsiness and lethargy, muscle weakness and aches, and tachycardia.
17. 60 bpm; 100 bpm.
18. Take prophylactic antibiotics.

Gastrointestinal System

Hiatal Hernia and Gastroesophageal Reflux Disease

A. Hiatal hernia is herniation of the stomach and other abdominal viscera through an enlarged esophageal opening in the diaphragm.
  1. Sliding hernia is the most common type, which accounts for 75% to 90% of adult hiatal hernias.
B. Gastroesophageal reflux disease (GERD) is the result of an incompetent lower esophageal sphincter that allows regurgitation of acidic gastric contents into the esophagus.
  1. Multiple factors determine whether GERD is present.
    a. Efficiency of antireflux mechanism
    b. Volume of gastric contents
    c. Potency of refluxed material
    d. Efficiency of esophageal clearance
    e. Resistance of the esophageal tissue to injury and the ability to repair tissue
  2. The client must have several episodes of reflux for GERD to be present.

Nursing Assessment (Data Collection)

A. Heartburn after eating
B. Feeling of fullness and discomfort after eating
C. Positive diagnosis determined by history and fluoroscopy or endoscopy

Analysis (Nursing Diagnoses)

A. Pain related to . . .
B. Deficient knowledge (specify) related to . . .
C. Anxiety related to . . .

Nursing Plans and Interventions

A. Determine eating pattern that alleviates symptoms.
  1. Encourage small, frequent meals.
  2. Encourage the client to eliminate foods that are determined to aggravate symptoms (these foods are client specific).
  3. Encourage the client to sit up while eating and remain in upright position for at least 1 hour after eating.
  4. Encourage the client to stop eating 3 hours before bedtime.
  5. Elevate the head of the bed on 6- to 8-inch blocks.

6. Assist with teaching about frequently prescribed medications (H_2 antagonists, antacids, and proton pump inhibitors [PPIs]).

> **HESI Hint** • A Fowler or semi-Fowler position is beneficial in reducing the amount of regurgitation and preventing the encroachment of the stomach tissue upward through the opening in the diaphragm.

B. Assist with the teaching plan for client/family that should include the following:
  1. Differentiate between the symptoms of hiatal hernia and MI.
  2. Be alert to the possibility of aspiration.
  3. Head of bed elevation increased by use of 6-inch blocks.
  4. Encourage weight loss if the client is overweight.

Peptic Ulcer Disease

Description: Peptic ulcer disease (PUD) is ulceration that penetrates the mucosal wall of any portion of the GI tract in contact with hydrogen chloride (HCl).
A. Gastric ulcers tend to occur in the lesser curvature of the stomach. Pain intensifies with food consumption.
B. Duodenal ulcers occur in the duodenum, often near the pylorus. Eating relieves pain.
C. Esophageal ulcers occur in the esophagus.
D. The etiology of some peptic ulcer disease is unknown. A significant number of gastric ulcers are caused by a bacteria, *Helicobacter pylori (H. pylori)*, and can be successfully treated with drug therapy. Risk factors for development of peptic ulcers include:
  1. Drugs (NSAIDs, corticosteroids)
  2. Alcohol
  3. Cigarette smoking
  4. Acute medical crisis or trauma
  5. Familial tendency
  6. Blood type O
E. Symptoms common to all types of ulcers include the following:
  1. Epigastric pain radiating to the back (not associated with the type of food eaten) and relieved by antacids
  2. Belching
  3. Bloating

Nursing Assessment (Data Collection)

A. Determine how food intake affects pain
B. History of antacid, histamine antagonist, or proton pump inhibitor use
C. Hematemesis
D. Melena (black, tarry stools)
E. Presence and/or location of peptic ulcers as determined by:
  1. Barium swallow
  2. Upper endoscopy
  3. Gastric analysis indicating increased levels of stomach acid
F. Potential complications:
  1. Hemorrhage
  2. Perforation (always demands surgery)
  3. Obstruction
  4. Cancer

Analysis (Nursing Diagnoses)

A. Pain related to . . .
B. Imbalanced nutrition: less than body requirements related to . . .
C. Deficient knowledge (specify) related to . . .
D. Risk for injury related to . . .
E. Risk for deficient fluid volume related to . . .

Nursing Plans and Interventions

A. Determine symptom onset and how symptoms are relieved.
B. Monitor color, quantity, consistency of stools and emesis, and test for occult blood.
C. Administer medications as prescribed, usually 1 to 2 hours after meals and at bedtime (Table 4-18, *Antiulcer Drugs*).

TABLE 4-18 Antiulcer Drugs

Drugs	Indications	Adverse Reactions	Nursing Implications
Antacids			
• Aluminum hydroxide/ magnesium hydroxide (Maalox, Mylanta, Riopan, Gelusil II)	• Treatment of peptic ulcers • Work by neutralizing or reducing acidity of stomach contents • Differences in absorption rate	• Constipation • Diarrhea • Drug interactions	• Need to take several times a day • Administer after meals • Review client's history of renal diseases when client is taking magnesium products; electrolyte readjustment occurs and can result in renal insufficiency and calcinosis
Histamine₂ Antagonists			
• Ranitidine HCL (Zantac) • Cimetidine (Tagamet) • Famotidine (Pepcid) • Nizatidine (Axid)	• Treatment of peptic ulcers • Prophylactic treatment for clients at risk for developing ulcers (those on steroids, or highly stressed)	• Multiple drug interactions	• Cigarette smoking interferes with drug action • Expensive
Mucosal Healing Agents			
• Sucralfate (Carafate)	• Treatment of peptic ulcers	• Constipation • Drug interaction with: • Tetracycline • Phenytoin sodium • Digoxin • Cimetidine	• Medication to be taken at least 1 hour before meals or other medications • Antacids interfere with absorption
Proton Pump Inhibitors			
• Lansoprazole (Prevacid) (PO only) • Pantoprazole (Protonix) (available oral and IV) • Esomeprazole (Nexium) (oral only) • Omeprazole (Prilosec) • Rabeprazole (Aciphex) • Dexlansoprazole (Kapidex)	• Treatment of erosive esophagitis associated with gastroesophageal reflux disease (GERD)	• Constipation • Heartburn • Anxiety • Diarrhea • Abdominal pain, hepatocellular damage, pancreatitis, gastroenteritis • Tinnitus, vertigo, confusion, H/A • Blurred vision, hypokinesia • Chest pain, dyspnea	• Taken before meals • Do not crush or chew • Pantoprazole IV: • Resume oral therapy as soon as feasible • Long-lasting effects of drug may inhibit absorption of other drugs • Not removed by hemodialysis • Monitor for indications of adverse reactions

HESI Hint • Gastric emptying can be delayed by withholding fluids with meals, by eating in a recumbent or semi-recumbent position, or by lying down after meals.

D. Administer mucosal healing agents at least 1 hour before meals, as prescribed (see Table 4-18, *Antiulcer Drugs*).
E. Encourage small, frequent meals with no bedtime snack. Avoid beverages containing caffeine or alcohol. Avoid "irritating" foods.
F. Prepare for surgery if uncontrolled bleeding, obstruction, or perforation occurs.
   1. Gastric resection
   2. Vagotomy
   3. Pyloroplasty
G. Anticipate dumping syndrome.
   1. Secondary to rapid entry of hypertonic food into jejunum (pulls water out of bloodstream).
   2. Occurs 5 to 30 minutes after eating.
   3. Characterized by vertigo, syncope, sweating, pallor, tachycardia, or hypotension.
   4. Provide small, frequent meals: high-protein, high-fat, low-carbohydrate diet.
   5. Avoid liquids with meals, and encourage client to lie down after eating.
   6. This syndrome can also be observed in clients on hypertonic tube feeding.
H. Reinforce the teaching plan related to the importance of avoiding medications that increase the risk for developing peptic ulcers.
   1. Salicylates
   2. Nonsteroidal anti-inflammatory drugs such as ibuprofen
   3. Corticosteroids in high doses
   4. Anticoagulants
I. Emphasize to the client the importance of informing all health care personnel of ulcer history.
J. Assist the client to recognize signs and symptoms of GI bleeding.
   1. Dark, tarry stools
   2. Coffee-ground emesis
   3. Bright red, rectal bleeding
   4. Fatigue
   5. Pallor
   6. Severe abdominal pain should be reported immediately (could denote perforation)
K. Emphasize the importance of smoking cessation and stress management.

HESI Hint • Stress can cause or exacerbate ulcers. Reinforce teaching about stress reduction methods and encourage those with a family history of ulcers to obtain medical surveillance for ulcer formation.

HESI Hint • CLINICAL MANIFESTATIONS OF GI BLEEDING
Pallor: conjunctival, mucous membranes, nail beds
Dark, tarry stools
Bright red or coffee-ground emesis
Abdominal mass or bruit
Decreased BP, rapid pulse, cool extremities (shock)

Inflammatory Bowel Diseases

Description: Inflammatory bowel diseases consist of Crohn disease and ulcerative colitis.

Crohn Disease (Regional Enteritis)

Description: Crohn disease (regional enteritis) is subacute, chronic inflammation extending throughout the entire intestinal mucosa (most frequently found in terminal ileum).

Nursing Assessment (Data Collection)

A. Abdominal pain (unrelieved by defecation)
B. Diarrhea and weight loss, with client becoming emaciated because of malabsorption
C. Constant fluid loss
D. Perforation of the intestine may occur because of severe inflammation and constitutes a medical emergency.

HESI Hint • The GI tract usually accounts for only 100 to 200 mL fluid loss per day, although it filters up to 8 liters per day. Large fluid losses can occur if vomiting and/or diarrhea occurs.

Ulcerative Colitis

Description: Ulcerative colitis is a disease that affects the superficial mucosa of the colon, causing the bowel to eventually narrow, shorten, and thicken due to muscular hypertrophy. It occurs in the large bowel and rectum.

Nursing Assessment (Data Collection)

A. Diarrhea
B. Abdominal pain (unrelieved by defecation), right lower quadrant
C. Intermittent tenesmus (anal contractions) and rectal bleeding
D. Liquid stools containing blood, mucous, and pus (may pass 10 to 20 liquid stools per day)
E. Weakness and fatigue
F. Anemia
G. Stress

Analysis (Nursing Diagnoses)

A. Risk for deficient fluid volume related to . . .
B. Pain related to . . .
C. Imbalanced nutrition, less than body requirements related to . . .

Nursing Plans and Interventions

A. Determine bowel elimination pattern and control diarrhea with diet and medication as indicated.
B. Provide a nutritious, well-balanced, low-residue, low-fat, high-protein, high-calorie diet. *No dairy products.*
C. Administer vitamin supplements and iron.
D. Encourage the client to avoid foods that are known to cause diarrhea, such as milk products and spicy food.
E. Encourage the client to avoid smoking, caffeinated beverages, pepper, and alcohol.
F. Provide complete bowel rest with IV total parenteral nutrition if necessary.
G. Administer medications as prescribed, often corticosteroids, antidiarrheals, sulfasalazine (Azulfidine), mesalamine (various brands), and infliximab (Remicade) or other biologic treatments, if there is no response to previous medications.
H. Monitor I&O and serum electrolytes.
I. Weigh at least twice a week.
J. Provide emotional support and encourage use of support groups such as local Ileitis and Colitis Foundation.
K. Encourage client to talk with the enterostomal therapists *before* surgery.
L. If ileostomy is performed, collaborate with RN to develop and implement a teaching plan for client/family about stoma care (see Stoma Care, p. 107).

> **HESI Hint** • Opiate drugs tend to depress gastric motility. However, they should be given with care, and those receiving them should be closely monitored because a distended intestinal wall accompanied by decreased muscle tone may lead to intestinal perforation.

Diverticular Diseases

Description: Diverticular diseases manifested in two clinical forms: diverticulosis and diverticulitis.
A. Diverticulosis: bulging pouches in the GI wall (diverticula) push the mucosa lining through the surrounding muscle.
B. Diverticulitis: inflamed diverticula (may cause obstruction, infection, and/or hemorrhage).

> **HESI Hint** • Diverticulosis is the presence of pouches in the wall of the intestine. There is usually no discomfort, and the problem goes unnoticed unless seen on radiologic examination (usually prompted by some other condition). Diverticulitis is an inflammation of the diverticula (pouches), which can lead to perforation of the bowel.

Nursing Assessment (Data Collection)

A. Left lower quadrant pain
B. Increased flatus
C. Rectal bleeding
D. Signs of intestinal obstruction:
   1. Constipation alternating with diarrhea
   2. Abdominal distention
   3. Anorexia
   4. Low-grade fever
E. Barium enema or colonoscopy positive for diverticular disease
F. Obstruction, ileus, or perforation confirmed with abdominal x-ray film. Barium enema not done during acute phase of illness.

Analysis (Nursing Diagnoses)

A. Ineffective gastrointestinal tissue perfusion related to . . .
B. Pain related to . . .
C. Imbalanced nutrition, less than body requirements related to . . .

Nursing Plans and Interventions

A. Provide a well-balanced, high-fiber diet unless inflammation is present, at which time client is NPO followed by low-residue, bland foods.

> **HESI Hint** • A client admitted with complaints of severe lower abdominal pain, cramping, and diarrhea is diagnosed with diverticulitis. What are the nutritional needs of this client throughout recovery?
> • Acute phase—NPO, graduating to liquids.
> • Recovery phase—No fiber or foods that irritate the bowel.
> • Maintenance phase—High-fiber diet, with bulk-forming laxatives to prevent pooling of foods in the pouches where they can become inflamed. Avoid small, poorly digested foods such as popcorn, nuts, seeds, and so on.

B. Include bulk-forming laxatives such as Metamucil in daily regimen.
C. Increase fluid intake to 3 liters/day.
D. Monitor I&O and bowel elimination; avoid constipation.
E. Observe for complications:
   1. Obstruction
   2. Peritonitis
   3. Hemorrhage (with ruptured diverticula, a temporary colostomy is performed and maintained for approximately 3 months to allow the bowel to rest)
   4. Infection

Intestinal Obstruction

Description: Partial or complete blockage of intestinal flow (fluids, feces, gas) that occurs mostly in the small intestines.

A. Mechanical causes of intestinal obstruction include:
1. Adhesions (most common cause)
2. Strangulated hernia
3. Volvulus (twisting of the gut)
4. Intussusception (telescoping of the gut within itself)
5. Tumors that develop slowly; usually mass of feces becomes lodged against the tumor
B. Neurogenic causes of intestinal obstruction:
1. Paralytic ileus (usually occurs in postoperative clients)
2. Spinal cord lesion
C. Vascular cause: mesenteric artery occlusion (leads to gut infarct)

HESI Hint • BOWEL OBSTRUCTIONS

Mechanical: Caused by disorders outside the bowel (hernia, adhesions); disorders within the bowel (tumors, diverticulitis); or blockage of the lumen in the intestine (intussusception, gallstone).

Nonmechanical: Paralytic ileus, which does not involve any actual physical obstruction but results from inability of the bowel to function.

Nursing Assessment (Data Collection)

A. Sudden onset of abdominal pain, tenderness, or guarding.
B. History of abdominal surgeries.
C. History of obstruction.
D. Distention.
E. Increased peristalsis when obstruction first occurs, then peristalsis becomes absent when paralytic ileus occurs. Assessed by listening to bowel sounds.
F. Bowel sounds are high-pitched with early mechanical obstruction and diminished to absent with neurogenic, or late, mechanical obstruction.
G. Nausea or vomiting.

Analysis (Nursing Diagnoses)

A. Impaired gastrointestinal tissue perfusion related to . . .
B. Deficient fluid volume related to . . .
C. Pain related to . . .

HESI Hint • Blood gas analysis will show an alkalotic state if the bowel obstruction is high in the small intestine where gastric acid is secreted. If the obstruction is in the lower bowel where base solutions are secreted, the blood will be acidic.

Nursing Plans and Interventions

A. NPO, IV fluids, and electrolyte therapy
B. I&O, Foley catheter to maintain strict output

C. Nasogastric intubation:
1. Attach to low suction (intermittent 80 mm Hg).
2. Document output q8 hours.
3. Irrigate with normal saline if policy dictates.
D. Cantor, Miller-Abbott, or Harris tubes are passed through the nose and into the stomach, usually by the health care provider.
1. Advance tube every 1 to 2 hours.
2. Do not secure to nose until tube reaches specified position.
3. Reposition client every 2 hours to assist with advancement of the tube.
4. Connect to suction as prescribed.
5. Irrigate with 20 to 30 mL of normal saline.
6. Label lumen of Miller-Abbott tube. Do *not* put anything with mercury in lumen.
7. Note amount, color, consistency, pH, and any unusual odor of drainage.
E. Document pain; medicate as prescribed.
F. Monitor abdomen regularly for distention, rigidity, change in status of bowel sounds.
G. If conservative medical interventions fail, surgery will be required to remove obstruction (see Perioperative Care in Chapter 3, *Advanced Clinical Concepts*, p. 46).

HESI Hint • A client admitted with complaints of constipation, thready stools, and rectal bleeding over the past few months is diagnosed with a rectal mass. What are the nursing priorities for this client?
• NPO
• NG tube (possibly an intestinal tube such as a Miller-Abbott)
• IV fluids
• Surgical preparation of bowel (if obstruction is complete)
• Teaching (preoperative, nutrition, etc.)

Cancer of the Colon

Description: Tumors occurring in the colon.

A. Cancer of the colon is the fourth most common cancer in the United States.
B. The estimated cure rate for cancer of the colon is 50%.
C. Forty-five percent of cancerous tumors of the colon occur in the rectal or sigmoid area, 25% in the cecum and ascending colon, and 30% in the remainder of the colon.
D. The highest incidence is in persons older than 60 years of age.
E. A diet of high-fiber, low-fat foods, including cruciferous vegetables, may be a factor in the prevention of colon cancer.

> **HESI Hint** • Diet recommended by the American Cancer Society to prevent bowel cancer:
> - Eat more cruciferous vegetables (from the cabbage family such as broccoli, cauliflower, Brussels sprouts, cabbage, and kale).
> - Increase fiber intake.
> - Maintain average body weight.
> - Eat less animal fat.

F. Early detection is important.

G. Usual treatment is surgical removal of the tumor with adjuvant radiation or antineoplastic chemotherapy.

H. Diagnosis is made by digital examination, flexible fiber-optic sigmoidoscopy with biopsy, colonoscopy, and barium enema.

I. Carcinoembryonic antigen serum level is used to evaluate effectiveness of treatment.

Nursing Assessment (Data Collection)

A. Rectal bleeding

B. Change in bowel habits

C. Sense of incomplete evacuation

D. Abdominal pain, nausea, vomiting

E. Weight loss, cachexia

F. Abdominal distention or ascites

G. Family history of cancer, particularly cancer of the colon

H. History of polyps

Analysis (Nursing Diagnoses)

A. Deficient knowledge (specify) related to . . .

B. Ineffective coping related to . . .

C. Disturbed body image related to . . .

Nursing Plans and Interventions

A. Treatment
  1. Prepare client for surgery (see Perioperative Care in Chapter 3, *Advanced Clinical Concepts*, p. 46).
  2. Bowel preparation may include laxatives and gut lavage with polyethylene glycol (GoLYTELY®).
  3. If colostomy is performed, collaborate with RN to develop and implement a teaching plan for client/family about stoma care (see Stoma Care, right).

B. Prevention
  1. Provide high-calorie, high-protein diet.
  2. Promote prevention of constipation with high-fiber diet.
  3. Encourage early detection by screening with Hemoccult (guaiac) tests.

> **HESI Hint** • American Cancer Society recommendations for early detection of colon cancer:
> - A digital rectal examination every year after 40.
> - A stool blood test every year after 50.

Continued

> - A colonoscopy or sigmoidoscopy examination every 10 years after the age of 50 in average-risk clients, or more often based on the advice of a physician.

Stoma Care

A. The more distal the stoma is, the greater the chance for continence.
  1. An ileostomy drains liquid material; peristomal skin is prone to breakdown from enzymes.
  2. As the stoma's location descends the GI tract, the effluence (stoma drainage) becomes more solid or formed.
  3. The greatest chance for continence is with a stoma created from the sigmoid colon on the left side of the abdomen.
  4. Consultation with an enterostomal therapist is essential.

B. Preoperative care
  1. Reinforce a teaching plan related to postoperative expectations of client and family.
  2. Proposed location of the stoma.
  3. Approximate size.
  4. What it will look like; provide a picture if indicated.
  5. Support for the family but emphasize that the client is ultimately responsible for his or her own care.

C. Pouch care
  1. Ostomates will often wear pouches.
  2. The adhesive-backed opening, designed to cover the stoma, should provide about ⅛-inch clearance from the stoma.
  3. Use rubber band or clip to secure the bottom of the pouch and prevent leakage.
  4. Use simple squirt bottle to remove effluence from the sides of the bag. Change pouch system every 3 to 7 days.
  5. Maintain an extra supply of pouches so they never run out.
  6. Change the pouch when bowel is inactive.
  7. Empty pouch when ⅓ to ½ full.

D. Irrigation
  1. Those with descending colon colostomies can irrigate to provide control over effluence.
  2. Irrigate at approximately the same time daily.
  3. Use warm water (cold or hot water will cause cramping).
  4. Wash around stoma with lukewarm water and a mild soap.
  5. Commercial skin barriers may be purchased for home use.
  6. Odor control:
     a. Commercial preparations are available.
     b. Eliminate foods in diet that cause offensive odors.

E. Diet
   1. Ileostomy
      a. Reinforce client instructions to chew food thoroughly.
      b. High-fiber foods can cause severe diarrhea and may need to be eliminated (popcorn, peanuts, unpeeled vegetables).
   2. Colostomy: reinforce client instructions to resume the regular diet gradually. Foods that were a problem preoperatively should be tried cautiously.

Cirrhosis

Description: Cirrhosis is damage to liver tissue, causing enlargement, fibrosis, scarring, and loss of effective hepatic functioning.

A. Etiology of cirrhosis includes the following:
   1. Chronic alcohol ingestion (Laennec cirrhosis)
   2. Viral hepatitis
   3. Exposure to hepatotoxins (including medications)
   4. Infections
   5. Congenital abnormalities
   6. Chronic biliary tree obstruction
   7. Chronic severe right heart failure (HF)
   8. Idiopathic
B. Initially, hepatomegaly occurs; later, the liver becomes hard and nodular. May be detectable upon palpation of right upper quadrant.

Nursing Assessment (Data Collection)

A. History of alcohol use, prescriptive and street drug use
B. Work history of exposure to toxic chemicals (pesticides, fumes, etc.)
C. Medication history of long-term use of hepatotoxic drugs
D. Family health history of liver abnormalities
E. Physical findings include the following:
   1. Weakness, malaise
   2. Anorexia, weight loss
   3. Palpable liver (early), abdominal girth increases as liver enlarges
   4. Jaundice
   5. Fetor hepaticus (fruity or musty breath)

HESI Hint • CLINICAL MANIFESTATIONS OF JAUNDICE
Yellow skin, sclera, and/or mucous membranes (bilirubin in skin)
Dark-colored urine (bilirubin in urine)
Chalky or clay-colored stools (absence of bilirubin in stools)

HESI Hint • Fetor hepaticus is a distinctive breath odor of chronic liver disease. It is characterized by a fruity or musty odor that results from the damaged liver's inability to metabolize and detoxify mercaptan, which is produced by the bacterial degradation of methionine, a sulfurous amino acid.

   6. Asterixis (hand-flapping tremor that often accompanies metabolic disorders)
   7. Mental and behavioral changes
   8. Bruising, erythema, or bleeding abnormalities
   9. Dry skin, spider angiomas
   10. Gynecomastia (breast development), testicular atrophy
   11. Ascites
   12. Peripheral neuropathy
   13. Hematemesis
   14. Palmar erythema (redness in palms of the hands)

HESI Hint • For treatment of ascites, paracentesis and peritoneovenous shunts (LeVeen and Denver shunts) may be indicated.

HESI Hint • Esophageal varices may rupture and cause hemorrhage. Immediate management includes insertion of an esophagogastric balloon tamponade—a Blakemore-Sengstaken or Minnesota tube. Other therapies include vasopressors, vitamin K, coagulation factors, and blood transfusions.

F. Alterations in laboratory findings include:
   1. Elevated bilirubin, AST, ALT, alkaline phosphatase, PT, and ammonia
   2. Decreased Hgb, Hct, electrolytes, and albumin

HESI Hint • Ammonia is not broken down as usual in the damaged liver; therefore, the serum ammonia level rises, which causes neurologic symptoms, including confusion. Due to possible altered mental state, the nurse should include safety precautions in the client's plan of care.

G. Complications include:
   1. Ascites, edema
   2. Portal hypertension
   3. Esophageal varices
   4. Encephalopathy
   5. Respiratory distress
   6. Coagulation defects

TABLE 4-19 Ammonia Detoxicant/Stimulant Laxative

Drug	Indications	Adverse Reactions	Nursing Implications
• Lactulose (Cephulac)	• Encephalopathy • Used to decrease ammonia levels and bowel pH	• Diarrhea	• Reinforce client instruction regarding need for medication • Observe for diarrhea • Monitor ammonia levels

Analysis (Nursing Diagnoses)

A. Excess fluid volume related to . . .
B. Risk for injury related to . . .
C. Pain related to . . .
D. Ineffective breathing pattern related to . . .
E. Imbalanced nutrition: less than body requirements related to . . .
F. Risk for infection related to . . .

Nursing Plans and Interventions

A. Eliminate causative agent (alcohol, hepatotoxin).
B. Administer vitamin supplements (A, B complex, C, K) and assist with teaching the client/family the need for continuing these supplements.
C. Monitor mental status frequently (at least every 2 hours); note any subtle changes.
D. Avoid initiating bleeding and observe for bleeding tendencies.
  1. Avoid injections whenever possible.
  2. Provide small-bore needles for IV insertion.
  3. Maintain pressure to venipuncture sites for at least 5 minutes.
  4. Use electric razor.
  5. Provide a soft-bristle toothbrush and encourage careful mouth care.
  6. Check stools and emesis for frank or occult blood.
  7. Prevent straining at stool.
    a. Administer stool softeners as prescribed.
    b. Provide high-fiber diet.
E. Provide special skin care.
  1. Avoid soap, rubbing alcohol, and perfumed products (which are drying to the skin).
  2. Apply moisturizing lotion or baby oil frequently.
  3. Observe skin for any lesions, including scratch marks.
  4. Turn frequently and apply lotion to exposed skin.
F. Monitor fluid and electrolyte status daily.
  1. I&O (accurate output may require Foley catheter).
  2. Observe for edema, pulmonary edema.
  3. Measure abdominal girth (determines increase or decrease of ascites).
  4. Weigh daily (determines increase or decrease of edema and ascites).
  5. Restrict fluids to 1500 mL/day (may help to reduce edema and ascites).
  6. Monitor dietary intake carefully, especially protein intake. Restrict protein if client has hepatic coma; otherwise, encourage foods with high biologic protein.
G. Reinforce teaching plan related to dietary restrictions: low-sodium, low-potassium, low-fat, high-carbohydrate.
H. If encephalopathy is present, lactulose is used (Table 4-19, *Ammonia Detoxicant/Stimulant Laxative*).
I. If esophageal varices are present, esophagogastric balloon tamponade (Blakemore tube), sclerotherapy, and/or portal systemic shunts may be used for treatment.

Hepatitis

Description: Hepatitis is widespread inflammation of liver cells, usually caused by a virus (Table 4-20, *Comparison of Three Types of Hepatitis*).

Nursing Assessment (Data Collection)

A. Known exposure to hepatitis
B. Recent transfusions or hemodialysis
C. Individuals at risk for contracting hepatitis:
  1. Homosexual males
  2. IV drug users (disease transmitted by dirty needles)
  3. Those who have recently had body piercings or tattoos (disease transmitted by dirty needles)
  4. Those living in crowded conditions
  5. Health care workers employed in high-risk areas:
    a. Labs
    b. Emergency rooms
    c. Critical care units
    d. Hemodialysis units
    e. Oncology
    f. Centers for care of the mentally challenged
D. Fatigue, malaise, weakness
E. Anorexia, nausea, and vomiting
F. Jaundice, dark urine, clay-colored stools
G. Myalgia (muscle aches), joint pain
H. Dull headaches, irritability, depression
I. Abdominal tenderness in right upper quadrant
J. Fever with hepatitis A
K. Elevations of liver enzymes (ALT, AST, alkaline phosphatase), bilirubin

Analysis (Nursing Diagnoses)

A. Activity intolerance related to . . .
B. Imbalanced nutrition: less than body requirements related to . . .
C. Risk for infection related to . . .

TABLE 4-20 Comparison of Three Types of Hepatitis

Characteristics	Hepatitis A	Hepatitis B	Hepatitis C
• Source of infection	• Contaminated food • Contaminated water	• Contaminated blood products • Contaminated needles or surgical instruments	• Contaminated blood products • Contaminated needles; IV drug use • Dialysis
• Route of infection	• Oral • Fecal • Parenteral	• Parenteral • Oral • Fecal • Direct contact • Breast milk • Sexual contact	• Parenteral • Sexual contact
• Incubation period	• 2 to 6 weeks	• 6 to 20 weeks	• Average: 6 to 7 weeks
• Onset	• Abrupt	• Insidious	• Insidious
• Seasonal variation	• Autumn • Winter	• All year	• All year
• Age group affected	• Children • Young adults	• Any age	• Any age
• Vaccine	• Yes	• Yes	• No
• Inoculation	• Yes	• Yes	• Yes
• Potential for chronic liver disease	• No	• Yes	• Yes
• Immunity	• Yes	• Yes	• No

Nursing Plans and Interventions

A. Observe and report client's response to activity and plan periods of rest after periods of activity.
B. Assist client with care as needed, and encourage client to get help with daily activities at home (caring for children, preparing meals, etc.).
C. Provide high-calorie, high-carbohydrate diet with moderate fats and proteins.
   1. Serve small, frequent meals.
   2. Provide vitamin supplements.
   3. Provide foods the client prefers.
D. Administer antiemetics as needed.

HESI Hint • PROVIDE AN ENVIRONMENT CONDUCIVE TO EATING
For clients who are anorexic and/or nauseated:
• Remove strong odors immediately; they can be offensive and increase nausea.
• Encourage client to sit up for meals; this can decrease the propensity to vomit.
• Serve small, frequent meals.

E. Emphasize to the client the importance of adhering to personal hygiene, using individual drinking and eating utensils, toothbrushes, and razors. Prevention of spread to others must also be emphasized.

F. Client should avoid hepatotoxic substances such as alcohol, aspirin, acetaminophen, and sedatives.

HESI Hint • Liver tissue is destroyed by hepatitis. Rest and adequate nutrition are necessary for regeneration of liver tissue being destroyed by the disease. Because many drugs are metabolized in the liver, drug therapy must be scrutinized carefully. Caution the client that recovery takes many months and that previously taken medications should not be resumed without the health care provider's directions.

Pancreatitis

Description: Pancreatitis is nonbacterial inflammation of the pancreas.
A. Acute pancreatitis occurs when there is digestion of the pancreas by its own enzymes, primarily trypsin.
B. Alcohol ingestion and biliary tract disease are major causes of acute pancreatitis.
C. Chronic pancreatitis is a progressive, destructive disease with permanent dysfunction.
D. Long-term alcohol use is the major factor in chronic pancreatitis.
E. Alcohol consumption should be avoided for both acute and chronic pancreatitis.

Nursing Assessment (Data Collection)

A. Acute pancreatitis
  1. Severe mid-epigastric pain radiating to back. Usually related to excessive alcohol ingestion or a fatty meal.
  2. Abdominal guarding; rigid, boardlike abdomen, and abdominal pain
  3. Nausea and vomiting
  4. Elevated temperature, tachycardia, decreased BP
  5. Bluish discoloration of flanks (Grey Turner sign) or periumbilical area (Cullen sign)
  6. Elevated amylase, lipase, and glucose levels
B. Chronic pancreatitis
  1. Continuous burning or gnawing abdominal pain
  2. Recurring attacks of severe upper abdominal and back pain
  3. Ascites
  4. Steatorrhea, diarrhea
  5. Weight loss
  6. Jaundice, dark urine
  7. Signs and symptoms of diabetes mellitus

Analysis (Nursing Diagnoses)

A. Pain related to . . .
B. Chronic pain related to . . .
C. Imbalanced nutrition, less than required related to . . .
D. Deficient fluid volume related to . . .

Nursing Plans and Interventions

A. Acute pancreatitis
  1. Nothing taken orally.
  2. Maintain nasogastric (NG) tube to suction; total parenteral nutrition given.
  3. Administer hydromorphone (Dilaudid) or fentanyl (Sublimaze) as needed.
  4. Administer antacids, histamine-2, receptor-blocking drugs, anticholinergics, proton pump inhibitors.
  5. Assist client to assume position of comfort on side with legs drawn up to chest.
  6. Reinforce teaching: avoid alcohol, caffeine, fatty and spicy foods.
  7. If severe, blood sugar monitoring and regular insulin coverage may be needed temporarily.
  8. Place in semi-Fowler position to decrease pressure on the diaphragm.
  9. Encourage client to cough and deep breathe; incentive spirometry.

HESI Hint • Acute pancreatic pain is located retroperitoneally. Any enlargement of the pancreas causes the peritoneum to stretch tightly. Therefore, sitting up or leaning forward will reduce the pain.

B. Chronic pancreatitis
  1. Administer analgesics such as hydromorphone (Dilaudid), fentanyl (Sublimaze), and morphine (narcotic tolerance and dependency may be a problem).
  2. Administer pancreatic enzymes such as pancreatin (Creon) or pancrelipase (Viokase) with meals or snacks. Powdered forms should be mixed with fruit juice or applesauce (mixing with proteins should be avoided).
  3. Monitor client's stools for number and consistency to determine effectiveness of enzyme replacement.
  4. Reinforce client/family instructions about eating a bland, low-fat diet and avoiding rich foods, alcohol, and caffeine.
  5. Monitor for signs and symptoms of diabetes mellitus.

Cholecystitis and Cholelithiasis

Description: Cholecystitis is an acute inflammation of the gallbladder. Cholelithiasis is the formation or presence of stones in the gallbladder.

A. Incidence of these diseases is greater in females who are multiparous and overweight.
B. Treatment for cholecystitis consists of IV hydration, administration of antibiotics, and pain control with morphine.
C. Treatment for cholelithiasis consists of nonsurgical removal of stones.
  1. Dissolution therapy (administration of bile salts, used rarely).
  2. Endoscopic retrograde cholangiopancreatography.
  3. Lithotripsy (not covered by many insurance carriers, thereby limiting its use).
D. Cholecystectomy is performed if stones are not removed nonsurgically and inflammation is *absent*. May be done through laparoscope.

HESI Hint • Following an endoscopic retrograde cholangiopancreatography, the client may feel sick. The scope is placed in the gallbladder, and the stones are crushed and left to pass on their own. These clients may be prone to pancreatitis.

Nursing Assessment (Data Collection)

A. Pain, anorexia, vomiting, and/or flatulence precipitated by ingestion of fried, spicy, or fatty foods
B. Fever, elevated WBC, and other signs of infection (cholecystitis)
C. Abdominal tenderness
D. Jaundice and clay-colored stools (blockage)
E. Elevated liver enzymes, bilirubin, and WBC
F. Biliary colic

Analysis (Nursing Diagnoses)

A. Pain related to . . .
B. Deficient knowledge (specify) related to . . .

Nursing Plans and Interventions

A. Administer analgesic for pain as needed.
B. Nothing taken orally.
C. Maintain NG tube to suction if indicated.
D. Monitor client's response to IV antibiotics.
E. Monitor intake and output (I&O).
F. Monitor electrolyte status regularly.
G. Collaborate with the RN to develop and implement a teaching plan for client or family about avoiding fried, spicy, or fatty foods and reducing intake of calories if indicated.

> **HESI Hint** • Nonsurgical management of the client with cholecystitis includes the following:
> * Low-fat diet
> * Medications for pain and clotting if required
> * Decompression of the stomach via NG tube

H. Provide preoperative and postoperative care if surgery is indicated (see Perioperative Care in Chapter 3, *Advanced Clinical Concepts*, p. 46).
I. Monitor T-tube drainage and safeguard the placement of the T-tube.

Review of Gastrointestinal System

1. List four nursing interventions for the client with a hiatal hernia.
2. List three categories of medications used in the treatment of peptic ulcer disease.
3. List the symptoms of upper and lower gastrointestinal bleeding.
4. What bowel sound disruptions occur with an intestinal obstruction?
5. List four nursing interventions for postoperative care of the client with a colostomy.
6. List the common clinical manifestations of jaundice.
7. What are the common food intolerances for clients with cholelithiasis?
8. List three classic initial signs of colorectal cancer.
9. In a client with cirrhosis, it is imperative to prevent further bleeding and observe for bleeding tendencies. List six relevant nursing interventions.
10. What is the main side effect of lactulose, which is used to reduce ammonia levels in clients with cirrhosis?
11. List four groups who have a high risk of contracting hepatitis.
12. How should the nurse administer pancreatic enzymes?

Answers to Review

1. Sit up while eating and for 1 hour after eating. Eat small, frequent meals. Eliminate foods that are problematic.
2. Antacids, histamine-2 receptor-blockers, mucosal healing agents, proton pump inhibitors.
3. Upper GI: melena, hematemesis, tarry stools. Lower GI: bloody stools, tarry stools. Similar: tarry stools.
4. Early mechanical obstruction: high-pitched sounds; late mechanical obstruction: diminished or absent bowel sounds.
5. Irrigate daily at same time; use warm water for irrigations; wash around stoma with mild soap and water after each ostomy bag change; pouch opening should extend at least ⅛ inch around the stoma.
6. Icteric sclerae or scleral icterus (yellow sclera), dark urine, chalky or clay-colored stools.
7. Fried, spicy, and/or fatty foods.
8. Rectal bleeding, change in bowel habits, sense of incomplete evacuation, abdominal pain with nausea, weight loss.
9. Avoid injections, use small-bore needles for IV insertion, maintain pressure for 5 minutes on all venipuncture sites, use electric razor, use soft-bristle toothbrush for mouth care, check stools and emesis for occult blood.
10. Diarrhea.
11. Homosexual males, IV drug users, those with recent piercing or tattooing, and health care workers.
12. Give with meals or snacks. Powder forms should be mixed with fruit juices.

Endocrine System

Hyperthyroidism (Graves Disease, Goiter)

Description: Hyperthyroidism (Graves disease, goiter) is excessive activity of thyroid gland, resulting in an elevated level of circulating thyroid hormones. Possibly long-term or lifelong treatment.

A. Hyperthyroidism can result from a primary disease state, from replacement hormone therapy, or from excess thyroid stimulating hormone (TSH) from anterior pituitary tumor.

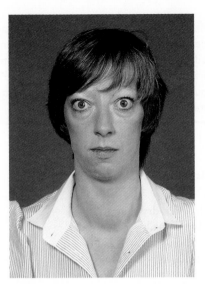

FIGURE 4-5 **Graves Disease.** This woman has a diffuse goiter and exophthalmos. Exophthalmos and goiter of Graves disease. (From Forbes CD, Jackson WF: *Colour atlas and text of clinical medicine*, ed 3, London, 2003, Mosby.)

B. Graves disease is thought to be an autoimmune process and accounts for most cases.
C. Diagnosis is made by evaluating serum hormone levels.
D. Common treatment for hyperthyroidism; goal is to create a euthyroid state.
   1. Thyroid ablation with medication
   2. Radiation
   3. Thyroidectomy
   4. Adenectomy of portion of anterior pituitary where TSH-producing tumor is located
E. *All* treatments leave the client in a hypothyroid state, requiring hormone replacement.

Nursing Assessment (Data Collection)

A. Enlarged thyroid gland
B. Acceleration of body processes:
   1. Weight loss
   2. Increased appetite
   3. Diarrhea
   4. Heat intolerance
   5. Tachycardia, palpitations, increased BP
   6. Diaphoresis, wet moist skin
   7. Nervousness, insomnia
C. Exophthalmos—abnormal protrusion of the eyes (Figure 4-5, *Graves Disease*)
D. T_3 elevated above 220 ng/dL
E. T_4 elevated above 12 mcg/dL
F. Radioactive iodine uptake (I_{131}) indicates presence of goiter.
G. Thyroid scan indicates presence of goiter.

Analysis (Nursing Diagnoses)

A. Decreased cardiac output related to . . .
B. Deficient knowledge (specify) related to . . .
C. Imbalanced nutrition: less than body requirements related to . . .
D. Risk for injury related to . . .

Nursing Plans and Interventions

A. Provide a calm, restful atmosphere.
B. Monitor for signs of thyroid storm (life-threatening, sudden oversecretion of thyroid hormone).

> **HESI Hint** • Thyroid storm is a life-threatening event that occurs with uncontrolled hyperthyroidism caused by Graves disease. Symptoms include fever, tachycardia, agitation, anxiety, and hypertension. Primary nursing interventions include maintaining an airway and adequate ventilation.
> Propylthiouracil (PTU) or methimazole (Tapazole) are antithyroid drugs used to treat thyroid storm. Propranolol (Inderal) may be given to decrease excessive sympathetic stimulation.

C. Collaborate with RN to develop and implement a teaching plan for client/family about the following:
   1. After treatment, resulting hypothyroidism will require daily hormone replacement.
   2. Client should wear medic alert jewelry in case of emergency.
   3. Signs of hormone replacement overdosage are the signs for hyperthyroidism (see Nursing Assessment under Hyperthyroidism).
   4. Signs of hormone replacement underdosage are the signs for hypothyroidism (see Nursing Assessment under Hyperthyroidism).
D. Reinforce the teaching plan related to the recommended diet: high-calorie, high-protein, low-caffeine, low-fiber diet if diarrhea is present.
E. Perform eye care for exophthalmos:
   1. Artificial tears to maintain moisture
   2. Sunglasses when in bright light
   3. Annual eye exams
F. Prepare client for treatment of hyperthyroidism.
   1. Thyroid ablation:
      a. Propylthiouracil (PTU) or methimazole (Tapazole) acts by blocking synthesis of T_3 and T_4.
      b. Dosage is calculated based on body weight and given over several months.
      c. Client should take medication exactly as prescribed so the desired effect can be achieved.
      d. The expected effect is to make the client euthyroid; often given to prepare the client for thyroidectomy.
   2. Radiation:
      a. Iodine$_{131}$ is given to destroy thyroid cells.
      b. Iodine$_{131}$ is very irritating to the GI tract.
      c. Clients often vomit (vomitus is radioactive).

d. Place client on radiation precautions. Use time, distance, and shielding as means of protection against radiation (see Reproductive System, p. 153).

> **HESI Hint** • **POSTOPERATIVE THYROIDECTOMY**
> Be prepared for the possibility of laryngeal edema. Put a tracheostomy set at bedside along with oxygen and a suction machine; Ca^{++} gluconate easily accessible in the event the parathyroid glands were removed.

3. Thyroidectomy:
   a. Monitor respirations.
   b. Check frequently for bleeding.
   c. Support the neck when moving client. (Do not hyperextend.)
   d. Watch for laryngeal edema damage by assessing for hoarseness or inability to speak clearly.
   e. Determine number of parathyroid glands that have been removed.
   f. Keep drainage devices compressed/empty.
4. Adenectomy: TSH-secreting pituitary tumors resected using transnasal approach (transsphenoidal hypophysectomy).

> **HESI Hint** • Normal serum calcium is 9 to 10.5 mEq/L. The best indicator of parathyroid problems is a decrease in the client's calcium compared with the preoperative value.

> **HESI Hint** • If two or more parathyroid glands have been removed, the chance of tetany increases dramatically:
> • Monitor serum calcium levels (9 to 10.5 mg/dL is normal range).
> • Check for tingling of toes and fingers and around the mouth.

Hypothyroidism (Hashimoto Disease, Myxedema)

Description: Hypothyroidism is a hypofunction of the thyroid gland with resulting insufficiency of thyroid hormone.
A. Early symptoms of hypothyroidism are nonspecific but gradually intensify.
B. Treated with hormone replacement.
C. Endemic goiters occur in individuals living in areas where there is deficit iodine. Iodized salt has helped to prevent this problem.

> **HESI Hint** • Myxedema coma can be precipitated by acute illness, withdrawal of thyroid medication, anesthesia, use of sedatives, or hypoventilation (with the potential for respiratory acidosis and carbon dioxide narcosis). The airway must be kept patent and ventilator support used as indicated.

Nursing Assessment (Data Collection)

A. Fatigue
B. Thin, dry hair; dry skin
C. Thick, brittle nails
D. Constipation
E. Bradycardia, hypotension
F. Goiter
G. Periorbital edema, facial puffiness
H. Cold intolerance
I. Weight gain
J. Dull emotions and mental processes
K. Diagnosed by:
   1. Low T_3 (below 70)
   2. Low T_4 (below 5)
   3. T_4 antibody present, indicating that T_4 is being destroyed by the body
L. Husky voice
M. Slow speech

Analysis (Nursing Diagnoses)

A. Deficient knowledge (specify) related to . . .
B. Noncompliance related to . . .
C. Activity intolerance related to . . .
D. Decreased cardiac output related to . . .
E. Ineffective breathing pattern related to . . .

Nursing Plans and Interventions

A. Collaborate with RN to develop and implement a teaching plan for client or family about:
   1. Medication regimen: daily dosage of prescribed hormone replacement
   2. Medication effects and side effects (Table 4-21, *Thyroid Preparations*)
   3. Ongoing follow-up with serum hormone levels
   4. Signs and symptoms of myxedema coma (hypotension, hypothermia, hyponatremia, hypoglycemia, respiratory failure)
B. Assist in the implementation of a bowel elimination plan to prevent constipation:
   1. Increase fluid intake to 3 liters per day.
   2. Encourage high-fiber diet, including fresh fruits and vegetables.
   3. Increase activity.
   4. Discourage use of enemas and laxatives.
C. Avoid sedation, which can lead to respiratory difficulties.

TABLE 4-21 Thyroid Preparations

Drugs	Indications	Adverse Reactions	Nursing Implications
• Levothyroxine (Synthroid) • Liothyronine sodium (Cytomel) • Desiccated thyroid (Armour Thyroid)	• Action is to increase metabolic rates • Synthetic T_4	• Anxiety • Insomnia • Tremors • Tachycardia • Palpitations • Angina • Dysrhythmias	• Check serum hormone levels routinely • Monitor BP and pulse regularly • Weigh daily • Report side effects to health care provider • Avoid foods and products containing iodine • Initiate cautiously in clients with cardio-vascular disease

TABLE 4-22 Corticosteroids

Drugs	Indications	Adverse Reactions	Nursing Implications
Steroids			
• Hydrocortisone • Prednisone • Dexamethasone • Methylprednisolone (Medrol)	• Hormone replacement • Severe rheumatoid arthritis • Autoimmune disorders	• Emotional lability • Impaired wound healing • Skin fragility • Abnormal fat deposition • Hyperglycemia • Hirsutism • Moon face • Osteoporosis • *All symptoms of Cushing's syndrome if overdosage occurs*	• Wean slowly (administer a high dose then taper off)—careful monitoring required during withdrawal • Monitor serum potassium, glucose (can become diabetic), and sodium • Weigh daily; report weight gain of more than 5 pounds per week • Administer with antiulcer drugs or food • Use care to prevent injuries • Reinforce the teaching plan related to the symptoms of Cushing's syndrome • Monitor BP and pulse closely

Addison's Disease (Primary Adrenocortical Deficiency)

Description: Addison's disease is an autoimmune process often found in conjunction with other endocrine diseases of an autoimmune nature—a primary disorder; hypofunction of the adrenal cortex.
A. Sudden withdrawal from corticosteroids may precipitate symptoms of Addison's disease (Table 4-22, *Corticosteroids*).
B. Addison's disease is characterized by lack of cortisol, aldosterone, and androgens.
C. Definitive diagnosis is made using an adrenocorticotropic hormone (ACTH) stimulation test.
D. If ACTH production failure by anterior pituitary is found, then it is considered secondary Addison's.

HESI Hint • People take steroids for a variety of conditions. Clients should be cautioned against suddenly stopping the medications and be informed that it is necessary to taper off taking steroids.

Nursing Assessment (Data Collection)
A. Fatigue, weakness
B. Weight loss, anorexia, nausea, vomiting
C. Postural hypotension
D. Hypoglycemia
E. Hyponatremia
F. Hyperkalemia
G. Hyperpigmentation of mucous membranes and skin (only if primary Addison's; not seen in secondary Addison's)
H. Signs of shock when in Addison's crises (see Shock in Chapter 3, *Advanced Clinical Concepts*, p. 27)
I. Loss of body hair
J. Hypovolemia, signs include:
  1. Hypotension
  2. Tachycardia
  3. Fever

Analysis (Nursing Diagnoses)
A. Risk for deficient fluid volume related to . . .
B. Deficient knowledge (specify) related to . . .

Nursing Plans and Interventions

A. Take vital signs frequently (every 15 minutes if in crisis).
B. Monitor I&O and weigh daily.
C. Instruct client to rise slowly because of the possibility of postural hypotension.
D. During Addison's crisis, monitor the client's response to intravenous glucose with parenteral glucocorticoids. This condition requires large fluid volume replacement.
E. Monitor serum electrolyte levels.
F. Collaborate with RN to develop and implement a teaching plan for client/family about:
   1. Need for lifelong hormone replacement
   2. Need for close medical supervision
   3. Need for medical alert jewelry
   4. Signs and symptoms of over- and underdosage of medication
   5. Diet: high-sodium, low-potassium, and high-carbohydrate (complex carbohydrates)
   6. Encourage fluid intake of at least 3 liters of fluid per day
G. Provide ulcer prophylaxis because of exogenous source of corticosteroid.

> **HESI Hint** • Addison's crisis is a *medical emergency* brought on by the sudden withdrawal of a steroid or by a stressful event (trauma, severe infection).
> - Vascular collapse: hypotension and tachycardia occur; administer IV fluids until stabilized.
> - Hypoglycemia: administer IV glucose.
> - Administer parenteral hydrocortisone: *essential to reversing the crisis.*
> - Aldosterone replacement: administer fludrocortisone acetate (Florinef) orally (only available as oral preparation) with simultaneous administration of salt (sodium chloride) if client has a sodium deficit.

Cushing's Syndrome

Description: Cushing's syndrome is excess adrenal corticoid activity.
A. Etiology is usually chronic administration of corticosteroids.
B. Cushing's syndrome can also be caused by adrenal, pituitary, or hypothalamus tumors.

Nursing Assessment (Data Collection)

A. Physical symptoms include:
   1. Moon face
   2. Truncal obesity
   3. Buffalo hump
   4. Abdominal striae
   5. Muscle atrophy
   6. Thinning of the skin
   7. Hirsutism in females
   8. Hyperpigmentation
   9. Amenorrhea
   10. Edema, poor wound healing, easy bruising
   11. Impotence
B. Hypertension
C. Susceptible to multiple infections
D. Osteoporosis
E. Peptic ulcer formation
F. Many false positives and false negatives in laboratory testing
G. Lab data often include the following findings:
   1. Hyperglycemia
   2. Hypernatremia
   3. Hypokalemia
   4. Decreased eosinophils and lymphocytes
   5. Increased plasma cortisol
   6. Increased urinary 17-hydroxycorticoids

Analysis (Nursing Diagnoses)

A. Excess fluid volume related to . . .
B. Risk for infection related to . . .
C. Disturbed body image related to . . .

Nursing Plans and Interventions

A. Protect from exposure to infection.
B. WASH HANDS; use good hand hygiene technique.
C. Monitor for signs of infection:
   1. Fever
   2. Oral candida
   3. Yeast infections
   4. Adventitious lung sounds
   5. Skin lesions
   6. Elevated WBCs
D. Collaborate with RN to develop and implement a teaching plan for client/family about safety measures.
   1. Position bed close to floor with call light within easy reach.
   2. Encourage use of side rails.
   3. Make sure walkways are unobstructed.
   4. Encourage wearing shoes when ambulating.
E. Provide low-sodium diet; encourage foods with vitamin D and calcium.
F. Provide good skin care.
G. Discuss weaning from steroids. (If weaning is done too quickly, Addison's disease symptoms will occur.)
H. Encourage selection of clothing that minimizes visible aberrations; encourage maintenance of normal physical appearance.
I. Monitor I&O and weigh daily.
J. Provide ulcer prophylaxis.

> **HESI Hint** • Instruct clients to take steroids with meals to prevent gastric irritation. They should never skip doses. If they have nausea or vomiting for more than 12 to 24 hours, they should contact the health care provider.

TABLE 4-23 Comparison of Type 1 and Type 2 Diabetes Mellitus (DM)

Variable	Type 1 DM	Type 2 DM
Prevalence	5% of U.S. population with DM	90% to 95% of U.S. population with DM
Pathology	Beta cell destruction leading to absolute insulin deficiency	Basic defect is insulin resistance and usually has relative rather than absolute insulin deficiency
Onset	Sudden	Gradual, insidious
Signs and Symptoms	• Polyuria • Polydipsia • Polyphagia • Weight loss	• Polydipsia • Polyuria • Polyphagia • Weight loss • Fatigue • Frequent infections • Blurred vision • Impotence
Age at Onset	Any age but mostly younger than 21	Any age but mostly adults
Weight	• Thin • Slender	• Overweight • Obese
Ketosis	Common	Rare
Pathology	• Autoimmune and viral component	• Obesity, CVD an equal comorbidity • Genetic predisposition
Lifestyle Management	• Medical nutrition therapy: Carbohydrate counting • Physical activity	• Medical nutrition therapy: Heart-healthy, portion-controlled diet • Physical activity

Pharmacologic Management	• Intensive insulin therapy	• Typically a stepwise approach:
		  1. Diet
		  2. Exercise
		  3. Oral agents
		  4. Oral agents and insulin

Diabetes Mellitus

Description: Diabetes mellitus is a metabolic disorder characterized by high levels of glucose resulting from defects in insulin secretion or insulin action or both.

A. Diabetes mellitus (DM) is characterized by hyperglycemia.

B. Diabetes mellitus affects the metabolism of protein, carbohydrate, and fat.

C. Four ways to diagnose DM:
   1. Fasting plasma glucose greater than or equal to 126 mg/dL
   2. Glycosylated Hgb greater than or equal to 6.5%
   3. Random blood glucose greater than or equal to 200 mg/dL in a client with classic symptoms of hyperglycemia
   4. Oral glucose tolerance test >200
      (Use plasma glucose, not fingersticks, to diagnose diabetes.)

D. The major classifications of diabetes are:

(See Table 4-23, *Comparison of Type 1 and Type 2 Diabetes Mellitus.*)
   1. Type 1: results from B-cell destruction
   2. Type 2: results from progressive secretory insulin deficit and/or defect in insulin uptake
   3. Other: transplant-related diabetes, cystic fibrosis–related diabetes, iatrogenic-induced diabetes (stress, hospital); steroid-induced diabetes
   4. Gestational diabetes
   5. Prediabetes: blood glucose levels when fasting are 100 mg/dL to 125 mg/dL or A1c of 5.7% to 6.4%

E. Many clients diagnosed with type 2 DM use insulin but retain some degree of pancreatic function.

F. Obesity is a major risk factor in type 2 DM.

Clinical Characteristics and Treatment of Diabetes Mellitus

A. Type 1
   1. Description: results from the progressive autoimmune-based destruction of beta cells.

a. Client can become hyperglycemic and ketosis prone relatively easily.

b. Precipitating factors for diabetic ketoacidosis (DKA) include infection and inadequate management or undermanagement of glucose.

2. Clinical characteristics of DKA:

a. Serum glucose of 250 and above

b. Ketonuria in large amounts

c. Arterial pH of <7.30 and HCO_3 <15 mEq/dL; nausea, vomiting, dehydration, abdominal pain; Kussmaul's respirations; acetone odor to breath

3. Treatment:

a. Usually with isotonic IV fluids 0.9% NaCl solution 1 L/hr until BP stabilized and urine output 30 to 60 mL/hr.

b. Slow IV infusion by IV pump of regular insulin; too-rapid infusion of insulin to lower serum glucose can lead to cerebral edema.

c. Careful replacement of potassium, based on lab data.

B. Type 2

1. Description: results from either the inadequate production of insulin by the body or lack of sensitivity to the insulin being produced.

a. Rare development of ketoacidosis

b. With extreme hyperglycemia, hyperosmolar hyperglycemia nonketotic syndrome develops.

2. Clinical characteristics:

a. Hyperglycemia >600 mg/dL

b. Plasma hyperosmolality

c. Dehydration

d. Changed mental status

e. Absent ketone bodies

3. Treatment:

a. Usually with isotonic IV fluid replacement and careful monitoring of potassium and glucose levels

b. Intravenous insulin given until blood glucose stable at 250 mg/dL

Nursing Assessment

A. Integument

1. Skin infections

2. Wounds that do not heal

3. Acanthosis

B. Oral cavity

1. Periodontal disease

2. Candidiasis (raised, white patchy areas on mucous membranes)

C. Eyes

1. Cataracts

2. Retinopathy

D. Cardiopulmonary system

1. Angina

2. Dyspnea

3. Hypertension

E. Periphery

1. Hair loss on extremities, indicating poor perfusion

2. Other signs of poor peripheral circulation:

a. Coolness

b. Skin shininess and thinness

c. Weak or absent peripheral pulses

d. Ulcerations on extremities

e. Pallor

f. Thick nails with ridges

F. Kidneys

1. Edema of face, hands, and feet

2. Symptoms of urinary tract infection (UTI)

3. Symptoms of renal failure: edema, anorexia, nausea, fatigue, difficulty in concentrating. Diabetic nephropathy is the primary cause of end-stage renal failure in the United States.

G. Neuromusculature

1. Neuropathies

2. Symptoms of neuropathies: numbness, tingling, pain, burning

H. Gastrointestinal disturbances

1. Nighttime diarrhea

2. Gastroparesis (faulty absorption)

I. Reproductive

1. Male impotence

2. Vaginal dryness, frequent vaginal infections

3. Menstrual irregularities

J. Psychosocial issues

1. Depression: persons with DM have a high rate of depression. Depression contributes to poor adherence to DM regimens, feelings of helplessness, and poor health outcomes.

2. Increased risk of developing anorexia nervosa and bulimia nervosa in women with type 1 DM.

Analysis (Nursing Diagnoses)

A. Readiness for enhanced knowledge related to . . .

B. Risk for injury related to . . .

C. Readiness for enhanced coping related to . . .

D. Deficit fluid volume related to . . .

E. Readiness for enhanced self-health management related to . . .

Nursing Plans and Interventions

A. Determine baseline lab data.

1. Serum glucose

2. Electrolytes

3. Creatinine

4. BUN

5. Cholesterol, both LDL and HDL

6. Triglycerides

7. ABGs as indicated

B. Reinforce teaching of injection technique and/or oral medication(s) (Table 4-24, *Oral Hypoglycemics*, and Table 4-25, *Types/Action of Insulin*).

1. Identify the prescribed dose and type of insulin.

TABLE 4-24 Oral Hypoglycemics

Drugs	Indications	Adverse Reactions	Nursing Implications
Sulfonylureas *First Generation* • Tolbutamide (Orinase) • Chlorpropamide (Diabinese) *Second Generation* • Glyburide (Micronase, DiaBeta) • Glipizide (Glucotrol) • Glimepiride (Amaryl)	• Lowers blood sugar by stimulating the release of insulin by the beta cells of the pancreas and causes tissues to take up and store glucose more easily • First generation is low potency and short acting • Second generation is high potency and longer acting	*First Generation* • Hypoglycemia • Nausea, heartburn, constipation, anorexia • Agranulocytosis • Allergic skin reactions *Second Generation* • Weight gain • Hypoglycemia, particularly in older adults	*First Generation* • Responsiveness may decline over time • Given once daily with first meal • Monitor blood sugar • Hard to detect hypoglycemia if older adult or also on beta-blockers *Second Generation* • Less likely to interact with other medications
Biguinides • Metformin (Glucophage)	• Lowers serum glucose levels by inhibiting hepatic glucose production and increasing sensitivity of peripheral tissue to insulin	• Abdominal discomfort • Diarrhea • Lactic acidosis	• Many drug–drug interactions • Extended-release tablets should be taken with the evening meal • Use cautiously with preexisting renal or liver disease or HF • Discontinue 48 hours before and wait 48 hours to restart dosage after diagnostic studies requiring IV iodine contrast media • Can lead to vitamin B_{12} deficiency
Alpha-Glucosidase Inhibitors • Acarbose (Precose) • Miglitol (Glyset)	• Lowers blood glucose by blunting sugar levels after meals	• Hypoglycemia	• Optimally, must be taken with the FIRST bite of each meal • May be taken with other classes of oral hypoglycemics • Monitor blood sugar • Use is controversial in IBD client
Thiazolidinediones • Rosiglitazone (Avandia) • Pioglitazone (Actos)	• Lowers blood sugar by decreasing the insulin resistance of the tissues	• Hypoglycemia • Increased total cholesterol, weight gain • Edema, anemia	• Many drug–drug interactions • Skip dose if meal skipped • No known drug interactions • Monitor liver function • Caution with use in CAD; may precipitate HF
Meglitindes • Repaglinide (Prandin) • Nateglinide (Starlix)	• Lowers blood sugar by stimulating beta cells in pancreas to release insulin; does this by closing K^+ channels and opening Ca^{++} channels	• Hypoglycemia • Angina, chest pain • Arthralgia, back pain • Nausea and vomiting, dyspepsia, constipation, or diarrhea	• May be used with metformin • Give before meals; if a meal is skipped, skip the dose • Monitor blood sugar

Continued

TABLE 4-24 Oral Hypoglycemics—cont'd

Drugs	Indications	Adverse Reactions	Nursing Implications
Incretin enhancer • Linagliptin (Tradjenta) • Saxagliptin (Onglyza) • Sitagliptin (Januvia)	• Lowers blood glucose by inhibiting degradation of incretins, which increases insulin secretion	• Hypoglycemia	• Not considered a first-line agent
Combinations • Glyburide and metformin (Glucovance) • Pioglitazone + metformin (Actoplus Met) • Rosiglitazone + glimepride (Avandaryl) • Rosiglitazone + metformin (Advanamet) • Glipizide + metformin (Metaglip)	• Lowers blood sugar by combining the advantages of two classes of hypoglycemics	• Note possible adverse reactions to both classes • Hypoglycemia (severe)	• Note implications of both classes of drugs

*Second-generation sulfonylureas are much more potent and have fewer drug-to-drug interactions than the first-generation agents.

TABLE 4-25 Types/Action of Insulin

Type	Name	Onset	Peak Action	Duration	Nursing Implications
• Rapid acting	• Human insulin lispro (Humalog) • Aspart (NovoLog) • Glulisine (Apidra)	• 0.5 to 1 hr • 5 to 15 min • 25 min	• 2 to 4 hr • 0.75 to 1.5 hr • 1 hr	• 4 hr • 3 to 5 hr • 2 to 3 hr	• Give within 15 min of a meal (Lispro and Aspart)
• Short acting	• Regular insulin (human) (Humulin R, Novolin R)	• 30 to 60 min	• 2 to 3 hr	• 5 to 7 hr	• Regular insulin may be given IV
• Intermediate acting	• Isophane insulin (human) (Humulin N, Novolin N)	• 1 to 2 hr	• 6 to 12 hr	• 18 to 28 hr	• Not to be given IV • Mixtures combine rapid-acting regular insulin with intermediate-acting NPH insulin in a 30% regular with 70% NPH proportion or at 50/50 combination
• Long acting	• Glargine (Lantus) • Detemir (Levemir)	• 4 to 8 hr • 1.1 hr	• 14 to 20 hr • 5 hr (some sources say there is no peak)	• 24 hr	• Not to be given IV • Recommended: give once daily, SE, at bedtime. In some cases, given two times a day. Acts as basal insulin. Caution: Solution is clear, but bottle is distinctly different shape from regular insulin. *Do not confuse insulins.* Do not shake solution. Do not mix other insulins with Lantus. Use cautiously if patient is NPO.

TABLE 4-25 Types/Action of Insulin—cont'd

Type	Name	Onset	Peak Action	Duration	Nursing Implications
• Premix	• Humalog 75/25 • Human 70/30 • NovoLog 70/30 • Humalog 50/50				• For all premixes: Offer when food readily available • 25% Lispro/75% Humulin N (NPH) • 30% Regular/70% NPH • 30% Aspart/70% NPH

Other Injectable Therapies

Drugs	Action/Indications	Adverse Reaction	Implications and Precautions
Exenatide (Byetta) (Victoza)	Stimulates release of insulin; ↓ glucagon secretion; ↑ satiety; ↓ gastric emptying; may facilitate weight loss (~3-5 kg) Indicated for clients with type 2 DM who are not adequately controlled with oral therapy; not indicated for clients with type 1 DM	Nausea, vomiting, hypoglycemia, diarrhea, headache	Not a substitute for insulin Not recommended for ESRD, pancreatitis, severe renal impairment, or severe gastrointestinal disease May slow absorption of other drugs
Pramlintide (Symlin)	Slows gastric emptying time, suppresses the release of glucagon, and appears to suppress appetite. Indicated as adjunct treatment in type 1 DM for clients who have not obtained adequate glycemic control with insulin therapy and for clients with type 2 DM who have not obtained adequate glycemic control with insulin with or without oral therapy	Nausea, vomiting, hypoglycemia, diarrhea, headache	Contraindicated for clients with diabetic gastroparesis. It is also avoided in clients who have exhibited significant hypoglycemic reactions or who are not able to recognize and manage hypoglycemic reactions

2. For insulin:
   a. Lift skin; use 90-degree angle. If very thin or using 5/16-inch needle, may need to use a 45-degree angle.
   b. May reuse syringes for same person. Recapping should only be done by the person using the syringe.
3. Rotate injection sites.
4. Draw regular insulin into syringe first when mixing insulins.

C. Reinforce teaching about medical nutrition therapy.
   1. Work with dietitian to reinforce specific meal plan.
   2. Overall goal is to make healthy nutritional choices, eat a varied diet, and maintain an exercise regimen.
   3. Encourage carbohydrate counting for those on complex insulin regimens.

4. Remind that meals should be timed according to medication (insulin) peak times.
5. Reinforce knowledge of diet regimen.
   a. 45% to 50% carbohydrates
   b. 15% to 20% protein
   c. 30% or less fat
   d. Foods high in complex carbohydrates, high in fiber, and low in fat, whenever possible
   e. Alcoholic beverages can be included in diet with proper planning.
6. Reinforce teaching about managing sick days (illness raises blood glucose).
   a. Teach client to keep taking insulin.
   b. Monitor glucose more frequently.
   c. Watch for signs of hyperglycemia.

D. Reinforce teaching about exercise regimen because exercise decreases blood sugar levels.

TABLE 4-26 Comparison of Hyperglycemia and Hypoglycemia

Hyperglycemia		Hypoglycemia	
Signs and Symptoms	Nursing Action	Signs and Symptoms	Nursing Actions
• Polydipsia • Polyuria • Polyphagia • Blurred vision • Weakness • Weight loss • Syncope	• Encourage water intake • Check blood glucose frequently • Assess for ketoacidosis: →Urine ketones →Urine glucose →Administer insulin as directed	• Headache • Nausea • Sweating • Tremors • Lethargy • Hunger • Confusion • Slurred speech • Tingling around mouth • Anxiety, nightmares	• Usually occurs rapidly and is potentially life-threatening; treat immediately with complex CHO. Example: graham cracker and peanut butter twice, and if no response, seek medical attention • Check blood glucose (may seize if less than 40).

1. Exercise after mealtimes; either exercise with someone or let someone know where exercise will take place to ensure safety.
2. A snack may be needed before or during exercise.
3. Monitor blood glucose before, during, and after exercise when beginning a new regimen.

E. Reinforce teaching signs and symptoms of hyperglycemia and hypoglycemia (Table 4-26, *Comparison of Hyperglycemia and Hypoglycemia*).

F. Reinforce teaching about foot care.
   1. Feet should be checked daily for changes; signs of injury and breaks in skin should be reported to health care provider.
   2. Feet should be washed daily with mild soap and warm water; soaking is to be avoided; feet should be dried well, especially between toes.
   3. Feet may be moisturized with a lanolin product, but not between the toes.
   4. Well-fitting leather shoes should be worn; going barefoot and wearing sandals are to be avoided.
   5. Clean socks should be worn daily.
   6. Garters and tight elastic-topped socks should never be worn.
   7. Corns and calluses should be removed by a professional.
   8. Nails should be cut or filed straight across.
   9. Warm socks should be worn if feet are cold.

G. Encourage regular health care follow-ups.
   1. Ophthalmologist
   2. Podiatrist
   3. Annual physical exam

H. Teach that immediate attention should be sought if any sign of infection occurs.

I. Refer client to the American Diabetes Association for additional information.

HESI Hint • Why do persons with DM have trouble with wound healing? High blood glucose contributes to damage of the smallest vessels: the capillaries. This damage causes permanent capillary scarring, which inhibits the normal activity of the capillary. This phenomenon causes disruption of capillary elasticity and promotes problems such as poor healing of breaks in the skin.

HESI Hint • **GLYCOSYLATED Hgb**
Indicates average blood glucose control over previous 2 to 3 months.

HESI Hint • **BLOOD GLUCOSE**
Indicates blood glucose at any one point in time.

HESI Hint • **DIABETES SELF-MANAGEMENT EDUCATION**
The goal is to assist the client to maintain good blood sugar control.

HESI Hint • The body's response to illness/stress is to produce glucose. Therefore, any illness or stressor results in hyperglycemia.

HESI Hint • If in doubt of whether a client is hyperglycemic or hypoglycemic, treat for hypoglycemia.

HESI Hint • **SELF-MONITORING BLOOD GLUCOSE**
• Provides data about blood glucose control.
• Good blood glucose control decreases long-term complications.
• Monitoring technique is specific to each meter.
• Monitor before meals, at bedtime, when symptoms occur, or as directed by health care provider.
• Record results and report to health care provider at time of visit.

Continued

Review of Endocrine System

1. What diagnostic test is used to determine thyroid activity?
2. What condition results from all treatments for hyperthyroidism?
3. State three symptoms of hyperthyroidism and three symptoms of hypothyroidism.
4. List five important teaching aspects for clients who are beginning corticosteroid therapy.
5. Describe the physical appearance of clients who are cushingoid.
6. Which type of diabetes always requires insulin replacement?
7. Which type of diabetes sometimes requires no medication?
8. List five symptoms of hyperglycemia.
9. List five symptoms of hypoglycemia.
10. Name the necessary elements to include in teaching the client with newly diagnosed diabetes.
11. A client has purchased a 3-month supply of insulin. Which bottles should be refrigerated?
12. Identify the peak action time of the following types of insulin: rapid-acting regular insulin, intermediate-acting, long-acting.
13. When preparing the diabetic client for discharge, the nurse teaches the client the relationship between stress, exercise, bedtime snacking, and glucose balance. State the relationship between each of these.
14. When making rounds at night, the nurse notes that an insulin-dependent client is complaining of a headache, slight nausea, and minimal trembling. The client's hand is cool and moist. What is the client most likely experiencing?
15. Identify five foot-care interventions that should be taught to the client with diabetes.

Answers to Review

1. T_3, T_4.
2. Hypothyroidism, requiring thyroid replacement.
3. Hyperthyroidism: weight loss, heat intolerance, diarrhea. Hypothyroidism: fatigue, cold intolerance, weight gain.
4. Continue medication until weaning plan is begun by physician; monitor serum potassium, glucose, and sodium frequently; weigh daily and report gain of more than 5 lb/wk; monitor BP and pulse closely; teach symptoms of Cushing's syndrome.
5. Moon face, obesity in trunk, buffalo hump in back, muscle atrophy, and thin skin.
6. Type 1, insulin-dependent diabetes mellitus.
7. Type 2, non–insulin-dependent diabetes mellitus.
8. Polydipsia, polyuria, polyphagia, weakness, weight loss.
9. Hunger, lethargy, confusion, tremors or shakes, sweating.
10. The underlying pathophysiology of the disease, its management/treatment regimen, meal planning, exercise program, insulin administration, sick day management, symptoms of hyperglycemia (not enough insulin), symptoms of hypoglycemia (too much insulin, too much exercise; not enough food).
11. All but the current bottle in use should be kept in the refrigerator.
12. Rapid-acting regular insulin: 1 to 4 hr. Immediate-acting insulin: 6 to 12 hr. Long-acting insulin: peakless.
13. Stress and stress hormones usually increase glucose production and increase insulin need; exercise can increase the chance for an insulin reaction; therefore the client should always have a sugar snack available when exercising (to treat hypoglycemia); a bedtime snack can prevent insulin reactions.
14. Hypoglycemia/insulin reaction.
15. Check feet daily and report any breaks, sores, or blisters to health care provider; wear well-fitting shoes; never go barefoot or wear sandals; never personally remove corns or calluses; cut or file nails straight across; wash feet daily with mild soap and warm water.

Musculoskeletal System

Rheumatoid Arthritis

Description: Rheumatoid arthritis is chronic, systematic, progressive deterioration of the connective tissue (synovium) of the joints characterized by inflammation.
A. The exact cause is unknown, but it is classified as an immune complex disorder.
B. Joint involvement is bilateral and symmetric.
C. Severe cases may require joint replacement (see Joint Replacement, p. 129).

> **HESI Hint** • A client comes to the clinic complaining of morning stiffness, weight loss, and swelling of both hands and wrists. Rheumatoid arthritis is suspected. Which methods of assessment might the nurse use and which methods would the nurse not use? Use inspection, palpation, and strength testing. Do not use range of motion (ROM). (This activity promotes pain because ROM is limited.)

Nursing Assessment (Data Collection)

A. Fatigue
B. Generalized weakness
C. Weight loss
D. Anorexia
E. Morning stiffness
F. Bilateral inflammation of joints with the following symptoms:
  1. Decreased range of motion
  2. Joint pain
  3. Warmth
  4. Edema
  5. Erythema
  6. Joint deformity

> **HESI Hint** • In the joint, the normal cartilage becomes soft, fissures and pitting occur, and the cartilage thins. Spurs form and inflammation sets in. The result is deformity marked by immobility, pain, and muscle spasm. The prescribed treatment regimen is corticosteroids for the inflammation; splinting, immobilization, and rest for the joint deformity; and NSAIDs for the pain.

G. Diagnosis confirmed by the following:
  1. Elevated erythrocyte sedimentation rate
  2. Positive rheumatoid factor
  3. Presence of antinuclear antibody
  4. Joint space narrowing indicated by arthroscopic exam (provides joint visualization)
  5. Abnormal synovial fluid (fluid in joint) indicated by arthrocentesis

> **HESI Hint** • Synovial tissues line the bones of the joints. Inflammation of this lining causes destruction of tissue and bone. Early detection of rheumatoid arthritis can decrease the amount of bone and joint destruction. Often the disease will go into remission. Decreasing the amount of bone and joint destruction will reduce the amount of disability.

Analysis (Nursing Diagnoses)

A. Chronic pain related to . . .
B. Impaired physical mobility related to . . .
C. Self-care deficit (specify) related to . . .
D. Ineffective coping related to . . .

Nursing Plans and Interventions

A. Implement pain relief measures:
  1. Use moist heat:
    a. Warm, moist compresses
    b. Whirlpool baths
    c. Hot shower in the morning
  2. Use diversionary activities:
    a. Imaging
    b. Distraction
    c. Self-hypnosis
    d. Biofeedback
  3. Administer medications and reinforce teaching about medications (Table 4-27, *Nonsteroidal Anti-Inflammatory Drugs [NSAIDs]*; see also Table 4-22, *Corticosteroids*).
B. Provide periods of rest after periods of activity.
  1. Encourage self-care to maximal level.
  2. Allow adequate time for the client to perform activities.
  3. Perform activities during time of day when client feels most energetic.
C. Do not overexert.
D. Encourage the client to maintain proper posture and joint position.

> **HESI Hint** • What activity recommendations should the nurse provide a client with rheumatoid arthritis?
> • Do not exercise painful, swollen joints.
> • Do not exercise any joint to the point of pain.
> • Perform exercises slowly and smoothly; avoid jerky movements.

E. Encourage use of assistive devices:
  1. Elevated toilet seat
  2. Shower chair
  3. Cane, walker, and/or wheelchair
  4. Reachers
  5. Adaptive clothing with Velcro closures
  6. Straight-backed chairs with elevated seat

TABLE 4-27 **Nonsteroidal Anti-Inflammatory Drugs (NSAIDs)**

Drugs	Indications	Adverse Reactions	Nursing Implications
• Aspirin (Anacin) • Ibuprofen (Motrin, Nuprin, Advil) • Ketorolac tromethamine (Toradol) • Celecoxib (Celebrex) • Etodolac (Lodine) • Diclofenac potassium (Voltaren) • Naproxen (Anaprox, Naprocin) • Piroxicam (Feldene)	• Used as anti-inflammatory • Antipyretic • Analgesic • Can be used with other agents	• GI irritation, bleeding, nausea, vomiting, constipation • Elevated liver enzymes • Prolonged coagulation time • Tinnitus • Thrombocytopenia • Fluid retention • Nephrotoxicity • Blood dyscrasias	• Reinforce teaching about taking with food or milk to reduce GI symptoms • Monitor serum salicylate level • Reinforce teaching about watching for signs of bleeding • Reinforce teaching about avoiding alcohol • Reinforce teaching about observing for tinnitus • Administer corticosteroids for severe rheumatoid arthritis (see Table 4-22) • NSAIDs reduce the effect of ACE inhibitors in hypertensive clients • Note name similarity of Celebrex with other drugs having one letter difference in spelling • Encourage routine appointments to check liver/renal labs and CBC

F. Collaborate with the RN in developing a teaching plan:
1. Medication regimen
2. Need for routine follow-up for evaluation of possible side effects
3. Range of motion and stretching exercises tailored to specific client needs
4. Safety tips/precautions on equipment use and environment

Lupus Erythematosus

Description: Lupus erythematosus is a systemic, inflammatory connective tissue disorder.
A. There are two classifications of lupus erythematosus:
1. Discoid lupus erythematosus (DLE) affects skin only.
2. Systemic lupus erythematosus (SLE).
B. SLE is more prevalent than DLE.
C. Lupus is an autoimmune disorder.
D. Kidney involvement is the leading cause of death in clients with lupus, followed by cardiac involvement.

> **HESI Hint** • Avoiding sunlight is key in management of lupus erythematosus. This is what differentiates it from other connective tissue diseases.

E. Factors that trigger lupus:
1. Sunlight
2. Stress
3. Pregnancy
4. Drugs

Nursing Assessment (Data Collection)

A. DLE: dry, scaly rash on face or upper body (butterfly rash)
B. SLE:
1. Joint pain and decreased mobility
2. Fever
3. Nephritis
4. Pleural effusion
5. Pericarditis
6. Abdominal pain
7. Photosensitivity
8. Hypertension

Analysis (Nursing Diagnoses)

A. Impaired skin integrity related to . . .
B. Chronic pain related to . . .
C. Disturbed body image related to . . .

Nursing Plans and Interventions

A. Reinforce instruction for client to avoid prolonged exposure to sunlight.
B. Reinforce instruction for client to clean the skin with mild soap.
C. Monitor and collaborate with RN to develop and implement a teaching plan for client/family about administration of steroids.

Degenerative Joint Disease

Description: Degenerative joint disease (DJD) is noninflammatory arthritis.

A. DJD is characterized by a degeneration of cartilage, a "wear and tear" process.
B. Usually affects one or two joints.
C. Occurs asymmetrically.
D. Obesity and overuse are predisposing factors.

> **HESI Hint** • Degenerative joint disease (DJD) and osteoarthritis are often described as the same disease, and indeed, they both result in hypertrophic changes in the joints. However, they differ in that osteoarthritis is an inflammatory disease and DJD is characterized by noninflammatory degeneration of the joints.

Nursing Assessment (Data Collection)

A. Joint pain, which increases with activity and improves with rest
B. Morning stiffness
C. Asymmetry of affected joints
D. Crepitus (grating sound in the joint)
E. Limited movement
F. Visible joint abnormalities indicated in x-ray films
G. Joint enlargement and bony nodules

Analysis (Nursing Diagnoses)

A. Chronic pain related to . . .
B. Impaired physical mobility related to . . .
C. Self-care deficit (specify) related to . . .
D. Deficient knowledge (specify) related to . . .

Nursing Plans and Interventions

See Rheumatoid Arthritis, p. 124.
A. Reinforce weight-reduction diet.
B. Remind client that excessive use of the involved joint aggravates pain and may accelerate degeneration.
C. Collaborate with RN to develop and implement a teaching plan for client/family about:
   1. Correct posture and body mechanics.
   2. Sleep with rolled terry cloth towel under cervical spine if neck pain is a problem.
   3. Encourage the client to relieve pain in fingers and hands, and wear stretch gloves at night.
   4. Keep joints in functional position.

Osteoporosis

Description: Osteoporosis is a metabolic disease in which bone demineralization results in decreased density and subsequent fractures.
A. Many fractures in older adults occur as a result of osteoporosis and often occur before the client falls, rather than the client sustaining a fracture caused by a fall.
B. The etiology of osteoporosis is unknown.
C. Postmenopausal women are at highest risk.

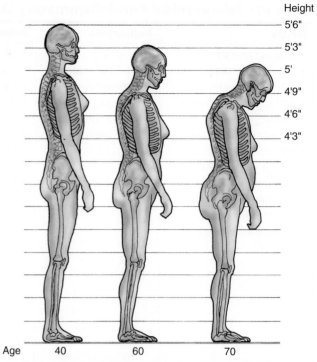

FIGURE 4-6 Normal Spine at 40 Years of Age and Osteoporotic Changes at 60 and 70 Years of Age. These changes can cause a loss of as much as 6 inches in height and can result in the so-called dowager hump (far right) in the upper thoracic vertebrae. (From Ignatavicius DD, Workman ML: *Medical-surgical nursing: patient-centered collaborative care*, ed 7, St. Louis, 2012, Saunders.)

Nursing Assessment (Data Collection)

A. Classic dowager hump or kyphosis of the dorsal spine (Figure 4-6).
B. Loss of height, often 2 to 3 inches.
C. Back pain, often radiating around the trunk.
D. Pathologic fractures, often occurring in the distal end of the radius and the upper third of the femur.
E. Compression fracture of spine can occur: assess ability to void and defecate.

> **HESI Hint** • Postmenopausal, thin, white women are at highest risk for development of osteoporosis. Encourage exercise, a diet high in calcium, and supplemental calcium.

Analysis (Nursing Diagnoses)

A. Risk for injury related to . . .
B. Impaired physical mobility related to . . .
C. Deficient knowledge (specify) related to . . .

Nursing Plans and Interventions

A. Create a hazard-free environment.
B. Keep bed in low position.
C. Encourage client to wear shoes or slippers when out of bed.

D. Encourage environmental safety.
1. Provide adequate lighting.
2. Keep floor clear.
3. Discourage use of throw rugs.
4. Clean spills promptly.
5. Keep side rails up at all times.

> **HESI Hint** • The main cause of fractures in older people, especially women, is osteoporosis. The main fracture sites seem to be the hip, vertebral bodies, clavicle, and forearm.

E. Provide assistance with ambulation.
1. May need walker or cane.
2. May need standby assistance when initially getting out of bed or chair.
F. Reinforce teaching plan regarding regular exercise program.
1. Range of motion several times a day.
2. Ambulate several times a day.
3. Use of proper body mechanics.
4. Regular weight-bearing exercises promote bone formation.
G. Provide diet that is high in protein, calcium, and vitamin D; discourage use of alcohol and caffeine.
H. Encourage preventive measures for females.
1. Estrogen replacement therapy after menopause for some women.
2. High calcium and vitamin D intake beginning in early adulthood.
3. Calcium supplementation after menopause (TUMS is an excellent source of calcium).
4. Weight-bearing exercise.
I. Bone density study as a baseline after menopause, with frequency as recommended by health care provider.

Fracture

Description: Any break in the continuity of the bone.
A. Fractures are described by type and extent of the break.
B. Fractures are caused by a direct blow, crushing force, sudden twisting motion, or disease such as cancer or osteoporosis.
1. Complete fracture: break across the entire cross section of the bone.
2. Incomplete fracture: break occurs across only part of the bone.
3. Closed fracture: does not produce a break in the skin.
4. Open fracture: extends through skin or mucous membranes (much more prone to infection).
C. Five types of fractures are:
1. Greenstick: one side of a bone is broken, and the other side is bent.

2. Transverse: Break occurs straight across the bone shaft.
3. Oblique: at an angle across the bone.
4. Spiral: twisting around the bone.
5. Comminuted: having more than three fragments (Table 4-28, *Common Types of Fractures*).

> **HESI Hint** • What type of fracture is more difficult to heal, an extracapsular fracture (below the neck of the femur) or an intracapsular fracture (in the neck of the femur)?
> The blood supply enters the femur below the neck of the femur. Therefore an intracapsular fracture is much harder to heal and has a greater likelihood of necrosis because it is cut off from the blood supply.

Nursing Assessment (Data Collection)

A. Signs and symptoms of fracture include:
1. Pain, swelling, tenderness
2. Deformity, loss of functional ability
3. Discoloration, bleeding at the site through an open wound
4. Crepitus: crackling sound between two broken bones
B. Fracture evident on x-ray film.
C. Therapeutic management is based on:
1. Reduction of the fracture
2. Maintenance of realignment by immobilization
3. Restoration of function

> **HESI Hint** • NCLEX-PN® questions focus on safety precautions. Improper use of assistive devices can be very risky. When using a nonwheeled walker, the client should lift and move the walker forward, then take a step into it. The client should avoid scooting the walker or shuffling forward into it, which takes more energy and is less stable than a single movement.

D. Observe client's use of assistive devices.
1. Crutches:
a. There should be two to three finger widths between axilla and the top of the crutch.
b. Three-point gait is most common. The client advances both crutches and the impaired leg at the same time. The client then swings the uninvolved leg to the crutches.
2. Cane:
a. Placed on the unaffected side.
b. Top of cane should be parallel to the greater trochanter.

TABLE 4-28 Common Types of Fractures

Description	Illustration	Description	Illustration
Burst: characterized by multiple pieces of bone; often occurs at bone ends or in vertebrae		Longitudinal: fracture line extends in the direction of the bone's longitudinal axis	
Comminuted: more than one fracture line; more than two bone fragments; fragments may be splintered or crushed		Nondisplaced: fragments aligned at fracture site	
Complete: break across the entire section of bone, dividing it into distinct fragments; often displaced		Oblique: fracture line occurs at degree angle across the longitudinal axis of the bone	
Displaced: fragments out of normal position at fracture site	Torsion	Spiral: fracture line results from twisting force; forms a spiral encircling the bone	
Incomplete: fracture occurs through only one cortex of the bone; usually nondisplaced		Stellate: fracture lines radiate from one central point	
Linear: fracture line is intact; fracture is caused by minor to moderate force applied directly to the bone		Transverse: fracture line occurs at a 90-degree angle to longitudinal axis of bone	
Avulsion: bone fragments are torn away from the body of the bone at the site of attachment of a ligament or tendon		Colles: fracture within the last inch of the distal radius; distal fragment is displaced in a position of dorsal and medial deviation	

TABLE 4-28 Common Types of Fractures—cont'd

Description	Illustration	Description	Illustration
Compression: bone buckles and eventually cracks as the result of unusual loading force applied to its longitudinal axis		Pott: fracture of the distal fibula, seriously disrupting the tibiofibular articulation; a piece of the medial malleolus may be chipped off as a result of rupture of the internal lateral ligament	
Greenstick: incomplete fracture in which one side of the cortex is broken and the other side is flexed but intact		Impacted: telescoped fracture, with one fragment driven into another	

Modified from Black JM, Hawks JH: *Medical-surgical nursing: clinical management for positive outcomes,* ed 8, St. Louis, 2009, Saunders.

3. Walker:
   a. Upper extremity and unaffected leg strength assessed and improved with exercises, if necessary, so that upper body is strong enough to use walker.
   b. Client lifts and advances the walker and steps forward.
E. See Chapter 5, *Pediatric Nursing,* p. 167, for cast care and care of the client in traction.

> **HESI Hint** • The risk of a fat embolism, a syndrome in which fat globules migrate into the bloodstream and combine with platelets to form emboli, is greatest in the first 36 hours after a fracture. It is more common in clients with multiple fractures, fractures of long bones, and fractures of the pelvis. The initial symptom of a fat embolism is confusion caused by hypoxemia. If an embolus is suspected, notify health care provider STAT, draw blood gases, administer oxygen, and assist with endotracheal intubation.

> **HESI Hint** • In clients with hip fractures, thromboembolism is the most common complication. Prevention includes passive range of motion exercises, elastic stocking use, elevation of the foot of the bed 25 degrees to increase venous return, and low-dose heparin therapy.

> **HESI Hint** • Clients with fractures, casts, or edema to the extremities need frequent neurovascular assessment distal to the injury. Skin color, temperature, sensation, capillary refill, mobility, pain, and pulses should be assessed.

> **HESI Hint** • Assess the "5 Ps" of neurovascular functioning: pain, paresthesia, pulse, pallor, and paralysis.

Joint Replacement

Description: A surgical procedure in which a mechanical device, designed to act as a joint, is used to replace a diseased joint.
A. Most commonly replaced joints include:
   1. Hip
   2. Knee
   3. Shoulder
   4. Finger
B. Prostheses may be ingrown or cemented.
C. Accurate fitting is essential.
D. Must have healthy bone stock for adequate healing.
E. Joint replacement provides excellent pain relief in 85% to 90% of the clients who have the surgery.
F. Infection is primary concern postoperatively.

Nursing Assessment (Data Collection)

A. Joint pathology:
   1. Arthritis
   2. Fracture
B. Pain not relieved with medication.
C. Poor range of motion in the affected joint.

Analysis (Nursing Diagnoses)

A. Risk for infection related to . . .
B. Pain related to . . .
C. Chronic pain related to . . .
D. Risk for injury to affected limb related to . . .

Nursing Plans and Interventions

A. Provide postoperative care for wound and joint.
   1. Monitor incision site.
      a. Monitor for bleeding and drainage.

HESI Hint • Orthopedic wounds have a tendency to ooze more than other wounds. A suction drainage device usually accompanies the client to the postoperative floor. Check drainage often.

    b. Observe suture line for erythema and/or edema.
    c. Determine proper functioning of drainage apparatus.
    d. Monitor client for signs of infection.

HESI Hint • NCLEX-PN questions about joint replacement focus on complications. A big problem after joint replacement is infection.

  2. Monitor functioning of extremity.
    a. Check circulation, sensation, and movement of extremity distal to replacement.
    b. Provide proper alignment of affected extremity (client will return from the operating room with alignment for initial postoperative period).
    c. Provide abductor appliance (hip replacement) or continuous passive motion device as prescribed.
B. Monitor intake and output (I&O) every shift, including suction drainage.

HESI Hint • Fractures of bone predispose the client to anemia, especially if long bones are involved. Check hematocrit every 3 to 4 days to monitor erythropoiesis.

C. Encourage fluid intake of 3 liters/day.
D. Encourage client to perform self-care activities at maximal level.
E. Support the rehabilitation plan: work closely with health care team to gradually increase client's mobility.
  1. Get client out of bed as soon as possible.
  2. Keep client out of bed as much as possible.
  3. Keep abductor pillow in place while client is in bed (hip replacement) as prescribed.
  4. Use elevated toilet seat and chairs with high seats for those who have had hip or knee replacement (prevents dislocation).
  5. Do not flex hip more than 90 degrees (hip replacement).

HESI Hint • Instruct the client not to lift the leg upward from a lying position or to elevate the knee when sitting. This upward motion can pop the prosthesis out of the socket.

F. Provide discharge planning to include rehabilitation on an outpatient basis as prescribed.

HESI Hint • Immobile clients are prone to complications: skin integrity problems, formation of urinary calculi (may limit milk intake), and venous thrombosis (may be on prophylactic anticoagulants).

Amputation

Description: Surgical removal of a diseased part or organ.
A. Causes for amputation include the following:
  1. Peripheral vascular disease, 80% (75% of these are clients with diabetes)
  2. Trauma
  3. Congenital deformities
  4. Malignant tumors
  5. Infection
B. Amputation necessitates major lifestyle and body image adjustments.

Nursing Assessment (Data Collection)

A. Before amputation, symptoms of peripheral vascular disease include:
  1. Cool extremity
  2. Absent peripheral pulses
  3. Hair loss on affected extremity
  4. Necrotic tissue and/or wounds
    a. Blue or blue-gray turning black
    b. Drainage possible, with or without odor
  5. Leathery skin on affected extremity
  6. Decrease of pain sensation in affected extremity
B. Inadequate circulation determined by the following:
  1. Arteriogram
  2. Doppler flow studies

Analysis (Nursing Diagnoses)

A. Pain related to . . .
B. Impaired physical mobility related to . . .
C. Self-care deficit (specify) related to . . .
D. Disturbed body image related to . . .

Nursing Plans and Interventions

A. Provide wound care.
  1. Monitor surgical dressing for drainage.
    a. Mark dressing for bleeding and check marking at least every 8 hours.
    b. Measure suction drainage every shift.
  2. Change dressing as needed (health care provider usually performs initial dressing change).
    a. Maintain aseptic technique.
    b. Observe wound color and warmth.
    c. Observe for wound healing.
    d. Monitor for signs of infection.

       (1) Fever
       (2) Tachycardia
       (3) Redness of incision area

B. Maintain proper body alignment in and out of bed.
C. Position client to relieve edema and spasms at residual limb (stump) site.
   1. Elevate residual limb (stump) the first 24 hours postoperatively.

> **HESI Hint** • The residual limb (stump) should be elevated on one pillow. If the residual limb (stump) is elevated too high, the elevation can cause a contracture.

   2. Do not elevate residual limb (stump) after 48 hours postoperatively.

   3. Keep residual limb (stump) in extended position and turn prone three times a day to prevent hip flexion contracture.
D. Be aware that phantom pain is *real*, eventually disappears, and responds to pain medication.
E. Handle affected body part gently and with smooth movements.
F. Provide passive range of motion until client is able to perform active range of motion.
G. Collaborate with rehabilitation team members for mobility improvement.
H. Encourage independence in self-care, allowing sufficient time for client to complete care and to have input into care.

Review of Musculoskeletal System

1. Differentiate between rheumatoid arthritis and degenerative joint disease in terms of joint involvement.
2. Identify the categories of drugs commonly used to treat arthritis.
3. Identify pain relief interventions for clients with arthritis.
4. What measures should the nurse encourage female clients to take to prevent osteoporosis?
5. What are the common side effects of salicylates?
6. What is the priority nursing intervention used with clients taking NSAIDs?
7. List three of the joints that are most commonly replaced.
8. Describe postoperative residual limb (stump) care (after amputation) for the first 48 hours.
9. Describe nursing care for the client who is experiencing phantom pain after amputation.
10. A nurse discovers that a client who is in traction for a long bone fracture has a slight fever, is short of breath, and is restless. What does the client most likely have?
11. What are the immediate nursing actions if fat embolization is suspected in a fracture/orthopedic client?
12. List three problems associated with immobility.
13. List three nursing interventions for the prevention of thromboembolism in immobilized clients with musculoskeletal problems.

Answers to Review

1. Rheumatoid arthritis occurs bilaterally. Degenerative joint disease occurs asymmetrically.
2. NSAIDs (nonsteroidal anti-inflammatory drugs) of which salicylates are the cornerstone of treatment, and corticosteroids (used when arthritic symptoms are severe).
3. Warm, moist heat (compresses, baths, showers), diversionary activities (imaging, distraction, self-hypnosis, biofeedback), and medications.
4. Estrogen replacement after menopause for some women, high-calcium and vitamin D intake beginning in early adulthood, calcium supplements after menopause, and weight-bearing exercise.
5. GI irritation, tinnitus, thrombocytopenia, mild liver enzyme elevation.
6. Administer or reinforce client teaching about taking drugs with food or milk.
7. Hip, knee, finger.
8. Elevate residual limb (stump) first 24 hours. Do not elevate residual limb (stump) after 48 hours. Keep residual limb (stump) in extended position and turn prone three times a day to prevent flexion contracture.
9. Be aware that phantom pain is real and will eventually disappear. Administer pain medication; phantom pain responds to medication.
10. Fat embolism, which is characterized by hypoxemia, respiratory distress, irritability, restlessness, fever, and petechiae.
11. Notify health care provider STAT, draw blood gases, administer oxygen according to blood gas results, assist with endotracheal intubation and treatment of respiratory failure.
12. Venous thrombosis, urinary calculi, skin integrity problems.
13. Passive range of motion exercises, elastic stockings, and elevation of foot of bed 25 degrees to increase venous return.

Neurosensory System

Glaucoma

Chronic open-angle glaucoma, which is also known as simple adult primary glaucoma, and primary open-angle glaucoma
Description: Condition characterized by increased intraocular pressure (IOP).

A. Gradual, painless vision loss.
B. Glaucoma may lead to blindness if untreated.
C. Glaucoma is the second leading cause of blindness in the United States.
D. There is an increased incidence in the older population.
E. Glaucoma usually occurs bilaterally in those who have a family history of the condition.
F. Aqueous fluid is inadequately drained from the eye.
G. Generally asymptomatic, especially in early stages.
H. Tends to be diagnosed during routine visual exams.
I. Cannot be cured but can be treated with success pharmacologically and surgically.

Nursing Assessment (Data Collection)

A. Early signs include:
1. Increase in intraocular pressure, greater than 22 mm Hg.
2. Decreased accommodation or ability to focus.

> **HESI Hint** • Glaucoma is often painless and symptom-free. It is usually diagnosed as part of a regular eye exam.

B. Late signs include:
1. Loss of peripheral vision
2. Halos around lights
3. Decreased visual acuity, not correctable with glasses
4. Headache or eye pain, which may be so severe as to cause nausea and vomiting (acute closed-angle glaucoma)
C. Diagnostic tests include the following:
1. Tonometer used to measure intraocular pressure.
2. Electronic tonometer used to detect drainage of aqueous humor.
3. Gonioscopy used to obtain a direct visualization of the lens.
D. Risk factors include the following:
1. Family history of glaucoma
2. Family history of diabetes
3. History of previous ocular problems
4. Medication use:
   a. Glaucoma is a side effect of many medications (e.g., antihistamines, anticholinergics).
   b. Glaucoma can result from the interaction of medications.

Analysis (Nursing Diagnoses)

A. Risk for injury related to . . .
B. Anxiety related to . . .
C. Disturbed visual sensory perception related to . . .
D. Ineffective health management related to . . .

Nursing Plans and Interventions

A. Administer eyedrops as prescribed (Table 4-29, *Treatment of Glaucoma*).

> **HESI Hint** • Eyedrops are used to cause pupil constriction because movement of the muscles to constrict the pupil also allows aqueous humor to flow out, thereby decreasing the pressure in the eye. Pilocarpine is often used. Caution client that vision may be blurred 1 to 2 hours after administration of pilocarpine and adaptation to dark environments is difficult because of papillary constriction (desired effect of the drug).

B. Orient client to surroundings.
C. Avoid nonverbal communication that requires visual acuity (e.g., facial expressions).
D. Collaborate with RN and implement a teaching plan.
1. Careful adherence to eyedrop regimen can prevent blindness.
2. Vision already lost cannot be restored.
3. Eyedrops are needed the rest of life.
4. Proper eyedrop instillation technique. Obtain a return demonstration.
   a. Wash hands and external eye.
   b. Tilt head back slightly.
   c. Instill drop into lower lid, without touching the lid with the tip of the dropper.
   d. Release the lid and sponge excess fluid from lid and cheek.
   e. Close eye gently and leave closed 3 to 5 minutes.
   f. Apply gentle pressure on inner canthus to decrease systematic absorption.
5. Safety measures to prevent injuries:
   a. Remove throw rugs.
   b. Adjust lighting to meet client's needs.
6. Avoid activities that may increase intraocular pressure:
   a. Emotional upsets
   b. Exertion: pushing, heavy lifting, shoveling
   c. Coughing severely or excessive sneezing; get medical attention before upper respiratory infection (URI) worsens
   d. Constrictive clothing: tight collar or tie; belt or girdle too tight
   e. Straining at stool or constipation

> **HESI Hint** • There is an increased incidence of glaucoma in the older population.

TABLE 4-29 **Treatment of Glaucoma**

Drugs	Indications	Adverse Reactions	Nursing Implications
Parasympathomimetics			
• Pilocarpine HCL (multiple brands available) 0.5% to 0.6% is the drug of choice	• Enhance papillary constriction (available in drops, gel, and time-release wafer)	• Bronchospasm • Nausea, vomiting, diarrhea • Blurred vision, twitching eyelids, eye pain with focusing	• Use cautiously with: →Pregnancy →Asthma →Hypertension • Reinforce teaching of proper drop instillation technique • Need for ongoing use of the drug at prescribed intervals • Blurred vision tends to decrease with regular use of this drug
Beta-Adrenergic Receptor-Blocking Agents			
• Timolol maleate optic (Timoptic Solution) • Carteolol (Ocupress) • Levobunolol (Betagan) • Betaxolol (Betoptic S) • Metipranolol (OptiPranolol)	• Inhibit formation of aqueous humor	• Side effects are insignificant • Hypotension	• Use cautiously with: →Hypersensitive →Asthmatic →Second- or third-degree heart block →HF →Congenital glaucoma →Pregnancy • Reinforce teaching of proper drop instillation technique • Need for ongoing use of the drug at prescribed intervals • Blurred vision tends to decrease with regular use of this drug
Carbonic Anhydrase Inhibitors			
• Acetazolamide (Diamox) • Brinzolamide (Azopt) • Dorzolamide (Trusopt)	• Reduce aqueous humor production	• Numbness, tingling hands and feet • Nausea • Malaise	• Administer orally or IV (Diamox) • Produces diuresis • Assess for metabolic acidosis
Alpha Agonists			
• Brimonidine (Alphagan P) • Apraclonidine (Iopidine)	• Lower intraocular pressure of glaucoma by decreasing fluid produced		
Prostaglandin Agonists			
• Latanoprost (Xalatan) • Travoprost (Travatan) • Bimatoprost (Lumigan)	• Lower intraocular pressure of glaucoma by increasing outflow of aqueous humor	• Local irritation • Foreign body sensation • Increased brown pigmentation of iris • Increased eyelash growth	

Nursing Plans and Interventions for the Nonseeing (Blind) Client

A. Upon entering room, announce your presence and identify yourself, address client by name.
B. Do not touch client unless he or she knows you are there.
C. Upon admission to hospital or nursing center, orient client thoroughly to surroundings:
   1. Demonstrate use of the call bell.
   2. Walk client around the room and acquaint him or her with all objects, including chairs, bed, TV, telephone, and bathroom.
D. Guide client when walking.
   1. Walk ahead of client and place his or her hand in the bend of your elbow.
   2. Describe where you are walking. Note if passageway is narrowing or if you are approaching stairs, curb, or an incline.
E. Always raise side rails for the "newly" sightless person, such as postoperative eye patch clients.
F. Assist with meal enjoyment by describing food and its placement in terms of face of a clock—for example, "meat is at 6 o'clock."
G. When administering medications, inform client of number of pills, and give only ½ glass of water (to avoid spills).

Cataract

Description: A cataract is a condition characterized by opacity of the lens. Cataracts are the leading cause of blindness in the world.

A. Aging accounts for 95% of cataracts (senile).
B. Remaining 5% are from trauma, toxic substances, or systemic diseases, or are congenital.
C. Safety precautions may reduce incidence of traumatic cataracts.
D. Surgical removal is done when vision impairment interferes with daily activities. Intraocular lens implants may be used.
E. Most surgeries are done under local anesthesia as outpatient surgery.

HESI Hint • The lens of the eye is responsible for projecting light, which enters onto the retina so that images can be discerned. Without the lens, which becomes opaque with cataracts, light cannot be filtered, and vision is blurred.

Nursing Assessment (Data Collection)

A. Early signs include:
   1. Blurred vision
   2. Decreased color perception
B. Late signs include:
   1. Diplopia

   2. Reduced visual acuity progressing to blindness
   3. Clouded pupil, progressing to a milky-white appearance
C. Diagnostic tests include the following:
   1. Ophthalmoscope
   2. Slit lamp biomicroscope

Analysis (Nursing Diagnoses)

A. Disturbed visual sensory perception related to . . .
B. Anxiety related to . . .

Nursing Plans and Interventions

A. Preoperative: reinforce teaching plan related to eye medication instillation.
B. Reinforce the postoperative teaching plan:
   1. Warn not to rub or put pressure on eye.
   2. Glasses or shaded lens should be worn during waking hours. Eye shield should be worn during sleeping hours.
   3. Avoid lifting objects over 5 pounds, bending, straining, coughing, or any activity that can increase intraocular pressure.
   4. Use stool softener to prevent straining at stool.
   5. Avoid lying on operative side.
   6. Need to keep water from getting into eye while showering or washing hair.
   7. Observe and report signs of increased intraocular pressure and infection (e.g., pain, changes in vital signs).

HESI Hint • When the cataract is removed, the lens is gone, making prevention of falls important. If the lens is replaced with an implant, vision is better than if a contact lens is used (some visual distortion) or if glasses are used (greater visual distortion—everything has a curved shape).

Eye Trauma

Description: Injury to the eye sustained from sharp or blunt trauma, chemicals, or heat.

A. Permanent visual impairment can occur.
B. Every eye injury should be considered an emergency.
C. Protective eye shields in hazardous work environments and during athletic sports may prevent injuries.

Nursing Assessment (Data Collection)

A. Determine type of injury and symptoms.
B. Diagnostic tests include the following:
   1. Slit lamp examination
   2. Fluorescein dye to detect corneal injury
   3. Visual acuity for medical documentation and legal protection

Analysis (Nursing Diagnoses)

A. Risk for injury related to . . .

B. Disturbed visual sensory perception related to . . .

C. Pain related to . . .

Nursing Plans and Interventions

A. Position the client relative to the type of injury; sitting position decreases intraocular pressure.

B. Remove conjunctival foreign bodies unless embedded.

C. Never attempt to remove a penetrating or embedded object. Do *not* apply pressure.

D. Apply cold compresses to eye contusion.

E. Irrigate the eye with copious amounts of water following chemical injuries.

F. Administer eye medications as prescribed.

G. Explain that an eye patch may be applied to rest the eye. Reading and watching TV may be restricted for 3 to 5 days.

H. Explain that sudden increase in eye pain should be reported.

Detached Retina

Description: A hole, tear, or separation of the sensory retina from the pigmented epithelium.

A. Can be result of increasing age, severe myopia, eye trauma, retinopathy (diabetic), cataract or glaucoma surgery, family or personal history.

B. Resealing is done by surgery:
   1. Cryotherapy—freezing
   2. Photocoagulation—laser
   3. Diathermy—heat
   4. Scleral buckling—most often used

Nursing Plans and Interventions

A. Position the client as ordered (thus allowing the agent being used to reattach the retina to the interior surface of the eye).

B. Eye patch over affected eye.

C. Eye prescription to inhibit accommodation and constriction. Cycloplegics to dilate (mydriatic): homatropine—an anticholinergic.

D. Postoperative for pain—Tylenol, oxycodone.

E. If gas bubble used (inserted in vitreous), position so bubble can "rise" against area to be reattached.

F. Reinforce client education about no heavy lifting, straining with bowel movement, or vigorous activity for several weeks postoperatively.

Hearing Loss

Conductive Hearing Loss

Description: Hearing loss in which sound does not travel well to the sound organs of the inner ear. The volume of sound is less, but the sound remains clear. If volume is raised, hearing is normal.

A. Hearing loss is the most common disability in the United States.

B. Usually results from cerumen (wax) impaction or middle ear disorders such as otitis media.

> **HESI Hint** • The ear consists of three parts: the external ear, the middle ear, and the inner ear. Inner ear disorders, or disorders of the sensory fibers going to the CNS, often are neurogenic in nature and may not be helped with a hearing aid. External and middle ear problems (conductive) may result from trauma, infection, or wax buildup. These types of disorders are treated more successfully with hearing aids.

Sensorineural Hearing Loss

Description: A form of hearing loss in which sound passes properly through the outer and middle ear but is distorted by a defect in the inner ear or damage to cranial nerve VIII, or both.

A. Perceptive loss, usually progressive and bilateral.

B. Involves damage to the eighth cranial nerve.

C. Detected easily by use of a tuning fork.

D. Common causes include:
   1. Infections
   2. Ototoxic drugs
   3. Trauma
   4. Neuromas
   5. Noise
   6. Aging process

Nursing Assessment (Data Collection)

A. Inability to hear a whisper from 1 to 2 feet away.

B. Inability to respond if nurse covers mouth when talking, indicating that client is lip reading.

C. Inability to hear a watch tick 5 inches from ear.

D. Shouting in conversation.

E. Straining to hear.

F. Turning head to favor one ear.

G. Answering questions incorrectly or inappropriately.

H. Raising volume of radio/TV.

Analysis (Nursing Diagnoses)

A. Disturbed auditory sensory perception related to . . .

B. Impaired verbal communication related to . . .

C. Social isolation related to . . .

Nursing Plans and Interventions

A. To enhance therapeutic communication with the hearing impaired client, the nurse will:
   1. Before starting conversation, reduce distraction as much as possible.
   2. Turn the television or radio down or off, close the door, or move to a quieter location.
   3. Devote full attention to the conversation; do not try to do two things at once.
   4. Look and listen during the conversation.

5. Begin with casual topics and progress to more critical issues slowly.
6. Do not switch topics abruptly.
7. If you do not understand, let the client know.
8. If the client is a lip reader, face them directly.
9. Speak slowly and distinctly; determine whether you were understood.
10. Allow adequate time for the conversation to take place; try to avoid hurried conversations.
11. Use active listening techniques.

> **HESI Hint** • NCLEX-PN questions often focus on communicating with older adults who are hearing impaired.
> Speak in a low-pitched voice, slowly, and distinctly.
> Stand in front of the person with the light source behind the client.
> Use visual aids if available.

B. Be sure to inform the health care staff of the client's hearing loss.
C. Helpful aids may include a telephone amplifier, earphone attachments for the radio and TV, and lights or buzzers in the most used rooms of the house that activate when the doorbell is rung.

Neurologic System

Altered State of Consciousness

Nursing Assessment (Data Collection)

A. Use agency neuro vital sign assessment tool. It sometimes contains a scale for scoring, such as the Glasgow Coma Scale, which objectively documents the client's level of consciousness (Table 4-30, *Glasgow Coma Scale*).
1. Maximum total is 15, minimum is 3.
2. A score of 7 or less indicates COMA.
3. Clients with low scores—3 to 4—have a high mortality and poor prognosis.
4. Clients with scores greater than 8 have a good prognosis for recovery.

> **HESI Hint** • Use of the Glasgow Coma Scale eliminates ambiguous terms to describe neurologic status such as *lethargic*, *stuporous*, or *obtunded*.

B. Neuro vital sign sheet will also address pupil size (with sizing scale), limb movement (with scale), and vital signs (blood pressure, temperature, pulse, respirations).
C. Monitor skin integrity and corneal integrity.

D. Check bladder for fullness, auscultate lungs, and monitor cardiac status.
E. Identify family's knowledge of client's clinical status, coping skills, and support needs.

Analysis (Nursing Diagnoses)

> **HESI Hint** • Almost every diagnosis in the NANDA format is applicable because severely neurologically impaired persons require total care.

A. Ineffective breathing pattern related to . . .
B. Ineffective airway clearance related to . . .
C. Impaired gas exchange related to . . .
D. Decreased cardiac output related to . . .
E. Risk for imbalanced body temperature related to . . .
F. Risk for injury related to . . .
G. Impaired physical mobility related to . . .
H. Risk for impaired skin integrity related to . . .
I. Anxiety related to . . .
J. Self-care deficit (specify dressing, grooming) related to . . .
K. Imbalanced nutrition: less than body requirements related to . . .
L. Impaired urinary elimination related to. . .

TABLE 4-30 Glasgow Coma Scale

Variable	Response	Score
Eye opening	Spontaneously	4
	To verbal command	3
	To pain	2
	No response	1
Motor response	To verbal command	6
	To painful stimuli	
	• Localizes pain	5
	• Flexes/withdraws	4
	• Flexor posturing (decorticate)	3
	• Extensor posturing (decerebrate)	2
	• No response	1
Verbal response	Oriented and converses	5
	Disoriented, converses	4
	Uses inappropriate words	3
	Incomprehensible sounds	2
	No response	1

HESI Hint • Clients with an altered state of consciousness are fed by enteral routes because the likelihood of aspiration with oral feedings is great. Residual feeding is the amount of previous feeding still in the stomach. The presence of 100 mL of residual in adults usually indicates poor gastric emptying, and the feeding should be held.

HESI Hint • Paralytic ileus is common in comatose clients. Gastric tubes aid in gastric decompression.

HESI Hint • Any client on bed rest or who is immobilized must have range of motion exercises often and very frequent position changes. Do not leave the client in any one position for longer than 2 hours. Any position that decreases venous return is dangerous—that is, sitting with dependent extremities for long periods.

Nursing Plans and Interventions

A. Maintain adequate respirations, airway, oxygenation:
   1. Document and report breathing pattern changes.
   2. Position for maximum ventilation: ¾ prone or semi-prone to prevent tongue from obstructing airway and slightly to one side with arms away from chest wall.
   3. Insert airway if tongue is obstructing or if client is paralyzed.
   4. Prepare for insertion of cuffed endotracheal tube.
   5. Keep airway free of secretions with suctioning (see Table 4-3, p. 68).
   6. Monitor arterial P_{O_2} and P_{CO_2}.
   7. Prepare for tracheostomy if prolonged ventilator support is needed.
   8. Provide chest physiotherapy as prescribed by health care provider.
   9. Hyperventilate with 100% O_2 before and after suctioning.

B. Provide nutritional and fluid and electrolyte support.
   1. Keep client NPO until responsive, and provide mouth care every 2 to 4 hours and as needed.
   2. Maintain calorie count.
   3. Administer feedings as prescribed (Box 4-1, *Unconscious Client*, p. 137).
   4. Monitor I&O.
   5. Record client's weight (weigh same time each day).

C. Prevent complications of immobility:
   1. Impairment in skin integrity:
      a. Turn every 2 hours and assess bony prominences.
      b. Use prescribed airflow therapy beds and mattresses.
      c. Use minimal amount of linens and under pads.
   2. Potential for thrombus formation:
      a. Monitor lower extremities for signs of thrombophlebitis.
      b. Perform passive ROM exercises to lower extremities every 4 hours.
      c. Use elastic hose; remove and reapply every 8 hours.
      d. Avoid positions that decrease venous return.
      e. Avoid pillows under knees or gatched bed.
   3. Urinary calculi:
      a. Increase fluid intake orally or through gastric tube.
      b. Monitor urine for high specific gravity (dehydration) and balance between intake and output.
   4. Contractures/joint immobility:
      a. Passive ROM every 4 hours.
      b. Sit client up in bed or chair if possible, or use neuro chair if necessary.

BOX 4-1 *Unconscious Client*

Gastric Gavage
- Begin feeding when GI peristalsis returns.
- Place client in high Fowler position.
- Place towel over chest.
- Connect gastrostomy tube to funnel or large syringe.
- Check gastric residual to assess absorption and client tolerance; return residual.
- Pour feeding into tilted funnel and unclamp tubing to allow feeding to flow by GRAVITY.
- Regulate flow by raising or lowering container. Feeding too fast causes diarrhea, gastric distention, pain. Feeding too slowly causes possible obstruction of flow.
- After feeding, irrigate tube with water (tepid) and clamp tube.
- Apply small dressing over tube opening, coil tube and attach to dressing. May cover with an abdominal binder.

- Get bowel history from reliable source.
- Establish specific time for evacuation. Regularity is essential.
  - In an unconscious client, can evacuate the bowel after the last tube feeding of day because the gastrocolic and duodenocolic reflexes are active after "meal."
  - Stimulate anorectal reflex with insertion of glycerin suppository 15 to 30 minutes before scheduled evacuation time. May need stronger suppository, such as bisacodyl (Dulcolax).
  - Ensure adequate fiber in tube feedings and adequate fluid intake of 2 to 4 liters/day.
  - May apply a rectal pouch to contain fecal material (ostomy bag with seal over anal opening).

    c. Reposition every 2 hours maintaining proper body alignment.

    d. Apply splints or other assistive devices to prevent foot drop, wrist drop, or other improper alignment.

D. Monitor and report the vital sign changes indicating changes in condition:

  1. Pulse: a pulse rate change to less than 60 can indicate increased intracranial pressure (ICP). Fast rate (more than 100 bpm) can indicate infection, thrombus formation, or dehydration.

  2. Blood pressure: rising BP or widening pulse pressure can indicate increased ICP.

  3. Temperature: report any abnormalities (temperature elevation can indicate worsening condition, damage to temperature regulating area of brain, and/or infection).

  4. Level of consciousness changes: active to somnolent.

  5. Pupillary changes: prompt to sluggish, increase in size.

HESI Hint • If temperature elevates, take quick measures to decrease it because fever increases cerebral metabolism and can increase cerebral edema.

HESI Hint • SAFETY FEATURES FOR IMMOBILIZED CLIENTS

- Prevent skin breakdown with frequent turning.
- Maintain adequate nutrition.
- Prevent aspiration with slow, small feedings or NG feedings.
- Monitor neurologic signs to detect the first signs that intracranial pressure may be increasing.
- Provide ROM exercises to prevent deformities.
- Prevent respiratory complications—frequent turning and positioning for optimal drainage.

E. Prevent injury/promote safety:

  1. Place bed in low position and keep side rails up at all times.

  2. Pad side rails if client is agitated or if there is a history of seizure activity.

  3. Restrain if client is trying to remove tubes or attempting to get out of bed.

  4. Touch gently and talk softly and calmly to the client, remembering that hearing is often intact.

HESI Hint • Restlessness may indicate a return to consciousness but can also indicate anoxia, distended bladder, covert bleeding, or increasing cerebral anoxia. Do not oversedate, and report any symptoms of restlessness.

---

  5. Avoid oversedating the client because sedatives/narcotics depress responsiveness and affect papillary

reaction (an important assessment in neuro vital signs).

  6. During all activities, tell the client what you are doing no matter what the client's level of consciousness is.

F. Maintain hygiene/cleanliness:

  1. Provide bathing, grooming, and dressing.

  2. Provide oral hygiene.

  3. Wash hair weekly.

  4. Provide nail care within agency guidelines.

G. Observe for bladder elimination problems:

  1. Insert indwelling catheter if prescribed.

  2. Remove indwelling catheter as soon as possible; use diaper or condom catheter.

H. Document and record bowel movements and report abnormal patterns of constipation or diarrhea.

  1. Rapid infusion of tube feedings may cause diarrhea, whereas lack of fiber/inadequate fluids may cause constipation.

  2. Initiate bowel program (see Box 4-1, *Unconscious Client*).

I. Prevent corneal injury/drying:

  1. Remove contact lenses if present.

  2. Irrigate eyes with sterile prescribed solution and instill ophthalmic ointment in each eye every 8 hours to prevent corneal ulceration.

J. See Seizures in Chapter 5, *Pediatric Nursing*, p. 167.

Head Injury

Description: Any traumatic damage to the head.

A. Open head injury occurs when there is a fracture of the skull or penetration of the skull by an object.

B. Closed head injury is the result of blunt trauma (more serious because of the chance of increased intracranial pressure in "closed" vault).

C. Increased intracranial pressure is the main concern in head injury related to edema, hemorrhage, impaired cerebral autoregulation, and hydrocephalus.

HESI Hint • The forces of impact influence the type of head injury. They include acceleration, injury, which is caused by the head in motion, and deceleration injury, which occurs when the head stops suddenly. Helmets are a *great* preventive measure for motorcyclists or bicyclists (Figure 4-7, *Head Movement During Acceleration-Deceleration Injury*).

Nursing Assessment (Data Collection)

A. Unconsciousness or disturbances in consciousness

B. Vertigo

C. Confusion, delirium, and/or disorientation

D. Symptoms of increased intracranial pressure (ICP)

  1. Change in level of responsiveness is the most important indicator of increased ICP.

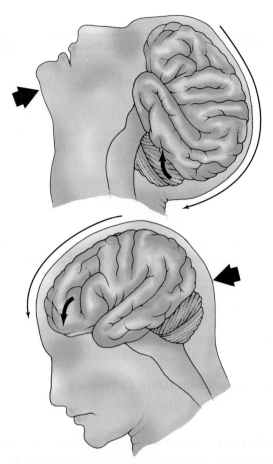

FIGURE 4-7 Head Movement During Acceleration-Deceleration Injury. Such movements are typically seen in motor vehicle accidents. (From Ignatavicius DD, Workman ML: *Medical-surgical nursing: patient-centered collaborative care*, ed 7, St. Louis, 2012, Saunders.)

> **HESI Hint** • Even subtle behavior changes, such as restlessness, irritability, or confusion, may indicate increased ICP.

    2. Changes in vital signs:
       a. Slowing of respirations or respiratory irregularities
       b. Increase or decrease in pulse
       c. Rising BP or widening pulse pressure
       d. Temperature rise
    3. Headache
    4. Vomiting (projectile)
    5. Pupillary changes reflecting pressure on optic/oculomotor nerves:
       a. Pupils decrease or increase in size or become unequal
       b. Lack of conjugate eye movement
       c. Papilledema
 E. Seizures
 F. Ataxia
 G. Abnormal posturing (decerebrate or decorticate)
 H. Cerebrospinal fluid (CSF) leakage through nose (rhinorrhea) or through ear (otorrhea). Usually unilateral.

> **HESI Hint** • CSF leakage carries the risk of meningitis and indicates a deteriorating condition. Because of CSF leakage, the usual signs of increased ICP may not occur. To verify presence of CSF, check drainage with adextrastix. The presence of glucose indicates CSF.

 I. Computed axial tomography (CAT) scan or magnetic resonance imaging (MRI) will show lesions such as epidural or subdural hematomas requiring surgery.
 J. EEG determines presence of seizure activity.

Analysis (Nursing Diagnoses)

 A. Ineffective cerebral tissue perfusion related to . . .
 B. Disturbed sensory perception (specify type) related to . . .
 C. Risk for injury related to . . .
 D. Ineffective family coping related to . . .

Nursing Plans and Interventions

 A. Maintain adequate ventilation/airway.
    1. Monitor Po_2 and Pco_2 for the development of hypoxia and hypercapnia.
    2. Position client semiprone or lateral recumbent to prevent aspiration.
    3. Turn from side to side to prevent lung secretion stasis.
 B. Keep head of bed elevated 30 to 45 degrees to aid venous return from the neck and decrease cerebral volume.
 C. Obtain neurologic vital signs as prescribed (at least every 1 to 2 hours) and maintain a continuous record of observations and Glasgow Coma Scale ratings.
 D. Notify RN and health care provider at *first* sign of deterioration or improvement in condition.
 E. Avoid activities that increase intracranial pressure such as:
    1. Change in bed position for caregiving, extreme hip flexion
    2. Endotracheal suctioning
    3. Compression of jugular veins (keep head straight and not to one side)
    4. Coughing, vomiting, or straining of any type (no Valsalva: increased intrathoracic pressure increases ICP)
 F. If temperature increases, take immediate measures to reduce it (e.g., aspirin, acetaminophen, cooling blanket) because increased temperature increases cerebral blood flow drastically; avoid shivering.
 G. Prepare for intracranial monitoring system, if available:
    1. Catheter inserted into lateral ventricle, sensor placed on the dura, or a screw inserted into the subarachnoid space attached to pressure transducer.
    2. Elevations of intracranial pressure greater than 20 mm Hg should be reported STAT.

TABLE 4-31 Osmotic Diuretic

Drug	Indications	Adverse Reactions	Nursing Implications
• Mannitol (Osmitrol)	• Acts on renal tubules by osmosis to prevent water reabsorption • In bloodstream, draws fluid from the extravascular spaces into the plasma	• Disorientation, confusion, and headache • Nausea and vomiting • Convulsions and anaphylactic reactions	• Use for short-term therapy ONLY • Never give to clients with cerebral hemorrhage • IV infusion is usually adjusted to urine output—filter and watch for crystals • Never give to clients with no urine output (anuria); if output is less than 30 mL/hr, accumulation can cause pulmonary edema and water intoxication

H. Administer and/or monitor medications prescribed by health care provider to reduce intracranial pressure:
   1. Hyperosmotic agents/diuretics: to dehydrate brain and reduce cerebral edema.
      a. Mannitol (Table 4-31, *Osmotic Diuretic*)
      b. Urea
   2. Steroids: dexamethasone (Decadron), methylprednisolone sodium/succinate (Solu-Medrol) to reduce brain edema.
   3. Barbiturates: to reduce brain metabolism and systemic blood pressure.
I. Insert indwelling Foley catheter to prevent restlessness caused by distended bladder and monitor balance between restricted fluid intake and output, especially if placed on osmotic diuretics.

HESI Hint • Try *not* to use restraints; they only increase restlessness. *Avoid* narcotics because they mask level of responsiveness.

J. Health care provider may order passive hyperventilation on ventilator: leads to respiratory alkalosis, which causes cerebral vasoconstriction, decreased cerebral blood flow, and therefore decreased ICP.
K. Continue seizure precautions. The health care provider may order prophylactic phenytoin (Dilantin).
L. Prevent complications of immobility (see Nursing Plans and Interventions for the Unconscious/Immobilized Client).
M. Reinforce teaching plan related to possible aftereffects of head injury:
   1. Posttraumatic syndrome: headache, vertigo, emotional instability, inability to concentrate, impaired memory
   2. Posttraumatic seizure disorder
   3. Posttraumatic neuroses/psychoses

Spinal Cord Injury

Description: Disruption in nervous system function, which may result in complete or incomplete loss of motor and sensory function. Changes occur in the function of all physiologic systems.

A. Injuries are described by location in the spinal cord. Most common sites are fifth, sixth, and seventh cervical (C-5, C-6, C-7), the twelfth thoracic (T-12), and the first lumbar (L-1).
B. Damage can range from contusion to complete transection.
C. Permanent impairment cannot be determined until spinal cord edema has subsided, usually by 1 week.

Nursing Assessment (Data Collection)

A. Monitor breathing pattern, auscultate lungs.

HESI Hint • Physical assessment should concentrate on respiratory status, especially in clients with injury at C-3 to C-5, as cervical plexus innervates diaphragm.

B. Check neuro vital signs frequently, especially sensory and motor functions.
C. Monitor cardiovascular status.
D. Monitor abdomen: girth, bowel sounds, lower abdomen for bladder distention.
E. Observe changes in temperature, remembering hyperthermia often occurs.
F. Identify psychosocial status.
G. Hypotension and bradycardia occur with any injury above T-6 because sympathetic outflow is affected.

Analysis (Nursing Diagnoses)

A. Ineffective breathing pattern related to . . .
B. Ineffective tissue perfusion (specify) related to . . .
C. Impaired skin integrity related to . . .
D. Self-care deficit (specify) related to . . .
E. Urinary retention related to . . .
F. Ineffective coping related to . . .

Nursing Plans and Interventions

A. Acute phase of spinal cord injury:
   1. See Nursing Plans and Interventions for the Unconscious/Immobilized Client.
   2. Maintain client in an extended position with cervical collar on during any transfer.
   3. Maintain a patent airway—*most important.*

4. In cervical injuries, skeletal traction is maintained by use of skull tongs or halo ring (Crutchfield tongs or Gardner-Wells fixation device).
5. High-dose corticosteroids are often given to help control edema during the first 8 to 24 hours.
6. Use a kinetic therapy treatment table (Roto-Rest bed), which provides continuous side-to-side motion.
7. Use Stryker frame or *very firm* mattress with board underneath.
8. Assess for respiratory failure, especially in clients with high cervical injuries.
9. Further loss of sensory/motor function below injury can indicate additional damage to cord from edema and should be reported immediately.
10. Evaluate for presence of spinal shock (a complete loss of all reflex, motor, sensory, and autonomic activity below the lesion). This is a MEDICAL EMERGENCY, which occurs immediately after the injury.
    a. Hypotension, bradycardia
    b. Complete paralysis and lack of sensation below lesion
    c. Bladder and bowel distention

> **HESI Hint** It is imperative to reverse spinal shock as quickly as possible. Permanent paralysis can occur if a spinal cord is compressed for 12 to 24 hours.

11. Observe for autonomic dysreflexia (exaggerated autonomic responses to stimuli), which occurs in clients with lesions at or above T-6.
12. Watch for acute paralytic ileus, lack of gastric activity.
    a. Assess bowel sounds frequently.
    b. Initiate gastric suction to reduce distention, prevent vomiting/aspiration.
    c. May use rectal tube to relieve gaseous distention.
13. Suction with caution to prevent vagus nerve stimulation, which can cause cardiac arrest.
14. Administer high-dose corticosteroids to decrease edema and reduce cord damage.
B. Rehabilitative phase:
    1. Encourage deep-breathing exercises.
    2. Chest physiotherapy.
    3. Kinetic bed to promote blood flow to extremities.
    4. Antiembolic stockings.
    5. Range-of-motion exercises.
    6. Mobilize to chair as soon as possible.
    7. Turn frequently.
    8. Keep client clean and dry.
    9. Observe for impending skin breakdown.
    10. Reinforce teaching about the importance of impeccable skin care.
    11. Intermittent catheterization every 4 hours. Collaborate with RN to develop and implement client/family teaching plan for catheterization.

12. Assist with teaching bladder-emptying techniques depending on level of injury and bladder muscle response.
    a. Upper motor neuron (spastic) bladder
    b. Lower motor neuron (flaccid) bladder
13. Collaborate with RN to develop and implement client/family teaching plan for I&O. Instruct client in I&O.

> **HESI Hint** A common cause of death after spinal cord injury is urinary tract infection. Bacteria grow best in alkaline media, so keeping urine dilute and acidic is prophylactic against infection. Also, keeping the bladder emptied assists in avoiding bacterial growth in urine that has stagnated in the bladder.

14. Reinforce bowel-training program.
15. Talk with client and family about permanence of disability.
16. Encourage rehabilitation facility staff to visit client.
17. Encourage client and family to visit rehabilitation facility.
18. Assist family to find support group, and assist with the referral process for community resources after dismissal from rehabilitation facility.

Brain Tumor

Description: Neoplasm occurring in the brain.
A. Primary tumors arise in any tissue of the brain.
B. Secondary tumors are a result of metastasis from other areas (most often from the lungs, followed by breast metastasis).
C. Without treatment, benign as well as malignant tumors lead to death.

> **HESI Hint** Benign tumors continue to grow and take up space in the confined area of the cranium, causing neural and vascular compromise for the brain, increased intracranial pressure, and necrosis of brain tissue; thus, even benign tumors must be treated because they may have malignant effects.

Nursing Assessment (Data Collection)

A. Headache that is more severe upon awakening
B. Vomiting not associated with nausea
C. Papilledema with visual changes
D. Behavioral and personality changes
E. Seizures
F. Aphasia, hemiplegia, ataxia
G. Cranial nerve dysfunction
H. Abnormal CT scan

Analysis (Nursing Diagnoses)

A. Ineffective tissue perfusion (cerebral) related to . . .
B. Pain related to . . .
C. Risk for injury related to . . .
D. Anxiety related to . . .

Nursing Plans and Interventions

A. Nursing plans and interventions are similar to those implemented for the head injury client with increased ICP.
B. Elevate the head of the bed 30 to 40 degrees; maintain head in neutral position.
C. Radiation therapy:
   1. Provide skin care with non–oil-based soap and water. Avoid alcohol, powder, or oils on the skin.
   2. Reinforce instructions for client not to wash off the lines drawn by the radiologist.
D. Chemotherapy: medications may be injected intraventricularly or intravenously.
E. Surgical removal (craniotomy):
   1. Preoperative: shave head
   2. Postoperative:
      a. Frequent neurologic and vital sign assessment.
      b. Position client with head of bed elevated per health care provider's recommendation. Position client off the operative site.
      c. Monitor dressings for signs of drainage (excess amount of cerebrospinal fluid [CSF]).
      d. Monitor respiratory status to prevent hypoventilation.
      e. Avoid activities that cause increased ICP.
      f. Monitor for seizure activity.
      g. Administer medications (see Head Injury, p. 138).

> **HESI Hint** • **CRANIOTOMY MEDICATIONS**
> - Corticosteroids to reduce swelling
> - Agents (atropine, Robinul) and osmotic diuretics to reduce secretions
> - Agents to reduce seizures (phenytoin)
> - Prophylactic antibiotics

Multiple Sclerosis

Description: Multiple sclerosis (MS) is a demyelinating disease resulting in the destruction of CNS myelin and consequent disruption in the transmission of nerve impulses.
A. Onset is insidious, with 50% of clients still ambulatory 25 years after diagnosis.
B. Diagnosis determined by combination of data:
   1. Presenting symptoms
   2. Increased white matter density seen on CT scan
   3. MRI shows presence of plaques
   4. CSF electrophoresis showing presence of oligoclonal (IgG) bands

C. Current thinking is that multiple sclerosis is autoimmune in origin.

> **HESI Hint** • Symptoms involving motor function usually begin in the upper extremities, with weakness progressing to spastic paralysis. Bowel and bladder dysfunction occurs in 90% of the cases. MS is more common in women. Progression is not "orderly."

Nursing Assessment (Data Collection)

A. Nursing history of client to include:
   1. History of symptoms
   2. Progression of illness
   3. Types of treatment received and the response
   4. Additional health problems
   5. Current medications
   6. Client's/family's perception of illness
   7. Community resources used by the client
B. Physical assessment to include:
   1. Optic neuritis (loss of vision or blind spots)
   2. Visual or swallowing difficulties
   3. Gait disturbances; intention tremors
   4. Unusual fatigue, weakness, and clumsiness
   5. Numbness, particularly on one side of face
   6. Impaired bladder and bowel control
   7. Speech disturbances
   8. Scotomas (white spots in visual field, diplopia)

Analysis (Nursing Diagnoses)

A. Risk for injury related to . . .
B. Impaired physical mobility related to . . .
C. Disturbed sensory perception (specify) related to . . .
D. Fatigue related to . . .
E. Impaired urinary elimination related to . . .
F. Impaired home maintenance related to . . .

Nursing Plans and Interventions

A. Allow hospitalized client to keep own routine.
B. Orient client to environment and teach strategies to maximize vision.
C. Encourage self-care and frequent rest periods.
D. With exercise programs, encourage client to work up to the point just short of fatigue.
E. For muscle spasticity, stretch-hold-relax exercises are helpful, as are riding a stationary bicycle and swimming; fall precautions.
F. Initially, work with client on a voiding schedule.
G. As incontinence worsens, the female may need to learn clean self-catheterization; the male may need a condom catheter.
H. Encourage adequate fluid intake, high-fiber foods, and a bowel regimen for constipation problems.
I. Encourage the client and the family to verbalize their concerns with ongoing care issues.

J. Encourage client to maintain contact with a support group.

K. Assist in the referral process for home health care services.

L. Encourage client to contact the local MS society for emotional and direct service support.

M. Steroid therapy and chemotherapeutic drugs are administered in acute exacerbations to shorten length of attack.

> **HESI Hint** • Drug therapy for MS clients: ACTH, cortisone, Cytoxan, and other immunosuppressive drugs. Nursing implications for administration of these drugs should focus on prevention of infection.

N. Biologic response modifiers such as interferon-B products have shown recent success in relapsing MS.

Myasthenia Gravis

Description: Myasthenia gravis is a disorder affecting the neuromuscular transmission of impulses in the voluntary muscles of the body.

A. Considered an autoimmune disease characterized by presence of acetylcholine receptor antibodies that interfere with neuronal transmission.

B. Usually affects females between ages 10 and 40 and males between ages 50 and 70.

Nursing Assessment (Data Collection)

A. Diplopia (double vision), ptosis (eyelid drooping).

B. Mask-like affect: sleepy appearance because of facial muscle involvement.

C. Weakness of laryngeal and pharyngeal muscles: dysphagia, choking, food aspiration, difficulty speaking.

D. Muscle weakness improved by rest, worsened by activity.

E. Advanced cases have respiratory failure, bladder and bowel incontinence.

F. Myasthenic crisis (attributed to disease worsening) symptoms associated with undermedication. Cholinergic crisis (attributed to anticholinesterase overdosage): diaphoresis, diarrhea, fasciculations, cramps, marked worsening of symptoms from overmedication.

> **HESI Hint** • Understand the symptoms associated with anticholinergic agent: impaired vision, dry mouth, dry eyes, orthostatic hypotension, constipation, and urinary retention.

> **HESI Hint** • In clients with myasthenia gravis, be alert for changes in respiratory status. The most severe involvement may result in respiratory failure.

Analysis (Nursing Diagnoses)

A. Ineffective airway clearance related to . . .

B. Ineffective breathing pattern related to . . .

C. Risk for injury related to . . .

D. Impaired physical mobility related to . . .

E. Risk for imbalanced nutrition: less than body requirements related to . . .

Nursing Plans and Interventions

A. If hospitalized, have tracheostomy kit available at bedside for possible myasthenic crisis.

B. Reinforce the teaching plan about the importance of wearing a medic alert bracelet.

C. Administer cholinergic drugs as prescribed (Table 4-32, *Treatment of Myasthenia Gravis*).

TABLE 4-32 Treatment of Myasthenia Gravis

Drug	Indications	Adverse Reactions	Nursing Implications
• Pyridostig-mine bromide (Mestinon)	• Inhibits the action of cholinesterase at the cholinergic nerve endings • To promote accumulation of acetylcholine at cholinergic receptor sites	• Cholinergic crisis can occur with overdose	• Atropine is antidote for drug-induced bradycardia • Take drug with milk/food to decrease GI side effects • Dosage regulation required; record keeping; side effects, drug response • Observe for symptoms of cholinergic crisis: →Fasciculations →Abdominal cramps, diarrhea, incontinence of stool or urine →Hypotension, bradycardia, respiratory depression →Lacrimation, blurred vision • Drug therapy is lifelong and requires family teaching and support

D. Schedule nursing activities to conserve energy—that is, complete daily hygiene activities, administration of medications, and treatments all at once, and allow rest periods. Plan activities during high-energy times, often in the early morning.
E. Instruct client to avoid situations that produce fatigue or physical/emotional stress (any type of stress can exacerbate symptoms).

HESI Hint • Bed rest often relieves symptoms. Bladder and respiratory infections are often a recurring problem. Remember need for health promotion teaching and reinforcement of teaching.

F. Encourage coughing and deep breathing every 4 to 6 hours. (Muscle weakness limits ability to cough up secretions, promotes upper respiratory infection [URI].)
G. If symptoms worsen, identify type of crisis: myasthenic or cholinergic crisis.

HESI Hint • Myasthenic crisis is associated with a positive edrophonium (Tensilon) test, whereas a cholinergic crisis is associated with a negative test.

Parkinson's Disease

Description: Parkinson's disease is a disorder affecting movement involving the basal ganglia and substantia nigra.

Nursing Assessment (Data Collection)
A. Rigidity of extremities
B. Mask-like facial expressions with associated difficulty in chewing, swallowing, and speaking
C. Drooling
D. Stooped posture and slow, shuffling gait
E. Tremors at rest, "pill rolling" movement
F. Emotional lability

HESI Hint • NCLEX-PN questions often focus on the features of Parkinson's disease: tremors (a coarse tremor of fingers and thumb on one hand that disappears during sleep and purposeful activity—also called "pill-rolling"), rigidity, hypertonicity, and stooped posture. Focus: SAFETY!

Analysis (Nursing Diagnoses)
A. Self-care deficit (specify) related to . . .
B. Impaired physical mobility related to . . .

C. Imbalanced nutrition: less than body requirements related to . . .
D. Impaired verbal communication related to . . .
E. Disturbed body image related to . . .

Nursing Plans and Interventions
A. Schedule activities later in the day to allow sufficient time for client to perform self-care activities without rushing.
B. Encourage activities and exercise. A cane or walker may be needed.
C. Eliminate environmental noise, and encourage the client to speak slowly and clearly, pausing at intervals.
D. Serve soft diet that is easy to swallow.
E. Administer antiparkinsonian drugs as prescribed (Table 4-33, *Antiparkinsonian Drugs*).

HESI Hint • An important aspect of Parkinson's treatment is drug therapy. Because the pathophysiology involves an imbalance between acetylcholine and dopamine, symptoms can be controlled by administering dopamine precursor (Levodopa).

Guillain-Barré Syndrome

Description: Guillain-Barré syndrome is a clinical syndrome of unknown origin involving peripheral and cranial nerves.
A. Usually preceded by a viral respiratory or gastrointestinal infection 1 to 4 weeks before the onset of neurologic deficits.
B. Constant monitoring of clients is required to prevent the life-threatening problem of acute respiratory failure.
C. Full recovery usually occurs within several months to a year after onset of symptoms.
D. About 10% to 20% of those diagnosed with Guillain-Barré syndrome are left with a residual disability. Death occurs in 5%.

Nursing Assessment (Data Collection)
A. Paresthesia (tingling and numbness)
B. Muscle weakness of legs progressing to the upper extremities, trunk, and face
C. Paralysis of the ocular, facial, and oropharyngeal muscles, causing marked difficulty in talking, chewing, and swallowing. Assess for the following:
  1. Breathlessness while talking
  2. Shallow and irregular breathing
  3. Use of accessory muscles while breathing
  4. Any change in respiratory pattern
  5. Paradoxic inward movement of the upper abdominal wall while in a supine position,

TABLE 4-33 **Antiparkinsonian Drugs**

Drugs	Indications	Adverse Reactions	Nursing Implications
Anticholinergics (Parasympatholytics)			
• Atropine sulfate (Atropisol) • Benztropine mesylate (Cogentin)	• Used to treat secondary cholinergic symptoms, such as drooling, sweating, tremors.	• Increased heart rate • Postural hypotension • Dry mouth • Constipation • Urinary retention	• Review client's history for glaucoma, urinary obstruction • Warn to avoid rapid position changes • Avoid extreme heat • Provide gum, hard candy, and frequent mouth care
Dopamine Agonist			
• Levodopa (Dopar) • Levodopa-carbidopa (Sinemet) Dopamine-releasing agents • Amantadine HCL (Symmetrel) Dopamine-receptor agonists • Bromocriptine mesylate (Parlodel) • Pramipexole (Mirapex) • Ropinirole (Requip)	• Stimulate dopamine production or increase sensitivity of dopamine receptors • Newer drugs require lower dosage	• Involuntary movements • Nausea • Vomiting	• Explain drugs may take months to achieve desired effects • Warn to avoid sudden position changes • Avoid foods high in vitamin B_6 (meats, liver—that is, high-protein foods) • If insomnia occurs, suggest taking last dose earlier in day • May initially cause drowsiness; teach to avoid driving until response is determined
Monoamine Oxidase Type B Inhibitor			
• Selegiline (Eldepryl) • Rasaliline (Azilect)	• Used with dopamine agonist when client symptoms do not respond	• Confusion, dizziness • Nausea, dry mouth • Insomnia	• Review drug–drug interaction carefully • Not an option if client on antidepressants (SSRIs or tricyclics)
Catechol-O-methyl Transferase (COMT) Inhibitor			
• Entacapone (Comtan) • Talcapone (Tasmar)	• Used with levodopa-carbidopa	• May increase levodopa-carbidopa side effects, including dyskinesias	• Levadopa dose may need to be decreased • Combination product may decrease pill burden

indicating weakness and impending paralysis of the diaphragm

D. Increasing pulse rate and disturbances in rhythm

E. Transient hypertension, orthostatic hypotension

F. Possible pain in the back and in calves of legs

G. Weakness or paralysis of the intercostal and diaphragm muscles may develop quickly.

Analysis (Nursing Diagnoses)

A. Ineffective breathing pattern related to . . .

B. Imbalanced nutrition: less than body requirements related to . . .

C. Impaired verbal communication related to . . .

Nursing Plans and Interventions

A. Monitor for respiratory distress and initiate mechanical ventilation if necessary.

B. See Nursing Plans and Interventions for the Unconscious/Immobilized Client.

Stroke/Brain Attack: Cerebral Vascular Accident (CVA)

Description: Stroke/brain attack: cerebral vascular accident (CVA) is the sudden loss of brain function resulting from a disruption of the blood supply to a part of the brain. Classified as thrombotic or hemorrhagic.

HESI Hint • CNS INVOLVEMENT RELATED TO CAUSE OF CVA

• Hemorrhagic—caused by a slow or fast hemorrhage into the brain tissue—often related to hypertension or ruptured aneurysm.

• Embolytic—caused by a clot that has broken away from some vessel and has lodged in one of the arteries of the brain, blocking the blood supply. It is often related to atherosclerosis and may recur.

A. Risk factors include the following:
1. Hypertension
2. Previous transient ischemic attacks
3. Cardiac disease: atherosclerosis, valve disease, history of dysrhythmias (particularly atrial flutter/fibrillation)
4. Advanced age
5. Diabetes
6. Oral contraceptives and hormone replacement therapy
7. Smoking
8. Alcohol: more than two drinks per day

HESI Hint • Atrial flutter/fibrillation has a high incidence of thrombus formation following dysrhythmia because of turbulence of blood flow through all valves/heart chambers.

B. Diagnosis is made by observation of clinical signs and confirmed by:
1. Cranial computed tomography (CT) scan
2. Magnetic resonance imaging (MRI)
3. Doppler flow studies
4. Ultrasound imaging
C. Presenting symptoms will relate to the specific area of the brain that has been damaged (Table 4-34, *Location of Disruption*).
D. Most common effects:
1. Motor loss, usually exhibited as hemiparesis or hemiplegia

2. Communication loss exhibited as dysarthria, dysphasia, aphasia, or apraxia
3. Perceptual disturbance that can be visual, spatial, and/or sensory
4. Impaired mental acuity or psychologic changes such as decreased attention span, memory loss, depression, lability, and hostility
E. Bladder dysfunction—may be either incontinence or retention
F. Rehabilitation is begun as soon as the client is stable.

HESI Hint • A woman who had a stroke 2 days ago has left-sided paralysis. She has begun to regain some movement in her left side. What can the nurse tell the family about the client's recovery period? "The quicker movement is recovered, the better the prognosis is for more or full recovery. She will need patience and understanding from her family as she tries to cope with the stroke. Mood swings can be expected during the recovery period, and bouts of depression and tearfulness are likely."

Nursing Assessment (Data Collection)

A. Change in level of consciousness
B. Paresthesia, paralysis
C. Aphasia, agraphia
D. Memory loss
E. Vision impairment
F. Bladder and bowel dysfunction
G. Behavioral changes

TABLE 4-34 Location of Disruption

Feature	Left Hemisphere	Right Hemisphere
• Language	• Aphasia • Agraphia	• May be alert and oriented
• Memory	• No deficit	• Disoriented • Cannot recognize faces
• Vision	• Unable to discriminate words and letters • Reading problems • Deficits in right visual field	• Visual/spatial deficits • Neglect of left visual fields • Loss of depth perception
• Behavior	• Slow • Cautious • Anxious when attempting a new task • Depression or catastrophic response to illness • Sense of guilt • Feeling of worthlessness • Worries over future • Quick anger and frustration	• Impulsive • Unaware of neurologic deficits • Confabulates • Euphoric • Constantly smiles • Denies illness • Poor judgment • Overestimates abilities • Impaired sense of humor
• Hearing	• No deficit	• Loses ability to hear tonal variations

H. Observe and report client's functional abilities, including:
  1. Mobility
  2. Activities of daily living (ADL)
  3. Elimination
  4. Communication
I. Collect data on the client's ability to swallow, eat, and drink without aspiration.

Analysis (Nursing Diagnoses)

A. Impaired physical mobility related to . . .
B. Self-care deficit (specify) related to . . .
C. Impaired urinary elimination related to . . .
D. Impaired verbal communication related to . . .
E. Ineffective coping related to . . .
F. Ineffective family coping related to . . .
G. Disturbed body image related to . . .

HESI Hint • **WORDS THAT DESCRIBE LOSSES FOR CVA**

1. **Apraxia:** inability to perform purposed movements in the absence of motor problems
2. **Dysarthria:** difficulty articulating
3. **Dysphasia:** impairment of speech and verbal comprehension
4. **Aphasia:** loss of the ability to speak
5. **Agraphia:** loss of the ability to write
6. **Alexia:** loss of the ability to read
7. **Dysphagia:** dysfunctional swallowing

Nursing Plans and Interventions

A. Control hypertension to help prevent future CVA.
B. Maintain proper body alignment while in bed. Use splints or other assistive devices (including bedrolls and pillows) to maintain functional position.
C. Position client to minimize edema, prevent contractures, and maintain skin integrity.
D. Perform full ROM four times a day. Follow up with program initiated by other team members.

E. Encourage client to participate in or manage own personal care.
F. Set realistic goals; add new tasks daily.
G. Include self-care activities for the hemiparetic person:
  1. Bathing
  2. Brushing teeth
  3. Shaving with electric razor
  4. Eating
  5. Combing hair
H. Encourage client to assist with dressing activities and modify them as necessary (client will wear street clothes during waking hours).
I. Monitor bladder elimination pattern.
  1. Offer bedpan or urinal according to client's particular pattern of elimination.
  2. Bladder control tends to be regained quickly.
J. Assist with follow-up speech program initiated by the speech/language therapist.
  1. Ensure consistency with this program.
  2. Reassure the client that regaining speech is a very slow process.
K. Do not cause sensory overload for the client—that is, give only one set of instructions at a time.
L. Encourage total family involvement in rehabilitation.
M. Encourage client/family to join a support group.
N. Encourage family members to allow the client to perform self-care activities as outlined by the rehabilitation team.
O. Coordinate outpatient follow-up or home health care.
P. Swallowing modifications may include pureed/soft diet, thickened liquids, and head positioning.

HESI Hint • Steroids are administered after a stroke to decrease cerebral edema and retard permanent disability. H_2 inhibitors are administered to prevent peptic ulcers.

Review of Neurosensory/Neurologic Systems

1. What are the classifications of the commonly prescribed eyedrops for glaucoma?
2. Identify two types of hearing loss.
3. Write four nursing interventions for the care of the blind person and four nursing interventions for the care of the deaf person.
4. In your own words, describe the Glasgow Coma Scale.
5. List four nursing diagnoses for the comatose client in order of priority. (Remember Maslow's Hierarchy of Needs to help you determine priority.)
6. State four independent nursing interventions to maintain adequate respirations, airway, and oxygenation in the unconscious client.
7. Who is at risk for cerebral vascular accidents?

8. Complications of immobility include the potential for thrombus development. State three nursing interventions to prevent thrombi.

9. List four rationales for the appearance of restlessness in the unconscious client.

10. What nursing interventions prevent corneal drying in a comatose client?

11. When can a comatose client on IV hyperalimentation begin to receive tube feedings instead?

12. What is the most important principle in a bowel management program for a neurologic client?

13. Define *cerebral vascular accident*.

14. A client with a diagnosis of CVA presents with symptoms of aphasia, right hemiparesis, but no memory or hearing deficit. In what hemisphere has the client suffered a lesion?

15. What are the symptoms of spinal shock?

16. What are the symptoms of autonomic dysreflexia?

17. What is the most important indicator of increased ICP?

18. What vital sign changes are indicative of increased ICP?

19. A neighbor calls the neighborhood nurse stating that he was knocked hard to the floor by his very hyperactive dog. He is wondering what symptoms would indicate the need to visit an emergency room. What should the nurse tell him to do?

20. What activities and situations should be avoided that increase ICP?

21. How do hyperosmotic agents (osmotic diuretics) that are used to treat intracranial pressure act?

22. Why should narcotics be avoided in clients with neurologic impairment?

23. Headache and vomiting are symptoms of many disorders. What characteristics of these symptoms would alert the nurse to refer a client to a neurologist?

24. How should the head of the bed be positioned for postcraniotomy clients with infratentorial lesions?

25. Is multiple sclerosis thought to occur because of an autoimmune process?

26. Is paralysis always a consequence of spinal cord injury?

27. What types of drugs are used in the treatment of myasthenia gravis?

Answers to Review

1. Parasympathomimetics for pupillary constriction, beta-adrenergic receptor-blocking agents to inhibit formation of aqueous humor, carbonic anhydrase inhibitors to reduce aqueous humor production, and prostaglandin agonists to increase aqueous humor outflow.

2. Conductive (transmission of sound to inner ear is blocked) and sensorineural (damage to eighth cranial nerve).

3. *Care of the blind client:* announce presence clearly, call by name, orient carefully to surroundings, guide by walking in front of client with his or her hand on your elbow. *Care of the deaf client:* reduce distraction before beginning conversation, look at and listen to client, give client full attention if he or she is a lip reader, face client directly.

4. An objective assessment of the level of consciousness based on a score of 3 to 15, with scores of 7 or less indicative of coma.

5. Ineffective breathing pattern, ineffective airway clearance, impaired gas exchange, and decreased cardiac output.

6. Position for maximum ventilation (prone or semiprone and slightly to one side), insert airway if tongue is obstructing; suction airway efficiently; monitor arterial Po_2 and Pco_2; and hyperventilate with 100% oxygen before suctioning.

7. Persons with history of hypertension, previous TIAs, cardiac disease (atrial flutter/fibrillation), diabetes, oral contraceptive use, and older adults.

8. Frequent range-of-motion exercises, frequent (every 2 hours) position changes, and avoidance of positions that decrease venous return.

9. Anoxia, distended bladder, covert bleeding, or a return to consciousness.

10. Irrigation of eyes as needed with sterile prescribed solution, application of ophthalmic ointment (every 8 hours), close assessment for corneal ulceration drying.

11. When peristalsis resumes, as evidenced by active bowel sounds; passage of flatus or bowel movement.

12. Establishment of regularity.

13. A disruption of blood supply to a part of the brain, which results in sudden loss of brain function.

14. Left.

15. Hypotension, bladder and bowel distention, total paralysis, and lack of sensation below lesion.

16. Hypertension, bladder and bowel distention, exaggerated autonomic responses, headache, sweating, goose bumps, and bradycardia.

17. A change in the level of responsiveness.

18. Increased BP, widening pulse pressure, increased or decreased pulse, respiratory irregularities, and temperature increase.

19. Call his health care provider now and inform him or her of the fall. Symptoms needing medical attention would include vertigo, confusion, or any subtle behavioral change; headache; vomiting; ataxia (imbalance); or seizure.

20. Change in bed position, extreme hip flexion, endotracheal suctioning, compression of jugular veins, coughing, vomiting, or straining of any kind.

21. Dehydrate the brain and reduce cerebral edema by holding water in the renal tubules to prevent reabsorption and by drawing fluid from the extravascular spaces into the plasma.

22. Narcotics mask the level of responsiveness as well as pupillary response.

23. Headache that is more severe upon awakening and vomiting not associated with nausea are symptoms of a brain tumor.

24. Supratentorial—elevated; infratentorial—flat.

25. Yes.

26. No.

27. Anticholinesterase drugs, which inhibit the action of cholinesterase at the nerve endings to promote the accumulation of acetylcholine at receptor sites, which should improve neuronal transmission to muscles.

Hematology/Oncology

Anemia

Description: Anemia is a deficiency of erythrocytes (red blood cells [RBCs]) reflected as decreased hematocrit (Hct), hemoglobin (Hgb), and RBCs.

Nursing Assessment (Data Collection)

A. Pallor, especially of the face (around the eyes) and nail beds; palmar crease; conjunctiva
B. Fatigue, exercise intolerance, lethargy, orthostatic hypotension
C. Tachycardia, heart murmurs, heart failure
D. Signs of bleeding such as hematuria, melena, menorrhagia
E. Dyspnea
F. Irritability, difficulty concentrating
G. Cool skin, cold intolerance
H. Risk factors:
   1. Diet lacking in iron, folate, and/or vitamin B_{12}
   2. Family history of genetic diseases such as sickle cell or congenital hemolytic anemia
   3. Medication history of anemia-producing drugs, such as salicylates, and thiazide diuretics
   4. Exposure to toxic agents such as lead or insecticides
I. Diagnostic tests indicate abnormally low results:
   1. Hgb below 10 g/dL
   2. Hct below 36%
   3. RBCs below 4×10^{12}
   4. Bone marrow aspiration positive for anemia
J. Blood loss, either acute or chronic
K. Medical history of kidney disorders

Analysis (Nursing Diagnoses)

A. Activity intolerance related to . . .
B. Anxiety related to . . .
C. Ineffective tissue perfusion (specify) related to . . .

Nursing Plans and Interventions

A. In accord with the scope of practice for the PN and agency guidelines, assist RN with administration of blood products as prescribed and monitor client's response to therapy (see Chapter 3, *Advanced Clinical Concepts*, p. 29, and Table 3-4, *Administration of Blood Products*, p. 31).
B. Alternate periods of activity with periods of rest
C. Reinforce diet teaching to include the following:
   1. Instruct in food selection and preparation to maximize intake:
      a. Iron (red meats, organ meats, whole wheat products, spinach, carrots)
      b. Folic acid (green vegetables, liver, citrus fruits)
      c. Vitamin B_{12} (glandular meats, yeast, green leafy vegetables, milk, and cheese)
   2. Reinforce teaching regarding need for vitamin/mineral supplements:
      a. Take iron on an empty stomach to enhance absorption, 1 hour before meals or 2 hours after meals. Give vitamin C to enhance absorption of iron.
      b. Give liquid iron through a straw, with oral care afterward, to prevent discoloring of teeth.
      c. Inform client that iron (oral) may turn stools black.
D. If parenteral iron is required, use Z-track method for administration to prevent staining of the skin (Table 4-35, *Administration of Iron*).

TABLE 4-35 Administration of Iron

Do's	Don'ts
• Use Z-track method of administration. • Use air bubble to avoid withdrawing medication into subcutaneous tissue.	• Do NOT use deltoid muscle. • Do NOT massage injection site.

E. Coordinate the referral process for genetic information if client has sickle cell or congenital hemolytic anemia.

F. Sickle cell crisis is precipitated by hypoxia:
1. Provide pain relief.
2. Provide adequate hydration.
3. Teach client to avoid activities that cause hypoxia.

G. Inform the client to report any unusual bleeding to health care professional

Leukemia

Description: Leukemia is malignant neoplasm of the blood-forming organs.

A. Leukemia is characterized by an abnormal overproduction of immature forms of any of the leukocytes. There is an interference with normal blood production, resulting in decreased erythrocytes and decreased platelets.
1. Anemia results from decreased RBC production and blood loss.
2. Immunosuppression occurs because of the large number of immature white blood cells or profound neutropenia.
3. Hemorrhage occurs because of thrombocytopenia.

B. Exact etiology of leukemia is unknown, but identified precipitating factors include:
1. Genetic abnormalities
2. Ionizing radiation (therapeutic or atomic)
3. Viral infections (human T cells, leukemia virus)
4. Exposure to certain chemicals or drugs
   a. Benzene
   b. Alkylating chemotherapeutic agents
   c. Immunosuppressants
   d. Chloramphenicol
   e. Phenylbutazone

C. Incidence is highest in children 3 to 4 years of age; declines until age 35, and then a steady increase occurs.

D. Diagnosis of leukemia is made by biopsy, bone marrow aspiration, lumbar puncture, and frequent blood counts.

E. Leukemia is treated with antineoplastics chemotherapy.

Types of Leukemia

A. Acute myelogenous leukemia
1. Inability of leukocytes to mature; those that do are abnormal.
2. Occurs throughout the life cycle.
3. Onset is insidious.
4. Prognosis is poor, 5-year survival of 20% overall, 50% for children.
5. Cause of death tends to be overwhelming infection.

B. Chronic myelogenous leukemia
1. Results from abnormal production of granulocytic cells.
2. Is a biphasic disease.
3. Chronic stage lasts approximately 3 years.
4. Acute phase tends to last 2 to 3 months.

5. Occurs in young to middle-aged adults.
6. Known causes include:
   a. Ionizing radiation
   b. Chemical exposure
7. Poor prognosis, 5-year survival rate of 37%—consecutive treatment if no allergenic transplant.

C. Acute lymphocytic leukemia
1. Abnormal leukocytes in blood-forming tissue.
2. Occurs in children (most common childhood cancer).
3. Favorable prognosis, 80% of children treated live 5 years or longer.

D. Chronic lymphocytic leukemia
1. Increased production of leukocytes and lymphocytes and proliferation of cells within the bone marrow, spleen, and liver.
2. Occurs after the age of 35, often in older adults.
3. Five-year survival rate of 73% overall.
4. Most clients are asymptomatic and are not treated.

> **HESI Hint** • A 24-year-old is admitted with large areas of ecchymosis on both upper and lower extremities. She is diagnosed with acute myelogenous leukemia. What are the expected laboratory findings for this client and what is the expected treatment?
> *Lab:* decreased Hgb, decreased Hct, decreased platelet count, altered WBC (usually quite high).
> *Treatment:* prevention of infection; prevention and/or control of bleeding; high-protein, high-calorie diet; assistance with ADL; drug therapy.

> **HESI Hint** • The care of the client with cancer by the practical nurse (PN) should be in accord with agency policy and the scope of practice for the PN.

Nursing Assessment (Data Collection)

A. Tendency to bleed:
1. Petechiae
2. Nosebleeds
3. Bleeding gums
4. Ecchymosis
5. Nonhealing skin abrasions

B. Anemia:
1. Fatigue
2. Pallor
3. Headache
4. Bone and joint pain
5. Hepatosplenomegaly

C. Infection:
1. Fever
2. Tachycardia
3. Lymphadenopathy (swollen lymph nodes)

4. Night sweats
5. Skin infection, poor healing
D. GI distress:
   1. Anorexia
   2. Weight loss
   3. Sore throat
   4. Abdominal pain
   5. Diarrhea
   6. Oral lesions, typically thrush

> **HESI Hint** • Infection in the immunosuppressed person may not be manifested with an elevated temperature. It is imperative, therefore, that the nurse performs a total and thorough assessment of the client frequently.

Analysis (Nursing Diagnoses)

A. Risk for infection related to . . .
B. Risk for injury related to . . .
C. Fatigue related to . . .
D. Anxiety related to . . .

Nursing Plans and Interventions for Immunosuppressed Clients and/or Clients with Bone Marrow Suppression

A. Monitor WBC count daily and inform health care provider of count.
B. Routinely examine oral cavity and genital area for signs of infection.
C. Monitor vital signs frequently:
   1. Note baseline.
   2. Report fever to health care provider as requested.
      a. Parameters for reporting tend to be lower than those of postoperative clients.
      b. Usually report temperatures of 100.5° F.
D. Administer antibiotics as prescribed, maintaining a strict schedule.
E. Notify health care provider if delay in administration occurs.
   1. Obtain trough and peak blood levels of antibiotics.
      a. Trough: draw blood sample shortly before administration of antibiotic.
      b. Peak: draw blood sample 30 minutes to 1 hour after administration of drug.
   2. Monitor blood levels of antibiotics for therapeutic dose range.
F. Reinforce family/client teaching about the importance of infection control.
   1. Wash hands using good hand-washing technique.
   2. Avoid contact with any infected person.
   3. Avoid crowds.
   4. Maintain daily hygiene to prevent spread of microorganisms.
   5. Avoid eating uncooked foods because they contain bacteria.
   6. Avoid water standing in cups, vases, and so forth because these are an excellent source of growth medium for microorganisms.
   7. Neutropenic and reverse isolation precautions PRN.
G. Institute an oral hygiene regimen.
   1. Use soft-bristle toothbrush to avoid bleeding gums.
   2. Use salt and baking soda mouth rinse.
   3. Perform oral hygiene after each meal and at bedtime.
   4. Lubricate lips with water-soluble gel.
   5. Avoid lemon-glycerin swabs; they dry oral mucosa.
H. Encourage coughing and deep breathing to prevent stasis of secretions in lungs.
I. Avoid rectal thermometers and suppositories to prevent further bleeding.
J. Monitor fluid status and balance; febrile clients dehydrate rapidly.
   1. Monitor I&O.
   2. Encourage fluid intake of at least 3 liters/day.
K. Encourage mobility to decrease pulmonary stasis.

> **HESI Hint** • Most oncologic drugs cause immunosuppression. Prevention of secondary infections is vital. Advise client to stay away from persons with known infections such as colds. In the hospital, maintain an environment as sterile and as clean as possible. These persons should not eat raw vegetables or fruits— only those that have been cooked to destroy any bacteria.

L. Protect the client from bleeding and injury.
   1. Handle the client gently.
   2. Avoid needle sticks. Use smallest-gauge needle possible, and apply pressure for 10 minutes after needle sticks.
   3. Encourage use of electric razor only for shaving.
   4. Instruct client to avoid blowing or picking nose.
   5. Assess for signs of bleeding.
   6. Avoid use of salicylates.

Hodgkin's Disease

Description: Hodgkin's disease is a malignancy of the lymphoid system that initiates in a single lymph node.

A. Hodgkin's disease is characterized by a generalized painless lymphadenopathy.
B. Incidence is higher in males and young adults.
C. Etiology is unknown.
D. Prognosis is good: 5-year survival rate of 90%; however, late recurrences after 5 to 10 years are not uncommon.
E. Diagnosis is made by excision of node for biopsy; characteristic cell called Reed-Stemberg.

F. Determination of stage of disease is done by surgical laparotomy.
   1. Stage I: involvement of single lymph node region or a single extralymphatic organ or site.
   2. Stage II: involvement of two or more lymph nodes on the same side of the diaphragm or localized involvement of an extralymphatic organ or site.
   3. Stage III: involvement of lymph node areas on both sides of the diaphragm to localized involvement of one extralymphatic organ, the spleen, or both.
   4. Stage IV: diffuse involvement of one or more extralymphatic organs with or without lymph node involvement.
G. Treatment:
   1. Radiotherapy
   2. Chemotherapy: nitrogen mustard, Adriamycin, vincristine, prednisone

Nursing Assessment (Data Collection)

A. Enlarged lymph nodes (one or more), usually cervical lymph nodes
B. Anemia, thrombocytopenia, elevated leukocytes, decreased platelets
C. Fever, increased susceptibility to infections
D. Anorexia, weight loss
E. Malaise, bone pain
F. Night sweats
G. Pruritus
H. Pain in affected lymph node after consuming alcohol

Analysis (Nursing Diagnoses)

A. Risk for infection related to . . .
B. Anxiety related to . . .
C. Imbalanced nutrition: less than body requirements related to . . .
D. Ineffective peripheral tissue perfusion related to . . .

Nursing Plans and Interventions

A. Protect from infection, monitor temperature carefully.
B. Observe for signs of anemia.
C. Provide adequate rest.
D. Provide preoperative and postoperative care for laparotomy and/or splenectomy.
E. Encourage high-nutrient foods.
F. Provide emotional support to client and family.

HESI Hint • Hodgkin's disease is one of the most curable of all adult malignancies. Emotional support is vital. Career development is often interrupted for treatment. Chemotherapy renders many male clients sterile. They may bank sperm before treatment, if desired.

General Oncology Content

A. Oncology terms:
   1. Cancer: disease characterized by uncontrolled growth of abnormal cells
   2. Neoplasm: new formation of tissue
   3. Carcinoma: malignant tumor arising from epithelial tissue
   4. Sarcoma: malignant tumor arising from nonepithelial tissue
   5. Differentiation: degree to which neoplastic tissue is different from parent tissue
   6. Metastasis: spread of cancer from the original site to other parts of the body
   7. Adjuvant therapy: supplemental therapy to the primary therapy
   8. Palliative procedure: relieves symptoms without curing the cause
B. Tumors identified by tissue of origin:
   1. Adeno: glandular tissue
   2. Angio: blood vessels
   3. Basal cell: epithelium (sun-exposed areas)
   4. Embryonal: gonads
   5. Fibro: fibrous tissue
   6. Lympho: lymphoid tissue
   7. Melano: pigmented cells of epithelium
   8. Myo: muscle tissue
   9. Osteo: bone
   10. Squamous cell: epithelium
C. Seven warning signs of cancer:
   1. Change in usual bowel and bladder function
   2. A sore that does not heal
   3. Unusual bleeding or discharge, hematuria, tarry stools, ecchymosis, bleeding mole
   4. Thickening or a lump in the breast or elsewhere
   5. Indigestion or dysphagia
   6. Obvious changes in a wart or mole
   7. Nagging cough or hoarseness

Review of Hematology/Oncology

1. List three potential causes of anemia.
2. Write two nursing diagnoses for the client suffering from anemia.
3. What is the only intravenous fluid compatible with blood products?
4. What actions should the nurse take if a hemolytic transfusion reaction occurs?

5. List three interventions for clients with a tendency to bleed.
6. Identify two sites that should be assessed for infection in immunosuppressed clients.
7. Name three food sources of vitamin B_{12}.
8. List three safety precautions for the administration of antineoplastic chemotherapy.
9. Describe the method of collecting the trough and peak blood levels of antibiotics.
10. List four nursing interventions for care of the client with Hodgkin's disease.
11. List four topics you would cover when assisting an RN with a teaching plan about infection control for an immunosuppressed client.

Answers to Review

1. Diet lacking in iron, folate, and/or vitamin B_{12}; use of salicylates, thiazides, diuretics; exposure to toxic agents such as lead or insecticides.
2. Activity intolerance and ineffective tissue perfusion.
3. Normal saline.
4. Turn off transfusion. Take temperature. Send blood being transfused to lab. Obtain urine sample. Keep vein patent with normal saline.
5. Use a soft toothbrush; avoid salicylates; do not use suppositories.
6. Oral cavity and genital area.
7. Glandular meats (liver), milk, green leafy vegetables.
8. Double-check order with another nurse. Check for blood return before administration to ensure that medication does not go into tissue. Use a new IV site daily for peripheral chemotherapy. Wear gloves when handling the drugs, and dispose of waste in special containers to avoid contact with toxic substances.
9. *Collection of trough:* draw blood 30 minutes before administration of antibiotic. *Collection of peak:* draw blood 30 minutes after administration of antibiotic.
10. Protect from infection. Observe for anemia. Encourage high-nutrient foods. Provide emotional support to client and family.
11. Hand-washing technique. Avoid infected persons. Avoid crowds. Maintain daily hygiene to prevent spread of microorganisms.

Reproductive System

Benign Tumors of the Uterus: Leiomyomas (Fibroids, Myomas, Fibromyomas, Fibromas)

Description: Benign tumors arising from the muscle tissue of the uterus.
A. Benign tumors are more common in black women than in white women.
B. Benign tumors are more common in women who have never been pregnant.
C. Most common symptom is abnormal uterine bleeding.
D. Tend to disappear after menopause.
E. Rarely become malignant.
F. Intervention for severe symptoms is hysterectomy:
   1. Vaginal hysterectomy
   2. Abdominal hysterectomy

Nursing Assessment (Data Collection)

A. Menorrhagia (hypermenorrhea: profuse or prolonged menstrual bleeding)
B. Dysmenorrhea (extremely painful menstrual periods)
C. Uterine enlargement
D. Low back pain and pelvic pain

> **HESI Hint** • Menorrhagia (profuse or prolonged menstrual bleeding) is the most important factor relating to benign uterine tumors. Assess for signs of anemia.

Uterine Prolapse, Cystocele, and Rectocele

Description: Uterine prolapse is downward displacement of the uterus. Cystocele is the relaxation of the anterior vaginal wall with prolapse of the bladder. Rectocele is the relaxation of the posterior vaginal wall with prolapse of the rectum.
A. Preventive measures:
   1. Postpartum perineal exercises
   2. Spaced pregnancies
   3. Weight control
B. Nonsurgical intervention (for uterine prolapse):
   1. Kegel exercises
   2. Knee-chest position
   3. Pessary use
C. Surgical intervention:
   1. Hysterectomy for complete prolapse
   2. Anterior and posterior vaginal repair (A&P repair)

> **HESI Hint** • What is the anatomic significance of a prolapsed uterus? When the uterus is displaced, it impinges on other structures in the lower abdomen. The bladder, rectum, and small intestine can protrude through the vaginal wall.

Nursing Assessment (Data Collection)

A. Predisposing conditions:
  1. Multiparity
  2. Pelvic tearing during childbirth
  3. Vaginal muscle weakness associated with aging
  4. Obesity
B. Symptoms associated with uterine prolapse:
  1. Dysmenorrhea
  2. Dragging sensation in pelvis and back
  3. Dyspareunia
C. Symptoms associated with cystocele:
  1. Incontinence or stress incontinence (dribbling with coughing or sneezing or any activity that increases intraabdominal pressure)
  2. Urinary retention
  3. Bladder infections (cystitis)
D. Symptoms associated with rectocele:
  1. Constipation
  2. Hemorrhoids
  3. Sense of pressure or need to defecate

Analysis (Nursing Diagnoses)

A. Pain related to . . .
B. Deficient knowledge (specify) related to . . .
C. Disturbed body image related to . . .

Nursing Plans and Interventions for Hysterectomy

A. Provide pre- and postoperative care (see Perioperative Care in Chapter 3, *Advanced Clinical Concepts,* p. 46).
B. Administer enema and douche as prescribed preoperatively.
C. Note amount and character of vaginal discharge. Postoperatively, there should be less than one saturated pad in 4 hours.
D. Avoid rectal thermometers or tubes, especially when A&P repair has been performed.
E. Check extremities for warmth and/or tenderness as indicators of thrombophlebitis.
F. Pain management postoperatively:
  1. Monitor character of pain and determine appropriate analgesic.
  2. Administer analgesics as needed and determine effectiveness.
G. Encourage ambulation as soon as possible.
H. Monitor urinary output (Foley catheter is usually inserted in surgery).
I. After catheter removal, monitor voiding patterns, catheterize every 6 to 8 hours if unable to void.
J. Observe incision for bleeding.
K. Abdominal distention may be a sign of gas (flatus) or internal bleeding.
L. Gradually increase diet from liquids to general.
M. Provide stool softeners before first bowel movement and thereafter as needed.
N. Reinforce instructions to client about follow-up care.
  1. Limit tampon use.
  2. Avoid douching.
  3. Refrain from intercourse until approved by health care provider (usually 3 to 6 weeks).
  4. Avoid heavy lifting (6 to 8 lb) or heavy housework for 4 to 6 weeks postoperatively.
O. Maintain adequate fluid intake (3 liters/day).
P. Notify health care provider of complications:
  1. Elevated temperature above 101° F
  2. Redness, pain, or swelling of suture line
Q. Encourage verbalization of feelings, especially with significant others.

Cancer of the Cervix

Description: Of cancers occurring in the cervix, 95% are squamous cell in origin. Some cervical cancers are directly linked to the human papillomavirus (HPV). Young women (between the ages of 9 and 26 years of age) are encouraged to be immunized with an intramuscular (IM) injection of quadrivalent human papillomavirus (types 6, 11, 16, 18) recombinant vaccine (Gardasil). All women should be tested for HPV.

A. Cancer of the cervix is easily detected early with the Papanicolaou test.
B. The precursor to cancer of the cervix is dysplasia.
C. Cancer of the cervix is subdivided into three stages:
  1. Early dysplasia can be treated in a variety of ways, including:
    a. Cryosurgery
    b. LEEP (Loop Electrocautery Excision Procedure)
    c. Laser
    d. Conization
    e. Hysterectomy

> **HESI Hint** • Laser therapy or cryosurgery is used to treat cervical cancer when the lesion is small and localized. Invasive cancer is treated with radiation, conization, hysterectomy, or pelvic exenteration (a drastic surgical procedure where the uterus, ovaries, fallopian tubes, vagina, rectum, and bladder are removed in an attempt to stop metastasis). Chemotherapy is not useful with this type of cancer.

  2. Early carcinoma can be treated with:
    a. Hysterectomy
    b. Intracavity radiation

3. Late carcinoma (the tumor size and stage of invasion of surrounding tissues increases) treatment often includes:
   a. External beam radiation along with hysterectomy
   b. Antineoplastic chemotherapy is of limited use for cancers arising from squamous cells.
   c. Pelvic exenteration

> **HESI Hint** • American College of Obstetricians and Gynecologists (ACOG) 2009 recommendations: Pap smears should begin at age 21, and women younger than 30 should be screened every 2 years; women 30 and older may be screened every 3 years after they have had three consecutive negative cervical cytology tests. Women ages 65 to 70 may stop Pap smears if they have three consecutive normal in a row and no abnormal Pap smears in the last 10 years. Women with high risk factors may need more frequent screenings.

Care of the Client with Radiation Implants

A. Radiation implants are used to treat disease by delivering high-dose radiation directly to the affected tissue.
B. The nurse must take certain precautions for protection of self as well as the client and visitors.
C. Follow specific guidelines provided by the agency. General care guidelines include:
   1. Remind the client that she is not radioactive; only the implants contain radioactivity.
   2. Remind the client that her isolation time is limited; isolation is not necessary indefinitely.
D. Assign client to a private room and place a "Caution: Radioactive Material" sign on the door.
E. Do not permit pregnant caretakers or pregnant visitors into the room.
F. Discourage visits by small children.
G. Keep a lead-lined container in the room for disposal of the implant should it become dislodged.
H. Client should remain in bed with as little movement as possible.
I. Be aware that *all* client secretions have the potential of being radioactive.
J. Wear latex gloves when handling potentially contaminated secretions.
K. Wear a radiation badge when providing care to clients with radiation implants.
   1. Badge is not to be worn out of doors.
   2. Badge is checked at regular intervals by health officials.
L. Provide nursing care in an efficient but caring manner.
   1. Plan care to limit overall time in the client's room.
   2. When in the room, stand at the greatest distances away from the client to minimize exposure.
   3. Stop by to check on the client from the door frequently.
M. Keep all supplies and equipment the client might need within reach.

Ovarian Cancer

Description: Cancer of the ovaries can occur at all ages, including infancy and childhood. Early diagnosis is difficult because no useful screening test exists at present.

Nursing Assessment (Data Collection)

A. Asymptomatic in early stages.
B. Laparotomy is primary tool for diagnosis and staging of the disease; ovarian cancer is surgically staged, rather than clinically staged.
C. Advanced clinical manifestations include:
   1. Pelvic discomfort
   2. Low back pain and leg pain
   3. Weight change
   4. Abdominal pain
   5. Nausea and vomiting
   6. Increased abdominal girth
   7. Constipation
   8. Urinary frequency

> **HESI Hint** • Ovarian cancer is the leading cause of death from gynecologic cancers in the United States. Growth is insidious, so it is not recognized until it is at an advanced stage.

Analysis (Nursing Diagnoses)

A. Anticipatory grieving related to . . .
B. Pain related to . . .
C. Self-care deficit (specify) related to . . .
D. Deficient knowledge (specify) related to . . .

Nursing Plans and Interventions

A. Care required for any major abdominal surgery following laparotomy.
B. Collaborate with RN to develop and implement client/family teaching plan about disease and follow-up treatment.
C. Offer supportive care to client and family throughout diagnosis and treatment.

> **HESI Hint** • The major emphasis in nursing management of cancers of the reproductive tract is early detection.

Breast Cancer

Description: Cancer originating in the breast.
A. Breast cancer is the most commonly occurring cancer in women in the United States.
B. One in eight women will develop breast cancer in her lifetime.

C. Early detection is important to successful treatment.

D. Men can develop breast cancer. They account for less than 1% of reported cases.

E. Of all breast cancers, 90% to 95% are discovered through breast self-examination.

F. Risk factors include:
1. Positive family history
2. Menarche before 12 years of age and/or menopause after age 50
3. Nulliparous, or those with first child after age 30
4. History of uterine cancer
5. Daily alcohol intake
6. Highest incidence in those age 40 to 49 and over 65

G. Breast cancer is generally adenocarcinoma originating in epithelial cells and occurs in the ducts or lobes.

H. Tumors tend to be located in the upper outer quadrant of the breast and more often in the left breast than the right.

I. Early detection is important.
1. Every woman should perform a breast self-examination monthly, preferably as soon as menstrual bleeding ceases or if postmenopausal the same day every month.
2. Mammography is very helpful with early detection of cancer of the breast.
   a. Baseline mammogram at approximately 35 to 40 years of age.
   b. Mammogram every 1 to 2 years for women in their 40s.
   c. Annual mammogram for women over 50 years of age.
   d. Advise not to use lotions, talc powder, or deodorant under arms before procedure (may mimic calcium deposits on x-ray).
3. Physical examination by a professional skilled in examination of the breast should be done annually.

J. Tumors less than 4 cm are deemed curable.

K. Larger tumors require much more aggressive treatment (cure is difficult).

L. Definitive diagnosis of cancer of the breast is made with biopsy.

M. Common sites of metastasis (spread) are the axillary, supraclavicular, or mediastinal lymph nodes followed by metastases to the lungs, liver, brain, and spine.

N. Bone metastasis is extremely painful.

O. Treatment is dependent on the stage of disease.
1. Mastectomy is commonly performed.
2. Adjuvant treatment consists of radiation (either external beam or implants), antineoplastic chemotherapy, and hormonal therapy.

> **HESI Hint** • The presence or absence of hormone receptors is paramount in selecting clients for adjuvant therapy.

Nursing Assessment (Data Collection)

A. Hard lump (not freely moveable and not painful)
B. Dimpling of skin
C. Retraction of nipple
D. Alterations in contour of breast
E. Change in skin color
F. Change in skin texture (peau d'orange)
G. Discharge from nipple
H. Pain and ulcerations (late signs)
I. Diagnostic tests include:
1. Mammogram
2. Biopsy and frozen section

Analysis (Nursing Diagnoses)

A. Disturbed body image related to . . .
B. Anticipatory grieving related to . . .
C. Acute or chronic pain related to . . .
D. Self-care deficit (specify) related to . . .

Nursing Plans and Interventions

A. Assess lesion:
1. Location
2. Size
3. Shape
4. Consistency
5. Fixation to surrounding tissues
6. Lymph node involvement

B. Preoperative:
1. Explore client's expectations of surgery and what the surgical site will look like postoperatively.
2. Discuss skin graft if one is possible and cosmetic reconstruction that might be implemented with mastectomy or at a later time.

C. Postoperative:
1. Monitor bleeding, check under dressing, Hemo Vac, and under client's back (bleeding will run to back).
2. Position arm on operative side on a pillow, slightly elevated.
3. Avoid BP measurements, injections, and venipuncture in affected arm.
4. Instruct client to avoid injury such as burns or scrapes to affected arm.
5. Encourage hand activity by squeezing a small rubber ball.
6. Encourage client to perform activities that will use arm, such as brushing hair.
7. Collaborate with RN to develop and implement a teaching plan for client/family about postmastectomy exercises (wall climbing with affected arm and rope turning).

D. Encourage client to verbalize concerns:
1. Cancer
2. Death
3. Loss of breast

E. Encourage client to discuss operation, diagnosis, feelings, concerns, and fears.

F. Be with client when she first looks at the operative site; offer emotional support.
G. Collaborate with RN and health care provider for Reach-to-Recovery visit, Y-me (prescription required).
H. Recognize the grief process.
  1. Allow client to cry, withdraw, and so on.
  2. Help client focus on the future while allowing discussions of loss.
I. If reconstruction was not discussed preoperatively, encourage client to discuss or explore these options postoperatively.
J. Discuss use of temporary and/or permanent prosthesis.

Testicular Cancer

Description: Cancer of the testes is the leading cause of death from cancer in males 15 to 35 years of age. If untreated, death usually occurs within 2 to 3 years. If detected and treated early, there is a 90% to 100% chance of cure.

Nursing Assessment (Data Collection)
A. Early signs are subtle and usually go unnoticed.
B. Feeling of heaviness or dragging sensation in lower abdomen and groin.
C. Lump or swelling (painless).
D. Late signs include:
  1. Low back pain
  2. Weight loss
  3. Fatigue

Analysis (Nursing Diagnoses)
A. Deficient knowledge (specify) related to . . .
B. Disturbed body image related to . . .
C. Anticipatory grieving related to . . .

HESI Hint • Men whose testes have not descended into the scrotum or whose testes descended after age 6 are at high risk for developing testicular cancer. The most common symptom is the appearance of a small, hard lump about the size of a pea on the front or side of the testicle. Testicular self-examination (TSE) should be done regularly at the same time each month by all males after age 14. It should be done after a shower by gently palpating the testes and cord to look for a small lump. Swelling may also be a sign of testicular cancer.

Nursing Plans and Interventions

A. Postoperative care following orchidectomy:
  1. Observe for hemorrhage.
  2. Active movement may be contraindicated.
B. Care for clients receiving radiation therapy.
C. Encourage genetic counseling (sperm banking is often recommended before surgery).

D. Reinforce teachings that sexual functioning is usually not affected because the remaining testis undergoes hyperplasia, producing sufficient testosterone to maintain sexual functioning. Though ejaculatory ability may be decreased, orgasm is still possible.

Cancer of the Prostate

Description: Prostate cancer rarely occurs before 40 years of age, but it is the second leading cause of death from cancer in American men. High-risk groups include those with a history of multiple sexual partners, STDs, or certain viral infections and family history.

Nursing Assessment (Data Collection)
A. Asymptomatic if confined to gland
B. Symptoms of urinary obstruction
C. With metastasis: low back pain, fatigue, aching in legs, and hip pain
D. Elevated prostate-specific antigen (PSA)
  1. PSA test should be conducted before a digital rectal exam so that manipulation of the prostate does not give a false positive reading.
  2. Serial blood screening should be done to observe trends. A rise in PSA or consistently high PSA is more reliable than a single assay.
  3. PSA levels can rise with inflammation, benign hypertrophy, or irritation, as well as in response to cancer.
E. Elevated prostatic acid phosphatase is an indication of metastasis to the bone.
F. Digital rectal examination reveals palpable nodule.
G. Transrectal ultrasound visualizes nonpalpable tumors.
H. Definitive diagnosis is made by biopsy.

Analysis (Nursing Diagnoses)
A. Deficient knowledge (specify) related to . . .
B. Disturbed body image related to . . .
C. Bowel incontinence related to . . .
D. Anticipatory grieving related to . . .

Nursing Plans and Interventions
A. Reinforce the importance of early detection.
B. Provide preoperative bowel preparation to prevent fecal contamination of operative site.
  1. Enemas and cathartics
  2. Sulfasalazine (Azulfidine) or neomycin
  3. Clear fluids only the day before surgery to prevent fecal contamination of operative site
C. Provide postoperative care:
  1. Monitor for urine leaks, hemorrhage, and signs of infection.
  2. Provide support dressing or supportive underwear to perineal incision.
  3. Use donut cushion to relieve pressure on incision site while sitting.

4. Avoid rectal manipulation (rectal thermometers, rectal tubes, and hard suppositories).
5. Provide low-residue diet until wound healing is advanced.
6. Institute measures to prevent bowel action in the first postoperative week to prevent contamination of incision.

Sexually Transmitted Infections

Description: Sexually transmitted infections (STIs) are diseases that may be transmitted during intimate sexual contact.
A. Sexually transmitted infections (STIs) are the most prevalent communicable diseases in the United States.
B. Most cases of STIs occur in adolescents and young adults.

> **HESI Hint** • STIs in infants and children usually indicate sexual abuse and should be reported. The nurse is legally responsible to report suspected cases of child abuse.

Nursing Assessment (Data Collection)
See Table 4-36, *Sexually Transmitted Infections (STIs)*.

Analysis (Nursing Diagnoses)
A. Deficient knowledge (specify) related to . . .
B. Anxiety related to . . .
C. Grieving related to . . .

> **HESI Hint** • Chlamydia is the most reported communicable disease in the United States.

Nursing Plans and Interventions
A. Use a nonjudgmental approach; be straightforward when taking history.
B. Reassure client that all information is strictly confidential. Obtain a complete sexual history that includes:
  1. The client's sexual orientation
  2. Sexual practices
    a. Penile-vaginal
    b. Penile-anal
    c. Penile-oral
    d. Oral-vaginal
    e. Anal-oral
  3. Type of protection (barrier) used
  4. Contraceptive practices
  5. Previous history of STIs
C. Collaborate with RN and implement the teaching plan that includes:
  1. Signs and symptoms of STIs.

  2. Mode of transmission of STIs. (Remember, not all persons practice sex in the same manner.)
  3. Sexual contact should be avoided with anyone while infected.
  4. Provide concise written instructions about treatment; request a return verbalization of these instructions to ensure the client has "heard" the instructions and understands them.
D. Encourage client to provide information regarding *all* sexual contacts.
E. Report incidents of STIs to appropriate health agencies/departments.
F. Instruct women of childbearing age about risks to newborns.
  1. Gonorrheal conjunctivitis
  2. Neonatal herpes
  3. Congenital syphilis
  4. Oral candidiasis

> **HESI Hint** • Pelvic inflammatory disease (PID) involves more than one of the pelvic structures. The infection can cause adhesions and eventually result in sterility. Manage the pain associated with PID with analgesics and warm sitz baths. Bed rest in a semi-Fowler position may increase comfort and promote drainage. Antibiotic treatment is necessary to reduce inflammation and pain.

G. Collaborate with RN to develop and implement a teaching plan about "safer sex."
  1. Reduce the number of sexual contacts.
  2. Avoid sex with those who have multiple partners.
  3. Examine genital area and avoid sexual contact if anything abnormal is present.
  4. Wash hands and genital area before and after sexual contact.
  5. Use a latex condom as a barrier.
  6. Use water-based lubricants rather than oil-based lubricants.
  7. Use a vaginal spermicidal gel.
  8. Avoid douching before and after sexual contact; douching increases risk of infections because the body's normal defenses are reduced or destroyed.
  9. Seek attention from health care provider immediately if symptoms occur.

> **HESI Hint** • A client comes into the clinic with a chancre on his penis. What is the usual treatment? IM dose of penicillin (such as Benzathine penicillin G 2.4 million units). Obtain a sexual history, including the names of his sex partners so they can receive treatment.

TABLE 4-36 **Sexually Transmitted Infections (STIs)**

STI	Symptoms	Treatment
Treponema Pallidum, Syphilis		
• Laboratory diagnosis: • VDRL, FTA-ABS	• *Primary (local):* up to 90 days post exposure • Chancre (red, painless lesions with indurated border) • Highly infectious • *Secondary (systemic):* 6 weeks to 6 months postexposure • Influenza-type symptoms • Generalized rash that affects palms of hands and soles of feet • Lesions contagious • *Tertiary:* 10 to 30 years postexposure • Cardiac and neurologic destruction	• Penicillin G IM (usually 2.4 to 4.8 million units) • If penicillin allergic (adults), alternatives: tetracycline, doxycycline, or ceftriaxone
Neisseria Gonorrhoeae, Gonorrhea		
• Laboratory diagnosis: • Smears, cultures	• Females: majority are asymptomatic • Males: dysuria, yellowish-green urethral discharge, urinary frequency	• Ceftriaxone sodium plus doxycycline hyclate or azithromycin • Cefixime plus doxycycline or azithromycin
Chlamydia Trachomatis, Chlamydia		
• Laboratory diagnosis: • Tissue culture, Chlamydiazine, Microtrak	• Females: many asymptomatic, but may exhibit dysuria, urgency, vaginal discharge • Males: leading cause of nongonococcal urethritis	• Doxycycline hyclate • Azithromycin
Trichomonas Vaginalis, Trichomoniasis		
• Laboratory diagnosis: • Wet slide	• Females: green, yellow, or white frothy foul-smelling vaginal discharge with itching • Males: asymptomatic	• Metronidazole (Flagyl) (male partners to be treated to prevent reinfection)
Candida Albicans, Candidiasis		
• Laboratory diagnosis: • Viral culture	• Females: odorless, white or yellow, cheesy discharge with itching • Males: asymptomatic	• Miconazole nitrate (Monistat) • Clotrimazole (Gyne-Lotrimin) • Nystatin (Mycostatin) • Fluconazole (Diflucan) PO single dose
Herpes Simplex Virus 2, Herpes		

	• Vesicles in clusters that rupture and leave painful erosions that cause painful urination
	• Characterized by remissions and exacerbations
	• May be contagious even when asymptomatic
		• Acyclovir (Zovirax) partially controls symptoms
		• Famciclovir
		• Valacyclovir
		• Palliative care
		  →Viscous lidocaine topically to ease pain
		  →Keep lesions clean and dry

Human Papillomavirus (HPV)		
	• Multiple strains (>70), some of which are implicated in cervical cancer • Alarming rate increase in adolescent population • Lesions may be small, wart-like, or clustered • May be flat or raised	• Routine vaccination is recommended for select populations before onset of sexual activity • Applied medications such as podophyllin (contraindicated in pregnancy) • Trichloroacetic acid (TCA) • Laser • Cryotherapy (freezing)
Human Immunodeficiency Virus (HIV), AIDS		
	• See HIV Infection in Chapter 3, *Advanced Clinical Concepts,* p. 49	

Review of Reproductive System

1. What are the indications for a hysterectomy in the client who has fibromas?
2. List the symptoms and conditions associated with cystocele.
3. What are the most important nursing interventions for the postoperative client who has had a hysterectomy with an A&P repair?
4. Describe the priority nursing care for the client who has had radiation implants.
5. What screening tool is used to detect cervical cancer? What are the American Cancer Society's recommendations for women ages 30 to 70 with three consecutive normal results?
6. Cite two nursing diagnoses for a client undergoing a hysterectomy for cervical cancer.
7. What are the three most important tools for early detection of breast cancer? How often should these tools be used?
8. Describe three nursing interventions to help decrease edema post mastectomy.
9. Name three priorities to include in a discharge plan for the client who has had a mastectomy.
10. What is the most common cause of nongonococcal urethritis?
11. What is the causative organism for syphilis?
12. Malodorous, frothy, greenish-yellow vaginal discharge is characteristic of which STI?
13. Which STI is characterized by remissions and exacerbations in both males and females?
14. Outline a teaching plan for the client with an STI.

Answers to Review

1. Severe menorrhagia leading to anemia, severe dysmenorrhea requiring narcotic analgesics, severe uterine enlargement causing pressure on other organs, and severe low back and pelvic pain.
2. Symptoms include incontinence/stress incontinence, urinary retention, and recurrent bladder infections. Conditions associated with cystocele include multiparity, trauma in childbirth, and aging.
3. Avoid rectal temps and/or rectal manipulation; manage pain; and encourage early ambulation.
4. Do not permit pregnant visitors or pregnant caretakers in room. Discourage visits by small children. Confine client to room. Nurse must wear radiation badge. Nurse limits time in room. Keep supplies and equipment within client's reach.
5. Pap smear. Women ages 30 to 70 with three consecutive normal results may have Pap smears every 3 years. Screened for HPV.
6. Altered body image related to uterine removal. Pain related to postoperative incision.
7. Breast self-exam monthly; mammogram baseline at age 35 followed by exams every 1 to 2 years in 40s and every year after age 50; physical examination by a health professional skilled in examination of the breast.
8. Position arm on operative side on pillow. Avoid BP measurements, injections, or venipunctures in operative arm. Encourage hand activity and use.
9. Arrange for Reach-to-Recovery visit. Discuss the grief process with the client. Have health care provider discuss with client the reconstruction options.
10. *Chlamydia trachomatis.*
11. *Treponema pallidum* (spirochete bacteria).
12. *Trichomonas vaginalis.*
13. Herpes simplex type II.
14. Signs and symptoms of STI. Mode of transmission. Avoid sex while infected. Provide concise written instructions regarding treatment and request a return verbalization to ensure the client understands. Collaborate with RN to develop and implement a teaching plan about "safer sex" practices.

Burns

Description: Tissue injury or necrosis caused by transfer of energy from a heat source to the body.

A. Categories:
   1. Thermal
   2. Radiation
   3. Electrical
   4. Chemical

B. Tissue destruction results from:
   1. Coagulation
   2. Protein denaturation
   3. Ionization of cellular contents

C. Critical systems affected include:
   1. Respiratory
   2. Integumentary
   3. Cardiovascular
   4. Renal

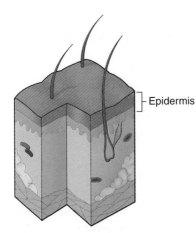

Superficial burns damage only the top layer of the skin—the epidermis. Healing occurs in 3-6 days.

Epidermis

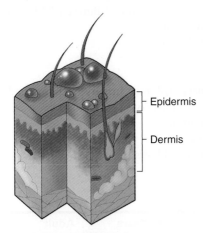

Superficial partial-thickness burns are those in which the entire epidermis and variable portions of the dermis layer of skin are destroyed. Uncomplicated healing occurs in 10-21 days.

Deep partial-thickness burns extend into the deeper layers of the dermis. Healing occurs in 2-6 weeks.

Epidermis

Dermis

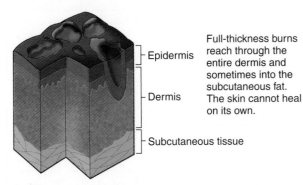

Full-thickness burns reach through the entire dermis and sometimes into the subcutaneous fat. The skin cannot heal on its own.

Epidermis

Dermis

Subcutaneous tissue

FIGURE 4-8 Tissues Involved in Burns of Various Depths. (From Ignatavicius DD, Workman ML: *Medical-surgical nursing: patient-centered collaborative care*, ed 7, St. Louis, 2012, Saunders.)

5. Gastrointestinal
6. Neurologic
D. Severity determined by burn depth (Figure 4-8, *Tissues Involved in Burns of Various Depths*).
   1. First degree:
      a. Superficial partial-thickness (e.g., sunburn)
      b. Injury to the epidermis
      c. Leaves skin pink or red, but no blisters
      d. Dry
      e. Painful (relieved by cooling)
      f. Slight edema
      g. No scarring, and skin grafts are not required

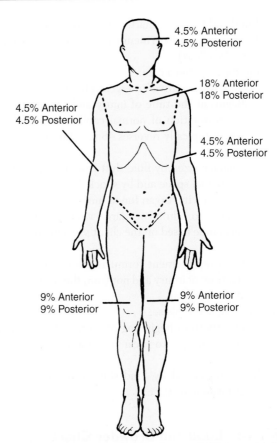

4.5% Anterior
4.5% Posterior

18% Anterior
18% Posterior

4.5% Anterior
4.5% Posterior

4.5% Anterior
4.5% Posterior

9% Anterior
9% Posterior

9% Anterior
9% Posterior

FIGURE 4-9 Estimation of Burn Injury in Children and Adults. (From Ignatavicius DD, Workman ML: *Medical-surgical nursing: patient-centered collaborative care*, ed 7, St. Louis, 2012, Saunders.)

2. Second degree:
   a. Deep partial-thickness destruction of epidermis and upper layers of dermis
   b. Injury to deeper portions of the dermis
   c. Painful (sensitive to touch and cold air)
   d. Appears red or white, weeps fluid, blisters
   e. Hair follicles remain intact—that is, hair does not pull out easily
   f. Very edematous

   g. Blanching followed by capillary refill
   h. Heals without surgical intervention; usually does not scar
3. Third degree:
   a. Full-thickness; deep full-thickness involves total destruction of dermis and epidermis.
   b. Skin cannot regenerate.
   c. Requires skin grafting.
   d. Underlying tissue (fat, fascia, tendon, bone) may be involved.
   e. Wound appears dry and leathery as eschar develops.
   f. Painless.
E. Severity is determined by extent of surface area burned:
   1. Rule of nines: head and neck 9%, upper extremities 9% each, lower extremities 18% each, front trunk 18%, back trunk 18%, perineal area 1% (for adults) (Figure 4-9, *Estimation of Burn Injury in Children and Adults*).

2. Lund and Browder chart: critical body areas are face, hands, feet, and perineum (Table 4-37, *Lund and Browder Chart*).

F. Three stages of burn care:
1. Stage I, resuscitative/emergent phase:
   a. Begins at the time of injury and concludes with the restoration of normal capillary permeability, which typically reverses 48 to 72 hours after the injury.
   b. Characterized by fluid shift from intravascular to interstitial space and by shock. Focus of care is to preserve vital organ functioning.
   c. Expect to administer large volumes of fluid in this phase based on the client's weight and extent of injury.
   d. Fluid replacement formulas are calculated from the time of injury and not from the time of arrival at the hospital.
2. Stage II, acute phase:
   a. Occurs from beginning of diuresis (48-72 hours after injury) to near completion of wound closure.
   b. Characterized by fluid shift from interstitial to intravascular space.
   c. Focus is on infection control, wound care and closure, pain management, nutritional support, and physical therapy.
3. Stage III, rehabilitation phase:
   a. Occurs from major wound closure to return to optimal level of physical and psychosocial adjustment (approximately 5 years).
   b. Characterized by grafting and rehabilitation specific to the client's needs.

Nursing Assessment (Data Collection)

A. Absence of bowel sounds indicating paralytic ileus.
B. Radically decreased urinary output in the first 72 hours after injury with increased specific gravity.
C. Radically increased urinary output (diuresis) 72 hours to 2 weeks after initial injury.
D. Signs of inadequate hydration:
   1. Restlessness
   2. Disorientation
   3. Decreased urinary volume, urinary sodium, and increased urine specific gravity
E. Signs of inhalation burn:
   1. Red or burned face
   2. Singed facial and nasal hairs

TABLE 4-37 Lund and Browder Chart

Area	1 Year	1 to 4 Years	5 to 9 Years	10 to 14 Years	15 Years	Adult
Head	19	17	13	11	9	7
Neck	2	2	2	2	2	2
Anterior trunk	13	13	13	13	13	13
Posterior trunk	13	13	13	13	13	13
Right buttock	2½	2½	2½	2½	2½	2½
Left buttock	2½	2½	2½	2½	2½	2½
Genitalia	1	1	1	1	1	1
Right upper arm	4	4	4	4	4	4
Left upper arm	4	4	4	4	4	4
Right lower arm	3	3	3	3	3	3
Left lower arm	3	3	3	3	3	3
Right hand	2½	2½	2½	2½	2½	2½
Left hand	2½	2½	2½	2½	2½	2½
Right thigh	5½	6½	8	8½	9	9½
Left thigh	5½	6½	8	8½	9	9½
Right leg	5	5	5½	6	6½	7
Left leg	5	5	5½	6	6½	7
Right foot	3½	3½	3½	3½	3½	3½
Left foot	3½	3½	3½	3½	3½	3½

3. Circumoral burns
4. Conjunctivitis
5. Sooty nasal mucous or bloody sputum
6. Hoarseness
7. Asymmetry of chest movements with respirations and use of accessory muscles indicative of pneumonia
8. Rales, wheezing, and rhonchi denoting smoke inhalation
9. Impaired speech and drooling indicating laryngeal edema

F. Description of physiologic responses to burns (Figure 4-10, *The Physiologic Actions of the Sympathetic Nervous System Compensatory Responses to Burn Injury [Early Phase]*).

G. Preexisting conditions/illnesses that may influence recovery.

HESI Hint · **ABC's OF ASSESSMENT**
• Airway
• Breathing
• Circulation

Analysis (Nursing Diagnoses)

A. Ineffective airway clearance related to . . .
B. Impaired gas exchange related to . . .
C. Decreased cardiac output related to . . .
D. Deficient fluid volume related to . . .
E. Ineffective tissue perfusion (specify) related to . . .
F. Impaired skin integrity related to . . .
G. Pain related to . . .
H. Disturbed body image related to . . .
I. Imbalanced nutrition: less than body requirements related to . . .
J. Risk for infection related to . . .
K. Impaired physical mobility related to . . .

Nursing Plans and Interventions

Emergent Phase. Efforts of the health care team are directed toward stabilization with ongoing assessment.

A. Provide admission care:
1. Extinguish source of burn (burning may continue with clothing attached to skin).
   a. Thermal: remove clothing, cool burns by immersion in tepid water, apply dry sterile dressings.
   b. Chemical: flush with water or saline.
   c. Electrical: separate client from electrical source.
2. Provide an open airway; intubation may be necessary if laryngeal edema is a risk.
3. Determine baseline data: vital signs, blood gases, weight.
4. Determine depth and extent of burn.

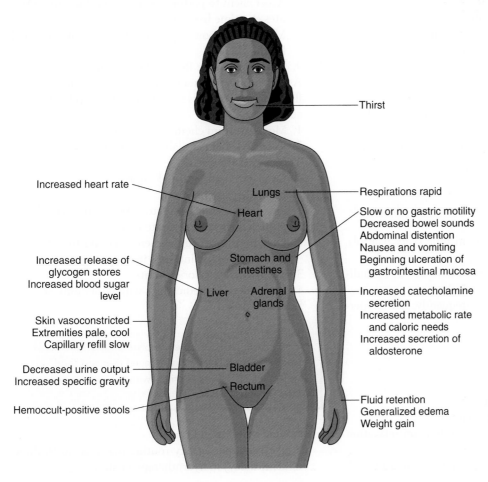

FIGURE 4-10 The Physiologic Actions of the Sympathetic Nervous System Compensatory Responses to Burn Injury (Early Phase). (From Ignatavicius DD, Workman ML: *Medical-surgical nursing: patient-centered collaborative care*, ed 7, St. Louis, 2012, Saunders.)

5. Administer tetanus toxoid.
6. Initiate fluid and electrolyte therapy: Ringer lactate with electrolytes and colloids adjusted according to lab results and fluid resuscitation formula used.

> **HESI Hint** Massive volumes of IV fluids are given. It is not uncommon to give over 1000 mL/hr during various phases of burn care. Hemodynamic monitoring must be closely observed to be sure the client is supported with fluid but is not overloaded.

7. Insert NG tube to prevent vomiting, abdominal distention, or gastric aspiration.
8. Monitor client's response to IV pain medication.
B. Monitor hydration status:
1. Record urinary output hourly (30 to 100 mL/hr is normal range).
2. Monitor IV fluids and assist RN in the titration to keep urine output at 30 to 100 mL/hr.
3. Accurately record I&O.
4. Weigh daily.
5. Observe for signs of inadequate hydration:
   a. Restlessness
   b. Disorientation
   c. Hypothermia
   d. Decreased urine output
C. Monitor respiratory functioning:
1. Provide care for the intubated client.
2. Suction endotrach or nasotrach.
3. Monitor ABGs.
4. Observe for cyanosis, disorientation.
5. Administer O_2.
6. Encourage use of incentive spirometer, coughing, and deep breathing.
7. Elevate the head of the bed to 30 degrees or more for burns of the face and head.
D. Provide wound care:
1. Use strict aseptic technique.
2. Débridement and dressing changes according to client's condition.
3. Change dressings in minimum time (very painful), premedicate.
4. Maintain room temperature above 90° F, humidified, and free of drafts.
5. Monitor body temperature frequently; have hyperthermia blankets available.
E. Monitor for paralytic ileus:
1. Absence of bowel sounds
2. Nausea and vomiting
3. Abdominal distention
F. Assist with management of pain:
1. Administer analgesics intravenously.
2. Reinforce teaching about distraction/relaxation techniques.
3. Reinforce teaching about use of guided imagery.

G. Monitor for circulatory compromise in burns that constrict body parts. Prepare client for escharotomy.

> **HESI Hint** Infection is a life-threatening risk for those with burns.

Acute Phase. Characterized by fluid shift from interstitial to intravascular (diuresis begins); occurs from 72 hours to 2 weeks after initial injury to near completion of wound closure.
A. Provide infection control, including the following:
1. Maintain protective isolation of entire burn unit.
2. Cover hair at all times.
3. Wear masks during dressing changes.
4. Use sterile technique for hydrotherapy, dressing change, and débridement.
5. Monitor client's response to IV antibiotics if indicated.
6. Live plants and flowers are prohibited.
B. Splint and position client to prevent contractures. Avoid use of pillows with neck bums.
C. Perform range of motion (ROM) exercises; will be painful for client.
1. Administer pain medication immediately before performing ROM.
2. Assist client to perform active ROM for 3 to 5 minutes at a time frequently during day.
3. Mobilize as soon as possible using splints designed for the client.
4. Encourage active ROM when up and about.
D. Assist the RN in monitoring the client's response to fluid therapy; colloids may be used to keep fluid in vascular space.
1. Monitor serum chemistries at all times.
2. Keep an IV site available; a saline lock is helpful.
3. Maintain strict I&O.
4. Encourage oral intake of fluids.
E. Provide adequate nutrition:
1. Provide high-calorie (up to 5000 calories/day), high-protein, high-carbohydrate diet.
2. Give nutritional supplements via NG tube feeding at night if caloric intake is inadequate.
3. Keep accurate calorie counts.
4. Administer all medications with either milk or juice.
5. Weigh daily.

> **HESI Hint** To ensure electrolyte balance, additional water is not given. These clients need to ingest food products or high-protein drinks with the highest biologic value rather than water.

F. Provide burn/wound care:
1. Cleansing per agency routine (daily or up to three times a day) in hydrotherapy or shower.

TABLE 4-38 Topical Antimicrobial Agents

Drugs	Indications	Adverse Reactions	Nursing Implications
• Mafenide acetate (Sulfamylon)	• Treatment of burns • Usually used with OPEN method of wound care	• Painful • Causes mild acidosis	• Administer pain medication before dressing changes • Penetrates wound rapidly
• Silver sulfadiazine (Silvadene)	• Treatment of burns • Usually used with OPEN method of wound care • Used to avoid acid-base complications • Keeps eschar soft making débridement easier	• Penetrates wound slowly	• Administer pain medication before dressing change • Is soothing to the burn

2. Wet-to-dry dressing changes two to three times a day to remove eschar.
3. Apply silver sulfadiazine (Silvadene) or mafenide acetate (Sulfamylon) to burn as prescribed (Table 4-38, *Topical Antimicrobial Agents*).
4. Cover (closed method) or leave open (open method) according to agency policy or health care provider's prescription.
5. Prepare client for grafting when eschar has been removed.
6. Prepare client for autografts (use of client's own skin for grafting).
7. Use heat lamp to donor site following graft to allow the area to reepithelialize.

HESI Hint • Having dressings changed is very painful. Medicate client before procedure.

HESI Hint • Preexisting conditions that might influence burn recovery are age, chronic illness (diabetes, cardiac problems, etc.), physical disabilities, disease, medications used routinely, and drug and/or alcohol abuse.

Rehabilitation Phase. Characterized by the absence of infection risk.
A. Collaborate with ongoing discharge planning.
B. May return home when the danger of infection has been eliminated.
C. High-protein fluids with vitamin supplement.
D. Pressure dressings such as Jobst garments may be worn continuously to prevent hypertrophic scarring and contractures.

Review of Burns

1. List four categories of burns.
2. Burn depth is a measure of severity. Describe the characteristics of superficial partial-thickness, deep partial-thickness, and full-thickness burns.
3. Describe fluid management in the emergent phase, acute phase, and rehabilitation phase of the burned client.
4. Describe pain management of the burned client.
5. Outline admission care of the burned client.
6. Nutritional status is a major concern when caring for a burned client. List three specific dietary interventions used with burned clients.
7. Describe the method of extinguishing each of the following burns: thermal, chemical, and electrical.
8. List four signs of an inhalation burn.
9. Why is the burned client allowed NO "free" water?
10. Describe an autograft.

Answers to Review

1. Thermal, radiation, chemical, and electrical.
2. Superficial partial-thickness: first degree = pink to red skin (i.e., sunburn), slight edema, and pain relieved by cooling. Deep partial-thickness: second degree = destruction of epidermis and upper layers of dermis; white or red, very edematous, sensitive to touch and cold air, hair does not pull out easily. Full-thickness: third degree = total destruction of dermis and epidermis; reddened areas do not blanch with pressure, not painful, inelastic, waxy, white skin to brown, leathery eschar.
3. Stage I (Emergent Phase): Replacement of fluids is titrated to urine output. Stage II (Acute Phase): Maintain patent infusion site in case supplemental IV fluids are needed; saline lock is helpful; may use colloids. Stage III (Rehabilitation Phase): No extra fluids are needed, but high-protein drinks are recommended.
4. Administer pain medication, especially before dressing wound. Reinforce distraction/relaxation techniques and use of guided imagery.
5. Provide a patent airway as intubation may be necessary. Determine baseline data. Initiate fluid and electrolyte therapy. Administer pain medication. Determine depth and extent of burn. Administer tetanus toxoid. Insert NG tube.
6. High-calorie, high-protein, high-carbohydrate diet. Medications with juice or milk; *no* "free" water. Tube feeding at night. Maintain accurate, daily calorie counts. Weigh client daily.
7. Thermal: remove clothing, immerse in tepid water. Chemical: flush with water or saline. Electrical: separate client from electrical source.
8. Singed nasal hairs, circumoral burns; sooty or bloody sputum, hoarseness, and pulmonary signs including asymmetry of respirations, rales, or wheezing.
9. Water may interfere with electrolyte balance. Client needs to ingest food products with highest biologic value.
10. Use of client's own skin for grafting.

5

PEDIATRIC NURSING

Growth and Development

Description: Growth and development follows an orderly yet individual pattern. Practical nurses (PNs) should determine growth and the emergence of developmental skills in all pediatric clients. Knowledge of cognitive abilities allows the nurse to interact with the child at the most appropriate level. Knowledge of appropriate toys and interests of children at different ages enables the nurse to use play to facilitate the child's development and minimize problems resulting from the hospitalization.

Birth to 1 Year

A. Developmental milestones:
1. Birth weight doubles by 6 months and triples by 12 months.
2. Birth length increases by 50% at 12 months.
3. Posterior fontanel closes by 8 weeks.
4. Social smile at 2 months.
5. Turns head to locate sounds at 3 months.
6. Moro reflex disappears around 4 months.
7. Achieves steady head control at 4 months.
8. Turns completely over at 5 to 6 months.
9. Plays peek-a-boo after 6 months.
10. Transfers objects hand to hand at 7 months.
11. Develops stranger anxiety at 7 to 9 months.
12. Sits unsupported at 8 months.
13. Crawls at 10 months.
14. Fine pincer grasp appears at 10 to 12 months.
15. Waves bye-bye at 10 months.
16. Walks with assistance at 10 to 12 months.
17. Says a few words in addition to "mama" or "dada" at 12 months.
18. Explores environment by motor and oral means.
B. Erikson's theory: developing a sense of trust (trust vs. mistrust)
C. Nursing implications:
1. During hospitalization, the infant's emerging skills may disappear.
2. If the parents are not able to be with the infant, the baby may experience separation anxiety.

> **HESI Hint** • The stages of separation anxiety consist of protest, despair, denial, and detachment.

3. The PN should encourage and plan to have the parents be part of the infant's care.
4. The infant's usual schedule at home should be respected.
5. Preparation and/or reinforcement of teaching should be directed to the family. However, the PN should always speak to the infant and console the infant, especially while performing painful or stressful procedures.
6. Toys for hospitalized infants include mobiles, rattles, squeaking toys, picture books, balls, colored blocks, and activity boxes.

> **HESI Hint** • Pediatric questions on the NCLEX-PN® examination often focus on the growth and development milestones of children. Some frequently tested content areas may include:
> - When does birth length double? Answer: By 4 years.
> - When does the child sit unsupported? Answer: 8 months.
> - When does a child achieve 50% of adult height? Answer: 2 years.
> - When does a child throw a ball overhand? Answer: 18 months.
> - When does a child speak two- to three-word sentences? Answer: 2 years.
> - When does a child use scissors? Answer: 4 years.
> - When does a child tie his/her shoes? Answer: 5 years.
> - Be aware that a girl's growth spurt during adolescence begins earlier than boys (as early as 10 years old).
> - Temper tantrums are common in the toddler and are considered "normal" behavior.
> - Be aware that adolescence is a time when the child forms his or her identity and that rebellion against family values is common for this age group.

HESI Hint • Normal growth and development knowledge is used to evaluate interventions and therapy. For example, "What behavior would indicate that thyroid hormone therapy for a 4-month-old is effective?" You must know what milestones are accomplished by a 4-month-old. One correct answer would be "Has steady head control," which is an expected milestone for a 4-month-old and indicates that replacement therapy is adequate for growth.

Toddler (1 to 3 Years)

A. Developmental milestones:
  1. Birth weight quadruples by 30 months.
  2. Achieves 50% of adult height by 2 years.
  3. Growth velocity slows.
  4. Appears to be bowlegged and potbellied.
  5. All primary teeth (20) are present.
  6. Anterior fontanel closes by 12 to 18 months.
  7. Throws a ball overhand at 18 months.
  8. Kicks a ball at 24 months.
  9. Feeds self with spoon and cup at 2 years.
  10. Daytime toilet training can usually be started around 2 years.
  11. Two- to three-word sentences at 2 years.
  12. Three- to four-word sentences by 3 years.
  13. States own first and last name by 2½ to 3 years.
  14. Temper tantrums common.
B. Erikson's theory: developing a sense of autonomy (autonomy vs. doubt and shame)
C. Nursing implications:
  1. Simple brief explanations should be given immediately before procedures because toddlers have limited concept of time.
  2. During hospitalization, enforced separation from parents is the greatest threat to the toddler's psychologic and emotional integrity.
  3. Security objects or favorite toys from home should be provided for toddler.
  4. Encourage parents to explain their plans to child—for example, "I will be back after your nap."
  5. Respect the child's routine.
  6. Expect regression—for example, bedwetting.
  7. Toys for the hospitalized toddler include board and mallet, push/pull toys, toy telephone, stuffed animals, and storybooks with pictures. Toddlers benefit from being taken to the hospital playroom when possible because mobility is very important to their development. Toddlers engage in parallel play where they play independently but among other children.
  8. Toddlers are learning to name body parts and are concerned about their bodies.
  9. Support autonomy by giving choices.

Preschool Child (3 to 5 Years)

A. Developmental milestones:
  1. Each year child gains about 5 pounds and grows 2½ to 3 inches.
  2. Stands erect with more slender posture.
  3. Learns to run, jump, skip, and hop.
  4. 3-year-olds ride a tricycle.
  5. Handedness is established.
  6. Uses scissors at 4 years.
  7. Ties shoelaces at 5 years.
  8. Learns colors, shapes.
  9. Visual acuity approaches 20/20.
  10. Thinking is egocentric and concrete.
  11. Uses sentences of 5 to 8 words.
  12. Learns sexual identity (curiosity and masturbation common).
  13. Imaginary playmates and fears are common.
  14. Aggressiveness at 4 years is replaced by more independence at 5 years.
B. Erikson's theory: developing a sense of initiative (initiative vs. guilt)
C. Nursing implications:
  1. Nursing care for hospitalized preschoolers needs to emphasize understanding of the child's egocentricity. Explain that he or she did not cause the illness and that painful procedures are not a punishment for misdeeds.
  2. The child's questions need to be answered at his or her level. Use simple words that will be understood by the child.
  3. Therapeutic play or medical play to allow the child to act out his or her experiences is helpful.
  4. Fear of mutilation from procedures is common. A Band-Aid may be helpful for restoring body integrity; children fear loss of blood because they are beginning to associate it with life.
  5. Toys and play for the hospitalized preschooler include coloring books, puzzles, cutting and pasting, dolls, building blocks, clay, and toys that allow the preschooler to work out hospitalization experiences. Preschoolers engage in associative play where they engage in similar activities and play together, but there is no organization, leadership, or group goals.
  6. The preschooler needs preparation for procedures. He or she needs to understand what is and what is not going to be "fixed." Simple explanations and basic pictures are helpful. Let child handle equipment or models of the equipment.

HESI Hint • Use facts and principles related to growth and development when reinforcing teaching interventions. For example: "What task could a 5-year-old boy with diabetes be expected to accomplish by himself?" One correct answer would be to pick the injection sites. This is possible for a preschooler to do and gives the child some sense of control.

School-Age Child (6 to 12 Years)

A. Developmental milestones:
1. Each year child gains 4 to 6 pounds and about 2 inches in height.
2. Girls may experience menarche.
3. Loss of primary teeth and eruption of most permanent teeth occur.
4. Fine and gross motor skills mature.
5. Able to write script at 8 years.
6. Dresses self completely.
7. Egocentric thinking is replaced by social awareness of others.
8. Learns to tell time and understands past, present, and future.
9. Learns cause-and-effect relationships.
10. Socialization with peers becomes important.
11. Molars (6-year) erupt.
B. Erikson's theory: developing a sense of industry (industry vs. inferiority)
C. Nursing implications:
1. The hospitalized school-age child may need more support from parents than the child wishes to admit.
2. Maintaining contact with peers and school activities is important during hospitalization.
3. Explanation of all procedures is important. Children can learn from verbal explanations, from pictures, from books, or from handling equipment.
4. Privacy and modesty are important and should be respected during hospitalization—for example, close curtains during procedures, allow privacy during baths, and so on.
5. Participation in care and planning with staff fosters a sense of involvement and accomplishment.
6. Toys for the school-age child include board games, card games, and hobbies such as stamp collecting, puzzles, and video games. School-age children engage in cooperative play where the play is organized, and they play with other children.

> **HESI Hint** • School-age children are in Erikson's stage of industry, meaning they like to do and accomplish things. Peers are also becoming important for children of this age.

Adolescence (12 to 19 Years)

A. Developmental milestones:
1. Girls' growth spurt during adolescence begins earlier than boys' (may begin as early as 9.5 years for girls).
2. Boys catch up around 14 and continue to grow.
3. Girls finish growth around 15, boys around 17.
4. Secondary sex characteristics develop.
5. Adult-like thinking begins around 15 years. They can problem solve and use abstract thinking.
6. Family conflicts develop.

B. Erikson's theory: developing a sense of identity (identity vs. role confusion)
C. Nursing implications:
1. Hospitalization of adolescents disrupts school and peer activities; they need to maintain contact with both.
2. Should share hospital room with other adolescents.
3. Illness, treatments, or procedures that alter the adolescent's body image can be viewed as being devastating by the adolescent.
4. Reinforcement of teaching about procedures should include time without parents present. It is important to direct questions to the adolescent when the parents are present.
5. Many hospitals require the adolescent's consent to treatment as well as the parents' consent to demonstrate that the adolescent understands the medical plan.
6. For prolonged hospitalizations, adolescents need to maintain identity—for example, their own clothing, posters, visitors. A teen room or teen night is very helpful.
7. Some assessment questions should be asked without parents' presence.
8. When reinforcing teaching adolescent about needs, the focus should be on the "here and now"—for example, "How will this affect me *today*?"

> **HESI Hint** • Age groups' concepts of bodily injury:
> - Infants: after 6 months, their cognitive development allows them to remember pain.
> - Toddlers: fear intrusive procedures.
> - Preschoolers: fear body mutilation.
> - School age: fear loss of control of their body.
> - Adolescent: major concern is change in body image.

> **HESI Hint** • Accidents are a major cause of deaths for children and adolescents. Collaborate with RN to develop a teaching plan for parents and children about developmentally appropriate safety/accident-prevention techniques.

Pain Assessment and Management in the Pediatric Client

Description: Historically, pain in the pediatric population has been unrecognized and/or undertreated. Research has shown that children, including neonates and infants, experience pain. Untreated pain may lead to complications such as delayed recovery, alterations in sleep patterns, and alterations in nutrition.
A. Pain assessment is often referred to as the fifth vital sign.
B. The PN collaborates with the registered nurse so as to determine the presence of pain and formulate

effective intervention to relieve such. The nurse is responsible to:

1. Ask about and observe for signs of pain.
2. Believe reports of pain as related by the child and/or family.
3. Assist in choosing appropriate pharmacologic and nonpharmacologic interventions.
4. Deliver timely, logical, and age-appropriate interventions.
5. Evaluate effectiveness of interventions.
6. Empower the child/family to achieve pain relief.

Nursing Assessment (Data Collection)

A. Verbal report by the child. Children as young as 3 years of age are able to report the location and degree of pain they are experiencing (Figure 5-1, *Wong-Baker FACES Pain Rating Scale*).
B. Observe for nonverbal signs of pain such as grimacing, irritability, restlessness, and difficulty with sleeping and/or feeding.
C. Include the child's parents in the assessment.
D. Observe for physiologic responses to pain, such as increased heart rate, increased respiratory rate, diaphoresis, and decreased oxygen levels.
E. Physiologic responses to pain are most often seen in response to acute pain, rather than in response to chronic pain.

Analysis (Nursing Diagnoses)

A. Acute pain related to …
B. Anxiety related to …
C. Disturbed sleep pattern related to …
D. Ineffective infant feeding pattern related to …

Nursing Plans and Interventions

A. Use a pain rating scale appropriate for the child's age and developmental level:
1. CRIES can to be used for infants 32 to 60 weeks of gestational age.
2. Pain Rating Scale (PRS) is to be used with children 1 to 36 months of age.
3. FACES Pain Rating Scale and the Poker Chip Scale can be used by children of preschool age and older.

4. Numeric Pain Scale can be used by children 9 years of age and older.
5. The Oucher Pain Scale is a scale used for children 3 to 12 years of age, with culturally specific photographs showing different levels of pain and discomfort.
6. Documentation of a child's self-report of pain is essential to effectively treating the child's pain.
7. A nonverbal child can be assessed using the FLACC pain assessment tool (Merkel et al, 1997). This tool has the nurse evaluate the child's facial expression, leg movement, activity, cry, and consolability.

B. Nonpharmacologic interventions:
1. They should be based on the child's age and developmental level.
2. Infants may respond best to pacifiers, holding, and rocking.
3. Toddlers and preschoolers may respond best to distraction. Distraction may be through books, music, television, and bubble blowing.
4. School-age children and adolescents may use guided imagery.
5. Other interventions may include massage, application of heat/cold, and deep-breathing exercises.

C. Pharmacologic interventions:
1. Prior to administering a pain medication to the pediatric client, verify that the prescribed dose is safe for the child, based on the child's weight.
2. Monitor the child's vital signs after administration of opioid medications.
3. Children as young as 5 years of age may be taught to use a patient-controlled analgesia pump.
4. Children may deny pain if they fear receiving an IM injection; therefore, intravenous pain medications are preferred over analgesia.

Child Health Promotion

Description: Immunization of children against communicable diseases is one of the greatest accomplishments of modern medicine. Protection against disease should begin in infancy according to the recommendations of the American Academy of Pediatrics and the United States Public Health Service (Figure 5-2, *Recommended Childhood and Adolescent Immunization Schedule, United States 2010*, and Table 5-1, *Screening for Tuberculosis*).

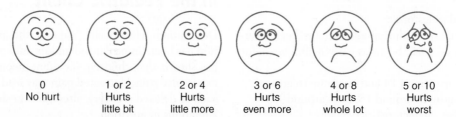

0	1 or 2	2 or 4	3 or 6	4 or 8	5 or 10
No hurt	Hurts little bit	Hurts little more	Hurts even more	Hurts whole lot	Hurts worst

FIGURE 5-1 FACES Pain Rating Scale. Explain to the child that each face is for a person who feels happy because he has no pain (hurt) or sad because he has some or a lot of pain. Ask the child to choose the face that best describes his or her own pain. (From Hockenberry MJ, Wilson D: *Wong's nursing care of infants and children*, ed 9, St. Louis, 2011, Mosby. Used with permission. Copyright Mosby.)

Figure 1. Recommended immunization schedule for persons aged 0 through 18 years – 2013.
(FOR THOSE WHO FALL BEHIND OR START LATE, SEE THE CATCH-UP SCHEDULE [FIGURE 2]).

These recommendations must be read with the footnotes that follow. For those who fall behind or start late, provide catch-up vaccination at the earliest opportunity as indicated by the green bars in Figure 1. To determine minimum intervals between doses, see the catch-up schedule (Figure 2). School entry and adolescent vaccine age groups are in bold.

Vaccines	Birth	1 mo	2 mos	4 mos	6 mos	9 mos	12 mos	15 mos	18 mos	19–23 mos	2-3 yrs	4-6 yrs	7-10 yrs	11-12 yrs	13–15 yrs	16–18 yrs
Hepatitis B¹ (HepB)	1ˢᵗ dose	←---- 2ⁿᵈ dose ----→			←-------------------- 3ʳᵈ dose --------------------→											
Rotavirus² (RV) RV-1 (2-dose series); RV-5 (3-dose series)			1ˢᵗ dose	2ⁿᵈ dose	See footnote 2											
Diphtheria, tetanus, & acellular pertussis³ (DTaP: <7 yrs)			1ˢᵗ dose	2ⁿᵈ dose	3ʳᵈ dose		←------ 4ᵗʰ dose ------→					5ᵗʰ dose				
Tetanus, diphtheria, & acellular pertussis⁴ (Tdap: ≥7 yrs)														(Tdap)		
Haemophilus influenzae type b⁵ (Hib)			1ˢᵗ dose	2ⁿᵈ dose	See footnote 5		3ʳᵈ or 4ᵗʰ dose, see footnote 5									
Pneumococcal conjugate⁶ᵃ,ᶜ (PCV13)			1ˢᵗ dose	2ⁿᵈ dose	3ʳᵈ dose		←------ 4ᵗʰ dose ------→									
Pneumococcal polysaccharide⁶ᵇ,ᶜ (PPSV23)																
Inactivated Poliovirus⁷ (IPV) (<18years)			1ˢᵗ dose	2ⁿᵈ dose	←-------------------- 3ʳᵈ dose --------------------→							4ᵗʰ dose				
Influenza⁸(IIV; LAIV) 2 doses for some : see footnote 8					Annual vaccination (IIV only)						Annual vaccination (IIV or LAIV)					
Measles, mumps, rubella⁹ (MMR)							←------ 1ˢᵗ dose ------→					2ⁿᵈ dose				
Varicella¹⁰ (VAR)							←------ 1ˢᵗ dose ------→					2ⁿᵈ dose				
Hepatitis A¹¹ (HepA)							←---- 2 dose series, see footnote 11 ----→				see footnote 13					
Human papillomavirus¹² (HPV2: females only; HPV4: males and females)														(3-dose series)		
Meningococcal¹³ (Hib-MenCY ≥ 6 weeks; MCV4-D≥9 mos; MCV4-CRM ≥ 2 yrs.)														1ˢᵗ dose		booster

Legend:
- Range of recommended ages for all children
- Range of recommended ages for catch-up immunization
- Range of recommended ages for certain high-risk groups
- Range of recommended ages during which catch-up is encouraged and for certain high-risk groups
- Not routinely recommended

This schedule includes recommendations in effect as of January 1, 2013. Any dose not administered at the recommended age should be administered at a subsequent visit, when indicated and feasible. The use of a combination vaccine generally is preferred over separate injections of its equivalent component vaccines. Vaccination providers should consult the relevant Advisory Committee on Immunization Practices (ACIP) statement for detailed recommendations, available online at http://www.cdc.gov/vaccines/pubs/acip-list.htm. Clinically significant adverse events that follow vaccination should be reported to the Vaccine Adverse Event Reporting System (VAERS) online (http://www.vaers.hhs.gov) or by telephone (800-822-7967).Suspected cases of vaccine-preventable diseases should be reported to the state or local health department. Additional information, including precautions and contraindications for vaccination, is available from CDC online (http://www.cdc.gov/vaccines) or by telephone (800-CDC-INFO [800-232-4636]).

This schedule is approved by the Advisory Committee on Immunization Practices (http://www.cdc.gov/vaccines/acip/index.html), the American Academy of Pediatrics (http://www.aap.org), the American Academy of Family Physicians (http://www.aafp.org), and the American College of Obstetricians and Gynecologists (http://www.acog.org).

NOTE: The above recommendations must be read along with the footnotes that accompany this schedule.

FIGURE 5-2 Recommended Childhood and Adolescent Immunization Schedule, United States 2013. See http://www.cdc.gov/vaccines/schedules/hcp/child-adolescent.html for footnotes that accompany this schedule and for any updates to the schedule. (From Department of Health and Human Services, Centers for Disease Control and Prevention, 2013)

FIGURE 2. Catch-up immunization schedule for persons aged 4 months through 18 years who start late or who are more than 1 month behind —United States • 2013

The figure below provides catch-up schedules and minimum intervals between doses for children whose vaccinations have been delayed. A vaccine series does not need to be restarted, regardless of the time that has elapsed between doses. Use the section appropriate for the child's age. Always use this table in conjunction with Figure 1 and the footnotes that follow.

Vaccine	Minimum Age for Dose 1	Minimum Interval Between Doses			
		Dose 1 to dose 2	Dose 2 to dose 3	Dose 3 to dose 4	Dose 4 to dose 5
Persons aged 4 months through 6 years					
Hepatitis B[1]	Birth	4 weeks	8 weeks and at least 16 weeks after first dose; minimum age for the final dose is 24 weeks		
Rotavirus[2]	6 weeks	4 weeks	4 weeks[2]		
Diphtheria, tetanus, pertussis[3]	6 weeks	4 weeks	4 weeks	6 months	6 months[3]
Haemophilus influenzae type b[5]	6 weeks	4 weeks if first dose administered at younger than age 12 months 8 weeks (as final dose) if first dose administered at age 12–14 months No further doses needed if first dose administered at age 15 months or older	4 weeks[5] if current age is younger than 12 months 8 weeks (as final dose)[5] if current age is 12 months or older and first dose administered at younger than age 12 months and second dose administered at younger than 15 months No further doses needed if previous dose administered at age 15 months or older	8 weeks (as final dose) This dose only necessary for children aged 12 through 59 months who received 3 doses before age 12 months	
Pneumococcal[6]	6 weeks	4 weeks if first dose administered at younger than age 12 months 8 weeks (as final dose for healthy children) if first dose administered at age 12 months or older or current age 24 through 59 months No further doses needed for healthy children if first dose administered at age 24 months or older	4 weeks if current age is younger than 12 months 8 weeks (as final dose for healthy children) if current age is 12 months or older No further doses needed for healthy children if previous dose administered at age 24 months or older	8 weeks (as final dose) This dose only necessary for children aged 12 through 59 months who received 3 doses before age 12 months or for children at high risk who received 3 doses at any age	
Inactivated poliovirus[7]	6 weeks	4 weeks	4 weeks	6 months[7] minimum age 4 years for final dose	
Meningococcal[13]	6 weeks	8 weeks[13]	see footnote 13	see footnote 13	
Measles, mumps, rubella[9]	12 months	4 weeks			
Varicella[10]	12 months	3 months			
Hepatitis A[11]	12 months	6 months			
Persons aged 7 through 18 years					
Tetanus, diphtheria; tetanus, diphtheria, pertussis[4]	7 years[4]	4 weeks	4 weeks if first dose administered at younger than age 12 months 6 months if first dose administered at 12 months or older	6 months if first dose administered at younger than age 12 months	
Human papillomavirus[12]	9 years	Routine dosing intervals are recommended[12]			
Hepatitis A[11]	12 months	6 months			
Hepatitis B[1]	Birth	4 weeks	8 weeks (and at least 16 weeks after first dose)		
Inactivated poliovirus[7]	6 weeks	4 weeks	4 weeks[7]	6 months[7]	
Meningococcal[13]	6 weeks	8 weeks[13]	see footnote 13		
Measles, mumps, rubella[9]	12 months	4 weeks			
Varicella[10]	12 months	3 months if person is younger than age 13 years 4 weeks if person is aged 13 years or older			

NOTE: The above recommendations must be read along with the footnotes of this schedule.

FIGURE 5-2, cont'd

TABLE 5-1 Screening for Tuberculosis

Tuberculosis (TB) skin testing • Offers screening for exposure to TB	• Screening usually done using one of the following: → Mantoux test with PPD (tuberculin purified protein derivative) injected intradermally on the fore-arm; standard method for identifying infection with *M. tuberculosis*. → Tine test (OT, Old Tuberculin), which consists of four prongs pressed into the forearm; these multiple puncture tests are unreliable and should not be used to determine the presence of a TB infection. • A positive reaction represents exposure to *M. tuberculosis*. • Screening can be initiated at 12 months. • Read at 48 to 72 hours; 15 cm induration is positive for a client with no known risk factor, 10 cm induration is positive for high-risk clients, and 5 cm induration is positive if the client is immunocompromised.

HESI Hint • Subcutaneous injection, rather than intradermal, invalidates the Mantoux test.

HESI Hint • The common cold is not a contraindication for immunization.

HESI Hint • Following immunization, what teaching should the nurse provide to the parents?
• Irritability, fever (<102° F), redness, and soreness at injection site for 2 to 3 days are normal side effects of DTaP and IPV administration.
• Call health care provider if seizures, high fever, or high-pitched crying occurs.
• A warm washcloth on the thigh injection site and "bicycling" the legs with each diaper change will decrease soreness.
• Acetaminophen (Tylenol) is administered orally every 4 to 6 hours (10 to 15 mg/kg).

HESI Hint • Pertinent history should be obtained before administering certain immunizations because reactions to previous immunizations or current health conditions may contraindicate current immunizations:
• DTaP: history of seizures, neurologic symptoms after previous vaccine, or systematic allergic reactions
• MMR: history of anaphylactic reaction to eggs or neomycin

HESI Hint • Pertussis fatalities continue to occur in unimmunized infants in the United States.

Common Communicable Diseases of Childhood

The nursing care of children with communicable diseases is virtually the same regardless of the particular disease.

A. **Rubeola (Measles)**
1. Incubation 10 to 20 days.
2. A highly contagious, viral disease that can lead to neurologic problems or death.
3. Transmitted by direct contact with droplets from infected persons.
4. It is contagious mainly during the prodromal period, which is characterized by fever and upper respiratory symptoms.
5. Classic symptoms include the following:
   a. Photophobia
   b. Koplik spots on the buccal mucosa
   c. Confluent rash that begins on the face and spreads downward

B. **Varicella Zoster (Chickenpox)**
1. Incubation 13 to 17 days.
2. Viral disease characterized by skin lesions.
3. Lesions begin on the trunk and spread to the face and proximal extremities.
4. Progresses through macular, papular, vesicular, and pustular stages.
5. Transmitted by direct contact, droplet spread, or freshly contaminated objects.
6. Communicability ends when scabs have formed.

C. **Rubella (German Measles)**
1. Incubation 14 to 21 days.
2. Common viral disease that has teratogenic effects on fetus during the first trimester of pregnancy.
3. Transmitted by droplet and direct contact with infected person.
4. Discrete red maculopapular rash starts on face and rapidly spreads to entire body.
5. Rash disappears within 3 days.

D. **Pertussis (Whooping Cough)**
1. Incubation 5 to 21 days.
2. An acute, infectious respiratory disease usually occurring in infancy.
3. Caused by a gram-negative bacillus.
4. Begins with upper respiratory symptoms.
5. Paroxysmal stage of the disease is characterized by prolonged coughing and crowing or whooping upon inspiration; lasts from 4 to 6 weeks.
6. Transmitted by direct contact, droplet spread, or freshly contaminated objects.

7. Treated with erythromycin and supportive care.

8. Complications include pneumonia, hemorrhage, and seizures.

E. **Paramyxovirus (Mumps)**

1. Incubation 14 to 21 days.

2. Symptoms include fever, headache, malaise, parotid gland swelling, and tenderness. The manifestations include submaxillary and sublingual infection, orchitis, and meningoencephalitis.

3. Transmitted by direct contact or droplet spread.

4. Use analgesics for pain and antipyretics for fever.

5. Maintain bed rest until swelling subsides.

F. Nursing care for children with communicable diseases:

1. Isolate child during period of communicability.

2. Treat fever with *nonaspirin* product because of risk of Reye syndrome.

3. Report occurrence to the health department.

4. Prevent child from scratching skin—that is, cut nails, apply mittens, and provide soothing baths.

5. Administer diphenhydramine HCl (Benadryl) as prescribed for itching.

6. *Wash hands* after caring for child and handling secretions or child's articles.

HESI Hint • Children with German measles pose a serious threat to their unborn siblings. The nurse should counsel all expectant mothers, especially those with young children, to be aware of the serious consequences of exposure to German measles during pregnancy.

HESI Hint • Common childhood problems are encountered by nurses caring for children in the community or hospital settings. The child's age directly influences the severity and management of these problems.

HESI Hint • Pediculosis is an infestation of lice on humans. The most common form is head lice, which affects the scalp and hair. Head lice appear as small white flakes along the shaft of the hair. Treatment is directed toward killing the adult lice, combing out the nits, and using a hair product containing permethrin or pyrethrin. Anything that is in direct contact of the infestation has to be treated to decrease spread of the lice.

Nutritional Assessment

Description: A profile of the child's and family's eating habits.

A. Iron deficiency occurs most often in children 12 to 36 months of age, adolescent females, and females during their childbearing years.

B. The vitamins most often consumed in less than appropriate amounts by preschool and school-age children are:

1. Vitamin A

2. Vitamin C

3. Vitamin B_6

4. Vitamin B_{12}

Nursing Plans and Interventions

A. Determine dietary history:

1. The 24-hour recall: ask the family to recall all food and liquid intake for the past 24 hours.

2. Food diary: ask the family to keep a 3-day record (2 weekdays and 1 weekend day) of all food and liquid intake.

3. Food frequency record: provide a questionnaire and ask family to record information regarding the number of times per day, week, or month a child consumes items from the four food groups.

B. Perform a clinical examination:

1. Observe skin, hair, teeth, gums, lips, tongue, and eyes.

2. Use of anthropometry: measurement of height, weight, head circumference in young children, proportion, skinfold thickness, and arm circumference.

   a. Height and head circumference reflect past nutrition.

   b. Weight, skinfold thickness, and arm circumference reflect present nutritional status (especially protein and fat reserves).

   c. Growth charts in which the child's weight, length, and head circumference are plotted and compared with those of the general population are often used to track growth. The charts are developed according to gender and age. Children who rank below the 5th or above the 95th percentile fall outside the norms of growth.

   d. Skinfold thickness provides a measurement of the body's fat content (one half of the body's total fat stores are directly beneath the skin).

3. Obtain biochemical analysis:

   a. Plasma, blood cells, urine, or tissues from liver, bone, hair, or fingernails can be used to determine nutritional status.

   b. Hemoglobin (Hgb), hematocrit (Hct), albumin, creatinine, and nitrogen laboratory testing are common laboratory procedures used to determine nutritional status.

C. Implement appropriate nursing interventions, and assist the RN and client/family to identify measures to correct identified nutritional deficits (Table 5-2, *Nutritional Assessment*).

Diarrhea

Description: Increased number or decreased consistency of stools.

A. Diarrhea can be a serious or *fatal* illness, especially in infancy.

B. Causes include, but are not limited to:
1. Infections: bacterial, viral. Rotavirus is the leading cause of serious gastroenteritis among children and is a significant hospital-acquired pathogen.
2. Malabsorption problems
3. Inflammatory diseases
4. Dietary factors
C. Conditions associated with diarrhea:
1. Dehydration
2. Metabolic acidosis
3. Shock

Nursing Assessment (Data Collection)

A. Usually occurs in infants.
B. History of exposure to pathogens, contaminated food, dietary changes.
C. Signs of dehydration:
1. Poor skin turgor
2. Absence of tears
3. Dry mucous membranes
4. Weight loss (5% to 15%)
5. Depressed fontanel
6. Decreased urinary output, increased specific gravity
D. Laboratory signs of acidosis:
1. Loss of bicarbonate (serum pH <7.33)
2. Loss of sodium and potassium through stools
3. Elevated Hct
4. Elevated blood urea nitrogen (BUN)
E. Signs of shock:
1. Decreased blood pressure (BP)
2. Rapid, weak pulse

TABLE 5-2   Nutritional Assessment

Nutrient	Signs of Deficiency	Food Sources	
Iron	• Anemia • Pale conjunctiva • Pale skin color • Atrophy of papillae on tongue • Brittle, ridged, spoon-shaped nails • Thyroid edema	• Iron-fortified formula • Infant high-protein cereal	• Infant rice cereal • Liver • Beef • Pork • Eggs
Vitamin B$_2$ (riboflavin)	• Redness and fissuring of eyelid corners; burning, itching, tearing eyes; photophobia • Tongue is magenta color; glossitis • Seborrheic dermatitis; delayed wound healing	• Prepared infant formula • Liver • Cow's milk • Cheddar cheese • Enriched cereals	• Some green leafy vegetables (broccoli, green beans, spinach)
Vitamin A (retinol)	• Dry, rough skin • Dull cornea; soft cornea; Bitot's spots • Night blindness • Defective tooth enamel • Retarded growth; impaired bone formation • Decreased thyroxine formation	• Liver • Sweet potatoes • Carrots • Spinach • Peaches • Apricots	
Vitamin C (ascorbic acid)	• Scurvy • Receding gums that are spongy and prone to bleeding • Dry, rough skin; petechiae • Decreased wound healing • Increased susceptibility to infection • Irritable, anorectic, apprehensive	• Strawberries • Oranges and orange juice • Tomatoes • Broccoli • Cabbage • Cauliflower • Spinach	
Vitamin B$_6$ (pyridoxine)	• Scaly dermatitis • Weight loss • Anemia • Irritability • Convulsions • Peripheral neuritis	• Meats, especially liver • Cereals (wheat and corn) • Yeast • Soybeans	• Peanuts • Tuna • Chicken • Bananas

HESI Hint • Reinforce teaching about proper cooking and storage to preserve potency—for example, cook vegetables in a small amount of liquid.

3. Mottled to gray skin color
4. Changes in mental status

Analysis (Nursing Diagnoses)

A. Diarrhea related to …
B. Risk for deficient fluid volume related to …

Nursing Plans and Interventions

A. Observe hydration status and vital signs frequently.
B. Monitor intake and output.
C. Do *not* take temperature rectally.
D. Rehydrate as prescribed with fluids and electrolytes.
E. Collect specimens to aid in diagnosis of cause as prescribed.
F. Check stools for pH, glucose, and blood.
G. Administer antibiotics as prescribed.
H. Check urine for specific gravity.
I. Institute careful isolation precautions, and wash hands.
J. Collaborate with health care team to provide a teaching plan to include:
  1. Oral rehydration solution such as Pedialyte or Lytren.
  2. May temporarily need lactose-free diet.
  3. Children should not receive antidiarrheals—for example, Imodium A-D.
  4. Do not give grape juice, orange juice, apple juice, cola, or ginger ale. These solutions have high osmolality and may cause diarrhea.

> **HESI Hint** • IV fluids containing potassium should be administered only with adequate urine output.

Burns

Description: Tissue injury caused by heat, electricity, chemicals, or radiation.

A. A leading cause of accidental death in children younger than 15 years.
B. It is estimated that 75% of burns are preventable.
C. Children younger than age 2 have a higher mortality rate because of:
  1. Greater body surface area.
  2. Greater fluid volume (proportionate to body size).
  3. Less effective cardiovascular responses to volume shifts.
D. In childhood, a partial-thickness burn is considered a major burn if it involves more than 25% of body surface. A full-thickness burn is considered major if it involves more than 10% of body surface.
E. Because of the changing proportions of the child, especially the infant, the rule of nines cannot be used to assess the percent of burn (see Figure 4-9, *Estimation of Burn Injury in Children and Adults*, p. 161). An assessment tool that takes into account the changing proportions of the child, such as the Lund-Browder chart, should be used.
F. Fluid needs should be calculated from the time of the burn.

G. The Parkland formula is a commonly used guideline for calculating fluid replacement and maintenance. It is based on the child's body surface area and should include volume for burn losses and maintenance.
H. Adequacy of fluid replacement is determined by evaluating urinary output.
I. Specific gravity should be less than 1.025.

> **HESI Hint** • Urinary output for infants and children should be 1 to 2 mL/kg/hour.

J. When children exhibit scald-type burns that have a glove or stocking distribution, child abuse should be considered.
K. See Burns in Chapter 4, *Medical-Surgical Nursing*, p. 160.

Child Maltreatment (Abuse)

Description: Includes physical and mental injury, sexual abuse, and emotional and physical neglect. This is a national problem from which 3000 to 5000 children die each year (see Abuse in Chapter 7, *Psychiatric Nursing*, p. 319).

Poisonings

Description: Ingesting, inhaling, or absorbing a toxic substance.

A. Poisoning, particularly by ingestion, such as lead and home remedies, is a frequent cause of childhood injury or illness.
  1. General signs of lead poisoning include anemia; acute, crampy abdominal pain; vomiting; constipation; anorexia; headache; lethargy; and impaired growth.
  2. Early CNS signs of lead poisoning include hyperactivity, aggression, impulsiveness, decreased interest in play, and irritability.
  3. Late CNS signs of lead poisoning include cognitive impairment, paralysis, blindness, convulsions, coma, and death.
B. Most poisonings occur in children younger than 6 years of age, with a peak at age 2 years.
C. The exploratory behavior, curiosity, and oral-motor activity of early childhood place the child at risk for poisonings.
D. Ninety percent of poisonings occur in the home.

Nursing Assessment (Data Collection)

A. Child found near the source of the poison
B. Gastrointestinal (GI) disturbance: nausea, abdominal pain, diarrhea, vomiting
C. Burns of mouth, pharynx
D. Respiratory distress
E. Seizures, changes in level of consciousness

F. Cyanosis
G. Shock

Analysis (Nursing Diagnoses)
A. Risk for injury related to …
B. Deficient knowledge (home safety) related to …

Nursing Plans and Interventions
A. Observe the child's respiratory, cardiac, and neurologic status.
B. Identify the poisonous agent quickly!
C. Instruct parent to bring any emesis, stool, and so on, and the poisonous agent to the emergency room.
D. Determine the child's age and weight.
E. Important parent education: reinforce to parents the need to notify pediatrician and/or Poison Control Help Line at 800-222-1222 if poisoning occurs in home.

HESI Hint • Use of syrup of ipecac is no longer recommended by the American Academy of Pediatrics. Teach parents that it is *not* recommended to induce vomiting in any way because it may cause more damage.

F. Poison removal or care may require gastric lavage, activated charcoal, or naloxone HCl (Narcan).
G. Collaborate with members of health care team to reinforce the following information:
1. Poisonproof/childproof the home:
   a. Identify location of poisons: under the sink (cleaning supplies, drain cleaners, bug poisons); medicine cabinets; storage rooms (paints, varnishes); garages (antifreeze, gasoline); poisonous plants (philodendron, dieffenbachia).
   b. Put locks on cabinets.
   c. Use safety containers: do not place poisonous materials in other, nonsafe containers. Always leave medications in their original containers so all information is readily available on the package.
   d. Safely discard unused medications.
   e. Make sure child is always under adult supervision.
2. Post phone number for local Poison Control Center by telephone.
3. Examine the environment from the child's viewpoint (the height that a 2- to 5-year-old can reach).
H. Coordinate referral to community health nurse or child welfare agency if necessary.

Review of Child Health Promotion

1. List two contraindications for live virus immunization.
2. List three classic signs and symptoms of measles.
3. List the signs and symptoms of iron deficiency.
4. Identify food sources for vitamin A.
5. What disease occurs with vitamin C deficiency?
6. What measurements reflect present nutritional status?
7. List the signs and symptoms of dehydration in an infant.
8. List the laboratory findings that can be expected in a dehydrated child.
9. How should burns in children be assessed?
10. How can the nurse *best* evaluate the adequacy of fluid replacement in children?
11. How should a parent be instructed to "childproof" a house?
12. What interventions should the nurse do *first* in caring for a child who has ingested a poison?
13. Name the early CNS signs of lead poisoning.

Answers to Review

1. Immunocompromised child or a child in a household with an immunocompromised individual.
2. Photophobia, confluent rash that begins on the face and spreads downward, and Koplik spots on the buccal mucosa.
3. Anemia, pale conjunctiva, pale skin color, atrophy of papillae on tongue, brittle/ridged/spoon-shaped nails, and thyroid edema.
4. Liver, sweet potatoes, carrots, spinach, peaches, and apricots.
5. Scurvy.
6. Weight, skinfold thickness, and arm circumference.
7. Poor skin turgor, absence of tears, dry mucous membranes, weight loss, depressed fontanel and decreased urinary output.
8. Loss of bicarbonate/decreased serum pH, loss of sodium (hyponatremia), loss of potassium (hypokalemia), elevated Hct, and elevated BUN.
9. Use the Lund-Browder chart, which takes into account the changing proportions of the child's body.

10. Monitor urine output.
11. Lock all cabinets, safely store all toxic household items in locked cabinets, and examine the house from the child's point of view.
12. Observe and report to RN the child's respiratory, cardiac, and neurologic statuses.
13. Early CNS signs of lead poisoning include hyperactivity, aggression, impulsiveness, decreased interest in play, and irritability.

Respiratory Disorders

Important Signs for Children

A. Normal pulse and respiratory rates (Table 5-3, *Normal Pulse and Respiratory Rates for Children*).
B. Signs of respiratory distress in children:
  1. Cardinal signs of respiratory distress:
    a. Restlessness
    b. Increased respiratory rate
    c. Increased pulse rate
    d. Diaphoresis
  2. Other signs of respiratory distress:
    a. Flaring nostrils
    b. Retractions
    c. Grunting
    d. Adventitious breath sounds (or absent breath sounds)
    e. Use of accessory muscles, head bobbing
    f. Alterations in blood gases: decreased P_{O_2}, elevated P_{CO_2}
    g. Cyanosis and pallor
C. Nursing implications:
  1. Pediatric clients often go into respiratory failure before cardiac failure.
  2. The PN should know the signs of respiratory distress.

Asthma

Description: Asthma is an inflammatory reactive airway disease that is often chronic.
A. The airways become edematous.
B. Airways become congested with mucus.
C. Smooth muscles of bronchi and bronchioles constrict.
D. Air trapping occurs in the alveoli.

Nursing Assessment (Data Collection)

A. History of asthma in the family
B. History of allergies
C. Home environment contains pets or other allergens
D. Tight cough (nonproductive cough)
E. Breath sounds: course, expiratory wheezing, rales, crackles
F. Chest diameter enlarges (late sign/symptom)
G. Increased number of school days missed during past 6 months
H. Signs of respiratory distress (see Respiratory Disorders and Important Signs for Children, p. XXX).

Analysis (Nursing Diagnoses)

A. Impaired gas exchange related to …
B. Ineffective breathing pattern related to …

Nursing Plans and Interventions

A. Monitor carefully for increasing respiratory distress.
B. Administer rapid-acting bronchodilators and steroids for acute attacks.
C. Maintain oral hydration and observe IV fluids.
D. Monitor blood gas values for signs of respiratory acidosis (see Fluid and Electrolyte Balance in Chapter 3, *Advanced Clinical Concepts*, p. 35).
E. Administer oxygen and/or nebulizer therapy as prescribed.
F. Monitor pulse oximetry as prescribed (usually more than 95% is normal).
G. Monitor beta-adrenergic agonists such as albuterol and levalbuteral (Xopenex), as well as anti-inflammatory corticosteroids such as budesonide, which are commonly used medications (Table 5-4, *Adrenergics*; and see Table 4-4).
H. Collaborate with health care team to develop and implement a teaching plan for a home care program:
  1. Identifying precipitating factors
  2. Reducing allergens in the home

TABLE 5-3 Normal Pulse and Respiratory Rates for Children

Age	Pulse	Respirations	Nursing Implications
Newborn	100 to 160	30 to 60	These ranges are averages only and vary with the gender, age, and condition of child; always note if the child is crying, febrile, or in some distress.
1 to 11 months	100 to 150	25 to 35	
1 to 3 years (toddler)	80 to 130	20 to 30	
3 to 5 years (preschooler)	80 to 120	20 to 25	
6 to 10 years (school age)	70 to 110	18 to 22	
10 to 16 years (adolescent)	60 to 90	16 to 20	

3. Using a metered-dose inhaler
4. Home monitoring of peak expiratory flow rate
5. Breathing exercises
6. Monitoring drug actions, dosages, and side effects
7. Instructing how to manage acute episode and when to seek emergency care

Cystic Fibrosis

Description: Cystic fibrosis is an autosomal recessive disease that causes dysfunction of the exocrine glands.
A. Tenacious mucus production obstructs vital structures.
B. Multiple problems result from the exocrine dysfunction:
   1. Lung insufficiency (most critical problem)
   2. Pancreatic insufficiency
   3. Increased loss of sodium and chloride in sweat

Nursing Assessment (Data Collection)

A. Usually white infant/child
B. Meconium ileus at birth (10% to 20% of cases)
C. Recurrent respiratory infection
D. Pulmonary congestion
E. Steatorrhea (excessive fat, greasy stools)
F. Foul-smelling, bulky stools
G. Delayed growth and poor weight gain
H. Skin tastes "salty" when kissed (caused by excessive secretions from sweat glands)
I. Later: cyanosis, nail bed clubbing, congestive heart failure (CHF)

Analysis (Nursing Diagnoses)

A. Ineffective airway clearance related to …
B. Imbalanced nutrition: less than body requirements related to …

Nursing Plans and Interventions

A. Monitor respiratory status.
B. Observe for signs of respiratory infection.

C. Administer pancreatic enzymes (pancrelipase [Cotazym-S, Pancrease]) (give with applesauce, rice, or cereal for infants, and give with regular meal for an older child).
D. Administer fat-soluble vitamins (A, D, E, K) in water-soluble form.
E. Administer oxygen/nebulizer treatments as prescribed (Box 5-1, *Respiratory Client*).
F. Observe for effectiveness of respiratory treatments.
G. Collaborate with health care team to enhance and reinforce a family teaching plan for percussion and postural drainage techniques.
H. Dietary recommendations include high calories, high protein, high fat (more calories per volume), and moderate to low carbohydrates (to avoid an increase in CO_2 drive).
I. Provide age-appropriate activities.

> **HESI Hint** • Child needs 150% of the usual calorie intake for normal growth and development.

BOX 5-1 *Respiratory Client*

Administration of Oxygen
- Oxygen hood: used for infants.
- Nasal prongs: provide low to moderate concentrations of oxygen.
- Tents: provide mist and oxygen. Monitor child's temperature. Keep edges tucked in. Keep child dry.

Measurement of Oxygenation
- Pulse oximetry measures oxygen saturation (SaO_2) of arterial hemoglobin noninvasively via a sensor that is usually attached to the finger or toe (infant: attach to sole of foot).
- Nurse should be aware of the alarm parameters signaling decreased SaO_2 (usually <95%).
- Blood gas evaluation is usually monitored in respiratory clients through arterial sampling.
- Norms: Po_2: 83 to 100; Pco_2: 35 to 45 for infants and children (not newborns).

TABLE 5-4 Adrenergics

Drugs	Indications	Adverse Reactions	Nursing Implications
Epinephrine HCl (Sus-Phrine)	• Rapid-acting bronchodilator • Drug of choice for acute asthma attack	• Tachycardia • Hypertension • Tremors • Nausea	• Give subcutaneous, IV, nebulizer • May be repeated in 20 minutes
Theophylline (Theo-Dur) Salmetrol (Serevent) Albuterol (Proventil HFA)	• Bronchodilator, used in asthma to reverse bronchospasm	• Tachycardia • Irritability • Palpitations • Hypotension • Nausea, vomiting	• Auscultate lungs before and after administration • Monitor blood levels

> **HESI Hint** • When calculating a pediatric dosage, the nurse must often change the child's weight from pounds to kilograms. *Hint:* Weight expressed in kilograms should always be a smaller number than weight expressed in pounds.

Epiglottitis

Description: Severe, life-threatening infection of the epiglottis.

A. Epiglottitis progresses rapidly, causing acute airway obstruction.
B. The organism usually responsible for epiglottitis is *Haemophilus influenzae* (*H. influenzae*, primarily type B).

Nursing Assessment (Data Collection)

A. Sudden onset
B. Restlessness
C. High fever
D. Sore throat, dysphagia
E. Drooling
F. Muffled voice
G. Child assumes upright sitting position with chin out and tongue protruding ("tripod" position)

Analysis (Nursing Diagnoses)

A. Ineffective breathing pattern related to …
B. Anxiety related to …

Nursing Plans and Interventions

A. Encourage prevention with Hib vaccine.
B. Maintain child in upright sitting position.
C. Prepare for intubation or tracheostomy.
D. Administer antibiotics as prescribed.
E. Prepare for hospitalization in ICU.
F. Restrain as needed to prevent extubation.
G. Employ measures to decrease agitation and crying.
H. Prevention: *H. influenzae* type B (see Figure 5-2).

HESI Hint • Do not examine the throat of a child with epiglottitis because of the risk of completely obstructing the airway—that is, do not put a tongue blade or any object in the throat.

Bronchiolitis

Description: A viral infection of the bronchioles characterized by thick secretions.

A. Bronchiolitis is usually caused by respiratory syncytial virus (RSV) and is found to be readily transmitted by close contact with hospital personnel, families, and other children.
B. Bronchiolitis occurs primarily in young infants.

Nursing Assessment (Data Collection)

A. History of upper respiratory symptoms
B. Irritable, distressed infant
C. Paroxysmal coughing
D. Poor eating
E. Nasal congestion
F. Nasal flaring
G. Prolonged expiratory phase of respiration
H. Wheezing; rales can be auscultated
I. Deteriorating condition that is often indicated by shallow, rapid respirations

Analysis (Nursing Diagnoses)

A. Impaired gas exchange related to …
B. Ineffective airway clearance related to …

Nursing Plans and Interventions

A. Isolate child in a separate room; maintain contact and standard precautions.
B. Use meticulous hand-washing technique.
C. Monitor respiratory status; observe for hypoxia.
D. Clear airway of secretions using a bulb syringe for suctioning.
E. Provide care in a mist tent; administer oxygen as prescribed.
F. Maintain hydration and observe IV fluids.
G. Monitor antiviral agent, if prescribed.
H. Observe response to respiratory therapy treatments.
I. Synagis (palivizumab) may be given to provide passive immunity against RSV in high-risk children (younger than 2 years of age with a history of prematurity, lung disease, or congenital heart disease).

HESI Hint • In planning and providing nursing care, patent airway is always a priority of care, regardless of age.

Otitis Media

Description: Otitis media is an inflammatory disorder of the middle ear.

A. Otitis media may be suppurative or serous.
B. Anatomic structure of the ear predisposes young child to ear infections.
C. There is a risk of conductive hearing loss if untreated or incompletely treated.

Nursing Assessment (Data Collection)

A. Fever, pain, infant may pull at ear
B. Enlarged lymph nodes
C. Discharge from ear (if drum is ruptured)
D. Upper respiratory symptoms
E. Vomiting, diarrhea

Analysis (Nursing Diagnoses)

A. Risk for infection related to …
B. Pain related to …

Nursing Plans and Interventions

A. Administer antibiotics if prescribed.
B. Reduce body temperature (can be very high, with risk of seizures).
   1. Tepid baths
   2. Acetaminophen if prescribed

C. Position child on affected side.

D. Comfort measure: warm compress on affected ear.

E. Collaborate with RN to enhance and reinforce a teaching plan for home care.

   1. Finish all prescribed antibiotics.

   2. Encourage follow-up visit.

   3. Monitor for hearing loss.

   4. Preventive care (exposure to tobacco smoke and bottle feeding in supine position are predisposing factors).

> **HESI Hint** • Respiratory disorders are the primary reason most children and their families seek medical care. Therefore, these disorders are frequently tested on the NCLEX-PN. Knowing the normal parameters for respiratory rates and the key signs of respiratory distress in children is essential.

Tonsillitis

Description: Inflammation of the tonsils.

A. Tonsillitis may be viral or bacterial.

B. Tonsillitis may be related to streptococcus infection.

C. If related to streptococcus, treatment is *very important* because of the risk of developing acute glomerulonephritis or rheumatic heart disease.

Nursing Assessment (Data Collection)

A. Sore throat

B. Fever

C. Enlarged tonsils (may have purulent discharge on tonsils)

D. Breathing may be obstructed (tonsils touching, called "kissing tonsils")

E. Throat culture to determine viral or bacterial etiology

> **HESI Hint** • The nurse should be sure a prothrombin time (PT) and partial thromboplastin time (PTT) have been determined before a tonsillectomy. More importantly, the nurse should ask if there has been a history of bleeding, prolonged/excessive, or if there is a history of any bleeding disorders in the family.

Analysis (Nursing Diagnoses)

A. Impaired swallowing related to …

B. Risk for injury related to …

Nursing Plans and Interventions

A. Collect throat culture if prescribed.

B. Implement instructions to parents for home care:

   1. Encourage warm saline gargles.

   2. Provide ice chips.

   3. Administer antibiotics if prescribed.

   4. Manage fever with acetaminophen.

C. Provide surgical care for tonsillectomy if indicated:

   1. Reinforce preoperative teaching and obtain assessment data.

   2. Monitor for signs of postoperative bleeding.

      a. Frequent swallowing

      b. Vomiting fresh blood

      c. Clearing throat

   3. Encourage soft foods and oral fluids (avoid red or purple fluids, which mimic signs of bleeding). *No straws.*

   4. Comfort measure: ice collar will help with pain and with vasoconstriction.

   5. Highest risk of hemorrhage is first 24 hours and 5 to 10 days after surgery.

Review of Respiratory Disorders

1. Describe the purpose of bronchodilators.

2. What are the physical assessment findings for a child with asthma?

3. What nutritional support should be provided for the child with cystic fibrosis?

4. Why is genetic counseling important for the cystic fibrosis family?

5. List seven signs of respiratory distress in a pediatric client.

6. Describe the care of a child in a mist tent.

7. What position does the child with epiglottitis assume?

8. Why are IV fluids important for the child with an increased respiratory rate?

9. Children with chronic otitis media are at risk for developing what problem?

10. What is the most common postoperative complication following a tonsillectomy? Describe the signs and symptoms of this complication.

Answers to Review

1. Reverse bronchospasm and open airways.

2. Expiratory wheezing, rales, tight cough, and signs of altered blood gases.

3. Pancreatic enzyme replacement, fat-soluble vitamins, and a moderate- to low-carbohydrate, high-protein, moderate-fat diet.

4. The disease is autosomal recessive in its genetic pattern.
5. Restlessness, tachycardia, tachypnea, diaphoresis, flaring nostrils, retractions, and grunting.
6. Monitor child's temperature. Keep tent edges tucked in. Keep clothing dry. Assess child's respiratory status. Look at child inside tent.
7. Upright, sitting, with chin out and tongue protruding ("tripod" position).
8. The child is at risk for dehydration and acid/base imbalance.
9. Hearing loss.
10. Hemorrhage; frequent swallowing, vomiting fresh blood, and clearing throat.

Cardiovascular Disorders

Congenital Heart Disorders

Description: Heart anomalies that develop in utero and manifest at birth or shortly thereafter.
A. Congenital heart disorders (CHD) occur in 4 to 10 children per 1000 live births.
B. May be categorized as:
 1. Acyanotic (VSD, ASD, PDA, coarctation of aorta, AS):
  a. Left to right shunts or increased pulmonary blood flow
  b. Obstructive defects
 2. Cyanotic (Tetralogy of Fallot, TA, TGV):
  a. Right to left shunts or decreased pulmonary blood flow
  b. Mixed blood flow
C. May use hemodynamic classification:
 1. Increased pulmonary blood flow defects (ASD, VSD, and PDA)
 2. Obstructive defects (coarctation of aorta, AS)
 3. Decreased pulmonary blood flow defects (Tetralogy of Fallot)
 4. Mixed defects (TGV, TA)

Acyanotic Heart Defects

Ventricular Septal Defect (VSD) (Increased Pulmonary Blood Flow)

A. Hole between the ventricles.
B. Oxygenated blood from left ventricle is shunted to right ventricle and re-circulated to the lungs.
C. Small defects may close spontaneously.
D. Large defects cause Eisenmenger syndrome or congestive heart failure and require surgical closures (Figure 5-3, *Ventricular Septal Defect*).

Atrial Septal Defect (ASD) (Increased Pulmonary Blood Flow)

A. Hole between the atria.
B. Oxygenated blood from the left atrium is shunted to the right atrium and lungs.
C. Most defects do not seriously compromise children.

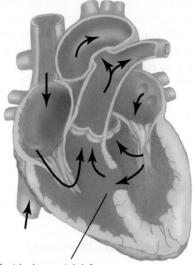

FIGURE 5-3 Ventricular Septal Defect. (From Price D, Gwin J: *Pediatric nursing: an introductory text*, ed 11, St. Louis 2012, Saunders.)

D. Surgical closure is recommended before school age. It can lead to significant problems such as congestive heart failure or atrial dysrhythmias later in life if not corrected (Figure 5-4, *Atrial Septal Defect*).

Patent Ductus Arteriosus (PDA) (Increased Pulmonary Blood Flow)

A. Abnormal opening between the aorta and pulmonary artery.
B. Usually closes within 72 hours after birth.
C. If it remains patent, oxygenated blood from the aorta returns to pulmonary artery.
D. Increased blood flow to the lungs causes pulmonary hypertension.
E. May require medical intervention with indomethacin (Indocin) administration or surgical closure (Figure 5-5, *Patent Ductus Arteriosus*).

Coarctation of the Aorta (Obstruction of Blood Flow from Ventricles)

A. An obstructive narrowing of the aorta.
B. The most common sites: aortic valve and aorta near ductus arteriosus.

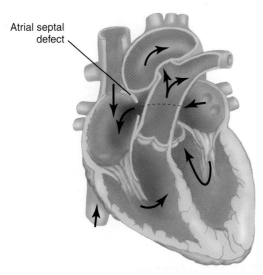

FIGURE 5-4 Atrial Septal Defect. (From James S, Ashwill J: *Nursing care of children: principles and practice*, ed 4, Philadelphia, 2013, Saunders.)

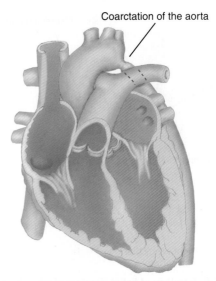

FIGURE 5-6 Coarctation of the Aorta. (From James S, Ashwill J: *Nursing care of children: principles and practice*, ed 4, Philadelphia, 2013, Saunders.)

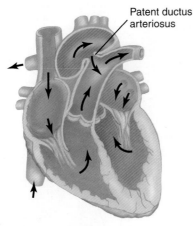

FIGURE 5-5 Patent Ductus Arteriosus. (From James S, Ashwill J: *Nursing care of children: principles and practice*, ed 4, Philadelphia, 2013, Saunders.)

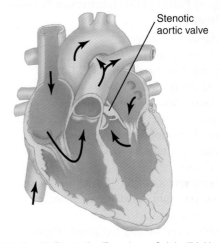

FIGURE 5-7 Aortic Stenosis. (From James S, Ashwill J: *Nursing care of children: principles and practice*, ed 4, Philadelphia, 2013, Saunders.)

C. Common finding: hypertension in the upper extremities and decreased or absent pulses in the lower extremities.

D. May require surgical correction (Figure 5-6, *Coarctation of the Aorta*).

Aortic Stenosis (AS) (Obstruction of Blood Flow from Ventricles)

A. An obstructive narrowing immediately before, at, or after the aortic valve (most commonly valvular).

B. Oxygenated blood flow from the left ventricle into systemic circulation is diminished.

C. Symptoms are caused by low cardiac output.

D. May require surgical correction (Figure 5-7, *Aortic Stenosis*).

Traditional Three Ts of Cyanotic Heart Disease

A. Tetralogy of Fallot: a combination of four defects:
   1. A ventricular septal defect (VSD)

2. An aorta placed over and above the ventricular septal defect (overriding aorta)

3. Pulmonary stenosis (PS) that obstructs right ventricular outflow

4. Right ventricular hypertrophy. The severity of the pulmonary stenosis is related to the degree of right ventricular hypertrophy and the extent of shunting.

B. Truncus arteriosus: one artery (truncus), rather than two arteries (aorta and pulmonary artery), arises from both ventricles.

C. Transposition of the great arteries: pulmonary artery leaves the left ventricle, and the aorta exits from the right ventricle.

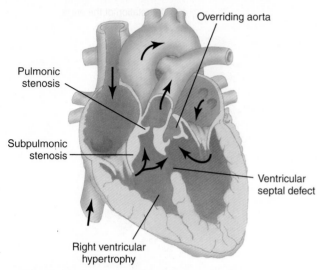

FIGURE 5-8 **Tetralogy of Fallot.** Tetralogy of Fallot showing the four defects: pulmonary stenosis, VSD, dextroposition of the aorta, and right ventricular hypertrophy (From James S, Ashwill J: *Nursing care of children: principles and practice,* ed 4, Philadelphia, 2013, Saunders.)

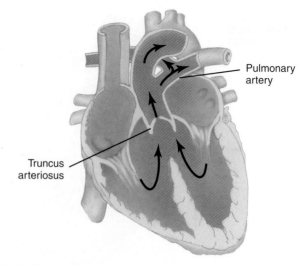

FIGURE 5-9 **Truncus Arteriosus.** (From James S, Ashwill J: *Nursing care of children: principles and practice,* ed 4, Philadelphia, 2013, Saunders.)

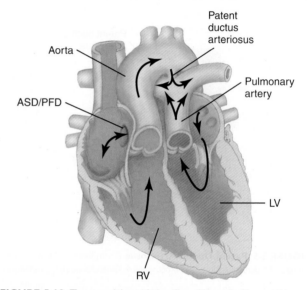

FIGURE 5-10 **Transposition of the Great Vessels.** Transposition of the great arteries (From James S, Ashwill J: *Nursing care of children: principles and practice,* ed 4, Philadelphia, 2013, Saunders.)

Tetralogy of Fallot (TOF; Decreased Pulmonary Blood Flow)

A. Consists of four defects:
1. Pulmonary stenosis (PS)
2. Ventricular septal defect (VSD)
3. Overriding aorta
4. Right ventricular hypertrophy
B. Cyanosis occurs because unoxygenated blood is pumped into the systemic circulation.
C. Decreased pulmonary circulation due to the pulmonary stenosis.
D. Child experiences "tet" spells, or hypoxic episodes; relieved by child squatting or being placed in knee-chest position.
E. Requires staged surgery to correct (Figure 5-8, *Tetralogy of Fallot*).

> **HESI Hint** • Polycythemia is common in children with cyanotic defects.

Truncus Arteriosus

A. Pulmonary artery and aorta do not separate.
B. One main vessel receives blood from the left and right ventricles together.
C. Blood mixes in right and left ventricles through a large ventricular septal defect (VSD), resulting in cyanosis.
D. Increased pulmonary resistance results in increased cyanosis.
E. This congenital defect requires surgical correction; only the presence of the large VSD allows for survival at birth (Figure 5-9, *Truncus Arteriosus*).

Transposition of the Great Vessels (Mixed Blood Flow)

A. The great vessels are reversed.
B. The pulmonary circulation arises from the left ventricle, and the systemic circulation arises from the right ventricle.
C. This is incompatible with life unless coexisting VSD, ASD, and/or PDA is present.
D. The diagnosis is a MEDICAL EMERGENCY. The child will receive prostaglandin E (PGE) to keep ducts open (Figure 5-10, *Transposition of the Great Vessels*).

Care of Children with Congenital Heart Disease (CHD)

Nursing Assessment (Data Collection)

A. Congenital heart disease manifestations:
1. Murmur (present or absent; thrill, or rub)

2. Cyanosis, clubbing of digits (usually after age 2 years)
3. Poor feeding, poor weight gain, failure to thrive
4. Frequent regurgitation
5. Frequent respiratory infections
6. Activity intolerance, fatigue

B. Assess for the following:
1. Heart rate and rhythm and heart sounds
2. Pulses (quality and symmetry)

> **HESI Hint** • For normal cardiac rates in children, see Table 5-3. The heart rate of a child increases with crying or fever.

3. Blood pressure (upper and lower extremities)
4. History of maternal infection during pregnancy

Analysis (Nursing Diagnoses)

A. Decreased cardiac output related to …
B. Activity intolerance related to …
C. Delayed growth and development related to …

Nursing Plans and Interventions

A. Provide care for the child with cardiovascular dysfunction:
1. Maintain nutritional status; feed small, frequent feedings. Provide high-calorie formula or fortified breast milk.

> **HESI Hint** • Infants may require tube feeding to conserve energy. Infants being tube fed need to continue to satisfy their sucking reflex.

2. Maintain hydration (polycythemia increases risk for thrombus formation).
3. Maintain neutral thermal environment.
4. Plan frequent rest periods.
5. Organize activities to disturb child only as indicated.
6. Administer digoxin/diuretics as prescribed.
7. Monitor for signs of deteriorating condition or congestive heart failure (CHF).
8. Collaborate with RN to enhance and reinforce a family teaching plan related to the need for prophylactic antibiotics before any dental or invasive procedures because of the risk of endocarditis.

B. Assist with diagnostic tests and support family during diagnosis:
1. ECG
2. Echocardiography

C. Prepare family and child for cardiac catheterization (conducted when surgery is probable or as an intervention for certain procedures):
1. Risks of catheterization are similar to those for a child undergoing cardiac surgery:
   a. Dysrhythmias
   b. Bleeding
   c. Perforation
   d. Phlebitis
   e. Arterial obstruction at the entry site
2. Child requires reassurance and close monitoring postcatheterization:
   a. Vital signs
   b. Pulses
   c. Incision site
   d. Cardiac rhythm
3. Prepare family and child (as able) for surgical intervention if necessary.

D. Prepare child as appropriate for age:
1. Give abbreviated tour of ICU.
2. Explain chest tubes, IVs, monitors, dressings, and ventilator.
3. Show family/child waiting area for families.
4. Use a doll or simple drawing for explanations.
5. Provide emotional support.

> **HESI Hint** • Basic difference between cyanotic and acyanotic defects:
> • Acyanotic: has abnormal circulation; however, all blood entering the systemic circulation is oxygenated.
> • Cyanotic: has abnormal circulation with unoxygenated blood entering systemic circulation.
> • CHF: congestive heart failure is more often associated with acyanotic defects.

Congestive Heart Failure

Description: Congestive heart failure (CHF) is a condition in which the heart is unable to effectively pump the volume of blood that is presented to it.

> **HESI Hint** • CHF is a common complication of congenital heart disease. It reflects the increased workload of the heart resulting from shunts or obstructions. The two objectives in treating CHF are to reduce the workload of the heart and to increase cardiac output.

Nursing Assessment (Data Collection)

A. Tachypnea, shortness of breath
B. Tachycardia
C. Difficulty feeding
D. Cyanosis
E. Grunting, wheezing, pulmonary congestion
F. Edema (face, eyes of infants), weight gain
G. Diaphoresis (especially head)
H. Hepatomegaly

Analysis (Nursing Diagnoses)

A. Decreased cardiac output related to …
B. Impaired gas exchange related to …

BOX 5-2 *Managing Digoxin*

Administration	Toxicity
• Prior to administering digoxin, nurse *must* take child's apical pulse for 1 minute to assess for bradycardia. Hold dose if pulse is below normal heart rate for child's age. • Collaborate with RN to maintain therapeutic blood levels of digoxin for child. • Collaborate with RN to teach families safe home administration of digoxin: • Administer on a regular basis; do *not* skip or make up for missed doses. • Give 1 hour before or 2 hours after meals. Do *not* mix with formula or food. • Take child's pulse prior to administration, and know when to call the caregiver. • Keep in safe place (e.g., a locked cabinet).	• Nurse must be acutely aware of the signs of digoxin toxicity. A small child or infant cannot describe feeling bad or nauseated. • Vomiting is a common early sign of toxicity. This symptom is often overlooked because infants commonly "spit up." • Other GI symptoms include anorexia, diarrhea, and abdominal pain. • Neurologic signs include fatigue, muscle weakness, and drowsiness. • Hypokalemia can increase digoxin toxicity.

Nursing Plans and Interventions

A. Monitor vital signs frequently and report signs of increasing distress.
B. Assess respiratory functioning frequently.
C. Elevate head of bed or use infant seat.
D. Administer oxygen therapy as prescribed.
E. Administer digoxin and diuretics as prescribed (Box 5-2, *Managing Digoxin*).
F. Weigh frequently (may be every shift for infants).
G. Maintain strict I&O, weigh diapers (1 g = 1 mL).
H. Report any unusual weight gains.
I. Provide low-sodium diet, formula, or breast milk.
J. Gavage feed infants if unable to get adequate nutrition by mouth.
K. Continue care for infant or child with a congenital defect as indicated.
L. See Nursing Plans and Interventions, Cyanotic Heart Defects, p. 183.

HESI Hint • When frequent weighings are required, weigh client on the same scale at the same time of day so that accurate comparisons can be made.

Rheumatic Fever

Description: Rheumatic fever is an inflammatory disease.
A. Rheumatic fever is the most common cause of acquired heart disease in children. It usually affects the aortic and mitral valves of the heart.
B. Rheumatic fever is associated with an antecedent beta hemolytic strep infection.
C. Rheumatic fever is a collagen disease that injures heart, blood vessels, joints, and subcutaneous tissue.

Nursing Assessment (Data Collection)

A. Chest pain, shortness of breath (carditis)
B. Tachycardia, even during sleep
C. Migratory large joint pain
D. Chorea (irregular, involuntary movements)
E. Rash (erythema marginatum)
F. Subcutaneous nodules over bony prominences
G. Fever
H. Lab findings:
   1. Elevated erythrocyte sedimentation rate
   2. Elevated ASO titer (antistreptolysin O)

Analysis (Nursing Diagnoses)

A. Decreased cardiac output related to …
B. Risk for injury related to …

Nursing Plans and Interventions

A. Monitor vital signs.
B. Observe for increasing signs of cardiac distress.
C. Encourage bed rest (as needed during febrile illness).
D. Assist with ambulation.
E. Reassure child/family that chorea is temporary.
F. Administer prescribed medications:
   1. Penicillin or erythromycin
   2. Aspirin for anti-inflammatory and anticoagulant actions
G. Collaborate with RN to enhance and reinforce a family teaching plan for a home care program:
   1. Explain the necessity for prophylactics.
     a. Antibiotics taken either orally or IM. Oral penicillin, as needed.
     b. IM penicillin G, each month (Table 5-5, *Anti-Infectives*).
   2. Inform dentist and other health care providers of diagnosis so they can evaluate the necessity for prophylactic antibiotics.

Kawasaki Disease (Mucocutaneous Lymph Node Syndrome)

Description: Kawasaki disease is an acute systemic vasculitis that can cause damage to vessels, including the coronary

TABLE 5-5 Anti-Infectives

Drugs	Indications	Adverse Reactions	Nursing Implications
Penicillin G (Bicillin)	Prophylaxis for recurrence of rheumatic fever	Allergic reactions ranging from rashes to anaphylactic shock and death	• Penicillin G is released very slowly over several weeks, giving sustained levels of concentration. • Have emergency equipment available wherever medication is administered. • *Always* determine existence of allergies to penicillin and cephalosporins; check chart/record and inquire of client/family.

arteries that supply blood flow to the heart. The disease can bring about permanent damage to the main arteries to the heart, resulting in the formation of an aneurysm of the coronary artery.

A. Cause of disease is unknown.
B. Usually seen in children younger than 5 years of age.
C. Has three phases: acute, subacute, and convalescent.
D. Leading cause of acquired heart disease in children.
E. Early treatment is essential to decrease chances of permanent heart damage.

Assessment (Data Collection)

A. Acute phase:
 1. High fever for more than 5 days
 2. Conjuctival redness, strawberry tongue
 3. Red, swollen hands and feet
B. Subacute phase includes peeling of hands and feet.
C. Convalescent (last) phase starts when all signs are gone and ends when lab values have returned to normal.
D. Extreme irritability is seen in the children during the disease process.

Analysis (Nursing Diagnoses)

A. Impaired skin integrity related to ...
B. Decreased cardiac output related to ...

Nursing Plan and Interventions

A. Assist RN to administer intravenous immunoglobulin (IVIG) as prescribed.
B. Treat high fevers with acetaminophen and aspirin (salicylate therapy) as prescribed.
C. Monitor cardiac status by documenting the child's:
 1. Intake and output
 2. Daily weights
D. Minimize skin discomfort with lotions and cool compresses.
E. Initiate meticulous mouth care.
F. Monitor intake of clear liquids and soft foods.
G. Support family as they comfort child during periods of irritability.
H. Assist RN with discharge teaching and home referral.

Review of Cardiovascular Disorders

1. Differentiate between a right-to-left and left-to-right shunt in cardiac disease.
2. List the four defects associated with Tetralogy of Fallot.
3. List the common signs of cardiac problems in an infant.
4. What are the two objectives in treating congestive heart failure?
5. Describe nursing interventions to reduce the workload of the heart.
6. What position would best relieve the child experiencing a "tet" spell?
7. What are common signs of digoxin toxicity?
8. List five risks of cardiac catheterization.
9. What cardiac complications are associated with rheumatic fever?
10. What medications are used to treat rheumatic fever?

Answers to Review

1. A left-to-right shunt moves oxygenated blood back through the pulmonary circulation. A right-to-left shunt bypasses the lungs and delivers unoxygenated blood to the systemic circulation, causing cyanosis.
2. VSD, overriding aorta, pulmonary stenosis, and right ventricular hypertrophy.
3. Poor feeding, poor weight gain, respiratory distress/infections, edema, and cyanosis.
4. Reduce the workload of the heart and increase cardiac output.
5. Small, frequent feedings or gavage feedings. Plan frequent rest periods. Maintain a neutral thermal environment. Organize activities to disturb child only as indicated.

6. Knee-chest position, or squatting.
7. Diarrhea, fatigue, weakness, and nausea and vomiting. The nurse should check for bradycardia before administration.
8. Dysrhythmia, bleeding, perforation, phlebitis, and obstruction of the arterial entry site.
9. Aortic valve stenosis and mitral valve stenosis.
10. Penicillin, erythromycin, and aspirin.

Neuromuscular Disorders

Down Syndrome

Description: Down syndrome is the most common chromosomal abnormality in children.
A. Down syndrome is evidenced by various physical characteristics and by cognitive impairment.
B. Down syndrome results from a trisomy of chromosome 21.
C. Down syndrome is associated with maternal age over 35 and with paternal factors, most often advanced paternal age.

Nursing Assessment (Data Collection)
A. Common physical characteristics (Figure 5-11, *Down Syndrome in an Infant*).
  1. Flat, broad nasal bridge
  2. Inner epicanthal eye folds
  3. Upward, outward slant of eyes
  4. Protruding tongue
  5. Short neck
  6. Transverse palmar crease (simian)
  7. Hyperextensible and lax joints (hypotonia)
B. Common associated problems:
  1. Cardiac defects
  2. Respiratory infections
  3. Feeding difficulties
  4. Delayed developmental skills
  5. Cognitive impairment
  6. Skeletal defects

Analysis (Nursing Diagnoses)
A. Delayed growth and development related to …
B. Risk for impaired parenting related to …

Nursing Plans and Interventions
A. Assist and support parents during the diagnostic process and management of associated problems.
B. Observe and monitor growth and development.

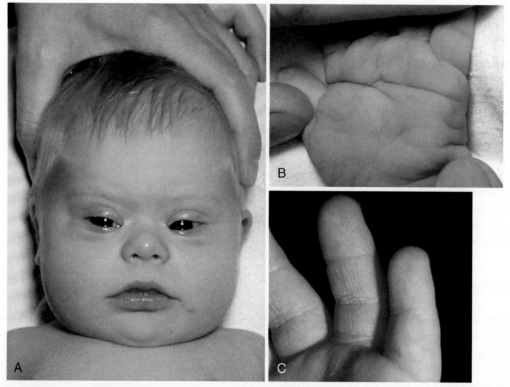

FIGURE 5-11 Down Syndrome in an Infant. Down syndrome. **A,** The typical facial appearance of an infant with Down syndrome shows the upward slant of the canthal folds of the eyes; protruding tongue; and short, thick neck. **B,** The straight simian crease in the palm of the hand is a typical finding in children with Down syndrome. **C,** The short fifth finger is a typical finding in children with Down syndrome. The tip of the fifth finger does not extend to the distal joint of the adjoining finger. (From Zitelli BL, Davis HW: *Atlas of pediatric physical diagnosis*, ed 6, St. Louis, 2012, Mosby.)

C. Collaborate with RN to develop and implement a family teaching plan for use of bulb syringe for suctioning nares.

D. Collaborate with RN to develop and implement a family teaching plan for signs of respiratory infection.

E. Assist family with feeding problems.

F. Feed to back and side of mouth.

G. Monitor for signs of cardiac difficulty or respiratory infection.

H. Coordinate with family and with an early intervention program.

> **HESI Hint** • The nursing goal in caring for a child with Down syndrome is to help the child reach his or her optimal level of functioning.

Cerebral Palsy

Description: Cerebral palsy (CP) is a nonprogressive injury to the motor centers of the brain causing neuromuscular problems of spasticity or dyskinesia (involuntary movements).

A. Associated problems may include cognitive impairment and seizures.

B. Etiology includes:
1. Anoxic injury before, during, or after birth
2. Maternal infections
3. Kernicterus (excessive bilirubin is deposited in brain cells, affecting neuron function and metabolism)
4. Low birth weight (major risk factor)

Nursing Assessment (Data Collection)

A. Persistent neonatal reflexes (Moro, tonic neck) after 6 months

B. Delayed developmental milestones

C. Apparent early preference for one hand

D. Poor suck, tongue thrust

E. Spasticity (may be described as "difficulty with diapering" by mother/caregiver)

F. Scissoring of legs is a common characteristic of spastic cerebral palsy (legs are extended and crossed over each other; feet are plantar flexed)

G. Involuntary movements

H. Seizures

Analysis (Nursing Diagnoses)

A. Delayed growth and development related to …

B. Imbalanced nutrition: less than body requirements related to …

Nursing Plans and Interventions

A. Observe for CP through follow-up of high-risk infants such as premature infants.

B. Coordinate with community-based agencies.

C. Coordinate with physical therapist, occupational therapist, speech therapist, nutritionist, orthopedic surgeon, and neurologist.

> **HESI Hint** • Feed infant or child with cerebral palsy using nursing interventions aimed at preventing aspiration. Position child upright and support the lower jaw.

D. Support family through grief process at diagnosis and throughout the child's life. Caring for severely affected children is very challenging.

E. Administer antiepileptic medications such as Dilantin, Tegretol, or Depakote if prescribed.

F. Administer baclofen (Lioresal) for muscle spasms if prescribed.

Attention Deficit Disorder/Attention Deficit Hyperactivity Disorder

Description: These disorders are currently classified in the *Diagnostic and Statistical Manual (of Mental Disorders)*, fourth edition (DSM-IV). However, recent studies indicate that these disorders are neurologic rather than psychiatric (see Childhood and Adolescent Disorders in Chapter 7, *Psychiatric Nursing*, p. 323).

Spina Bifida

Description: Spina bifida is a malformation of the vertebrae and spinal cord resulting in varying degrees of disability and deformity (Figure 5-12, *Midline Defects of Osseous Spine with Varying Degrees of Neural Herniations*).

A. Spina bifida occulta is a defect of vertebrae only. No sac is present, and it is usually a benign condition, although bowel and bladder problems may occur.

B. With meningocele and myelomeningocele, a sac is present at some point along the spine.

C. Meningocele contains only meninges and spinal fluid and has less neurologic involvement than a myelomeningocele.

D. Myelomeningocele is more severe than meningocele because the sac contains spinal fluid, meninges, and nerves.

E. The severity of neurologic impairment is determined by the anatomic level of the defect.

F. All children with a history of spina bifida should be screened for latex allergies.

G. Prevention: folic acid 0.4 mg beginning at least 3 months before pregnancy.

Nursing Assessment (Data Collection)

A. Spina bifida occulta: dimple with/without hair tuft at base of spine

B. Presence of sac in myelomeningocele is usually lumbar or lumbosacral

C. Flaccid paralysis and limited or no feeling below the defect

D. Head circumference at variance with norms on growth grids

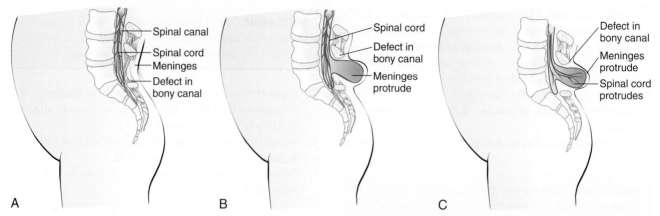

FIGURE 5-12 Midline Defects of Osseous Spine with Varying Degrees of Neural Herniations. Types of spina bifida. **A,** Spina bifida occulta. There is a defect in the bony canal. The meninges and spinal cord are normal. **B,** Spina bifida cystica meningocele. The spinal cord is normal, but there is a defect in the bony canal. The meninges protrude through this defect. **C,** Spina bifida cystica meningomyelocele. There is a defect in the bony canal. The meninges protrude, and the spinal cord protrudes through the defect. (From Leifer G: *Introduction to maternity & pediatric nursing,* ed 6, St. Louis, 2011, Saunders.)

E. Associated problems:
   1. Hydrocephalus (90% with myelomeningocele)
   2. Neurogenic bladder, poor anal sphincter tone
   3. Congenital dislocated hips
   4. Club feet
   5. Skin problems associated with anesthesia below the defect
   6. Scoliosis

Analysis (Nursing Diagnoses)

A. Risk for infection related to …
B. Impaired urinary elimination related to …
C. Impaired physical mobility related to …

Nursing Plans and Interventions

A. Preoperative:
   1. Keep sac free of stool and urine.
   2. Cover sac with moist sterile dressing.
   3. Place child in prone position with partial side lying position not causing undesirable hip flexion or tension on defect.
   4. Measure head circumference at least every 8 hours/every shift; check fontanel.
   5. Observe neurologic function.
   6. Monitor for signs of infection.
   7. Empty bladder using Credé method, or catheterize if needed.
   8. Promote parent-infant bonding.
B. Postoperative:
   1. Same as preoperative.
   2. Observe incision for drainage/infection.
   3. Observe neurologic function.
C. Long-term care:
   1. Collaborate with RN to enhance and reinforce a family teaching plan for a catheterization program when child is young.
   2. Help older children learn self-catheterization.

3. Administer propantheline (Pro-Banthine) or bethanechol (Urecholine) as prescribed to improve continence.
4. Collaborate with RN to enhance and implement a bowel program:
   a. High-fiber diet
   b. Increased fluids
   c. Regular fluids
   d. Suppositories, as needed
5. Observe skin condition frequently; provide latex-free environment.
6. Assist with ROM exercises, ambulation, and bracing, if client is able.
D. Support independent functioning of child.
E. Assist family to make realistic developmental expectations of child.

Hydrocephalus

Description: Hydrocephalus is a condition characterized by an abnormal accumulation of cerebral spinal fluid (CSF) within the ventricles of the brain.

A. Usually caused by an obstruction in the flow of CSF between the ventricles.
B. Hydrocephalus is most often associated with spina bifida; can be a complication of meningitis.

> **HESI Hint** The signs of increased intracranial pressure (ICP) are the opposite of those of shock.
> • Shock: increased pulse, decreased blood pressure
> • Increased ICP: decreased pulse, increased blood pressure

Nursing Assessment (Data Collection)

A. Older children show classic signs of increased intracranial pressure (ICP):
   1. Change in level of consciousness (LOC)

2. Irritability
3. Vomiting
4. Headache on awakening
5. Motor dysfunction
6. Unequal pupil response
7. Seizures
8. Decline in academics
9. Change in personality

B. Signs of increased ICP in infants:
1. Irritable, lethargic
2. Increasing head circumference
3. Bulging fontanels
4. Widening suture lines
5. "Sunset" eyes
6. High-pitched cry

> **HESI Hint** • Baseline data on the child's USUAL behavior and level of development is essential so changes associated with increased ICP can be detected EARLY.

Analysis (Nursing Diagnoses)

A. Delayed growth and development related to …
B. Risk for injury related to …

Nursing Plans and Interventions

A. Prepare infant/family for diagnostic procedures.
B. Monitor for signs of increased ICP.
C. Maintain seizure precautions.
D. Elevate head of bed.
E. Assist with preparation of parents for surgical procedure.
   1. Shunt is inserted into ventricle.
   2. Tubing is tunneled through skin to peritoneum, where it drains excess CSF.
F. Postoperative care:
   1. Observe for signs of shunt malfunction.
   2. Observe for signs of infection (meningitis).
   3. Monitor I&O closely.

> **HESI Hint** • Do not pump shunt unless specifically prescribed. The shunt is made up of delicate valves, and pumping changes pressures within the ventricle.

G. Collaborate with RN to enhance and reinforce a family teaching plan for a home care program:
   1. Watch for signs of increased ICP or infection.
   2. Child will eventually outgrow shunt and show symptoms of difficulty with level of consciousness (LOC).
   3. Child will need shunt revision.
   4. Anticipatory guidance for potential problems with growth and development.

Seizures

Description: An uncontrolled electrical discharge of neurons in the brain.

A. Seizures are more common in children younger than 2 years of age.
B. Seizures can be associated with immaturity of the central nervous system (CNS), fevers, infections, neoplasms, cerebral anoxia, and metabolic disorders.
C. Seizures are categorized as generalized or partial.
   1. Generalized seizures are:
      a. Tonic-clonic (grand mal); consciousness is lost.
         (1) Tonic phase—generalized stiffness of entire body
         (2) Clonic phase—spasm followed by relaxation
      b. Absence (petit mal); momentary loss of consciousness, posture is maintained; has minor face, eye, hand movements.
      c. Myoclonic; sudden, brief contracture of a muscle or muscle groups, no postictal state, may or may not be symmetric or include loss of consciousness.
   2. Partial seizures arise from a specific area in the brain and cause limited symptoms. Examples: focal and psychomotor seizures.

Nursing Assessment (Data Collection)

A. Tonic-clonic (grand mal):
   1. Aura (a warning sign of impending seizure)
   2. Loss of consciousness
   3. Tonic phase is characterized by generalized stiffness of entire body
   4. Apnea, cyanosis
   5. Clonic phase is characterized by spasms followed by relaxation
   6. Pupils dilated and nonreactive to light
   7. Incontinence
   8. Postseizure: disoriented, sleepy
B. Absence seizures (petit mal):
   1. Onset between 4 and 12 years
   2. Lasts 5 to 10 seconds
   3. Child appears inattentive, "daydreaming"
   4. Poor performance in school

> **HESI Hint** • Medication noncompliance is the most common cause of increased seizure activity.

Analysis (Nursing Diagnoses)

A. Risk for injury related to …
B. Risk for trauma related to …
C. Noncompliance (medication) related to …

Nursing Plans and Interventions

A. Maintain airway during seizure: turn on side to aid ventilation.
B. Do not restrain.

C. Protect from injury during seizure and support head (avoid neck flexion).
D. Document seizure, noting all data observed.
E. Maintain seizure precautions:
1. Reduce environmental stimuli as much as possible.
2. Pad side rails or crib rails.
3. Have suction equipment and oxygen quickly accessible.
4. Tape oral airway to the head of the bed.

HESI Hint • Do *not* use tongue blade, padded or not, during a seizure. It can cause traumatic damage to mouth/oral cavity.

F. Support during diagnostic tests: EEG, CT scan.
G. Support during workup for infections such as meningitis.
H. Administer anticonvulsant medications as prescribed.
1. For tonic-clonic seizures: phenytoin (Dilantin), carbamazepine (Tegretol), phenobarbital (Luminal), and Cerebyx (fosphenytoin)-IV
2. For absence seizures: ethosuximide (Zarontin), valproic acid (Depakene) (Table 5-6, *Anticonvulsants*)
I. Monitor therapeutic drug levels.
J. Collaborate with RN to develop and implement a family teaching plan about drug administration: dosage, action, and side effects.

TABLE 5-6 Anticonvulsants

Drugs	Indications	Adverse Reactions	Nursing Implications
• Phenobarbital (Luminal)	• Tonic-clonic and partial seizures • Is the longest acting of common barbiturates • Usually combined with other drugs	• Drowsiness • Nystagmus • Ataxia • Paradoxic excitement	• Therapeutic levels; 15 to 40 mcg/mL
• Phenytoin (Dilantin)	• Tonic-clonic and partial seizures	• Gingival hyperplasia • Dermatitis • Ataxia • Nausea, anorexia • Bone marrow depression • Nystagmus	• Therapeutic levels 10 to 20 mcg/mL • Monitor any drug interactions • Meticulous oral hygiene • Monitor CBC • Report to MD if any rash develops • Do not administer with milk
• Fosphenytoin sodium (Cerebyx)	• Generalized convulsive status epilepticus • Prevention/treatment of seizures during neurosurgery • Short-term parenteral replacement for phenytoin oral (Dilantin)	• Rapid IV infusion (greater than rate of 15 mg PE/minute) can cause hypotension • Severe: ataxia, CNS toxicity, confusion, gingival hyperplasia, irritability, lupus erythematosus, nervousness, nystagmus, paradoxic excitement, Stevens-Johnson syndrome, toxic epidural necrosis	• Used for short-term parenteral (IV infusion or IM injection) only • Should always be prescribed and dispensed in phenytoin sodium equivalents (PE)
• Valproic acid (Depakene)	• Absence seizures • Myoclonic seizures	• Hepatotoxicity, especially in children younger than 2 years of age • Prolonged bleeding times	• Monitor liver function studies • Potentiates phenobarbital and Dilantin, altering blood levels
• Carbamazepine (Tegretol)	• Tonic-clonic, mixed seizures	• Hepatitis • Agranulocytosis • Drowsiness	• Monitor liver function tests while on therapy • Therapeutic level: 6 to 12 mcg/mL
• Levetiracetam (Keppra) PO/IV	• Partial seizures • Myoclonic seizures • Tonic-clonic seizures	• Depression • Dizziness	• Monitor for depression • Do not abruptly discontinue drug • Monitor liver function, CBC, and renal function periodically
• Clonazepam (Klonopin)	• Absence seizures • Myoclonic seizures	• Drowsiness • Hyperactivity • Agitation • Increased salivation	• Therapeutic levels 20 to 80 mcg/mL • Do not abruptly discontinue drug • Monitor liver function tests, CBC, and renal function tests periodically

Bacterial Meningitis

Description: Bacterial inflammatory disorder of the meninges that covers the brain and spinal cord.

A. Meningitis is usually caused by *Haemophilus influenzae*, type B (less prevalent); *Streptococcus pneumonia*; or *Neisseria meningitidis*.

B. The usual route of bacterial invasion is from the middle ear or nasopharynx.

C. Other sources of bacterial invasion are related to wounds, including fractures of the skull, lumbar punctures, or shunts.

D. Exudate covers the brain, and cerebral edema occurs.

E. Lumbar puncture shows:
   1. Increased white blood cell count.
   2. Decreased glucose.
   3. Elevated protein.
   4. Increased ICP.
   5. Positive culture for meningitis.

Nursing Assessment (Data Collection)

A. Older children:
   1. Classic signs of increased ICP (see Hydrocephalus, p. 190)
   2. Fever, chills
   3. Neck stiffness, opisthotonus
   4. Photophobia
   5. Positive Kernig sign (inability to extend leg when thigh is flexed anteriorly at hip)
   6. Positive Brudzinski sign (neck flexion causes adduction and flexion movements of lower extremities)

B. Infants:
   1. Absence of classic signs
   2. Ill, with generalized symptoms
   3. Poor feeding
   4. Vomiting, irritability
   5. Bulging fontanel (an important sign)
   6. Seizures

Analysis (Nursing Diagnoses)

A. Disturbed sensory perception related to …

B. Risk for injury (specify) related to …

Nursing Plans and Interventions

A. Administer antibiotics (usually ampicillin, ceftriaxone, and/or chloramphenicol) and antipyretics as prescribed.

B. Isolate for at least 24 hours.

C. Monitor vital signs and neuro signs.

D. Keep environment quiet and darkened to prevent overstimulation.

E. Implement seizure precautions.

F. Position for comfort: head of the bed slightly elevated, with client on side if prescribed.

G. Measure head circumference daily in infants.

H. Monitor I&O closely.

I. Hib vaccine to protect against *H. influenzae* infection.

HESI Hint • Monitor hydration status carefully. With meningitis, there may be inappropriate antidiuretic hormone (ADH) secretions causing fluid retention (cerebral edema) and dilutional hyponatremia.

Reye Syndrome

Description: Reye syndrome is acute, rapidly progressing encephalopathy and hepatic dysfunction.

A. Etiology includes antecedent viral infections such as influenza or chickenpox.

B. Etiology is often associated with aspirin usage; aspirin is often found in OTC products, necessary to check labels.

C. Disease is staged by the clinical manifestations to reflect the severity of the condition.

Nursing Assessment (Data Collection)

A. Usually occurs in school-age children

B. Lethargy, rapidly progressing to deep coma (marked cerebral edema)

C. Vomiting

D. Elevated AST, ALT, lactate dehydrogenase, serum ammonia, decreased PT

E. Hypoglycemia

Analysis (Nursing Diagnoses)

A. Excess fluid volume related to …

B. Ineffective breathing pattern related to …

Nursing Plans and Interventions

A. Assist with critical care early in syndrome.

B. Monitor neurologic status: frequent noninvasive assessments and invasive ICP monitoring.

C. Maintain ventilation.

D. Monitor cardiac parameters.

E. Monitor I&O accurately.

F. Care for Foley catheter.

G. Provide family with emotional support.

Brain Tumors

Description: The second most common cancer in children.

A. Most pediatric brain tumors are infratentorial, making them difficult to excise surgically.

B. Tumors usually occur close to vital structures.

C. Gliomas are the most common childhood brain tumors.

Nursing Assessment (Data Collection)

A. Headache

HESI Hint • Headache upon awakening is the most common presenting symptom of brain tumors.

B. Vomiting (usually in the morning) often without nausea
C. Loss of concentration
D. Change in behavior or personality
E. Vision problems, tilts head
F. In infants: widening sutures, increasing frontal occipital circumference, tense fontanel
G. In older children, changes in gait
H. Changes in previously acquired skills

Analysis (Nursing Diagnoses)

A. Ineffective tissue perfusion (cerebral) related to …
B. Risk for injury related to …
C. Risk for infection related to …

Nursing Plans and Interventions

A. Identify baseline neurologic functioning.
B. Support child/family during diagnostic workup and treatment.
C. If surgery is treatment of choice, reinforce preoperative teaching:
   1. Explain that head will be shaved.
   2. Describe ICU, dressings, IVs, and so on.
   3. Identify child's developmental level, and plan teaching accordingly.
D. Observe family's response to the diagnosis, and treat family appropriately.
E. After surgery, position client as prescribed by the health care provider.

> **HESI Hint** • Most postoperative clients with infratentorial tumors are prescribed to lie flat and turn to either side. A large tumor may require that the child not be turned to the operative side.

F. Monitor intake and output carefully. Overhydration can cause cerebral edema and increased ICP.
G. Administer steroids as prescribed.
H. Support child/family to promote optimum functioning postoperatively.

> **HESI Hint** • Suctioning, coughing, straining, and/or turning causes increased ICP.

Muscular Dystrophy

Description: Muscular dystrophy is an inherited disease of the muscles, causing muscle atrophy and weakness.
A. Most serious and most common of the dystrophies is Duchenne muscular dystrophy, an X-linked recessive disease affecting primarily males.
B. Duchenne muscular dystrophy appears in early childhood (ages 3 to 5 years). It rapidly progresses, causing respiratory or cardiac complications and death, usually by 25 years of age.

Nursing Assessment (Data Collection)

A. Waddling gait, lordosis
B. Increasing clumsiness, muscle weakness
C. Gowers' sign: difficulty rising to standing position; has to "walk" up legs using hands
D. Pseudohypertrophy of muscles (especially noted in calves) because of fat deposits
E. Muscle degeneration, especially the thigh and fatty infiltrates (detected with muscle biopsy). Cardiac muscle is also involved.
F. Delayed cognitive development
G. Elevated creatine phosphokinase (CPK) and ALT/AST
H. Later in disease, scoliosis, respiratory difficulty, and cardiac difficulties occur.
I. Child is eventually wheelchair dependent and then confined to bed.

Analysis (Nursing Diagnoses)

A. Impaired, physical mobility related to …
B. Chronic low self-esteem related to …

Nursing Plans and Interventions

A. Provide supportive care.
B. Provide exercises (active and passive).
C. Prevent exposure to respiratory infection.
D. Encourage a balanced diet to avoid obesity.
E. Support family's grieving process.
F. Support participation with Muscular Dystrophy Association.

Review of Neuromuscular Disorders

1. What are the physical features of a child with Down syndrome?
2. Describe "scissoring."
3. What are two nursing priorities for a newborn with myelomeningocele?
4. List the signs and symptoms of increased ICP in older children.
5. What teaching should parents of a newly shunted child receive?
6. State the three main goals in providing nursing care for a child experiencing a seizure.
7. What are the side effects of Dilantin?
8. Describe the signs and symptoms of a child with meningitis.

9. What antibiotics are usually prescribed for bacterial meningitis?
10. How is a child usually positioned after brain tumor surgery?
11. What nursing interventions increase intracranial pressure?
12. Describe the mechanism of inheritance for Duchenne muscular dystrophy.
13. What is "Gowers' sign"?

Answers to Review

1. Simian creases of palms, hypotonia, protruding tongue, and upward/outward slant of eyes.
2. A common characteristic of spastic cerebral palsy in infants. The legs are extended and crossed over each other; feet are plantar flexed.
3. Prevention of infection of the sac and monitoring for hydrocephalus (measure head circumference; check fontanel; assess neurologic functioning).
4. Irritability, change in LOC, motor dysfunction, headache, vomiting, unequal pupil response, and seizures.
5. Signs of infection and increased ICP (see Signs of Increased ICP and Meningitis; shunt should not be pumped. Child will need revisions because of growth. Provide guidance for growth and development.
6. Maintain patent airway, protect from injury, and observe carefully.
7. Gingival hyperplasia of the gums, dermatitis, ataxia, GI distress.
8. Fever, irritability, vomiting, neck stiffness, opisthotonus, positive Kernig sign, positive Brudzinski sign. Infant does not show all classic signs but is very ill.
9. Ampicillin, ceftriaxone, and/or chloramphenicol.
10. Flat on his or her side.
11. Suctioning and positioning/turning.
12. Duchenne muscular dystrophy is inherited as an X-linked recessive trait.
13. Gowers' sign is an indicator of muscular dystrophy. The child has to "walk" up legs using hands to stand.

Renal Disorders

Acute Glomerulonephritis

Description: Acute glomerulonephritis (AGN) is an immune complex response to an antecedent beta-hemolytic streptococcal infection of skin or pharynx. Antigen-antibody complexes become trapped in the membrane of the glomeruli, causing inflammation and decreased glomerular filtration.

Nursing Assessment (Data Collection)
A. Recent streptococcal infection
B. Mild to moderate edema (often confined to face)
C. Irritable, lethargic
D. Hypertension
E. Dark-colored urine (hematuria)
F. Slight to moderate proteinuria (protein in the urine)
G. Elevated antistreptolysin (ASO) titer, elevated BUN, and creatinine

Analysis (Nursing Diagnoses)
A. Excess fluid volume related to …
B. Risk for injury related to …

Nursing Plans and Interventions
A. Provide supportive care.
B. Monitor vital signs (especially BP) frequently.
C. Monitor I&O closely.
D. Weigh daily.
E. Provide low-sodium diet with *no* added salt; low potassium, if oliguric.
F. Encourage bed rest during acute phase (usually 4 to 10 days).
G. Administer antihypertensives if prescribed.
H. Monitor for seizures (hypertensive encephalopathy).
I. Monitor for signs of congestive heart failure (CHF).
J. Monitor for signs of renal failure (uncommon).

HESI Hint • Decreased urinary output is *first* sign of renal failure. A constant urine specific gravity is also an indication of renal failure. (Kidneys can no longer regulate the concentration of the urine.)

Nephrotic Syndrome

Description: A disorder in which the basement membrane of the glomeruli becomes permeable to plasma proteins. Most often idiopathic in nature.

TABLE 5-7 A Comparison of Acute Glomerulonephritis (AGN) and Nephrotic Syndrome

Variable	Acute Glomerulonephritis (AGN)	Nephrotic Syndrome
Etiology	• Follows streptococcal infection	• Usually idiopathic
Edema	• Mild, usually around eyes	• Severe, generalized
Blood pressure	• Elevated	• Normal
Urine	• Dark, tea-colored (hematuria) • Slight/moderate proteinuria	• Dark, frothy yellow • Massive proteinuria
Blood	• Normal serum protein • Positive ASO titer	• Decreased serum protein • Negative ASO titer

A. Usually occurs between ages 2 to 3 years.
B. Course may have exacerbations and remissions over several years (Table 5-7, *A Comparison of Acute Glomerulonephritis [AGN] and Nephrotic Syndrome*).

Nursing Assessment (Data Collection)

A. Edema that begins insidiously and becomes severe and generalized
B. Lethargy
C. Anorexia
D. Pallor
E. Frothy-appearing urine
F. Massive proteinuria (protein present in the urine)
G. Decreased serum protein (hypoproteinemia)
H. Elevated serum lipids

Analysis (Nursing Diagnoses)

A. Excess fluid volume related to …
B. Imbalanced nutrition: less than body requirements related to …

Nursing Plans and Interventions

A. Provide supportive care.
B. Monitor temperature, assess for signs of infection.
C. Protect from persons with infections.
D. Provide skin care (edematous areas are vulnerable).
E. Maintain bed rest during edematous phase.
F. Administer steroids such as prednisone as prescribed (Table 5-8, *Medications Used with Renal Disorders*).
G. Monitor I&O.
H. Measure abdominal girth daily.

I. Administer cyclophosphamide (Cytoxan) if prescribed (used if nonresponsive to prednisone).
J. Provide small, frequent feedings of a normal protein, low-salt diet.
K. Collaborate with RN to enhance and reinforce a family teaching plan for home care:
  1. Weigh child daily
  2. Medication side effects
  3. Signs of relapse (see Nursing Assessment, [Data Collection])
  4. Prevention of infection

Urinary Tract Infection

Description: A urinary tract infection (UTI) is a bacterial infection anywhere along the urinary tract (most are ascending).

Nursing Assessment (Data Collection)

A. In infants:
  1. Vague symptoms
  2. Fever
  3. Irritability
  4. Poor food intake
  5. Diarrhea, vomiting, jaundice
  6. Strong-smelling urine
B. In older children:
  1. Urinary frequency
  2. Hematuria
  3. Enuresis
  4. Dysuria
  5. Fever
C. Urine cultures often reveal presence of *Escherichia coli*.

Analysis (Nursing Diagnoses)

A. Impaired urinary elimination related to …
B. Deficient knowledge (medications) related to …

Nursing Plans and Interventions

A. Suspect and assess for UTI in infants who are ill.
B. Assess for recurrent urinary tract infections. In infants and young boys, UTI may indicate structural abnormalities of the urinary system.
C. Collect clean voided or catheterized specimen, as prescribed (Table 5-9, *Collection of Urine Specimens*).
D. Administer antibiotics as prescribed.
E. Collaborate with RN to develop and implement family teaching plan for a home program:
  1. Finish all prescribed medication.
  2. Follow-up specimens are needed.
  3. Avoid bubble baths.
  4. Increase acidic oral fluids—for example, apple, cranberry juices.
  5. Void frequently.
  6. Clean genital area from front to back.
  7. Symptoms of recurrence (Nursing Assessment [Data Collection]).

TABLE 5-8 Medications Used with Renal Disorders

Drugs	Indications	Adverse Reactions	Nursing Implications
• Bethanechol chloride (Urecholine)	• Cholinergic used to treat: →Urinary retention →Neurogenic bladder →Gastric reflux	• Orthostatic hypotension • Flushing • Asthmatic reaction • GI distress	• Do not give IV or IM (may cause circulatory collapse) • Monitor vital signs • Preferably give on empty stomach
• Prednisone (Deltasone)	• Adrenocorticosteroid used to treat: →Immunosuppression (acts as an anti-inflammatory) →Edema (promotes diuresis in nephrotic syndrome)	• Mood changes • Increased susceptibility to infection • Cushingoid appearance (moon face and buffalo hump) • Acne • GI distress • Thrombocytopenia • Edema • Potassium loss • Growth failure in children	• In children, every other day administration is best to avoid growth failure when drug is taken long term • Discontinuing this drug requires tapering dose • Avoid live virus vaccines in children receiving prednisone
• Oxybutynin (Ditropan) • Tolterodine (Detrol) • Solifenacin (Vesicare) • Trospium (Sanctura) • Darifenacin (Enablex)	• Genitourinary smooth muscle relaxants (antispasmodics) used to treat: →Uninhibited neurogenic bladder →Reflex urogenic bladder, which are characterized by voiding symptoms of urgency, frequency, nocturia, and incontinence	• Increased susceptibility to urinary tract infection (UTI) • GI distress • Dry eyes • Dry mouth • Vision changes • Dizziness • Chest pain • Drowsiness	• Administered orally; available in extended-release forms • Do not administer with other medications that have anticholinergic effects • May exacerbate reflux esophagitis • Contraindicated in clients with untreated glaucoma or any GI narrowing (GI obstruction may occur) • Safety for use with children has not been established

TABLE 5-9 Collection of Urine Specimens

Method	Description for Children/Infants
Clean catch	• Best obtained using a urine bag to catch the specimen. • Apply from side to side or back to front; diaper should be applied over the bag. • Check child frequently to note urination.
Catheterization	Sterile feeding tube is often used to catheterize small children and infants.
Sterile specimen	In small infants it is best collected by the physician performing a bladder tap; urine is aspirated through a needle inserted directly into bladder. The nurse is responsible for making sure infant is appropriately hydrated and restrained during the procedure.

Vesicoureteral Reflex

Description: Vesicoureteral reflex results from valvular malfunction and backflow of urine into the ureters (and higher) from the bladder. Severe cases are associated with hydronephrosis.

Nursing Assessment (Data Collection)
A. Recurrent UTI
B. Reflux common with neurogenic bladder
C. Reflux noted on VCUG (voiding cystourethrogram)

Analysis (Nursing Diagnoses)
A. Risk for infection related to …
B. Risk for injury related to …

Nursing Plans and Interventions
A. Collaborate with RN to develop a family teaching plan for a home program for prevention of UTI.
B. Collaborate with RN to enhance and reinforce a family teaching plan about the importance of medication compliance, which usually leads to resolution of mild cases.
C. Provide support for children requiring surgery and their families.
D. Reinforce the goal of ureteral reimplantation: stop reflux and prevent kidney damage.
E. Monitor postoperative urinary drainage (may be suprapubic and/or urethral).
1. Measure output from *each* catheter.
2. Observe dressing/incision for drainage.
3. Restrain child's hands as necessary.
F. Maintain hydration.

G. Manage pain relief postoperatively:
  1. Surgical pain
  2. Bladder spasms

Wilms Tumor (Nephroblastoma)

Description: A malignant renal tumor.
A. Wilms tumor is embryonic in origin.
B. This tumor is encapsulated.
C. Occurs in young, preschool children.
D. With early detection, surgery, adjuvant chemotherapy, and radiation therapy postoperatively, the prognosis is good.

Nursing Assessment (Data Collection)

A. Mass in the flank area, confined to *midline*
B. Parents often discover mass when bathing child
C. Fever
D. Pallor, lethargy
E. Elevated BP (excess renin secretion)
F. Hematuria (rare)

Analysis (Nursing Diagnoses)

A. Risk for injury related to …
B. Fear related to …

Nursing Plans and Interventions

A. Support family during diagnostic period.
B. Protect child from injury; place a sign on bed stating, "NO ABDOMINAL PALPATION."
C. Assist with preparation of family and child for imminent nephrectomy.
D. Provide postoperative care:
  1. Monitor for increased BP.
  2. Monitor kidney function: I&O, urine specific gravity.
  3. Provide care for abdominal surgery client.
    a. Maintain nasogastric (NG) tube.
    b. Check for bowel sounds.
  4. Support child/family during chemotherapy and/or radiation therapy.

Hypospadias

Description: Hypospadias is a congenital defect of the urethral meatus in males. The urethra opens on the ventral side of the penis behind the glans.

> **HESI Hint** Surgical correction for hypospadias is usually done before preschool years to avoid any complications associated with achieving sexual identity, castration anxiety, and toilet training.

Nursing Assessment (Data Collection)

A. Abnormal placement of meatus
B. Altered voiding stream
C. Presence of chordee
D. Undescended testes and inguinal hernia may occur concurrently.

Analysis (Nursing Diagnoses)

A. Impaired urinary elimination related to …
B. Disturbed body image related to …

Nursing Plans and Interventions

A. Assist with preparation of child and family for surgery (no circumcision before surgery).
B. Observe circulation to tip of penis postoperatively.
C. Monitor urinary drainage after urethroplasty:
  1. Foley catheter
  2. Suprapubic tube
  3. Urethral stent
D. Restrain child's arms and legs as necessary.
E. Maintain hydration (IV and oral fluids).
F. Collaborate with RN to enhance and reinforce family teaching plan for home care:
  1. Care of catheters
  2. How to empty drainage bag
  3. Prevention of catheter displacement or blockage
  4. Increase oral fluids
  5. Signs of infection

Review of Renal Disorders

1. Compare the signs and symptoms of acute glomerulonephritis (AGN) with nephrosis.
2. What antecedent event occurs with acute glomerulonephritis?
3. Compare the dietary interventions for acute glomerulonephritis and nephrosis.
4. What is the physiologic reason for the lab finding of hypoproteinemia in nephrosis?
5. Describe safe monitoring of prednisone administration and withdrawal.
6. What interventions can be taught to prevent urinary tract infections in children?
7. Describe the pathophysiology of vesicoureteral reflux.
8. What are the priorities for a client with Wilms tumor?
9. Explain why hypospadias correction is done before the child reaches preschool age.

Answers to Review

1. AGN: gross hematuria, recent streptococcus infection, hypertension, and mild edema. Nephrosis: Severe edema, massive proteinuria, frothy-appearing urine, and anorexia.
2. Beta-hemolytic streptococcus infection.
3. AGN: low-sodium diet with no added salt. Nephrosis: high-protein, low-salt diet.
4. Hypoproteinemia occurs because the glomeruli are permeable to serum proteins.
5. Long-term prednisone should be given every other day. Signs of edema, mood changes, and GI distress should be noted and reported. The drug should be tapered, not discontinued suddenly.
6. Avoid bubble baths; void frequently; drink adequate fluids, especially acidic fluids such as apple or cranberry juice; and clean genital area from front to back.
7. A malfunction of the valves at the end of the ureters allowing urine to reflux out of the bladder into the ureters and possibly the kidneys.
8. Protect the child from injury to the encapsulated tumor. Prepare the family/child for surgery.
9. Preschoolers fear castration, are achieving sexual identity, and are acquiring independent toileting skills.

Gastrointestinal Disorders

Cleft Lip and/or Palate

Description: Malformations of the face and oral cavity, which seem to be multifactorial in inheritance (Figure 5-13, *Variations in Clefts of Lip and Palate at Birth*).
A. Cleft lip is readily apparent.
B. Cleft palate may not be identified until the infant has difficulty with feeding.
C. Initial closure of cleft lip is performed when infant weighs approximately 10 pounds and has a hemoglobin (Hgb) of 10 g/dL.

D. Closure of palate defect is usually performed at 1 year of age to minimize speech impairment.

Nursing Assessment (Data Collection)
A. Failure of fusion of the lip and/or palate
B. Difficulty sucking and swallowing
C. Parent reaction to facial defect

Analysis (Nursing Diagnoses)
A. Imbalanced nutrition: less than body requirements related to …
B. Impaired parenting related to …

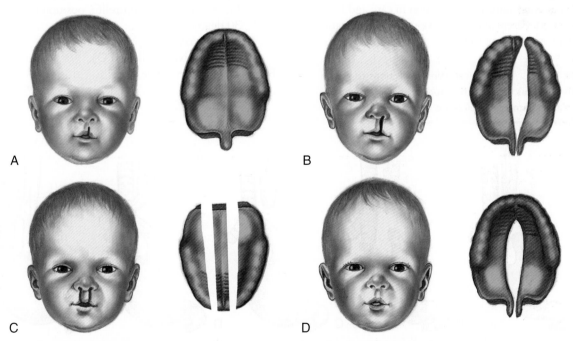

FIGURE 5-13 Variations in Clefts of Lip and Palate at Birth. **A,** Notch in vermilion border. **B,** Unilateral cleft lip and cleft palate. **C,** Bilateral cleft lip and cleft palate. **D,** Cleft palate. (From Hockenberry MJ, Wilson D: *Wong's nursing care of infants and children*, ed 9, St. Louis, 2012, Mosby.)

Nursing Plans and Interventions

A. Promote family bonding and grieving during newborn period.
B. Reinforce to the family that successful corrective surgery is available.
C. In newborn period, assist with feeding.
  1. Feed in upright position.
  2. Feed slowly with frequent bubbling.
  3. Use soft, large nipples; lamb's nipple; prosthetic palate; or rubber-tipped Asepto syringe.
  4. Support mother in decision to breastfeed if possible.
  5. Consider ESSR method:
    a. Enlarge nipple opening.
    b. Suck.
    c. Swallow.
    d. Rest.
D. Provide postoperative care:
  1. Maintain patent airway and proper positioning:
    a. Cleft lip—on side or upright in infant seat (not prone)
    b. Cleft palate—on side or abdomen
    c. Remove oral secretions carefully with bulb syringe.
  2. Protect surgical site:
    a. Apply elbow restraints.
    b. Minimize crying to prevent strain on lip suture line.
    c. Maintain "Logan Bow" to lip if applied.
  3. Provide care for restrained child:
    a. Remove one restraint at a time, and do range-of-motion exercises.
    b. Provide age-appropriate stimulation.
  4. Resume feeding as prescribed. Cleanse suture site after feeding; formula sitting on suture line may impede healing, lead to infection.
  5. Encourage family participation in care and feeding.
  6. Report parent/family reaction and participation in care and feeding to RN.

> **HESI Hint** • Typical parent/family reactions to a child with an obvious malformation such as cleft lip/palate are guilt, disappointment, grief, sense of loss, and anger.

Esophageal Atresia with Tracheoesophageal Fistula

Description: Esophageal atresia with tracheoesophageal fistula (TEF) is a congenital anomaly in which the esophagus does not fully develop (Figure 5-14, *Five Most Common Types of Esophageal Atresia and Tracheoesophageal Fistula*).

A. Most common: upper esophagus ends in a blind pouch with the lower part of the esophagus connected to the trachea.
B. This condition is a CLINICAL AND SURGICAL EMERGENCY.

Nursing Assessment (Data Collection)

A. Three Cs of TEF in the newborn:
  1. Choking
  2. Coughing
  3. Cyanosis
B. Excess salivation
C. Increased respiratory rate, effort, and adventitious breath sounds

Analysis (Nursing Diagnoses)

A. Risk for aspiration related to …
B. Imbalanced nutrition: less than body requirements related to …

Nursing Plans and Interventions

A. Provide preoperative care:
  1. Monitor respiratory status.
  2. Remove excess secretions (suction is usually continuous to blind pouch).
  3. Elevate infant into antireflux position of 30 degrees.
  4. Provide oxygen as prescribed.
  5. Nothing given orally (NPO).
B. Provide postoperative care:
  1. NPO.
  2. Monitor I&O.

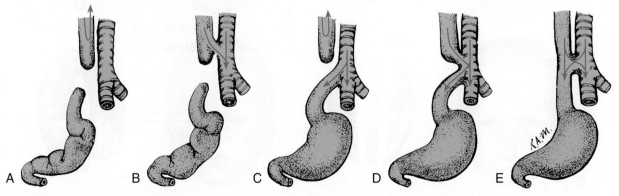

FIGURE 5-14 Five Most Common Types of Esophageal Atresia and Tracheoesophageal Fistula. (From Hockenberry MJ, Wilson D: *Wong's nursing care of infants and children*, ed 9, St. Louis, 2012, Mosby.)

3. Provide gastrostomy tube care and feedings as prescribed.
4. Provide pacifier to meet developmental needs.
5. Monitor child for postoperative stricture of the esophagus.
C. Promote parent-infant bonding for high-risk infant.

Pyloric Stenosis

Description: Pyloric stenosis is a narrowing of the pyloric sphincter. The circular muscle of the pylorus hypertrophies to twice the normal size.

Nursing Assessment (Data Collection)

A. Usually occurs in firstborn males
B. Vomiting (free of bile) usually begins after 14th day of life and becomes projectile
C. Hungry, fretful infant
D. Weight loss, failure to gain weight
E. Dehydration with decreased sodium and potassium
F. Metabolic alkalosis (decreased serum chloride, increased pH and bicarbonate or CO_2 content)
G. Palpable olive-shaped mass in upper right quadrant of the abdomen
H. Visible peristaltic waves

Analysis (Nursing Diagnoses)

A. Imbalanced nutrition: less than body requirements related to …
B. Deficient fluid volume (actual) related to …

> **HESI Hint** • Children with cleft lip/palate and those with pyloric stenosis both have a nursing diagnosis of "Nutrition: less than body requirements, altered."
> • Cleft lip/palate is related to decreased ability to suck.
> • Pyloric stenosis is related to frequent vomiting.

Nursing Plans and Interventions

A. Preoperative care:
   1. Observe for dehydration.
   2. Weigh daily, monitor I&O.
   3. Provide small, frequent feedings if prescribed.
B. Assist with preparation of family for surgery by teaching that:
   1. Hypertrophied muscle will be split.
   2. Prognosis is excellent.
C. Postoperative care:
   1. Provide small oral feedings with electrolyte solutions or glucose (usually 4 to 6 hours postoperative).
   2. Position on *right* side in semi-Fowler position after feeding.
   3. Burp frequently—do not want stomach to become distended and put pressure on surgical site.
   4. Weigh daily, monitor I&O.

Intussusception

Description: Telescoping of one part of the intestine into another part of the intestine, usually the ileum into the colon (called *ileocolic*).
A. Partial to complete bowel obstruction occurs.
B. Blood vessels become trapped in the telescoping bowel, causing necrosis.

Nursing Assessment (Data Collection)

A. Child under 1 year of age
B. Acute, intermittent abdominal pain
C. Screaming with legs drawn up to abdomen
D. Vomiting
E. "Currant jelly" stools (mixed with blood and mucus)
F. Sausage-shaped mass in upper right quadrant, while lower right quadrant is empty (dance sign)

Analysis (Nursing Diagnoses)

A. Ineffective tissue perfusion (bowel) related to …
B. Risk for deficient fluid volume related to …

Nursing Plans and Interventions

A. Monitor vital signs carefully for shock or bowel perforation. Report decreased blood pressure, increased pulse, increased respirations to RN.
B. Monitor I&O.
C. Assist with preparation of family for emergency intervention.
D. Assist with preparation of child for barium enema (which provides hydrostatic reduction). Two out of three cases respond to this treatment; if not, surgery is necessary.
E. Provide postoperative care for infants who require abdominal surgery.

> **HESI Hint** • Nutritional needs and fluid and electrolyte balance are key problems for children with GI disorders. The younger the child, the more vulnerable he or she is to fluid and electrolyte imbalances and the greater the need for caloric intake required for growth.

Congenital/Aganglionic Megacolon (Hirschsprung Disease)

Description: Congenital absence of autonomic parasympathetic ganglion cells in a distal portion of the colon and rectum.
A. Lack of peristalsis in the area of the colon where the ganglion cells are absent.
B. Fecal contents accumulate above the aganglionic area of the bowel.
C. Correction usually involves a series of surgical procedures:
   1. A temporary colostomy
   2. Later, a reanastomosis and closure of the colostomy

Nursing Assessment (Data Collection)

Analysis (Nursing Diagnoses)

A. Constipation related to …
B. Diarrhea related to …
C. Imbalanced nutrition: less than body requirements related to …

Nursing Plans and Interventions

A. Provide preoperative care.
 1. Begin preparation for abdominal surgery; usually not begun until bowel perforation ruled out.
 2. Provide bowel cleansing program as prescribed.
 3. Insert rectal tube if prescribed.
 4. Observe for symptoms of bowel perforation:
  a. Abdominal distension—measure abdominal girth.
  b. Vomiting.
  c. Increased abdominal tenderness.
  d. Irritability.
  e. Dyspnea and cyanosis.
 5. Collaborate with RN to develop and initiate preoperative teaching regarding colostomy.
B. Provide postoperative care:
 1. Check vital signs, axillary temperature.

> **HESI Hint** • Take axillary temperature on children with congenital megacolon.

 2. Monitor I&O.
 3. Care for NG tube with connection to intermittent suction.
 4. Check abdominal/perineal dressings.
 5. Assess bowel sounds.
C. Collaborate with RN to enhance and reinforce a family teaching plan for home care:
 1. Contribute to the plan of teaching skin care and colostomy care.
 2. Coordinate referral of family to enterostomal therapist and social services.
D. Collaborate with RN to enhance and reinforce a family teaching plan for closure of temporary colostomy.
E. After closure, encourage family to be patient with child when toileting.
F. Begin toilet training after age 2 years.

Anorectal Malformations

Description: Congenital malformation of the anorectal section of the GI tract (imperforate anus).

A. Often associated with a fistula.
B. May also be associated with urinary tract anomalies.
C. Type and level of rectal anomaly determines surgical procedure and degree of bowel control possible.

Nursing Assessment (Data Collection)

A. An unusual-appearing anal dimple.
B. Newborn who does not pass meconium stool within 24 hours.
C. Meconium appearing from perineal fistula or in urine.

Analysis (Nursing Diagnoses)

A. Bowel incontinence related to …
B. Deficient knowledge (colostomy home program) related to …

Nursing Plans and Interventions

A. Determine newborn's first temperature; axillary or tympanic temperature is used for first reading unless hospital policy indicates otherwise.
B. Observe newborn for passage of meconium.
C. Assist family's ability to cope with diagnosis.
D. Provide preoperative care to infant:
 1. Assess vital signs.
 2. Monitor I&O.
E. Provide postoperative care for anal reconstruction:
 1. Keep perineal site clean.
 2. Position side-lying prone with hips elevated (decreased pressure on perineal sutures).
 3. Provide colostomy care if needed.
 4. No rectal temperatures postoperative.
F. Home care:
 1. Collaborate with RN to enhance and reinforce a family teaching plan for home care of colostomy if necessary.
 2. With high-level defects, long-term follow-up is required.
 3. Toilet training is delayed, and full continence may not be achieved.

Review of Gastrointestinal Disorders

1. Describe feeding techniques for the child with cleft lip or palate.
2. List the signs and symptoms of esophageal atresia with TEF.
3. What nursing actions are initiated for the newborn with suspected esophageal atresia with TEF?
4. Describe the postoperative nursing care for an infant with pyloric stenosis.
5. Describe why a barium enema is used to treat intussusception.
6. Describe the preoperative nursing care for a child with Hirschsprung disease.

7. What care is needed for the child with a temporary colostomy?
8. What are the signs of anorectal malformation?
9. What are the priorities for a child undergoing abdominal surgery?

Answers to Review

1. Lamb's nipple or prosthesis. Feed child upright with frequent bubbling.
2. Choking, coughing, cyanosis, and excess salivation.
3. NPO immediately and suction secretions.
4. Maintain IV hydration. Provide small, frequent oral feedings of glucose and/or electrolyte solutions within 4 to 6 hours. Gradually increase to full-strength formula. Position on right side in semi-Fowler position after feeding.
5. A barium enema reduces the telescoping of the intestine through hydrostatic pressure without surgical intervention.
6. Check vital signs and take axillary temperatures. Provide bowel cleansing program and teach about colostomy. Observe for bowel perforation; measure abdominal girth.
7. Family needs education about skin care and appliances. Referral to an enterostomal therapist is appropriate.
8. A newborn who does not pass meconium within 24 hours, meconium appearing from a fistula or in the urine, or an unusual-appearing anal dimple.
9. Maintain fluid balance (I&O, NG suction, monitor electrolytes), monitor vital signs, care of drains if present, assess bowel function, prevent infection of incisional area and other postoperative complications, and support child/family with appropriate teaching.

Hematologic Disorders

Iron Deficiency Anemia

Description: Hemoglobin levels below normal range because of the body's inadequate supply, intake, or absorption of iron.
A. Iron deficiency anemia is the leading hematologic disorder in children.
B. The need for iron is greater in children than adults because of accelerated growth.
C. Anemia may be caused by the following:
 1. Inadequate stores during fetal development
 2. Deficient dietary intake
 3. Chronic blood loss
 4. Poor use of iron by the body

Nursing Assessment (Data Collection)
A. Pallor, paleness of mucous membranes
B. Tiredness, fatigue
C. Usually seen in infants 6 to 24 months old (times of growth spurt). Toddlers and female adolescents most affected.
D. Dietary intake low in iron
E. Milk intake greater than 32 oz/day
F. Pica habit (eating nonfood substances)
G. Lab values:
 1. Decreased hemoglobin (Hgb)
 2. Low serum iron level
 3. Elevated total iron binding capacity

HESI Hint *Remember the Hgb norms:*
- Newborn: 14 to 24 g/dL
- Infant: 10 to 15 g/dL
- Child: 11 to 16 g/dL

Analysis (Nursing Diagnoses)
A. Ineffective tissue perfusion (specify) related to …
B. Activity intolerance related to …

Nursing Plans and Interventions
A. Support child's need to limit activities.
B. Provide rest periods.
C. Administer oral iron (ferrous sulfate) as prescribed.

HESI Hint Reinforce family teaching about administration of oral iron:
- Give on empty stomach (as tolerated for better absorption).
- Give with citrus juices (vitamin C) for increased absorption.
- Use dropper or straw to avoid discoloring teeth.
- Stools will become tarry.
- Iron can be fatal in severe overdose; keep away from children.
- Do not give with dairy products.

D. Assist RN by enhancing and reinforcing a family teaching plan concerning iron deficiency.
  1. Limit milk intake to less than 32 oz/day.
  2. Encourage dietary sources of iron:
     a. Meat
     b. Green leafy vegetables
     c. Fish
     d. Liver
     e. Whole grains
     f. Legumes
     g. For infants: iron-fortified cereals and formula
  3. Teach appropriate nutrition for age.
E. Be aware of family's income and cultural food preferences.
F. Coordinate with a nutritionist and Women, Infants and Children's nutrition program, if available to family.

Hemophilia

Description: Hemophilia is an inherited bleeding disorder.
A. Transmitted by an X-linked recessive chromosome. (The mother is the carrier; her sons may express the disease.)
B. A normal individual has between 50% and 200% factor activity in blood; the hemophiliac has from 0% to 25% activity.
C. The affected individual usually is missing either factor VIII (classic, 75% of cases) or factor IX.

Nursing Assessment (Data Collection)

A. Male child: first "red flag" may be prolonged bleeding following circumcision or after vitamin K injection
B. Prolonged bleeding with minor trauma
C. Hemarthrosis (most frequent site of bleeding)
D. Spontaneous bleeding into muscles and tissues (less severe cases have fewer bleeds)
E. Loss of motion in joints
F. Pain
G. Lab values:
  1. PTT is prolonged.
  2. Factor assays are less than 25%.

Analysis (Nursing Diagnoses)

A. Risk for injury related to …
B. Deficient knowledge (home care) related to …

Nursing Plans and Interventions

A. RN will administer infusions, which help to replace the clotting factors that are missing or low, as prescribed by health care provider.
B. Administer pain medication as prescribed (analgesics containing no aspirin).
C. Collaborate with RN to enhance and reinforce a client/family teaching plan for home care:
  1. Recognize early signs of bleeding into joints.

  2. Local treatment for minor bleeds (pressure, splinting, ice)
  3. Administration of factor replacement
  4. Dental hygiene: soft toothbrushes
  5. Protective care: soft toys, padded bed rails
  6. Wear medic alert identification.
D. Support family seeking genetic counseling.
E. Support child/family during periods of growth and development when increased risk for bleeding occurs (i.e., learning to walk, tooth loss).

> **HESI Hint** ● Inherited bleeding disorders (hemophilia and sickle cell anemia) are often used to test knowledge of genetic transmission patterns. Remember:
> - Autosomal recessive: both parents must be heterozygous, or carriers of the recessive trait, for the disease to be expressed in their offspring. With each pregnancy, there is a 1:4 chance of the infant having the disease. However, all children of such parents *can* get the disease—*not* just 25% of them. This is the transmission for sickle cell anemia, cystic fibrosis, and phenylketonuria.
> - X-linked recessive trait: the trait is carried on the X chromosome; therefore, it usually affects male offspring—for example, hemophilia. With each pregnancy of a woman who is a carrier, there is a 25% chance of having a child with hemophilia. If the child is male, he has a 50% chance of having hemophilia. If the child is female, she has a 50% chance of being a carrier.

Sickle Cell Anemia

Description: Inherited autosomal recessive disorder of hemoglobin.
A. Occurs primarily in blacks and persons of eastern Mediterranean descent. One in 12 black persons is a carrier of the heterozygous gene HgbAS. Therefore, the risk of two black parents having a child with sickle cell disease is 0.7%.
B. Usually appears after 6 months of age.
C. Hemoglobin S (HgbS) replaces all or part of the normal hemoglobin, which causes the red blood cells to sickle when oxygen is released to the tissues.
  1. Sickled cells cannot flow through capillary beds.
  2. Dehydration promotes sickling.

> **HESI Hint** ● Hydration is very important in the treatment of sickle cell disease because it promotes hemodilution and circulation of red cells through the blood vessels.

D. An HgbS has a less than normal lifespan (less than 40 days), which leads to chronic anemia.

E. Tissue ischemia causes widespread pathologic changes in the spleen, liver, kidney, bones, and central nervous system.

> **HESI Hint** • Important terms:
> - Heterozygous gene (HgbAS) sickle cell trait
> - Homozygous gene (HbSS) sickle cell disease
> - Abnormal hemoglobin (HgbS) disease and trait

Nursing Assessment (Data Collection)

A. Black child, usually older than 6 months of age
B. Parents with sickle cell trait or sickle cell anemia
C. Lab diagnosis: Hgb electrophoresis (differentiates *trait* from disease)
D. Frequent infections (nonfunctional spleen)
E. Tiredness
F. Chronic hemolytic anemia
G. Delayed physical growth
H. Vasoocclusive crisis is the classic sign
   1. Fever
   2. Severe abdominal pain
   3. Hand-foot syndrome (infants): Painful edematous hands and feet
   4. Arthralgia
I. Leg ulcers (adolescents)
J. Cerebrovascular accidents (increased risk with dehydration)

Analysis (Nursing Diagnoses)

A. Acute pain related to …
B. Risk for infection related to …
C. Deficient knowledge (crisis prevention) related to …

Nursing Plans and Interventions

A. Collaborate with RN to enhance and reinforce family/client teaching plan for the prevention of crisis (hypoxia):
   1. Avoid strenuous exercise.
   2. Avoid high altitudes.
   3. Avoid infection and seek care at first sign of infection.
   4. Use of prophylactic penicillin if prescribed.
   5. Keep child well hydrated (more than 125 mL/kg/day).
   6. Enuresis is a complication of treatment and disease; do not withhold fluids at night.
B. For child hospitalized with a vasoocclusive crisis:
   1. Monitor IV fluids (one to two times maintenance) and electrolytes, as prescribed, to increase hydration and treat acidosis.
   2. Monitor I&O.
   3. Assist with administration of blood products as prescribed.
   4. Administer analgesics, including parenteral morphine, for severe pain as prescribed.
   5. Use warm compresses—not ice.
   6. Administer prescribed antibiotics to treat infection.

C. Administer pneumococcal vaccine, meningococcal vaccine, and Haemophilus B vaccine as prescribed.
D. Administer hepatitis B vaccine as prescribed (for child at risk from transfusions).
E. Help family to coordinate with genetic counseling.
F. Support child/family experiencing chronic disease.

> **HESI Hint** • Supplemental iron is not given to clients with sickle cell anemia. The anemia is not caused by iron deficiency. Folic acid is given orally to stimulate RBC synthesis.

Acute Lymphocytic Leukemia

Description: Acute lymphocytic leukemia is a cancer of the blood-forming organs.
A. Acute lymphocytic leukemia accounts for about 80% of childhood leukemia.
B. Noted by the presence of lymphoblasts (immature lymphocytes) replacing normal cells in the bone marrow.
C. Blast cells are also seen in the peripheral blood count.
D. Acute lymphocytic leukemia is classified by whether it is:
   1. T lymphocyte.
   2. B lymphocyte.
   3. Null cell (neither T cell nor B cell).
E. Over 75% of children with acute lymphocytic leukemia have null cells, which has the best prognosis.
F. Signs and symptoms of leukemia result from replacement of normal cells by leukemic cells in the bone marrow and extramedullary sites.
G. Treatment has four phases:
   1. Induction
   2. Sanctuary
   3. Consolidation
   4. Maintenance

Nursing Assessment (Data Collection)

A. Pallor, tiredness, weakness, lethargy caused by anemia
B. Petechia, bleeding, bruising caused by thrombocytopenia
C. Infection, fever caused by neutropenia
D. Bone joint pain caused by leukemic infiltration of bone marrow
E. Enlarged lymph nodes; hepatosplenomegaly
F. Headache and vomiting (signs of central nervous system involvement)
G. Anorexia, weight loss
H. Lab data: bone marrow aspiration reveals 80% to 90% immature blast cells

Analysis (Nursing Diagnoses)

A. Risk for infection related to …
B. Fear related to …
C. Deficient knowledge (disease process and chemotherapy) related to …

Nursing Plans and Interventions

A. Recommend private room.
B. Reverse isolation if prescribed.
C. Reinforce information to child with age-appropriate explanations for diagnostic tests, treatments, and nursing care.
D. Observe child for infection of skin, needle stick site, and dental problems.
E. Assist with administration of blood products as prescribed.
F. Assist with administration of antineoplastic chemotherapy.
G. Observe for side effects of chemotherapeutic agents.
  1. Vincristine (induction)
  2. L-asparaginase (induction)
  3. Methotrexate (sanctuary and maintenance)
  4. Mercaptopurine (6-MP) (maintenance)

> **HESI Hint** • Have epinephrine and oxygen readily available to treat anaphylaxis when administering l-asparaginase.

H. Provide care directed toward managing side effects and toxic effects of antineoplastic agents.
  1. Administer antiemetics as prescribed.
  2. Monitor fluid balance.
  3. Monitor for signs of infection.
  4. Monitor for signs of bleeding.
  5. Monitor for cumulative toxic effects of drugs: hepatic toxicity, cardiac toxicity, renal toxicity, and neurotoxicity.
  6. Provide oral hygiene.
  7. Provide small, appealing meals; increase calories and protein; refer to nutritionist.
  8. Promote self-esteem and positive body image if child has alopecia, severe weight loss, or other disturbance in body image.
  9. Provide care to prevent infection.
I. Provide emotional support for family in crisis.
J. Encourage family and child's input and control in plans and treatment.

> **HESI Hint** • Prednisone is frequently used in combination with antineoplastic drugs to reduce the mitosis of lymphocytes. Allopurinol, a xanthine-oxidase inhibitor, is also administered to prevent renal damage from uric acid.

Review of Hematologic Disorders

1. Describe what information families should be given when a child is receiving oral iron preparations.
2. List dietary sources of iron.
3. Explain why hydration is a priority in treating sickle cell disease.
4. What should families and clients do to avoid triggering sickling episodes?
5. Nursing interventions and medical treatment for the child with leukemia are based on what three physiologic problems?

Answers to Review

1. Give oral iron on an empty stomach and with vitamin C. Use straws to avoid discoloring teeth. Tarry stools are normal. Increase dietary sources of iron.
2. Meat, green leafy vegetables, fish, liver, whole grains, legumes.
3. Hydration promotes hemodilution and circulation of the red cells through the blood vessels.
4. Keep child well hydrated. Avoid known sources of infections. Avoid high altitudes. Avoid strenuous exercise.
5. Anemia (decreased erythrocytes). Infection (neutropenia). Bleeding thrombocytopenia (decreased platelets).

Metabolic and Endocrine Disorders

Congenital Hypothyroidism

Description: A congenital condition resulting from inadequate thyroid tissue development in utero. Cognitive impairment and growth failure occur if it is not detected and treated in early infancy.

Nursing Assessment (Data Collection)

A. Newborn screening: low T4 (thyroxine) and high TSH (thyroid stimulating hormone)
B. Symptoms in the newborn:
  1. Long gestation (over 42 weeks)
  2. Large hypoactive infant
  3. Delayed meconium passage
  4. Feeding problems (poor suck)

5. Prolonged physiologic jaundice
6. Hypothermia
C. Symptoms in early infancy:
   1. Large, protruding tongue
   2. Coarse hair
   3. Lethargic, sleepy
   4. Flat expression
   5. Constipation

> **HESI Hint** • An infant with hypothyroidism is often described as a "good, quiet baby" by the parents.

Analysis (Nursing Diagnoses)

A. Delayed growth and development related to …
B. Deficient knowledge (medication program) related to …

Nursing Plans and Interventions

A. Perform newborn screening programs before discharge.
B. Observe newborn for signs of congenital hypothyroidism.
C. Collaborate with RN to enhance and reinforce a family teaching plan for replacement therapy with thyroid hormone.
   1. Lifelong need.
   2. Give single dose in morning.
   3. Constipation.
   4. Check pulse daily before giving thyroid medication.
   5. Signs of overdose include rapid pulse, irritability, fever, weight loss, and diarrhea.
   6. Signs of underdose include lethargy, fatigue, constipation, and poor feeding.
   7. Necessary for periodic thyroid testing.

Phenylketonuria

Description: Phenylketonuria (PKU) is an autosomal recessive disorder in which the body cannot metabolize the essential amino acid phenylalanine.
A. The buildup of serum phenylalanine leads to CNS damage, most notably cognitive impairment.
B. Decreased melanin (produces light skin and blond hair).

Nursing Assessment (Data Collection)

A. Newborn screening using the Guthrie test is positive when serum phenylalanine is 4 mg/dL
B. Must be at least 24 hours old; if early discharge, the test will need to be repeated by 2 weeks of age
C. Frequent vomiting, failure to gain weight
D. Irritability, hyperactivity
E. Musty urine odor

> **HESI Hint** • Early detection of hypothyroidism and phenylketonuria is essential in preventing cognitive impairment in infants. Knowledge of normal growth and development is important because a lack of attainment can be used to detect the existence of these metabolic/endocrine disorders and attainment can be used for evaluating the treatment's effect.

Analysis (Nursing Diagnoses)

A. Delayed growth and development related to …
B. Deficient knowledge (disease and diet) related to …

Nursing Plans and Interventions

A. Perform newborn screening at birth and again within 3 weeks of age.
B. Collaborate with RN to enhance and reinforce a family teaching plan for dietary management.
   1. Stress importance of strict adherence to prescribed low-phenylalanine diet.
   2. Provide special formulas for infants: Lofenalac, PKU 1.
   3. Provide Phenyl-free (milk substitute) after age 2 years.
   4. Avoid dietary sources high in phenylalanine: high-protein foods, such as meat, milk, dairy products, and eggs.
   5. Offer foods low in phenylalanine: vegetables, fruits, juices, cereals, breads, and starches.
   6. Work with nutritionist.
   7. Diet must be maintained at least until brain growth is complete (age 6 to 8 years).
C. Support family seeking genetic counseling.

> **HESI Hint** • NutraSweet (aspartame) contains phenylalanine and therefore should not be given to a child with phenylketonuria.

Type 1 Diabetes (Insulin-Dependent Diabetes Mellitus)

Description: Type 1 diabetes is a metabolic disorder in which the insulin-producing cells of the pancreas are nonfunctioning as a result of some insult (see Diabetes Mellitus in Chapter 4, *Medical-Surgical Nursing*, p. 117, for additional data).
A. Heredity, viral infections, and autoimmune processes are implicated in diabetes mellitus.
B. Diabetes causes altered carbohydrate, protein, and fat metabolism.
C. Insulin replacement and lifestyle management (diet, exercise, and stress management) are the treatment.

Nursing Assessment (Data Collection)

A. Classic three "Ps":
   1. Polydipsia
   2. Polyphagia
   3. Polyuria, enuresis (bedwetting) in previously continent child
B. Irritability, fatigue
C. Weight loss
D. Abdominal complaints, nausea, and vomiting
E. Usually occurs in school-age children, but can occur even in infancy

F. See Table 4-23, *Comparison of Hyperglycemia and Hypoglycemia*, p. 117

Analysis (Nursing Diagnoses)

A. Imbalanced nutrition: less than body requirements related to …
B. Deficient knowledge (diabetes self-care management) related to …

> **HESI Hint** • Diabetes mellitus (DM) in children typically has been diagnosed as type 1 until recently. A marked increase in type 2 DM (noninsulin-dependent diabetes mellitus [NIDDM]), known as type 2, has occurred in the United States, particularly among Native American, African-American, and Hispanic children and adolescents. Average age at diagnosis is 13.7 years, with overweight or obesity being a major concern. Diabetes self-care management is difficult for adolescents because their growth is rapid and they feel the need to be like peers. Diet and exercise are the cornerstones for good glycemic control with type 2.
> Remember to consider the child's age, cognitive level of development, and psychosocial development when answering NCLEX-PN questions.

Nursing Plans and Interventions

(See Diabetes Mellitus, Chapter 4, p. 117.)
A. If child is in ketoacidosis, provide care in collaboration with RN and other health care providers for seriously ill child (may be unconscious).
   1. Monitor vital signs and neuro status.
   2. Monitor blood glucose, pH, and serum electrolytes.
   3. Observe hydration status.
   4. Maintain strict I&O.

C. Reinforce home teaching program involving both child and family.
   1. Medications:
      a. Type 1: insulin administration either two or more injections per day or insulin pump
      b. Type 2: oral medication or insulin or a combination of the two
   2. Dietary management (carbohydrate counting, may use plate or exchange method)
      a. Meals and snacks
      b. Growth and exercise needs
      c. Basic four food groups, no concentrated sweets
      d. Refer to nutritionist
   3. Exercise:
      a. Regular, planned activity
      b. Diet modification; snacks before or during exercise
   4. Home glucose monitoring and urine testing
   5. Signs and symptoms of hyperglycemia and hypoglycemia
   6. Medical follow-up
D. Reinforce teaching program for school-age child, as appropriate:
   1. Identify issues specific to school:
      a. Physical education class/exercise
      b. Scheduled mealtimes and snacks
      c. Cooperation with teachers and school nurse
      d. Need to be like peers
   2. School-age child should be responsible for most management.
   3. Wear medic alert ID bracelet.

> **HESI Hint** • There has been an increase in the number of children diagnosed with type 2 diabetes. The increasing rate of obesity in children is thought to be a contributing factor. Other contributing factors include lack of physical activity and a family history of type 2 diabetes.

Review of Metabolic and Endocrine Disorders

1. How is congenital hypothyroidism diagnosed?
2. What are the symptoms of congenital hypothyroidism in early infancy?
3. What are the outcomes of untreated congenital hypothyroidism?
4. What are the metabolic effects of PKU?
5. What two formulas are prescribed for infants with PKU?
6. List foods high in phenylalanine content.
7. What are the three classic signs of diabetes?
8. Differentiate between signs of hypoglycemia and hyperglycemia.
9. Describe the nursing care of a child with ketoacidosis.
10. Describe developmental factors that would impact the school-age child with diabetes.
11. What is the relationship between hypoglycemia and exercise?

Answers to Review

1. Newborn screening revealing a low T4 and high TSH.
2. Large, protruding tongue; coarse hair; lethargy; sleepiness; and constipation.
3. Cognitive impairment and growth failure.
4. CNS damage, cognitive impairment, and decreased melanin.
5. Lofenalac and PKU 1.
6. Meat, milk, dairy products, and eggs.
7. Polydipsia, polyphagia, and polyuria.
8. Hypoglycemia: tremors, sweating, headache, hunger, nausea, lethargy, confusion, slurred speech, anxiety, tingling around mouth, nightmares. Hyperglycemia: polydipsia, polyuria, polyphagia, blurred vision, weakness, weight loss, and syncope.
9. Provide care for an unconscious child, monitor blood gas values, and maintain strict I&O.
10. Need to be like peers. Assuming responsibility for own care. Modification of diet, snacks, and exercise in school.
11. During exercise, insulin uptake is increased and the risk of hypoglycemia occurs.

Skeletal Disorders

Fractures

Description: Traumatic injury to bone.
A. Fractures can be classified according to types (see Table 4-28, *Common Types of Fractures*, p. 128).
  1. Complete fractures: bone fragments completely separate.
  2. Incomplete fractures: bone fragments remain attached (e.g., greenstick, bends, buckle).
  3. Comminuted fractures: bone fragments from the fractured shaft break free and lie in the surrounding tissue; this type of fracture is rare in children.
  4. Open fracture (compound fracture): fracture with an open wound through which the bone is or has protruded.
B. Fractures that occur in the epiphyseal plate (growth plate) may affect growth of the limb.

> **HESI Hint** • Fractures in older children are common because they fall during play and are injured in motor vehicle accidents.
> • Spiral fractures (caused by twisting) and fractures in infants may be related to child abuse.
> • Fractures involving the epiphyseal plate (growth plate) can have serious consequences in terms of growth of the affected limb.

Nursing Assessment (Data Collection)
A. General condition:
  1. Visible bone fragments
  2. Pain
  3. Swelling
  4. Contusions
  5. Child guarding or protecting the extremity

B. May be able to use fractured extremity due to intact periosteum
C. The five "Ps" (may indicate the presence of ischemia)
  1. Pain
  2. Pallor
  3. Pulselessness
  4. Paresthesia
  5. Paralysis

Analysis (Nursing Diagnoses)
A. Ineffective tissue perfusion (peripheral) related to ...
B. Acute pain related to ...

Nursing Plans and Interventions
A. Obtain baseline data and frequently perform neurovascular observation:
  1. Pulses: check pulses distal to the injury to assess circulation.
  2. Color: check injured extremity for pink, brisk, capillary refill.
  3. Movement and sensation: check injured extremity for nerve impairment; compare symmetry to uninjured extremity (child may guard injury).
  4. Temperature: check extremity for warmth.
  5. Swelling: check for an increase in swelling (elevate extremity to prevent swelling).
  6. Pain: monitor for severe pain that is not relieved by analgesics.
B. Report abnormal assessment PROMPTLY! Compartment syndrome may occur, which results in permanent damage to nerves and vasculature of the injured extremity caused by compression.
C. Maintain traction if prescribed. Note bed position, type of traction, weights, pulleys, pins, pin sites, adhesive strips, ace wraps, splints, and casts.
  1. Skin traction: force applied to skin:

> **HESI Hint** • Skin traction for fracture reduction should *not* be removed unless prescribed by health care provider.

a. Buck extension traction: lower extremity, legs extended, no hip flexion
b. Dunlop traction: two lines of pull on the arm
c. Russell traction: two lines of pull on the lower extremity, one perpendicular, one longitudinal
d. Bryant traction: both lower extremities flexed 90 degrees at hips (rarely used because extreme elevation of lower extremities causes decreased peripheral circulation)
2. Skeletal traction: pin or wire applies pull directly to the distal bone fragment:
a. 90-degree—90-degree traction: 90-degree flexion of hip and knee; lower extremity is in a boot cast. Can also be used on upper extremities (Figure 5-15, *"90-90" Traction*).
b. Dunlop traction may be used as skeletal traction.

> **HESI Hint** • Pin sites can be a source of infection. Monitor for signs of infection. Clean and dress pin sites as prescribed.

D. Maintain child in proper body alignment, restrain if necessary.
E. Monitor for problems of immobility.
F. Provide age-appropriate play/toys.
G. Prepare child for cast application. Use age-appropriate terms when explaining procedures.
H. Provide routine cast care following application; petal cast edges.
I. Collaborate with RN to enhance and reinforce a client/family teaching plan for home cast care:
1. Neurovascular assessment of casted extremity.

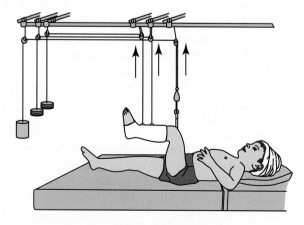

90-90 femoral traction

FIGURE 5-15 "90-90" Traction. (From McKinney ES, James S, Murray SS, Nelson K, Ashwill J: *Maternal-child nursing*, ed 4, St. Louis, 2013, Saunders.)

2. Do not get cast wet.
3. Do not stick anything under cast.
4. Keep small objects, toys, and food out of cast.
5. Modify diapering and toileting to prevent cast soilage.
6. Hip spica: may use Bradford frame under small child to help with toileting. *Do not* use abduction bar to turn child.
7. Follow-up care with health care provider.

Congenital Dislocated Hip (Developmental Dysplasia of Hip)

Description: Abnormal development of the femoral head in the acetabulum.
A. Conservative treatment consists of splinting.
B. Surgical intervention is necessary if splinting is not successful.

Nursing Assessment (Data Collection)
A. Infant:
1. Positive Ortolani sign ("clicking" with abduction)
2. Unequal folds of skin on buttocks and thigh
3. Limited abduction of affected hip
4. Unequal leg lengths
B. Older child:
1. Limp on affected side
2. Trendelenburg sign

Analysis (Nursing Diagnoses)
A. Impaired physical mobility related to …
B. Deficient knowledge (home care) related to …

Nursing Plans and Interventions
A. Review newborn assessment, at birth.
B. Apply abduction device/splint (Pavlik harness; Frejka or Von Rosen splint) as prescribed. Therapy involves positioning legs in flexed, abducted position.
C. Collaborate with RN to development and implement a family teaching plan for home care:
1. Application/removal of device (worn 24 hours/day)
2. Skin care and bathing (health care provider may allow parents to remove device for bathing)
3. Diapering
4. Follow-up care: frequent adjustments due to growth
D. Provide care for infant in Bryant traction (used if splinting is ineffective):
1. Maintain hips in 90-degree flexion.
2. Elevate buttocks off bed.
3. Monitor circulation to feet.
4. Meet developmental needs for immobilized infant.
5. Incorporate family in care.
6. Prepare family for spica cast application.
E. Provide nursing care for a child requiring surgical correction:
1. Reinforce preoperative teaching of child and family, including cast application.

2. Postoperative care:
   a. Assess vital signs.
   b. Check cast for drainage and bleeding.
   c. Observe extremities for neurovascular integrity.
   d. Promote respiratory hygiene.
   e. Administer narcotic analgesics as prescribed.
   f. Collaborate with RN to develop and implement a family teaching plan for cast care when child is discharged home.

> **HESI Hint** • Children do not like injections and will deny pain to avoid "shots."

Scoliosis

Description: Scoliosis is lateral curvature of the spine.
A. If severe, affects thoracic growth and inhibits cardiopulmonary function.
B. Surgical correction with spinal fusion or instrumentation may be required if conservative treatment is ineffective.

Nursing Assessment (Data Collection)

A. Occurs most frequently in adolescent females (10 to 15 years old).
B. Elevated shoulder or hip.
C. Head and hips not aligned.
D. While bending forward, a rib hump is apparent. (Ask child to bend forward from the hips with arms hanging free, and examine child for a curve of the spine, rib hump, and hip asymmetry; Figure 5-16, *Defects of Spinal Column.*)

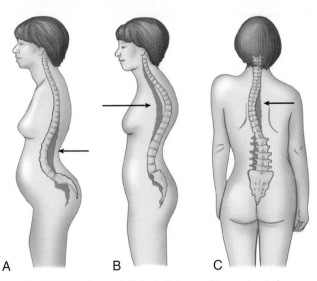

FIGURE 5-16 Defects of Spinal Column. Abnormal spinal curvatures. **A,** Lordosis, known as "sway back," is commonly seen during pregnancy. **B,** Kyphosis, known as "hunchback," is an increased roundness in the thoracic curve commonly found in the elderly. **C,** Scoliosis, an abnormal side-to-side curvature of the spine, is commonly found in adolescents. (From Patton KT, Thibodeau GA: *Anatomy & physiology,* ed 7, St. Louis, 2010, Mosby.)

Analysis (Nursing Diagnoses)

A. Impaired physical mobility related to …
B. Disturbed body image related to …

Nursing Plans and Interventions

A. Assist RN with screening adolescent children, especially females, during "growth spurt."
B. Assist with preparation of child/family for conservative treatment such as use of brace.
   1. Collaborate with RN to develop and implement a family teaching plan about application of Milwaukee brace:
      a. Wear 23 hours/day.
      b. Wear T-shirt under brace to decrease skin irritation.
      c. Check skin for areas of irritation or breakdown.
   2. Suggest clothing modifications to camouflage brace.
   3. Reinforce prescribed exercise regimen for back and abdominal muscles.
   4. Plan with adolescent to increase self-concept.
   5. Reinforce teaching to family that severe, untreated scoliosis can cause respiratory difficulty.

> **HESI Hint** • A brace does not correct the curve of a child with scoliosis but only stops or slows progression.

C. Collaborate with RN to enhance and reinforce a client/family teaching plan to prepare child/family for surgical correction if required:
   1. Teach child and family log-rolling technique.
   2. Practice respiratory hygiene.
   3. Orient to ICU.
   4. Discuss "postoperative tubes": Foley, NG tube, and chest tube (if anterior fusion is performed).
   5. Describe postoperative pain management; patient-controlled analgesic (PCA) may be used.
   6. Obtain a baseline neurologic assessment.
D. Provide postoperative care:
   1. Perform frequent neurologic assessments.
   2. Log-roll for number of days prescribed by HCP (Box 5-3, *Log Rolling*).
   3. Monitor IV fluids and analgesics as prescribed.
   4. Oral hygiene (client NPO).

> **BOX 5-3 *Log Rolling***
>
> - Usually requires two or more persons, depending on the size of the client.
> - Client is carefully moved on a draw sheet to the side of the bed away from which he or she is to be turned (moved to the left if the client is to face to the right).
> - Client is then turned in a simultaneous motion (log-rolled), maintaining the spine in a straight position.
> - Pillows are arranged for support and comfort, and they assist the client to maintain alignment.

5. Monitor NG tube and bowel sounds.
6. Assist with ambulation, provide body jacket; progressively ambulate.
7. Reinforce teaching to child/family that body jacket will be worn for several months until the bone fusion is stable.
8. Determine the need for a homebound teacher.
9. Encourage child's participation in care to promote self-esteem.

Juvenile Rheumatoid Arthritis

Description: Chronic inflammatory disorder of the joint synovium.
A. Single or multiple joints may be involved.
B. May also have systemic presentation.
C. Occurs between ages 2 to 5 years and 9 to 12 years.

Nursing Assessment (Data Collection)

A. Joint swelling and stiffness (usually large joints)
B. Painful joints
C. Generalized symptoms: fever, malaise, and rash
D. Periods of exacerbations and remissions
E. Varying severity: may be mild and self-limiting or severe and disabling
F. Lab data: latex fixation test (usually negative) and elevated erythrocyte sedimentation rate
G. Poorest prognosis:
   1. Positive rheumatoid factor
   2. Polyarticular systemic onset

Analysis (Nursing Diagnoses)

A. Impaired physical mobility related to …
B. Chronic pain related to …

Nursing Plans and Interventions

A. Reinforce instructions for home program of prescribed exercise, splinting, and activity.
B. Assist with identifying adaptations in routine—for example, Velcro fasteners, frequent rest periods, and so on.
C. Support maintaining school schedule and activities appropriate for age.
D. Collaborate with team to enhance and reinforce a client/family teaching plan for medication regimen: combination drugs are used (see Chapter 4, *Medical-Surgical Nursing*, p. 61).
   1. Nonsteroidal anti-inflammatory drugs:
      a. Tolmetin sodium
      b. Ibuprofen
      c. Naproxen
   2. Antirheumatic drugs (gold salts)
   3. Corticosteroids (prednisone)
   4. Cytotoxic drugs (cyclophosphamide, methotrexate)
E. Collaborate with team to enhance and reinforce a client/family teaching plan about side effects and toxic effects of prescribed drugs.
F. Reinforce to child/family that optimum anti-inflammatory effects from drugs may take a month to achieve.
G. Encourage periodic eye exams for early detection of iridocyclitis to prevent vision loss.
H. Encourage family to allow child's independence.

> **HESI Hint** • Corticosteroids are used short term in low doses during exacerbations. Long-term use is avoided due to side effects and their adverse effect on growth.

Review of Skeletal Disorder

1. List normal findings in a neurovascular assessment.
2. What is compartment syndrome?
3. What are the signs and symptoms of compartment syndrome?
4. Why are fractures of the epiphyseal plate a special concern?
5. How is skeletal traction applied?
6. What discharge instructions should be included for a child with a spica cast?
7. What are the signs and symptoms of congenital dislocated hip in infants?
8. How would the nurse conduct scoliosis screening?
9. What instructions should the child with scoliosis receive about the Milwaukee brace?
10. What care is indicated for a child with juvenile rheumatoid arthritis?

Answers to Review

1. Warm extremity, brisk capillary refill, free movement, normal sensation of the affected extremity, and equal pulses.
2. Damage to nerves and vasculature of an extremity due to compression.
3. Abnormal neurovascular assessment: severe pain, cold extremity, inability to move the extremity, and poor capillary refill.
4. Fractures of the epiphyseal plate (growth plate) may affect the growth of the limb.

5. Skeletal traction is maintained by pins or wires applied to the distal fragment of the fracture.

6. Check circulation. Keep cast dry. Do not stick anything under cast. Prevent cast soilage during toileting or diapering. Do not turn with abductor bar.

7. Unequal skin folds of the buttocks, Ortolani sign (performed by HCP), limited abduction of the affected hip, and unequal leg lengths.

8. Ask the child to bend forward from the hips with arms hanging free. Examine the child for a curve of the spine, rib hump, and hip asymmetry.

9. Wear the brace 23 hours per day. Wear T-shirt under brace. Check skin for irritation. Perform back and abdominal exercises. Modify clothing. Encourage the child to maintain normal activities as able.

10. Prescribed exercise to maintain mobility, splinting of affected joints, and teaching medication management and side effects of drugs.

6

MATERNITY NURSING

Anatomy and Physiology of Reproduction

The Menstrual Cycle

Description: Composed of four (4) phases. The normal cycle is 21 to 45 days in length. The mean age for menarche (first menstruation) in the United States is 12.87 years or 1 to 3 years after breast budding. Pregnancy can occur from the very first menstrual cycle. Most women have ovulatory cycles within 24 months after menarche (Figure 6-1, *Menstrual Cycle: Hypothalamic-Pituitary, Ovarian, and Endometrial*).

Phases of the Menstrual Cycle

A. Menstrual phase—Days 1 to 5 of cycle. Shedding of the endometrium occurs as uterine bleeding, approximately 60 ml (less than 2 ounces).

> **HESI Hint** • The menstrual phase varies in length for most women, usually lasting 2 to 8 days.

B. Proliferative (follicular) phase—day 5 to ovulation. Endometrium is restored under primary hormone influence of estrogen. In this preovulatory phase, FSH (follicle stimulating hormone) is secreted by the anterior pituitary. Preovulatory surge of LH (luteinizing hormone) affects one follicle, and ovulation occurs.
C. Secretory (luteal) phase—ovulation to approximately 3 days before menstruation begins. Estrogen levels level off, and progesterone levels increase.
D. Ischemic phase—if fertilization does not occur, the corpus luteum degenerates and estrogen and progesterone levels drop off, causing the endometrium to become "blood starved," leading to menstruation.

> **HESI Hint** • From ovulation to the beginning of the next menstrual cycle is usually 14 days. In other words, ovulation occurs 14 days before the next menstrual period.

> **HESI Hint** • Sperm live approximately 3 days (but some sperm may remain viable for as long as 5 days), and eggs live about 24 hours. A couple must avoid unprotected intercourse for several days before the anticipated ovulation and for 3 days after ovulation to prevent pregnancy.

Fertilization

A. Indications of ovulation:
   1. Slight drop in temperature 1 day before ovulation with a 0.5° F to 1° F rise in temperature at ovulation. Temperature remains elevated for approximately 10 to 12 days.
   2. Cervical mucus is abundant, watery, clear, and more alkaline.
   3. Cervical os dilates slightly, softens, and rises in the vagina.
   4. Spinnbarkeit (egg white stretchiness of cervical mucus).
   5. Ferning under microscope.
B. Conditions for fertilization:
   1. Postcoital test demonstrates live, motile, normal sperm present in cervical mucus.
   2. Fallopian tubes patent.
   3. Endometrial biopsy indicates adequate progesterone and secretory endometrium.
   4. Semen is supportive to pregnancy: 2 mL semen; at least 20 million sperm/mL; more than 60% normal; and more than 50% motile (moving forward).
C. Implantation:
   1. Fertilization takes place in ampulla (outer one third) portion of the fallopian tube.
   2. Zygote (fertilized ovum) takes 3 to 4 days to enter the uterus.
   3. Takes 7 to 10 days to complete the process of nidation (implantation).
D. Fetal development:
   1. Zygote:
      a. 12 to 14 days after fertilization
      b. From the time the ovum is fertilized until it is implanted in the uterus

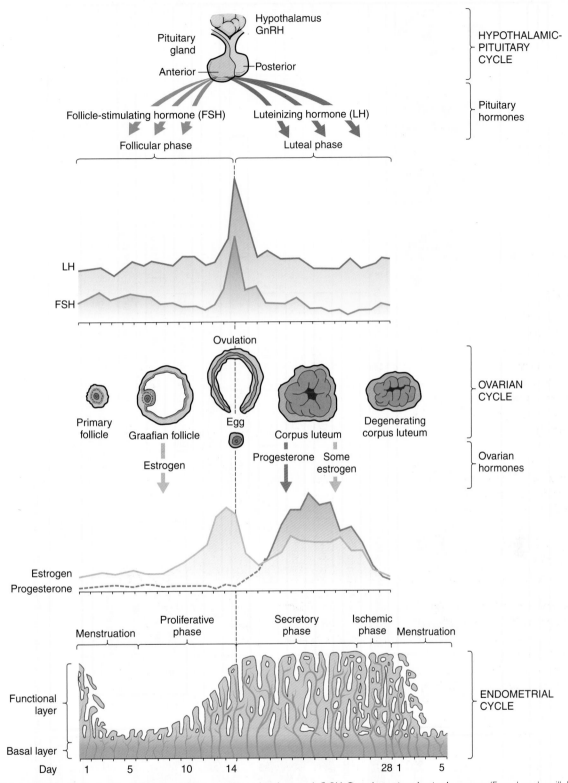

FIGURE 6-1 Menstrual Cycle. Hypothalamic-pituitary, ovarian, and endometrial. *GnRH,* Gonadotropin-releasing hormone. (From Lowdermilk DL, Perry SE, Cashion MC: *Maternity & women's health care,* ed 10, St. Louis, 2012, Mosby.)

2. Embryo:
   a. 15 days to 8 weeks after fertilization
   b. During this period, embryo is most vulnerable to teratogens: viruses, drugs, radiation, or infections can cause MAJOR congenital anomalies

3. Fetus:
   a. 9 weeks from fertilization to term (38+ weeks)
   b. Teratogen influence during fetal period results in fewer major anomalies (Figure 6-2, *The Sensitive or Critical Periods in Human Prenatal Development*)

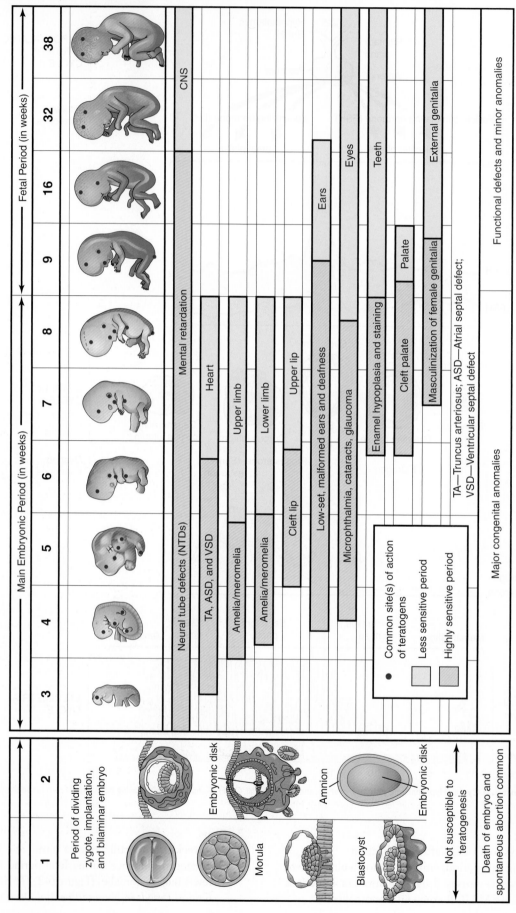

FIGURE 6-2 The Sensitive or Critical Periods in Human Prenatal Development. Dark color denotes highly sensitive periods; light color indicates stages that are less sensitive to teratogens. (From Moore KL, Persaud TVN: *The developing human: clinically oriented embryology,* ed 9, Philadelphia, 2011, Saunders.)

Maternal Physiologic Changes During Pregnancy

A. Pregnancy length is counted from the first day of last menstrual period (LMP):
 1. 280 days (approximately)
 2. 40 weeks
 3. 10 lunar months (perfect 28-day months)
 4. 9 calendar months
B. Pregnancy is divided into three 13-week trimesters:
 1. First trimester: from the first day of LMP through 13 weeks
 2. Second trimester: 14 weeks through 26 weeks
 3. Third trimester: 27 weeks to 40 weeks

> **HESI Hint** • Because some women experience implantation bleeding or spotting, they do not know they are pregnant.

Fetal/Maternal Changes

8 Weeks

A. Fetal development:
 1. Rapid development.
 2. Heart begins to pump blood.
 3. Limb buds are well developed.
 4. Facial features discernible.
 5. Major divisions of brain discernible.
 6. Ears develop from skin folds.
 7. Tiny muscles are formed beneath this skin embryo.
 8. Weighs 2 grams.
B. Maternal changes:
 1. Nausea persists up to 12 weeks.
 2. Uterus changes from pear to globular shape.
 3. Hegar sign (softening of the isthmus of cervix).
 4. Goodell sign (softening of cervix).
 5. Cervix flexes.
 6. Leukorrhea increases.
 7. Ambivalence about pregnancy may occur.
 8. No noticeable weight gain.
 9. Chadwick sign (bluing of vagina) appears as early as 4 weeks' gestation.
C. Nursing interventions:
 1. Collaborate with RN to enhance and reinforce a teaching plan about prevention of nausea.
  a. Suggest eating dry crackers before getting out of bed in the morning.
  b. Suggest eating small, frequent meals; avoiding fatty foods; and avoiding skipping meals.
 2. Collaborate with RN to enhance and reinforce a teaching plan about safety.
  a. Avoid hot tubs, saunas, and steam rooms throughout pregnancy (increases risk of neural tube defects in first trimester; hypotension may cause fainting).
  b. Reinforce prenatal nutrition guidelines.

 3. Prepare for pregnancy:
  a. Discuss attitudes toward pregnancy.
  b. Discuss the value of early pregnancy classes that focus on what to expect during pregnancy.
  c. Reinforce information about childbirth preparation classes.
  d. Include father/family in preparation for childbirth (expectant fathers experience many of the same feelings/conflicts experienced by expectant mothers).

12 Weeks

A. Fetal development:
 1. Embryo becomes a fetus.
 2. Heart discernible by ultrasound.
 3. Lower body develops.
 4. Sex determinable.
 5. Kidneys produce urine.
 6. Fetus weighs 19 to 28 grams (less than 1 ounce).
B. Maternal changes:
 1. Uterus rises *above* pelvic brim.
 2. Braxton Hicks contractions possible (continue throughout pregnancy).
 3. Potential for urinary tract infection (UTI) increases (exists throughout pregnancy).
 4. Weight gain 2½ to 4 pounds during first trimester.
 5. Placenta fully functioning and producing hormones.
C. Nursing interventions:
 1. Collaborate with RN to enhance and reinforce a teaching plan about prevention of urinary tract infections:
  a. Adequate fluid intake, 3 liters/day.
  b. Void frequently (every 2 hours while awake).
  c. Void before and after intercourse.
  d. Wipe from front to back.
 2. Reinforce teaching plan about nutrition and exercise:
  a. Increase caloric intake by 300 calories/day.
  b. Stress value of regular exercise.
  c. Stress well-balanced diet.
  d. Reinforce importance of prenatal vitamins with folic acid.
 3. Reinforce possible effects of pregnancy on sexual relationship:
  a. Recognize father's role as he labors to incorporate the parental role into his self-identity.

20 Weeks

A. Fetal development:
 1. Vernix protects body.
 2. Lanugo (fine hair) covers body, protects body.
 3. Eyebrows, eyelashes, head hair develops.
 4. Fetus sleeps, sucks, and kicks.
 5. Fetus weighs 200 to 400 grams (11 to 14 ounces).
 6. Fetus may survive outside of uterus: called the age of viability.
B. Maternal changes:
 1. Fundus reaches level of umbilicus.

2. Breasts begin secreting colostrums, areola darken.
3. Amniotic sac holds approximately 400 mL fluid.
4. Postural hypotension may occur.
5. Fetal movement felt (quickening); pregnancy becomes "real."
6. Nasal stuffiness may begin.
7. Leg cramps may begin.
8. Varicose veins may develop.
9. Constipation may develop.

C. Nursing interventions:
1. Collaborate with RN to enhance and reinforce a teaching plan about comfort measures:
    a. Remain active.
    b. Sit with feet elevated when possible.
    c. Avoid pressure on lower thighs.
    d. Use of support stockings may be helpful.
    e. Dorsiflex foot to relieve leg cramps.
    f. Apply heat to muscles affected by cramps.
    g. Cool-air vaporizer or saline nasal spray may help with nasal stuffiness.
2. Collaborate with RN to enhance and reinforce a teaching plan about measures to avoid constipation:
    a. Eat raw fruits, raw vegetables, cereals with bran.
    b. Drink 3 liters fluid/day.
    c. Exercise frequently.

28 Weeks

A. Fetal development:
1. Fetus can breathe, swallow, regulate temperature.
2. Surfactant forms in lungs.
3. Fetus can hear.
4. Fetus's eyelids open.
5. Period of greatest fetal weight gain begins.
6. Fetus weighs 1100 grams (2½ pounds).

B. Maternal changes:
1. Fundus halfway between umbilicus and xiphoid process.
2. Thoracic breathing replaces abdominal breathing.
3. Fetal outline palpable.
4. Woman becomes more introspective and concentrates interest on the unborn child.
5. Heartburn may begin.
6. Hemorrhoids may develop.

C. Nursing interventions:
1. Reinforce teaching of hemorrhoid treatment:
    a. Sitz baths.
    b. Suppositories as prescribed.
    c. Topical anesthetic agents as prescribed.
    d. Stool softeners as prescribed.
2. Collaborate with RN to enhance and reinforce a teaching plan about comfort measures:
    a. Elevate legs when sitting.
    b. Assume side-lying position when resting.
3. Collaborate with RN to enhance and reinforce a teaching plan about measures to avoid heartburn:
    a. Eat small, frequent meals.

b. Avoid fatty foods.
c. Avoid lying down after meals.
d. Take antacids as prescribed.
e. Avoid sodium bicarbonate.
4. Prepare parents for delivery of baby and parenthood:
    a. Discuss mother's/father's/family's expectations of labor and delivery.
    b. Discuss mother's/father's/family's expectations of caring for infant at home.
    c. Start childbirth preparation classes.

32 Weeks

A. Fetal development:
1. Brown fat deposits develop beneath skin to insulate baby following birth.
2. Fetus is 15 to 17 inches in length.
3. Begins storing iron, calcium, and phosphorus.
4. Fetus weighs 1800 to 2200 grams (4 to 5 pounds).

B. Maternal changes:
1. Fundus reaches xiphoid process.
2. Breasts full and tender.
3. Urinary frequency returns.
4. Swollen ankles may occur.
5. Sleeping problems may develop.
6. Dyspnea may develop.

C. Nursing interventions:
1. Collaborate with RN to enhance and reinforce a teaching plan about measures to decrease edema:
    a. Elevate legs 1 to 2 times/day for approximately 1 hour.
2. Collaborate with RN to enhance and reinforce a teaching plan about comfort measures:
    a. Wear well-fitting supportive bra.
    b. Maintain proper posture.
    c. Use semi-Fowler position at night for dyspnea.
3. Prepare parents for birth of child:
    a. Review signs of labor.
    b. Discuss plans for other children (if any).
    c. Discuss plans for transportation to agency.
    d. Assess father's and family member's role during childbirth.

36 to 40 Weeks

A. Fetal development:
1. Fetus occupies entire uterus; activity is restricted.
2. Maternal antibodies are transferred to fetus (provides immunity for approximately 6 months, until infant's own immune system can take over).
3. Fetus weighs 3200+ grams (7+ pounds).

B. Maternal changes:
1. Lightening occurs.
2. Placenta weighs approximately 20 ounces.
3. Mother eager for birth, may have burst of energy.
4. Backaches increase.
5. Urinary frequency increases.

6. Braxton Hicks contractions intensify (cervix and lower uterine segment prepare for labor).

C. Nursing interventions:
   1. Collaborate with RN to enhance and reinforce a teaching plan about safety measures:
      a. Wear low-heeled shoes or flats.
      b. Avoid heavy lifting.
      c. Sleep on side to increase blood flow to the placenta.
   2. Prepare for delivery:
      a. Continue pelvic tilt exercises.
      b. Pack a suitcase for delivery.
      c. Encourage couple to tour labor and delivery area.
      d. Discuss postpartum: circumcision, rooming-in, possibility of postpartum "blues," birth control, need for adequate rest, father's role.

Antepartum Nursing Care

Psychosocial Response to Pregnancy

Maternal Responses

A. First trimester:
   1. Ambivalence: whether pregnancy is planned or unplanned, ambivalence is normal.
   2. Financial worries about increased responsibility are normal.
   3. Career concerns are common.
B. Second trimester:
   1. Quickening occurs, and pregnancy becomes real.
   2. Pregnant woman accepts pregnancy.
   3. Ambivalence wanes.
C. Third trimester:
   1. Pregnant woman becomes introverted and self-absorbed.
   2. Pregnant woman begins to ignore partner (may strain the relationship).
D. Throughout pregnancy:
   1. Wide mood swings (joy, anticipation, fear) occur.
   2. Pregnant woman is ultrasensitive.
   3. Strained relationship may occur with partner.

> **HESI Hint** • Look for signs of maternal-fetal bonding during pregnancy. For example, talking to fetus in utero, massaging abdomen, and nicknaming fetus are all healthy psychosocial activities.

Paternal Responses

A. Announcement phase, acceptance of the biologic fact of pregnancy:
   1. At the confirmation of pregnancy, men may react with joy or dismay, depending on whether the pregnancy is desired or unplanned or unwanted.
   2. Ambivalence in the early stages of pregnancy is common.
   3. Some men experience pregnancy-like symptoms, such as nausea, weight gain, and other physical symptoms, which is known as the *couvade syndrome*.
   4. May last from a few hours to a few weeks
B. Moratorium phase, the period of adjustment to the reality of pregnancy:
   1. Accepts the pregnancy.
   2. May put conscious thought of the pregnancy aside for a time and become more introspective by engaging in many discussions about his philosophy of life, religion, childbearing, and child rearing practices and relationships with family members, particularly with his father.
   3. This phase may be relatively short or may persist until the last trimester, depending on the father's readiness for the pregnancy.
C. Focusing phase, active involvement in both the pregnancy and his relationship with his child:
   1. Negotiates with the mother the role he is to play in labor and to prepare for parenthood.
   2. Concentrates on his experience of the pregnancy and begins to think of himself as a father.
   3. Begins in the last trimester.

Activities During First Prenatal Visit

A. Obtain history:
   1. Medical history
   2. Obstetric history can be determined by two common methods:
      a. Two digits: G/P only records the gravida and para of a client.
      b. Five digits: GTPAL (Gravidity, Term Births, Preterm Births, Abortions & Miscarriages, and Living Children) provides information on the client's obstetric history but does *not* refer to para.
   3. History and status of current pregnancy
B. Determine gravidity (G) and parity (P):
   1. *Gravida* refers to the number of times one has been pregnant (regardless of the outcome).
   2. *Para* refers to the number of pregnancies that have reached 20 weeks' or greater gestation and before birth.
      a. Any pregnancy loss occurring before 20 weeks is counted as an abortion (whether spontaneous or elective termination) and adds only to a client's gravidity, not parity.
      b. When calculating parity, multiple births count only as (1) after pregnancy has reached 20 weeks and before birth.
C. Assist with physical examination.
D. Calculate gestational age: estimated date of birth (EDB) using Nägele's rule:
   1. Count back 3 months from the first day of the last normal menstrual period, and add 7 days.
   2. For example: if the LMP was March 23, the EDB would be December 30.

E. Vital signs:
1. BP should increase no more than 30 points systolic and 15 points diastolic from baseline normal. Average BP is 90 to 140 mm Hg systolic and 60 to 90 mm Hg diastolic.
2. Average pulse is 60 to 90 beats per minute (bpm).
3. Average respiration is 16 to 24 breaths per minute (breaths/min).
4. Average temperature is 97°F to 100°F.
F. Future office visits:
1. Low-risk client's schedule is:
   a. Every 4 weeks until 28 weeks.
   b. Every 2 weeks from 28 weeks until 36 weeks.
   c. Every week from 36 weeks until delivery.
2. High-risk client's schedule is determined by client's needs; visits are scheduled as necessary.
G. Obtain laboratory data as ordered (Appendix A, p. 338):
1. Hgb: values during pregnancy >11
2. Hct: values during pregnancy >33
3. WBC and differential
4. Hgb electrophoresis (sickle cell)
5. Pap smear and cytology (gonorrhea and chlamydia)
6. Antibody screens
   a. HIV
   b. Hepatitis B
   c. Toxoplasmosis
   d. Rubella (>1:10 = immunity)
   e. Syphilis (RPR, VDRL)
   f. Cytomegalovirus
7. Tuberculin skin testing (PPD)
8. Rh and blood type
9. Urinalysis

> **HESI Hint** • For many women, *battering* (emotional or physical abuse) begins during pregnancy. Women should be assessed for abuse in private, away from the partner, by a nurse who knows local resources and how to determine the safety of the client.

> **HESI Hint** • Practice determining gravidity and parity. A woman who is 6 weeks pregnant has the following maternal history:
> • Has a 2-year-old, healthy daughter.
> • Had a miscarriage at 10 weeks, 3 years ago.
> • Had an elective abortion at 6 weeks, 5 years ago.
> With this pregnancy, she is a gravida 4, para 1 (only 1 delivery after 20 weeks' gestation).

> **HESI Hint** • Practice calculating EDB (estimated date of birth). If the first day of a woman's last normal menstrual period was October 17, what is her EDB using Nägele's rule? Count back 3 months and add 7 days (always give February 28 days).

> **HESI Hint** • At approximately 28 to 32 weeks' gestation, the maximum plasma volume increase of 25% to 40% occurs, resulting in normal hemodilution of pregnancy and Hct values of 32% to 42%. High Hct values may look "good," but in reality, they represent a gestational hypertension disorder and a depleted vascular space.

> **HESI Hint** • Hgb/Hct data can be used to evaluate nutritional status. Example: A 22-year-old primigravida at 12 weeks' gestation has an Hgb of 9.6 g/dL and an Hct of 31%. She has gained 3 pounds during the first trimester.
> A weight gain of 2 to 4 pounds during the first trimester is recommended, and this client is anemic. Supplemental iron and a diet higher in iron are needed.
> Foods high in iron:
> • Fish and red meats
> • Cereal and yellow vegetables
> • Green leafy vegetables and citrus fruits
> • Egg yolks and dried fruits

Activities During Subsequent Visits

A. Check urine for:
1. Albumin (protein): no more than a trace for a normal finding (related to preeclampsia).
2. Glucose: no more than 1+ for a normal finding (related to gestational diabetes).
B. Graph weight gain:
1. 2 to 4 pounds in the first trimester is considered normal.
2. 0.9 pound per week thereafter (more than 2 lb/wk related to preeclampsia-edema).
3. Total weight gain during the pregnancy for normal-weight woman should be between 25 and 35 pounds.
C. Check fundus height (Figure 6-3, *Fundal Height Assessment*):
1. 12 to 13 weeks: fundus rises above symphysis.
2. 20 weeks: fundus at umbilicus.
3. 24 weeks: fundus height is measured in centimeters (cm), with the number of cm above the symphysis equal to the number of weeks' gestation, until 36 weeks' gestation.

> **HESI Hint** • As pregnancy advances, the uterus presses on abdominal vessels (vena cava and aorta). Reinforce teaching that a side-lying or knee-chest position increases perfusion to the uterus, placenta, and fetus.

D. Check fetal heart rate:
1. 10 to 12 weeks detectable using Doppler.
2. 15 to 20 weeks detectable by using fetoscope.
3. 110 to 160 beats per minute (bpm) is normal range.

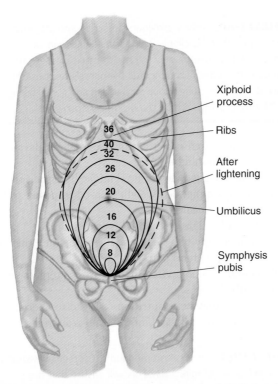

FIGURE 6-3 Fundal Height Assessment. Height of the fundus of the uterus during pregnancy. The numbers represent the weeks of gestation, and the circles represent the height of the fundus expected at that stage of gestation. The dotted line at the 40th week indicates that lightening has occurred. (From Murray SS, McKinney ES: *Foundations of maternal-newborn and women's health nursing,* ed 5, Philadelphia, 2010, Saunders.)

Labels: Xiphoid process, Ribs, After lightening, Umbilicus, Symphysis pubis. Numbers: 36, 40, 32, 26, 20, 16, 12, 8.

> **HESI Hint** • Fetal well-being is determined by assessing fundal height, fetal heart tones/rate, fetal movement, and uterine activity (contractions). Changes in fetal heart rate are the first and most important indicator of compromised blood flow to the fetus, and these changes require action! Remember, the normal fetal heart rate (FHR) is 110 to 160 bpm.

E. Emphasize importance of continuing prenatal care.
F. Reinforce teaching plan that includes anticipatory guidance—first trimester:
1. Discomforts such as nausea, fatigue, and urinary frequency subside after 13 weeks.
2. Sleep needs increase to 8 hr/day.
3. Plan rest periods.
4. May exercise as long as the woman is able to converse easily while exercising. If not, she should slow down.
5. May work if no hazardous chemical/toxin exposure.
6. May bathe until membranes rupture (usually within hours of delivery).
7. May travel by car, but woman will need frequent breaks and must wear seat belt.

8. Air travel: policies vary by airline. Remain well hydrated. Move about frequently to minimize risk of thrombophlebitis.
9. Best to ingest no medications and no alcohol and to stop smoking.
G. Reinforce teaching plan that includes anticipatory guidance—second trimester:
1. Sexual needs/desires may change for better/worse. Encourage communication with partner regarding adjustments.
2. Have regular checkups/dental hygiene (gum hypertrophy common). Delay x-rays and major dental work if possible.
H. Reinforce teaching plan that includes anticipatory guidance—third trimester:
1. Schedule childbirth classes.
2. Note that urinary frequency and dyspnea may occur.
3. Review interventions for leg cramps (dorsiflex foot), nasal stuffiness, varicose veins, and constipation.
4. Reinforce teaching about safety related to balance.
5. Position with pillows for comfort.
6. Round ligament pain will occur.
7. Instruct client to come to hospital when contractions are occurring regularly 5 minutes apart for 1 hour.
8. Reinforce information on feeding methods.
9. Encourage choosing a pediatrician/clinic.
10. Reinforce nutritional needs because third trimester is a period of rapid fetal growth.
11. Reinforce the risks/symptoms of preterm labor.

> **HESI Hint** • **DANGER SIGNS DURING PREGNANCY.**
> Reinforce teaching about immediately reporting any of the following danger signs. Early intervention can optimize maternal and fetal outcome.
> **Possible indications of preeclampsia/eclampsia:**
> • Visual disturbances
> • Swelling of face, fingers, or sacrum
> • Severe, continuous headache
> • Persistent vomiting
> **Signs of infection:**
> • Chills
> • Temperature greater than 100.4° F
> • Dysuria
> • Pain in abdomen or back
> • Fluid discharge from vagina (anything other than normal leukorrhea)
> • Change in fetal movement

Nutrition

Nursing Assessment (Data Collection)

A. Diet:
1. Ask client to recall diet for last 24 hours.

2. Use a questionnaire to determine individual deficiencies.
3. Note symptoms of malnutrition:
   a. Glossitis
   b. Cracked lips
   c. Dry, brittle hair
B. Dental caries, periodontitis
C. Weight (those who weigh less than 100 lb or greater than 200 lb are at risk)

Analysis (Nursing Diagnoses)

A. Imbalanced nutrition: less than body requirements related to …
B. Imbalanced nutrition: more than body requirements related to …
C. Deficient knowledge (specify) related to …

Nursing Plans and Interventions

A. Collaborate with RN to enhance and reinforce a teaching plan about minimum nutritional increases.
   1. Increase of 300 calories above basal and activity needs.
   2. Increase intake of iron (30+ mg) and folic acid (800 to 1000 mcg) with diet and supplementation.
   3. Increase intake of vitamin A, vitamin C, and calcium with diet.

> **HESI Hint** Most providers prescribe prenatal vitamins to ensure that the client receives an adequate intake of vitamins. However, only the health care provider can prescribe prenatal vitamins. It is the nurse's responsibility to reinforce teaching about proper diet and about taking vitamins as prescribed by the health care provider.

   4. Drink a total of 8 to 10 glasses of fluid/day; 4 to 6 glasses should be water.
   5. Evaluate adequacy of fluid intake by urine color.
B. Relate recommended weight gain by trimester to fetal growth/fetal health.
   1. Record weight at each visit, using graph.
C. Provide a copy of a healthy daily food guide that considers cultural food patterns.
D. Encourage taking vitamin and iron supplements as prescribed.
E. Reinforce that poor nutrition can lead to anemia, preterm labor, obesity, and intrauterine growth restriction.

> **HESI Hint** It is recommended that pregnant women drink 1 quart of milk a day. This will ensure that the daily calcium needs are met and will help to alleviate the occurrence of leg cramps.

Review of Anatomy and Physiology of Reproduction and Antepartum Nursing Care

1. State the objective signs that signify ovulation.
2. Ovulation occurs how many days before the next menstrual period?
3. State three ways to identify the chronologic age of a pregnancy (gestation).
4. What maternal position provides optimum fetal maternal/placental perfusion during pregnancy?
5. Name the major discomforts of the first trimester and one suggestion for amelioration of each.
6. If the first day of a woman's last normal menstrual period was May 28, what would be the estimated date of birth (EDB) using Nägele's rule?
7. At 20 weeks' gestation, the fundal height would be _____, and the fetus would weigh approximately _____ and would look like _____.
8. State the normal psychosocial responses to pregnancy in the second trimester.
9. Hemodilution of pregnancy peaks at _____ weeks and results in a/an _____ _____ in a woman's Hct.
10. State three principles relative to the pattern of weight gain in pregnancy.
11. Fetal heart rate can be auscultated by Doppler at _____ weeks' gestation.
12. Describe the schedule for prenatal visits for a low-risk pregnant woman.

Answers to Review

1. Abundant, thin, clear cervical mucus; spinnbarkeit (egg white stretchiness) of cervical mucus; open cervical os; slight drop in basal body temperature (BBT) and then 0.5° F to 1° F rise; ferning under the microscope.
2. 14 days.
3. 10 lunar months, 9 calendar months consisting of three trimesters of 3 months each, 40 weeks, 280 days.
4. The knee-chest position, but the ideal position of *comfort* for the mother, which supports fetal/maternal/placental perfusion, is the side-lying position off the abdominal vessels (vena cava, aorta).

5. Nausea and vomiting: crackers before rising. Fatigue: teach the need for rest periods/naps and 7 to 8 hours of sleep at night.
6. Count back 3 months and add 7 days: March 7. (Always give February 28 days.)
7. At the umbilicus; 300 to 400 grams; a "baby" with hair, lanugo, and vernix, but without any subcutaneous fat.
8. Ambivalence wanes, and acceptance of pregnancy occurs; pregnancy becomes "real"; signs of maternal-fetal bonding occur.
9. 28 to 32 weeks, decrease.
10. Total weight gain during pregnancy for a normal-weight woman should be 25 to 35 pounds. Gain should be consistent throughout pregnancy. An average of 1 lb/week should be gained in the second and third trimesters.
11. 10 to 12.
12. Once a month until 28 weeks, then once every 2 weeks until 36 weeks, and then weekly until delivery.

Fetal/Maternal Assessment Techniques

Description: Techniques used to obtain data regarding fetal and maternal physiologic status.
A. Maternal risk factors include, but are not limited to:
   1. Age younger than 17 or older than 34.
   2. High parity: more than 5.
   3. Recent pregnancy (3 months since last delivery).
   4. Hypertension, preeclampsia in current pregnancy.
   5. Anemia, history of hemorrhage, or current hemorrhage.
   6. Multiple gestations.
   7. Rh incompatibility.
   8. History of dystocia or previous operative delivery.
   9. Under 60 inches (5 feet) in height.
   10. Malnutrition (15% under ideal weight) or extreme obesity (20% over ideal weight).
   11. Medical disease in pregnancy (diabetes, hyperthyroidism, hyperemesis, clotting disorders, such as thrombocytopenia).
   12. Infection in pregnancy: toxoplasmosis and other diseases: rubella, cytomegalovirus infections, herpes simplex, syphilis (TORCH diseases); influenza; herpes-type virus (HTV); chlamydia; human papilloma virus (HPV).
   13. History of family violence, lack of social support.
B. Various techniques are used to determine fetal/maternal well-being.

> **HESI Hint** • In some states, the screening for neural tube defects through either maternal serum alpha-fetoprotein (AFP) levels or amniotic fluid AFP levels is mandated by state law. This screening test is highly associated with both false positives and false negatives.

Ultrasonography

Description: Ultrasonography consists of high-frequency sound waves that are beamed on the pregnant abdomen; echoes are returned to a machine, which records the "object's" location and size.

A. Used in the first trimester to determine:
   1. Number of fetuses
   2. Presence of fetal cardiac movement/rhythm
   3. Uterine abnormalities
   4. Assessment of gestational age
B. Used in the second and third trimesters to determine:
   1. Fetal viability/gestational age
   2. Size/date discrepancies
   3. Amniotic fluid volume
   4. Placental location/maturity
   5. Uterine anomalies/abnormalities
   6. Used routinely with amniocentesis
C. Findings:
   1. Fetal heart activity as early as 6 to 7 weeks' gestation.
   2. Serial evaluation of biparietal diameter and limb length can differentiate between wrong dates and true intrauterine growth restriction (IUGR).
   3. Biophysical profile for fetal well-being:
      a. Five variables assessed: fetal breathing movements, gross body movements, fetal tone, reactivity of fetal heart rate, and amniotic fluid volume.
      b. A score of 2 or 0 can be obtained on each variable. An overall score of 10 designates that the fetus is "well" the day of the examination.

> **HESI Hint** • Gestational age is best determined by an early sonogram rather than a later one.

D. Nursing care:
   1. Instruct woman to drink 3 to 4 glasses of water before coming for exam and not to urinate before exam. When the fetus is very small (in the first or second trimesters), the client's bladder must be full for the uterus to be supported for imaging. (A full bladder is not needed if ultrasound is done transvaginally instead of abdominally or in the third trimester.)
   2. Position woman with pillows under neck and knees to keep pressure off bladder; late in the third trimester, place wedge under right hip to displace uterus to the left.
   3. Position display so woman can watch if she wishes.
   4. Have bedpan or bathroom immediately available.

E. Complications:
1. No known complications.
2. Controversy regarding routine use of ultrasound in pregnancy.

Chorionic Villi Sampling

Description: In chorionic villi sampling (CVS), a small piece of villi is removed from the fetal portion of the placenta between 8 and 12 weeks' gestation under ultrasound guidance (cannot replace amniocentesis completely because no sample of amniotic fluid can be obtained for alpha-fetoprotein or Rh disease testing).
A. Findings:
1. Determines genetic diagnosis early in the first trimester.
2. Results obtained in 1 week.
B. Nursing care:
1. Informed consent needed before any procedure.
2. Place woman in lithotomy position using stirrups (if CVS done trancervically).
3. Warn of slight sharp pain upon catheter insertion.
4. Abnormal results should *not* be given over the phone.
C. Complications:
1. Spontaneous abortion (5%)
2. Controversy regarding fetal anomalies

Amniocentesis

Description: Amniocentesis is the removal of an amniotic fluid sample from the uterus as early as 14 to 16 weeks.
A. Used to determine:
1. Fetal genetic diagnosis (usually in the first trimester)
2. Fetal maturity (last trimester)
3. Fetal well-being
B. Performed only when uterus rises above the symphysis (between 12 and 13 weeks) and amniotic fluid has formed (see Figure 6-3, *Fundal Height Assessment*).
C. Usually takes 10 days to 2 weeks to develop cultured-cell karyotype. Therefore, could be well into second trimester before diagnosis is made, making choice for abortion more dangerous at that time.
D. Findings:
1. Genetic disorders:
   a. Karyotype: determines Down syndrome (trisomy 21), other trisomies, and sex chromatin (sex-linked disorders).
   b. Alpha-fetoprotein (AFP): elevations may be associated with neural tube defects; low levels may indicate trisomy 21.
2. Fetal maturity:
   a. L/S ratio (lecithin/sphingomyelin): 2:1 ratio indicates fetal lung maturity unless mother is diabetic, mother has Rh disease, or fetus is septic.
   b. L/S ratio and presence of phosphatidylglycerol (PG): most accurate determination of fetal maturity. PG present after 35 weeks' gestation.
   c. Lung maturity is the best predictor of extrauterine survival.
3. Fetal well-being:
   a. Meconium in amniotic fluid may indicate fetal stress.
E. Nursing care:
1. Obtain baseline vital signs and fetal heart rate (FHR).
2. Place client in supine position with hands across chest.
3. If prescribed, shave area and scrub with Betadine (povidone/iodine).
4. Draw maternal blood sample for comparison with postprocedure blood sample to determine maternal bleeding.
5. Provide emotional support, reinforce explanation of procedure, stay with the client (do not leave alone).
6. Label samples; if bilirubin test is prescribed, darken room and immediately cover the tubes with aluminum foil or use opaque tubes.
7. After specimen is drawn, wash abdomen, assist woman to empty bladder. A full bladder can irritate the uterus and cause contractions.
8. Monitor FHR for 1 hour after procedure and observe for uterine contractions/irritability.
9. Instruct woman to report any contractions, change in fetal movement, or fluid leaking from vagina.
F. Complications:
1. Spontaneous abortion (1%)
2. Fetal injury
3. Infection

> **HESI Hint** When an amniocentesis is done in early pregnancy, the bladder must be full to help support the uterus and help push the uterus up in the abdomen for easy access. When an amniocentesis is done in late pregnancy, the bladder must be empty to avoid puncturing the bladder.

Electronic Fetal Monitoring

Variables Measured with Fetal Monitoring

A. Contractions:
1. Depicts the beginning, peak, and end of each contraction.
2. Duration (length) of each contraction from beginning to end.
3. Frequency: beginning of one contraction to beginning of another. Must measure at least three to five contractions.

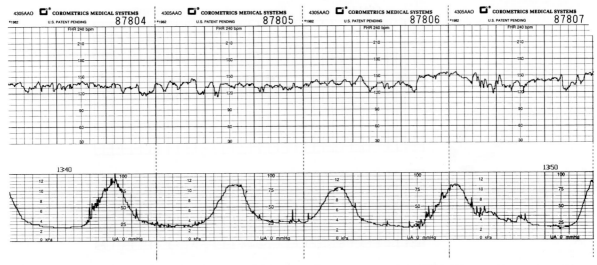

FIGURE 6-4 Normal (Reassuring) Fetal Heart Rate (FHR) Pattern. Upper grid represents the FHR, and lower grid represents uterine contractions. The FHR is in the normal range of 110 to 160 beats/minute. Note the saw-toothed appearance of the FHR tracing, which indicates variability. (From Leifer G: *Introduction to maternity & pediatric nursing*, ed 6, St. Louis, 2011, Saunders. Courtesy GE Healthcare, Milwaukee, Wisconsin.)

4. Intensity: strength not measured by external monitoring, measured in mm Hg by internal (intrauterine) monitoring after amniotic membranes are ruptured. Range from 30 (mild) to 70 (strong) mm Hg at peak.

B. Baseline fetal health rate:
  1. The range of FHR (average 110 to 160 bpm) between contractions, monitored over a 10-minute period.
  2. The balance between parasympathetic and sympathetic impulses usually produces no observable changes in the FHR during uterine contractions (with a *healthy* fetus, *healthy* placenta, and *good* uteroplacental perfusion) (Figure 6-4, *Normal [Reassuring] Fetal Heart Rate [FHR] Pattern*).

Nursing Actions Based on Fetal Heart Rate

A. Baseline fetal heart rate:
  1. Normal rhythmicity
  2. Average FHR 110-160 bpm
  3. Potential causes:
    a. The FHR results from the balance between the parasympathetic and sympathetic branches of the autonomic nervous system.
    b. The most important indicator of fetal central nervous system health.

B. Baseline variability:
  1. Variability describes constant changes, fluctuations, or normal irregularity in the FHR.
  2. Variability, with external or internal monitoring, has undulating wavelike movements that average 6 to 10 changes per minute. (Example: the heart rate may average 140 bpm, but changes from 136 to 147 bpm during that minute.) The FHR has a fine sawtooth appearance, denoting variability with internal monitoring (fetal scalp electrode) and denoting the changes in the FHR from one beat to the next.
  3. Variability has four characteristics: absent, minimal, moderate, or marked.

C. Nursing actions:
  1. Observe contractions using monitor strip.
  2. Observe FHR for normal baseline range and variability.
  3. If variability is not present, report finding to RN and health care provider.

D. Periodic changes:
  1. FHR changes in relation to uterine contractions.
  2. Potential causes:
    a. Accelerations (Figure 6-5, *Review of Fetal Variability*).
      (1) Caused by sympathetic fetal response.
      (2) Occur in response to fetal movement.
      (3) Indicative of a reactive, healthy fetus if increase is 15 bpm for at least 15 seconds.
    b. Early decelerations (see Figure 6-5, *Review of Fetal Variability*).
      (1) Benign pattern caused by parasympathetic response (head compression).
      (2) Heart rate slowly and smoothly decelerates at beginning of contraction and returns to baseline at end of contraction.

E. Nursing actions for early decelerations:
  1. No nursing interventions required except to monitor for progress of labor.
  2. Document the processes of labor.

Nonreassuring Warning Signs

A. Variability (see Figure 6-5, *Review of Fetal Variability*):
  1. FHR is absent or minimal.
  2. Potential causes:
    a. Hypoxia (asphyxia)

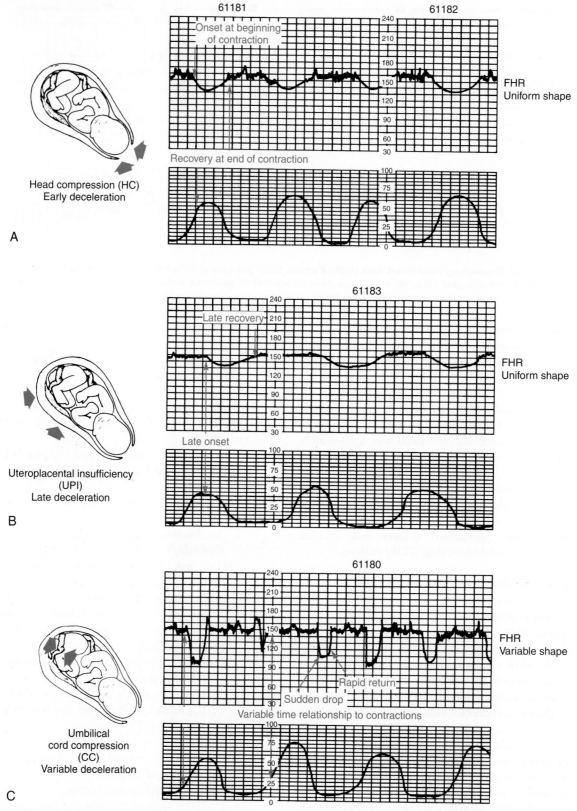

FIGURE 6-5 Review of Fetal Variability. Fetal heart rate (FHR) stress patterns showing early deceleration **(A)**, late deceleration **(B)**, and variable deceleration **(C)**. *UC,* uterine contractions. (From Miller L, Tucker S: *Mosby's pocket guide to fetal monitoring and assessment,* ed 7, St. Louis, 2013, Mosby.)

b. Acidosis

c. Maternal drug ingestion (narcotics, CNS depressants such as MgSO_4)

d. Fetal sleep

B. Bradycardia:

1. Baseline FHR below 110 bpm for 10 minutes (between contractions to differentiate from periodic change)

2. Potential causes:

a. Late manifestation of fetal hypoxia

b. Medication-induced (narcotics, MgSO_4)

c. Maternal hypotension

d. Fetal heart block

e. Prolonged umbilical cord compression

C. Tachycardia:

1. Baseline FHR above 160 bpm (assessed between contractions)

2. Potential causes:

a. Early sign of fetal hypoxia

b. Fetal anemia

c. Dehydration

d. Maternal infection/maternal fever

e. Maternal hyperthyroid disease

f. Medication-induced (atropine, terbutaline, hydroxyzine)

D. Nursing actions for decreased variability, bradycardia, and tachycardia:

1. Assist in treating based on cause.

E. Variable deceleration pattern (see Figure 6-5, *Review of Fetal Variability*).

1. Most common periodic pattern.

2. Characterized by an abrupt transitory decrease in the FHR that is *variable* in duration, depth of fall, and timing relative to the contraction cycle.

3. Occasional variable is usually benign.

4. Potential cause: occurs in 40% of all labors and is caused mainly by cord compression, but can also indicate rapid fetal descent.

F. Nursing actions for variable decelerations:

1. Change maternal position.

2. Stimulate fetus if indicated.

3. Discontinue oxytocin if infusing.

4. Administer oxygen at 10 liters by tight face mask.

5. Report findings to the RN and/or the health care provider and document.

Nonreassuring/Ominous Signs

E. Severe variable decelerations:

1. FHR below 70 bpm lasting longer than 30 to 60 seconds

2. Slow return to baseline

3. Decreasing or absent variability

F. Late decelerations (see Figure 6-5, *Review of Fetal Variability*):

1. Ominous/potentially disastrous, *nonreassuring* sign.

2. Indicative of uteroplacental insufficiency.

3. The shape of the deceleration is uniform, and the FHR returns to baseline after the contraction is over.

4. Depth of deceleration does not indicate severity, rarely falls below 100 bpm.

G. Nursing actions:

1. Immediately turn client to side.

2. Administer O_2 at 10 liters by tight face mask.

3. Turn off oxytocin if infusing.

4. Monitor intravenous line, and, if possible, elevate legs to increase venous return.

5. Correct any underlying hypotension.

6. Determine presence of FHR variability.

7. Assist with fetal blood sampling if indicated.

8. Notify RN and health care provider.

9. Document pattern and response to each nursing action.

HESI Hint Early decelerations, caused by head compression and fetal descent, usually occur between 4 and 7 cm and in the second stage. Check for labor progress if early decelerations are noted (see Figure 6-5, *Review of Fetal Variability*).

HESI Hint If cord prolapse is detected, the examiner should position the mother to relieve pressure on the cord (i.e., knee-chest position) or push the presenting part off the cord until *immediate* cesarean delivery can be accomplished.

HESI Hint Late decelerations indicate uteroplacental insufficiency and are associated with conditions such as postmaturity, preeclampsia, diabetes mellitus, cardiac disease, and abruptio placentae.

HESI Hint When deceleration patterns (late or variable) are associated with decreased or absent variability and tachycardia, the situation is *ominous* (potentially disastrous) and requires immediate intervention and fetal assessment.

HESI Hint A decrease in uteroplacental perfusion results in late decelerations; cord compression results in a pattern of variable decelerations (see Figure 6-5, *Review of Fetal Variability*). Nursing interventions should include changing maternal position, discontinuing oxytocin (Pitocin) infusion, administering oxygen, and notifying the health care provider.

Additional Antepartum Tests

A. Nonstress test:
1. Description:
   a. Used to determine fetal well-being in high-risk pregnancy, especially useful in postmaturity (notes response of the fetus to his/her own movements).
   b. A healthy fetus usually responds to own movement by FHR acceleration of 15 beats lasting for at least 15 seconds after the movement twice in a 20-minute period.
   c. The fetus that responds with the 15/15 acceleration is considered "reactive" and healthy.
2. Nursing care:
   a. Apply fetal monitor, ultrasound, and tocodynamometer to maternal abdomen.
   b. Give mother handheld event marker and reinforce instruction for her to push the button whenever fetal movement is felt or recorded "FM" on the fetal heart rate strip.
   c. Monitor client for 20 to 30 minutes, observing for reactivity.
   d. Suspect fetus is sleeping if no fetal movement. Stimulate fetus, or have mother move fetus around and begin test again.

> **HESI Hint** • The danger of nipple stimulation lies in controlling the "dose" of oxytocin stimulated from the posterior pituitary. The chance of hyperstimulation or tetany (contractions over 90 seconds or contractions with less than 30 seconds in between) is increased.

B. Biophysical profile:
1. Description:
   a. Ultrasonography used to evaluate fetal health by assessing five variables:
      (1) Fetal breathing movements
      (2) Gross body movements
      (3) Fetal tone
      (4) Reactive fetal heart rate (nonstress test)
      (5) Qualitative amniotic fluid volume
   b. Each variable receives 2 points for a normal response or 0 points for an abnormal or absent response.
2. Nursing care:
   a. Prepare client for procedure.
   b. Reinforce information about the purpose for exam.
   c. Provide psychologic support, especially if testing will continue throughout the pregnancy.
   d. Reinforce information to the client that a low score may indicate fetal compromise, which would warrant more detailed investigation.

Fetal PH Blood Sampling

A. Description:
1. This technique is only performed in the intrapartum period when the fetal blood from the presenting part (breech or scalp) can be taken—that is, when membranes are ruptured and the cervix is dilated 2 to 3 cm.
2. Used to determine true acidosis when nonreassuring fetal heart rate is noted (e.g., late decelerations, severe variable decelerations unresponsive to treatment, decreased variability unrelated to nonasphyxial causes, tachycardia unrelated to maternal variables).
3. Because fetal blood gas values vary rapidly with transient circulatory changes, this is usually done only in tertiary centers with the capabilities of repetitive sampling and rapid results.
B. Nursing care:
1. Client in lithotomy position at end of labor bed and prepare with perineal cleansing and sterile draping.
2. PN may assist the health care provider with sterile supplies and provides ice in cup or emesis basin to carry pipette filled with blood to unit pH machine or to lab.

> **HESI Hint** • Percutaneous umbilical blood sampling can be done during pregnancy under ultrasound for prenatal diagnosis and therapy. Hemoglobinopathies, clotting disorders, sepsis, and some genetic testing can be done using this method.

> **HESI Hint** • The most important determinant of fetal maturity for extrauterine survival is the L/S ratio (2:1 or higher).

Review of Fetal/Maternal Assessment Techniques

1. Name five maternal variables associated with diagnosis of a high-risk pregnancy.
2. Is one ultrasound examination useful in determining the presence of intrauterine growth retardation (IUGR)?
3. What does the biophysical profile determine?
4. List three necessary nursing actions to be taken before an ultrasound exam for a woman in the first trimester of pregnancy.

5. State the advantage of CVS over amniocentesis.
6. Why are serum and amniotic AFP levels done prenatally?
7. What is the most important determinant of fetal maturity for extrauterine survival?
8. Name the three most common complications of amniocentesis.
9. Name the four periodic changes of the fetal heart rate, their causes, and one nursing treatment for each.
10. What is the most important indicator of fetal autonomic nervous system integrity/health?
11. Name four causes of decreased FHR variability.
12. State the most important action to take when a cord prolapse is determined.
13. What is a "reactive" nonstress test?
14. What are the dangers of the nipple-stimulation stress test?

Answers to Review

1. Age (younger than 17 years or older than 34 years of age), parity (over 5), less than 3 months between pregnancies, diagnosis of preeclampsia, diabetes mellitus, or cardiac disease.
2. No, serial measurements are needed to determine IUGR.
3. Fetal well-being.
4. Have client fill bladder. Do not allow client to void. Position supine with uterine wedge.
5. Can be done between 8 and 12 weeks' gestation with results returned within 1 week, which allows for decision about termination while still in first trimester.
6. To determine whether alpha-fetoprotein levels are elevated, which may indicate the presence of neural tube defects, or are low, which may indicate trisomy 21.
7. L/S ratio (lung maturity, lung surfactant development).
8. Spontaneous abortion, fetal injury, infection.
9. *Accelerations:* caused by burst of sympathetic activity; they are reassuring and require no treatment. *Early decelerations:* caused by head compression, are benign, and caution the nurse to monitor for labor progress and fetal descent. *Variable decelerations:* caused by cord compression; change of position should be tried first. *Late decelerations:* caused by uteroplacental insufficiency and should be treated by placing client on her side and administering O_2.
10. Fetal heart rate variability.
11. Hypoxia, acidosis, drugs, fetal sleep.
12. Examiner should position mother to relieve pressure on the cord or push the presenting part off the cord with fingers until emergency delivery is accomplished.
13. FHR acceleration of 15 beats per minute for 15 seconds in response to fetal movement.
14. The inability to control "oxytocin" dosage and the chance of tetany/hyperstimulation.

Intrapartum Nursing Care

Description: Begins with true labor and consists of four steps:

Stage I: from the beginning of regular contractions or rupture of membranes to 10 cm of dilation and effacement (Table 6-1, *First Stage of Labor*).

Stage II: 10 centimeters to delivery.

Stage III: delivery of the placenta.

Stage IV: first 1 to 4 hours following delivery (recovery).

HESI Hint • In some states or local areas, the PN's scope of practice may be limited in Labor and Delivery settings and may include only assisting the RN and/or the health care provider. Assessments, diagnostic techniques, and medication administration may not be within the scope of the PN in your area. The PN should check the State Board of Nursing website where he or she is practicing to clarify the scope of practice in the state.

HESI Hint • Be able to differentiate true labor from false labor.

TRUE LABOR
- Pain in lower back that radiates to abdomen
- Accompanied by regular, rhythmic contractions
- Contractions that intensify with ambulation
- Progressive cervical dilation and effacement

Continued

Continued

TABLE 6-1 **First Stage of Labor**

Phase	Description	Psychologic/Physical Responses
Latent	From beginning of true labor until 3 to 4 centimeters cervical dilation	• Mildly anxious, conversant • Able to continue usual activities • Contractions mild, initially 10 to 20 minutes apart, 15 to 20 seconds duration; later 5 to 7 minutes apart, 30 to 40 seconds duration
Active	From 4 to 7 centimeters cervical dilation	• Increased anxiety • Increased discomfort • Unwillingness to be left alone • Contractions moderate to severe, 2 to 3 minutes apart, 30 to 60 seconds duration
Transition	From 8 to 10 centimeters cervical dilation	• Changed behavior • May have sudden nausea, hiccups • Extreme irritability and unwillingness to be touched although desirous of companionship • Contractions severe, 1½ minutes apart, 60 to 90 seconds duration

FALSE LABOR
- Discomfort is localized in abdomen
- No lower back pain
- Contractions decrease in intensity and/or frequency with ambulation
- No cervical changes

Initial Examination

Nursing Assessment (Data Collection)

A. Prodromal labor signs include the following:
   1. Lightening (fetus drops into true pelvis)
   2. Braxton Hicks contractions (practice contractions)
   3. Cervical softening and slight effacement
   4. Bloody show or expulsion of mucus plug
   5. Burst of energy, "nesting instinct"
B. Determine the following:
   1. Gravidity and parity: parity greater than 5 (grand multiparity)
   2. Gestational age: 38 to 40 weeks (term gestation)
   3. FHR: best heard over fetal back (Box 6-1 and Figure 6-6, *Leopold's Maneuvers*).
   4. Maternal vital signs
   5. Contraction frequency, intensity, and duration
   6. Any vaginal bleeding
C. Assist with vaginal exam to determine (unless active vaginal bleeding):
   1. Fetal presentation and position
   2. Cervical dilation, effacement, position, and consistency
   3. Fetal station
D. Observe the client for:
   1. Status of membranes (ruptured or intact). If ruptured, time of spontaneous rupture of membrane (SROM) and color of fluid.
   2. Urine glucose and albumin data
   3. Comfort level
   4. Labor/delivery preparation

BOX 6-1 *Leopold's Maneuvers*

Description: Leopold maneuvers are abdominal palpations used to determine fetal presentation, lie, position, and engagement.
A: With client in supine position, place both cupped hands over fundus and palpate to determine whether breech (soft, immovable, large) or vertex (hard, moveable, small).
B: Place one hand firmly on side and palpate with other hand to determine presence of small parts or fetal back. (Fetal heart rate is heard best through fetal back.)
C: Facing client, grasp the area over the symphysis with the thumb and fingers and press to determine the degree of descent of the presenting part. (A ballot table or floating head can be rocked back and forth between the thumb and fingers.)
D: Facing the client's feet, outline the fetal presenting part with the palmar surface of both hands to determine the degree of descent and attitude of the fetus. (If cephalic prominence is located on the same side as small parts, assume the head is flexed.)

   5. Presence of support person
   6. Presence of true or false labor

Assist with Vaginal Exam

A. Preceded by antiseptic cleansing with client in modified lithotomy position.
   1. Obtain sterile gloves.
   2. Exams are not done routinely. Sharply curtailed after membranes rupture to prevent infection.
   3. Exams are done:
      a. Before analgesia/anesthesia
      b. To determine progress of labor
      c. To determine whether second stage pushing can begin
B. Purpose of vaginal exam is to determine:
   1. Degree of cervical dilation: cervix opens from 0 to 10 centimeters.

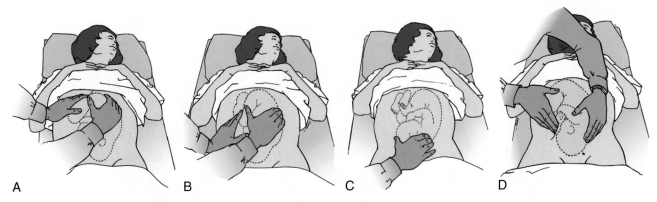

A   **B**   **C**   **D**

FIGURE 6-6 Performing Leopold's Maneuvers. (From Perry S, Hockenberry MJ, Lowdermilk DL, Wilson D: *Maternal child nursing care*, ed 4, St. Louis, 2010, Mosby.)

2. Cervical effacement: cervix is taken up into the upper uterine segment; expressed in percent from 0% to 100%; cervix is "shortened" from 3 cm to less than 0.5 cm in length; often called "thinning of the cervix" (misnomer).
3. Cervical position: cervix can be directly anterior and palpated easily or posterior and difficult to palpate.
4. Cervical consistency: firm to soft.

C. Fetal station: location of presenting part in relation to midpelvis or ischial spines. Expressed as centimeters above or below the spines (Figure 6-7, *Stations of Presenting Part*).
1. Station 0 is "engaged."
2. Station 2 is 2 cm above the ischial spines.

D. Fetal presentation: part of the fetus that presents to the inlet (Figure 6-8, *Types of Breech Presentations*).
1. Vertex (head, cephalic)
2. Shoulder (acromion)
3. Breech (buttocks)
4. Other variations include brow (sinciput), chin (mentum), face

E. Fetal position: the relationship of the point of reference (occiput sacrum, acromion) on the fetal presenting part (vertex, breech, shoulder) to the mother's pelvis. Most common is LOA (left occiput anterior). The point of reference on the vertex (occiput) is pointed up toward the symphysis and directed toward the left side of the maternal pelvis (Figure 6-9, *Fetal Positions*).

F. Fetal lie: the relationship of the long axis (spine) of the fetus to the long axis (spine) of the mother. It can be either longitudinal (up and down), transverse (perpendicular), or oblique (slated) (see Figure 6-8).

G. Fetal attitude:
1. Relationship of the fetal parts to one another
2. Flexion or extension
3. Flexion is desired so that the smallest diameters of the presenting part move through the pelvis

Analysis (Nursing Diagnoses)

A. Deficient knowledge (specify) related to …
B. Acute pain related to …
C. Anxiety related to …

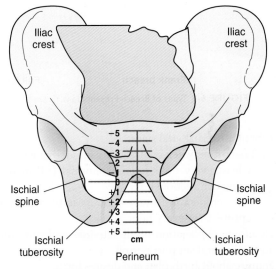

FIGURE 6-7 Stations of Presenting Part (Degree of Engagement). In this diagram, the presenting part has reached the +1 station. The lower pelvis, from the ischial spines to the pelvic floor, represents positive stations (+1, +2, +3), and the upper pelvis, from the inlet or pelvic brim to the ischial spines, represents negative stations (−3, −2, −1). (From Perry SE, Hockenberry MJ, Lowdermilk DL, Wilson D: *Maternal child nursing care*, ed 4, St. Louis, 2010, Mosby.)

HESI Hint • Know normal findings for clients in labor:
- Normal FHR in labor: 110 to 160 bpm
- Normal maternal BP: less than 140/90
- Normal maternal pulse: less than 100 bpm
- Normal maternal temperature: less than 100.4° F
- Slight elevation is often due to dehydration and the work of labor. Anything higher indicates infection and must be reported immediately.

Nursing Plans and Interventions

A. Observe fetal heart rate (auscultation schedule):
1. FHR every 30 minutes in early latent stage
2. FHR every 15 to 30 minutes in midactive stage
3. FHR every 15 minutes in transition stage

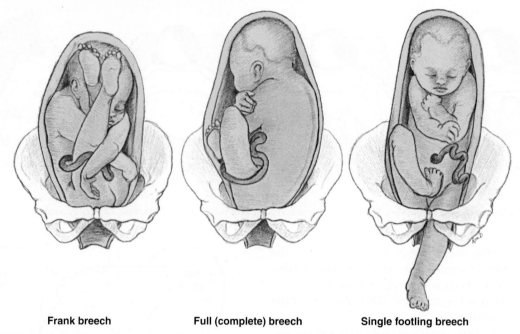

Frank breech **Full (complete) breech** **Single footling breech**

FIGURE 6-8 Types of Breech Presentations. (From Leifer G: *Introduction to maternity & pediatric nursing*, ed 6, St. Louis, 2011, Saunders.)

B. Obtain maternal vital signs:
   1. Take BP, between contractions, in side-lying position at least every hour unless abnormal (BP increases during contractions).
   2. Take temperature every 4 hours until membranes rupture, then every hour.
C. Reinforce explanation of all activities and procedures to mother and support person.
D. Inquire about birth plan and desires for:
   1. Analgesia and anesthesia
   2. Delivery situation

HESI Hint • ADMISSION PROCEDURES
- Vulvar/perineal shave (optional)

ENEMA
- Enema may be refused by woman because of prelabor diarrhea or recent, large bowel movement.
- An enema should not be administered to a client in active labor.
- If fetal head is floating, watch for cord prolapse.

E. Monitor urinary output.
F. Observe contractions when assessing fetal heart rate:
   1. Frequency: time contractions from beginning of one contraction to beginning of the next (measured in minutes apart).
   2. Duration: length of the entire contraction (from beginning to end).
   3. Strength: intensity of strongest part (peak) of contraction. Measured by clinical estimation of indentability of the fundus (use gentle pressure of fingertips to determine):
      a. Very indentable (mild)

   b. Moderately indentable (moderate)
   c. Unindentable (firm)
   4. Norms: contraction frequency, duration, and intensity vary with the stage of labor.
G. If membranes or bag of waters (BOW) ruptured:
   1. Nitrazine paper turns black or dark blue.
   2. Vaginal fluid "ferns" under microscope.
   3. Note color, amount of amniotic fluid.
   4. Allow woman to ambulate during labor only if the FHR is within a normal range and if the fetus is engaged (zero station). If fetus is not engaged, there is an increased risk for a prolapsed cord to occur.
H. Begin graph of labor progress (Friedman graph) (Figure 6-10, *Labor Graph*):
   1. Prolonged latent phase lasts more than 20 hours in primigravida, more than 14 hours in multipara.
   2. Primigravidas dilate an average of 1.2 cm/hr in the midactive phase, multiparas 1.5 cm/hr

---

HESI Hint • Meconium-stained fluid is yellow-green or gold-yellow and may indicate fetal stress.

I. Take client to bathroom or offer bedpan at least every 2 hours during labor unless client has an epidural. (Full bladder can impede labor progress.)
J. Assist woman with coping techniques such as breathing exercises and effleurage (abdominal massage).

HESI Hint • Breathing techniques such as deep chest, accelerated, and cued are not prescribed by the stage and phase of labor but by the discomfort level of the laboring woman. If coping is decreasing, switch to a new technique.

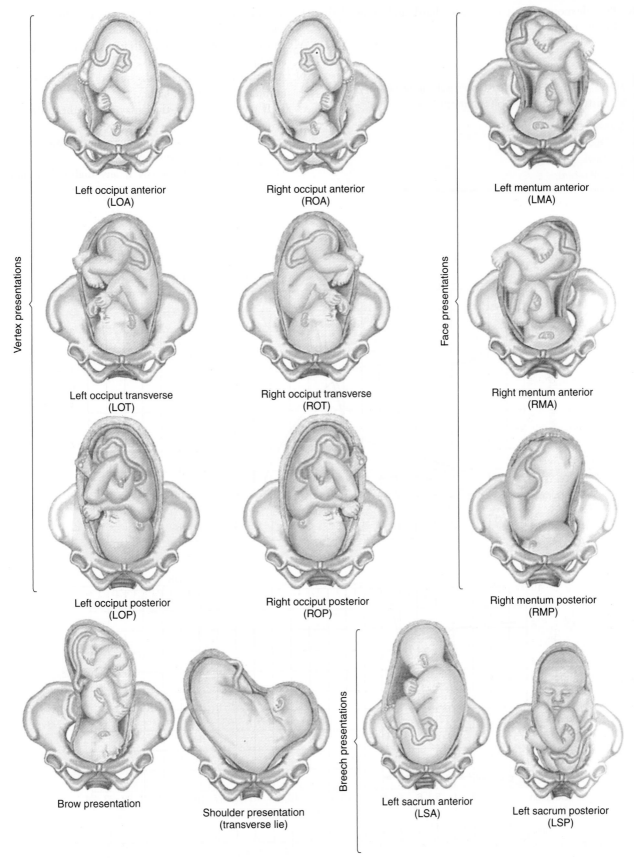

Vertex presentations

Left occiput anterior
(LOA)

Right occiput anterior
(ROA)

Left occiput transverse
(LOT)

Right occiput transverse
(ROT)

Left occiput posterior
(LOP)

Right occiput posterior
(ROP)

Face presentations

Left mentum anterior
(LMA)

Right mentum anterior
(RMA)

Right mentum posterior
(RMP)

Brow presentation

Shoulder presentation
(transverse lie)

Breech presentations

Left sacrum anterior
(LSA)

Left sacrum posterior
(LSP)

FIGURE 6-9 Fetal Positions. Various presentations. (From McKinney ES, James SR, Ashwill JW, Murray SS: *Maternal-child nursing,* ed 4, Philadelphia, 2013, Saunders.)

K. Provide mouth care, ice chips, and hard candy as needed for dry mouth.

HESI Hint • Hyperventilation results in respiratory alkalosis due to blowing off too much CO_2.

SYMPTOMS INCLUDE:
- Dizziness
- Tingling of fingers
- Stiff mouth

L. Maintain asepsis in labor by frequent perineal care and changing of linen and underpads.
M. Allow sips of clear fluid if *no* general anesthesia is anticipated.
N. Assist with anesthesia/analgesia, if desired by the client, in midactive phase of labor.
   1. If given too early, they may retard the progress of labor.
   2. If given too late, narcotics increase the risk of neonatal respiratory depression.
O. Monitor fetus continuously if any high-risk situation occurs.

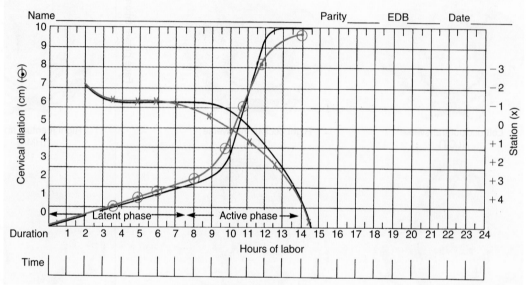

A

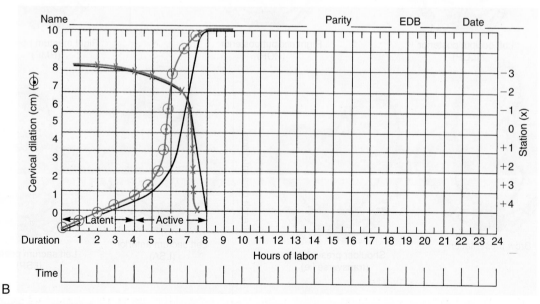

B

FIGURE 6-10 Labor Graph. Partogram for assessment of patterns of cervical dilation and descent. Individual woman's labor patterns (*colored*) are superimposed on prepared labor graph (*black*) for comparison. **A,** Nulliparous labor. **B,** Multiparous labor. The rate of cervical dilation is indicated by the symbol "O." A line drawn through the symbols depicts the slope of the curve. Station is indicated with an X. A line drawn through the Xs reveals the pattern of descent. (From Lowdermilk DL, Perry SE: *Maternity nursing,* ed 8, St. Louis, 2011, Mosby.)

P. Notify health care provider if any of the following occurs:
1. Labor progress is retarded.
2. Maternal vital signs are abnormal.
3. Fetal distress is noted.

Second Stage of Labor

Description: Involuntary need to push, 10 centimeters of cervical dilation, rapid fetal descent, and birth.

A. The second stage of labor averages 1 hour for the primigravida, 15 minutes for the multipara.
B. The addition of abdominal force to the uterine contraction force enhances the cardinal movements of the fetus: engagement, descent, flexion, internal rotation, extension, restitution, and external rotation (Figure 6-11, *Mechanisms of Normal Labor*).

Nursing Assessment (Data Collection)
A. Obtain BP and pulse every 5 to 15 minutes.

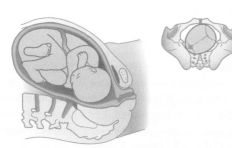

1. Head floating, before engagement

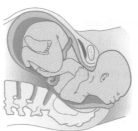
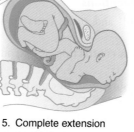

5. Complete extension

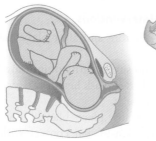

2. Engagement, flexion, descent

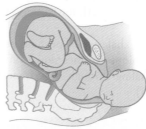
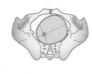

6. Restitution, external rotation

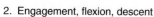
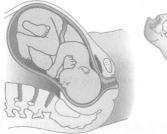

3. Further descent, internal rotation

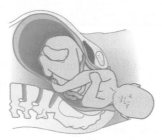

7. Delivery of anterior shoulder

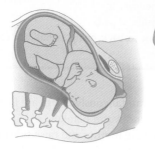

4. Complete rotation, beginning extension

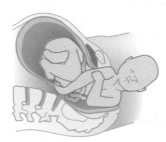

8. Delivery of posterior shoulder

FIGURE 6-11 Mechanisms of Normal Labor in a Left Occipitoanterior Vertex Position. 1, Head floating before engagement. 2, Engagement, flexion, and descent occur as the head moves toward the pelvic inlet; descent continues. 3, Descent and internal rotation to occiput anterior (OA) position. 4, Complete rotation and beginning extension as the head reaches the pelvic floor. 5, The head is born by complete extension. 6, Restitution and external rotation, returning to left OA (LOA) position and alignment with the shoulders. 7, Delivery of the anterior shoulder. 8, With delivery of the posterior shoulder, expulsion occurs as the body of the baby is rapidly born. (From Matteson P: *Women's health during the childbearing years: a community-based approach,* St. Louis, 2001, Mosby.)

B. Determine FHR with every contraction.
C. Observe perineal area for the following:
1. Increase in bloody show
2. Bulging perineum and anus
3. Visibility of the presenting part
D. Palpate bladder for distention.
E. Assess amniotic fluid for color and consistency.

Analysis (Nursing Diagnoses)

A. Pain related to …
B. Risk for injury related to …
C. Deficient knowledge (specify) related to …

Nursing Plans and Interventions

A. Document maternal BP and pulse every 15 minutes between contractions.
B. Monitor FHR with each contraction or by continuous fetal monitoring.
C. Continue comfort measures: mouth care, linen change, positioning.
D. Decrease outside distractions.
E. Support mother in positions such as squatting, side-lying, or high-Fowler/lithotomy for pushing.
F. Encourage mother to hold breath for *no longer* than 10 seconds during pushing.
G. Encourage mother to exhale when pushing or to use "gentle" pushing technique (pushes down on vagina, while constantly exhaling through open mouth, followed by deep breath).

> **HESI Hint** • In many settings, the PN may only assist the RN and the health care provider with the delivery of the neonate.

H. If delivering in another room/setting:
1. Transfer multipara at 8 to 9 centimeters, +2 station.
2. Transfer primigravida at 10 centimeters with presenting part visible between contractions *and* during contractions.
I. Set up delivery table, including bulb syringe, cord clamp, and sterile supplies.
J. Perform perineal cleansing.
K. Make sure client and support person can visualize birth if so desired. If sibling(s) present, make sure closely accompanied by support person, giving explanations that mother is okay.
L. Record *exact* delivery time (complete delivery of baby).

Third Stage of Labor

Description: From complete expulsion of the baby to complete expulsion of the placenta.
A. Average length of third stage of labor is 5 to 15 minutes.
B. The longer the third stage of labor, the greater the chance that uterine atony or hemorrhage might occur.

Nursing Assessment (Data Collection)

A. Signs of placental separation:
1. Lengthening of umbilical cord outside vagina
2. Gush of blood
3. Uterus changes from oval (discoid) shaped to globular
B. Mother describes "full" feeling in vagina.
C. Continued firm uterine contractions.

Analysis (Nursing Diagnoses)

A. Risk for imbalance related to …
B. Anxiety related to …

> **HESI Hint** • Oxytocin (Pitocin) may be given after the placenta is delivered because the drug causes the uterus to contract. If the oxytocic drug is administered before the placenta is delivered, it may result in a retained placenta, which predisposes the client to hemorrhage and infection (Table 6-2, Uterine Stimulants)

Nursing Plans and Interventions

A. Take maternal BP before and after placental separation.
B. Monitor patency and site integrity of infusing IV.
C. Observe for blood loss and ask health care provider for estimate of blood loss.
D. Dry and suction infant, place blanket on mother's abdomen, or allow skin-to-skin contact with mother after delivery. Initiate breastfeeding ASAP.
E. Place stockinette cap on newborn's head or cover head to prevent heat loss.
F. Allow father/support person to hold infant during repair of episiotomy.
G. Allow sibling(s), if present, to hold new family member.
H. Gently cleanse vulva and apply sterile perineal pad.

> **HESI Hint** • **APPLICATION OF PERINEAL PADS AFTER DELIVERY**
> • Place two on perineum.
> • DO NOT touch inside of pad.
> • DO apply from front to back, being careful not to drag pad across the anus.

I. Remove both legs simultaneously if legs are in stirrups.
J. Provide clean gown and warm blanket.
K. Lock bed before moving mother and raise side rails during transfer.

Fourth Stage of Labor

Description: The fourth stage of labor is the first 1 to 4 hours after delivery of placenta.

TABLE 6-2 Uterine Stimulants

Drug	Indications	Adverse Reactions	Nursing Implications
Oxytocin synthetic (Pitocin, Syntocinon)	Uterine atony	• Severe afterpains in multipara • Hypertension	• Give immediately after delivery of placenta to avoid "trapped" placenta • 10 to 20 units added to remaining IV fluid (at least 50 mL) • May stimulate let-down milk reflex and flow of milk when engorged
Methylergono-vine maleate (Methergine)	Uterine atony	• Hypertension	• Usual dose: 0.2 mg IM followed by tabs of 0.2 mg every 4 to 6 hours • Use with caution in clients with elevated BP or preeclampsia • Take BP before administration and if 140/90 or above, withhold and notify physician
Carboprost (prosta-glandin F$_2$) (Hemabate)	Uterine atony	• Headache • Nausea and vomiting • Fever • Bronchospasm, wheezing	• Contraindicated for clients with asthma • Dose: 0.25 IM every 15 to 90 minutes; up to 8 doses • May be given intramyometrially by provider • Check temperature every 1 to 2 hours • Auscultate breath sounds frequently

HESI Hint • Methergine is *not* given to clients with hypertension owing to its vasoconstrictive action. Pitocin is given with caution to those with hypertension.

HESI Hint • Never give Methergine or Hemabate to the client while she is in labor or before delivery of the placenta.

Nursing Assessment (Data Collection)

A. Review antepartum and labor and delivery records for possible complications:
  1. Postpartum hemorrhage
  2. Uterine hyperstimulation
  3. Uterine overdistention
  4. Dystocia
  5. Antepartum hemorrhage
  6. Magnesium sulfate therapy
  7. Bladder distention
B. Maternal/infant bonding

Analysis (Nursing Diagnoses)

A. Risk for deficient fluid volume related to …
B. Risk for injury related to …
C. Risk for impaired parenting related to …

Nursing Plans and Interventions

A. Maintain bed rest for at least 2 hours to prevent orthostatic hypotension.
B. Monitor BP, pulse, and respirations every 15 min × 1 hr, then every 30 min until stable (BP less than 140/90, pulse less than 100, and respiration less than 24).
C. Obtain temperature at beginning of fourth stage and before discharge to postpartum room. If more than 100.4° F, report to health care provider and monitor hourly per agency protocol.

D. Observe fundal firmness and height, bladder, lochia, and perineum every 15 min × 1 hr, then every 30 min × 2 hr.
  1. **Fundus:** firm, midline, at or below the umbilicus. Massage if soft or boggy. Suspect full bladder if above umbilicus and up to the right side of abdomen.
  2. **Lochia:** rubra (red), moderate, and clots less than 2 cm to 3 cm. Suspect undetected laceration if fundus firm and bright red blood continues to trickle. Always check perineal pad *and* under buttocks.
  3. **Perineum:** intact, clean, and slightly edematous. Suspect hematomas if very tender, discolored, or pain is disproportionate to vaginal delivery.

HESI Hint • Full bladder is one of the most common reasons for uterine atony and/or hemorrhage in the first 24 hours after delivery. If the nurse finds the fundus soft, boggy, and displaced above and to the right of the umbilicus, what action should be taken first? First, perform fundal massage; then have the client empty her bladder. Recheck fundus every 15 min × 4 (1 hr); every 30 min × 2 hr.

E. Report to RN and/or health care provider:
  1. Abnormal vital signs
  2. Uterus does not become firm with massage
  3. Second perineal pad soaked in 15 min
  4. Signs of hypovolemic shock: pale, clammy, tachycardia, lightheaded, hypotension

F. Change perineal pads and cleanse vulva/perineum at each change.
G. Prevent discomfort of afterpains:
1. Keep bladder empty. Catheterize only if absolutely necessary.
2. Place warm blanket on abdomen.
3. Administer analgesics as prescribed (usually codeine, acetaminophen, or ibuprofen).

HESI Hint • If narcotic analgesics are given, raise side rails and place call light within reach. Instruct client not to get out of bed or ambulate without assistance. Caution client about drowsiness as a side effect.

H. Offer oral fluids when client is alert and able to swallow.
I. Apply ice pack to perineum to minimize edema, especially if third- or fourth-degree episiotomy or if lacerations are present.
J. Support parental emotional needs and promote bonding:
1. Allow extended time with newborn.
2. Openly share in the joy and excitement of childbirth, as well as grieve with parents experiencing loss.
3. Encourage initiation of breastfeeding.
4. Provide a warm, darkened environment so newborn will open eyes.
5. Withhold eye prophylaxis for up to 2 hours.
6. Perform newborn admission/routine procedures in room with parents.

HESI Hint • A first-degree tear involves only the epidermis. A second-degree tear involves dermis, muscle, and fascia. A third-degree tear extends into the anal sphincter, and a fourth-degree tear extends up the rectal mucosa. Tears cause pain and swelling. Avoid rectal manipulations.

Newborn Care (Delivery Room)

Description: Care provided to newborn for transition and initial assessment, usually performed by the registered nurse.

Nursing Assessment (Data Collection)
A. Maternal history/labor data indicating potential problems with newborn
B. Apgar scores
C. Findings of brief physical examination performed in delivery room

Analysis (Nursing Diagnoses)
A. Ineffective airway clearance related to …
B. Risk for injury related to …
C. Ineffective thermoregulation related to …

Nursing Plans and Interventions
A. Immediately dry infant under warmer or facilitate skin-to-skin contact with mother, suction mouth and nose with bulb syringe, keep head slightly lower than body, and assess airway status.
1. Observe for five symptoms of respiratory distress:
a. Retractions
b. Tachypnea (rate greater than 60)
c. Dusky color/circumoral cyanosis
d. Expiratory grunt
e. Flaring nares
2. Do not hyperextend the newborn's neck at any time (may close glottis). Place infant in "sniff" position (neck slightly extended as if sniffing the air) to open airway.
B. Assist in obtaining Apgar score at 1 and 5 minutes (Table 6-3, *Apgar Scoring System*).
C. Observe for maternal/parent bonding.
D. Keep neonate's head covered.

TABLE 6-3 Apgar Scoring System

- Performed at exactly 1 and 5 minutes after birth.
- Cannot just eyeball, must have hands-on examination.
- Score:
  → 7 to 10, Good
  → 4 to 6, Needs moderate resuscitative efforts
  → 0 to 3, Severe need for resuscitation

Five Criteria	Scoring
Heart rate	Absent = 0; Under 100 = 1; 100 or higher = 2
Respiratory effort	No cry = 0; Weak cry = 1; Vigorous cry = 2
Muscle tone	Flaccid = 0; Some flexion = 1; Total flexion = 2
Reflex irritability	No response to foot tap = 0; Slight response to foot tap (grimace) = 1; Quick foot removal = 2
Color	Dusky, cyanotic = 0; Acrocyanotic = 1; Totally pink = 2

HESI Hint • Do *not* wait until a 1-minute Apgar is assigned to begin resuscitation of the compromised neonate.

HESI Hint • Apgar scores of 6 or less at 5 minutes require an additional Apgar assessment at 10 minutes.

From Leifer S. *Maternity nursing: an introductory text*, ed 11, St. Louis, 2012, Saunders.

E. Assist with quick gestational age assessment (Table 6-4, *Gestational Age Assessment*):
1. Sole creases
2. Breast tissue bud
3. Skin, vessels, and peeling
4. Genitalia
5. Resting posture
F. Observe cord for presence of three vessels (two arteries, one vein), and document.
G. Make sure cord blood is collected for analysis and sent to lab.
H. Document passage of meconium or urine after delivery in the newborn.
I. Place two identibands on neonate and one on mother. Place infant security device per institutional policy.
J. Obtain newborn footprints and maternal thumb/fingerprint. Follow institutional policy regarding identification procedures.

TABLE 6-4 Gestational Age Assessment

28 Weeks	• No nipple bud
	• Testes in the inguinal canal
	• Labia majora widely separated with labia minora prominent, open, and equal in size
	• Vernix (cheesy coating) over the entire body
	• Lanugo (fine, downy hair) over the entire body
	• Full extension of extremities in resting posture
40 Weeks	• Raised nipple with a tissue bud underneath
	• Decreased testes with large rugae (folds) on the scrotum
	• Labia majora large and covering the minora
	• Vernix only in the creases
	• Lanugo perhaps only over the shoulders
	• Hypertonic flexion of extremities in resting posture

K. Observe newborn:
1. Check for gross anomalies: spina bifida, hydrocephaly, and cleft lip/palate.
2. Elicit several reflexes: Moro (startle).
3. Examine cord clamp for closure, no oozing of blood from cord; again check for presence of three vessels.
L. May instill eye prophylaxis in delivery room (Table 6-5, *Newborn Prophylactic Eye Care*).

HESI Hint • If it was documented that the fetus passed meconium in utero or the nurse noted *late* passage of meconium in delivery room, the neonate *must* be attended by a pediatrician, neonatologist, and/or nurse practitioner to determine, through endotracheal tube observation and suction, the presence of meconium below the vocal cords. It can result in pneumonitis/meconium aspiration syndrome, which will necessitate a sepsis workup including a chest x-ray early in the transitional newborn period.

Labor with Analgesia/Anesthesia

A. Analgesia/anesthesia in labor is usually withheld until the midactive phase:
1. If given in the early latent phase of the first stage of labor, it may retard the progress of labor.
2. If given late in transition or in second stage, it may depress the newborn (some narcotic analgesics).
B. Most drugs used for systematic pain relief/relaxation cause central nervous system (CNS) depression, which can slow labor and harm fetus.
C. Regional blocks (epidural, caudal, and subarachnoid) cause a temporary interruption of nerve impulses (especially pain) but also cause vasodilation in area below block, causing pooling of blood and hypotension.

TABLE 6-5 Newborn Prophylactic Eye Care

Drugs	Indications	Adverse Reactions	Nursing Implications
Ointments Erythromycin Tetracycline	Prevention of ophthalmia, neonatorum, and *Chlamydia trachomatis* conjunctivitis	• Most commonly used agents • None known, except puffy eyes from manipulation	• Place a thin line of ointment along the entire lower lid in conjunctival sac • Use only one tube per baby and *discard* afterward • Manipulate upper lid to ensure complete eye coverage • After 1 minute, may wipe excess from around eye
Silver nitrate	Prevention of ophthalmia neonatorum from gonorrhea exposure through the birth canal in a vaginal delivery	• Chemical conjunctivitis (red, puffy eyes) • Staining of skin if contact occurs	• Eye prophylaxis is mandatory in the United States • May not kill other organisms such as *Chlamydia* • Instill 2 gtt in lower conjunctival sac, making sure drops spread over entire eye • *Do not* irrigate eyes following instillation

Nursing Assessment (Data Collection)

A. Acute pain experienced in active labor.
B. Birth plan; includes use of analgesic/anesthetic agents.
C. Decreased coping and increased anxiety.
D. Assist the RN in obtaining the following data:
   1. Vital signs and fetal heart rate
   2. Labor progress—that is, cervical dilation and effacement, fetal position, and lie
   3. Last time and amount of food/fluids ingested
   4. Lab values (Hgb, Hct, clotting time)
   5. Hydration status
   6. Signs/symptoms of infection

Analysis (Nursing Diagnoses)

A. Acute pain related to …
B. Ineffective coping related to …
C. Risk for injury related to …

Nursing Plans and Interventions

A. Assist with administration of analgesic drugs in labor:
   1. Document baseline maternal vital signs and fetal heart rate before administration of narcotics or sedatives (Table 6-6, *Analgesics*).
   2. Observe phase/stage of labor.
   3. Obtain health care provider's prescription for medication.
   4. Determine client/family desires regarding analgesics, and verbally praise informed choice.
   5. Do *not* give oral medications. Labor retards gastrointestinal activity and absorption.
   6. Reinforce the explanation of the purpose of the drug to the laboring woman, but do not promise results.
B. After drug administration:
   1. Record the woman's response and level of pain relief.
   2. Monitor maternal vital signs, FHR, and characteristics of uterine contractions every 15 minutes for 1 hour after administration.
   3. Monitor bladder for distention/retention (medication can decrease perception of bladder filling).
   4. Decrease environmental stimuli; darken room, reduce number of visitors, turn off TV.
   5. Note time between drug administration and birth of baby on delivery record.
C. General anesthesia is rarely used in today's obstetric units. It might be used in emergency deliveries or when regional block anesthesia is contraindicated or refused.
   1. Assist in administering drugs to reduce gastric secretions such as famotidine (Pepcid) or clear (nonparticulate) antacids to neutralize gastric acid.
   2. Assist with speedy delivery. (General anesthesia may depress fetus if delivery is not accomplished quickly.)
   3. Observe closely for uterine atony; check fundal firmness and uterine contraction. (General anesthesia is associated with postpartum uterine atony.)

TABLE 6-6 Analgesics

Drugs	Indications	Adverse Reactions	Nursing Implications
• Fentanyl (Sublimaze) • Morphine sulfate (MS Contin)	• Opioid agonists • Narcotic used to produce analgesia, euphoria, and sedation in labor • Analgesia during labor	• Respiratory depression • Fetal narcosis/distress • Hypotension • Fetus receives normeperidine, which is linked to fetal compromise • Itching • Urinary retention • Respiratory depression	• Store in narcotics cabinet • Record use accurately • Do *not* administer if respirations less than 12/min • Have narcotic antagonist available (Narcan) • Monitor respirations, pulse, BP closely • (see Table 6-21)
• Butorphanol tartrate (Stadol) • Nalbuphine (Nubain)	• Opioid agonist/antagonists • Provision of analgesia in labor • Narcotic analgesic	• Woman with preexisting narcotic dependency will experience withdrawal symptoms immediately (abstinence syndrome)	• Give IV or IM • Obtain drug history before administration • Monitor respirations, pulse
• Naloxone HCl (Narcan)	• Narcotic antagonist used to counteract narcotic effects on mother/fetus	• Decreased respirations rarely occur	• Monitor respirations closely because drug action is shorter than the narcotic (may need to readminister) • Pain returns after administration to mother • Can be administered to newborn after delivery (0.01 mg/kg body weight) to counteract narcotic depression

Regional Block Anesthesia

A. Local anesthesia:
1. Used for pain relief during episiotomy and perineal repair.
2. Safe for mother and infant.
B. Regional blocks:
1. Used for relief of perineal and uterine pain.
2. Usually safe for mother and infant unless severe hypotension occurs.
3. Types of regional blocks:
   a. Pudendal block: given in second stage to deaden pudendal nerve plexus, which deadens perineum and vagina.
      (1) Has no effect on pain of uterine contractions.
      (2) Safe for mother and baby.
   b. Peridural (epidural, caudal) block: given in first or second stage of labor and blocks nerve impulses from T10 to S5, thereby deadening pain of contractions.
      (1) Used in conjunction with local or pudendal for delivery or a delivery dose is given to deaden perineum for delivery.
      (2) May be given in single dose or continuously through catheter threaded into epidural space.
      (3) Moderately associated with hypotension, which can cause maternal and fetal distress.
      (4) Epidural block associated with prolonged second stage because of decreased effectiveness of pushing.
   c. Intradural (subarachnoid, spinal) block; given in second stage of labor to deaden uterine and perineal pain.
      (1) Rapid onset but highly associated with maternal hypotension, which can cause maternal and fetal distress.
      (2) Client must remain flat for 6 to 8 hours after delivery.
C. Contraindications to subarachnoid and peridural blocks include:
1. Client's refusal or fear.
2. Anticoagulant therapy or presence of bleeding disorder.
3. Presence of antepartum hemorrhage causing acute hypovolemia.
4. Infection or tumor at injection site.
5. Allergy to-caine drugs.
6. CNS disorders, previous back surgery, or spinal anatomic abnormality.

> **HESI Hint** • Pudendal block and subarachnoid (saddle block) are used only for second stage of labor.

Nursing Assessment (Data Collection)

A. No contraindications to regional block anesthesia.
B. Experiencing severe pain.

C. Possible need for cesarean delivery.
D. BP before block greater than 100/70.
E. Status of maternal-fetal unit.

Analysis (Nursing Diagnoses)

A. Risk for injury (fetus/client) related to …
B. Risk for urinary retention related to …

Nursing Plans and Interventions

A. Ensure that the health care provider has explained procedures, the risks, the benefits, and the alternatives.
B. Assist with prehydration of client to counteract possible hypotension; 500 to 1000 mL IV fluid (isotonic) infused over 20 to 30 minutes before initiation of regional block.
C. Place client in a modified Sims position or sitting on side of bed with head flexed.
D. Ask client to describe symptoms after test dose of medication is given:
1. Metallic taste in mouth/ringing in ears denotes possible injection of medication into bloodstream.
2. Nausea/vomiting is one of first signs of hypotension.

> **HESI Hint** • The first sign of a block's effectiveness is usually warmth and tingling in the ball of the foot or the big toe.

E. Monitor BP every 1 to 2 min for 15 min after injection of anesthetic drug and initiate continuous fetal monitoring.
F. Monitor BP every 15 min during continuous regional block infusion.
G. Assist client to keep bladder empty.
H. Observe level of pain relief with sharp/dull technique and record return of pain sensation. Change positions frequently to help ensure a complete block.
I. Report return of pain sensation, incomplete anesthesia, or uneven anesthesia to anesthesiologist.
J. If hypotension occurs, DO the following:
1. Immediately turn client to left side.
2. Begin O_2 at 10 L/min by face mask.
3. Notify RN and/or health care provider STAT.
4. Obtain FHR.
K. Assist client in pushing technique once complete dilation is achieved.

> **HESI Hint** • **REGIONAL BLOCK ANESTHESIA AND FETAL PRESENTATION**
> - Internal rotation is harder to achieve when the pelvic floor is relaxed by anesthesia, resulting in persistent occiput posterior position of fetus.
> - Monitor for fetal position. REMEMBER, mother cannot tell you she has back pain, which is the cardinal sign of persistent posterior fetal position.

Continued

• Regional blocks, especially epidural and caudal, often result in assisted (forceps or vacuum) delivery because of the inability to push effectively in second stage, even with adequate coaching.

HESI Hint • Nerve block anesthesia (spinal or epidural) during labor blocks motor as well as nerve fibers. Vasodilation below the level of the block results in blood pooling in the lower extremities and maternal hypotension.

Review of Intrapartum Nursing Care

1. List five prodromal signs of labor the nurse might teach the client.
2. How is true labor discriminated from false labor?
3. State two ways to determine whether the membranes have truly ruptured (ROM).
4. Are breathing techniques prescribed for use by the stage and phase of labor?
5. Describe maternal changes that characterize the transition phase of labor.
6. When should a laboring client be examined vaginally?
7. Define cervical effacement.
8. Where is the fetal heart rate best heard?
9. Normal fetal heart rate in labor is _____. Normal maternal BP in labor is _____. Normal maternal pulse in labor is _____. Normal maternal temperature in labor is _____.
10. List three signs of placental separation.
11. When should the postpartum dosage of Pitocin be administered? Why is it administered?
12. State five symptoms of respiratory distress in the newborn.
13. If signs of meconium were observed in the amniotic fluid during ROM, what action must the nurse take in the delivery room?
14. What score is considered a "good" Apgar score?
15. What is the purpose of eye prophylaxis for the newborn?
16. What is the danger associated with regional blocks?
17. What is the major cause of maternal death when general anesthesia is administered?
18. Why are oral medications avoided in labor?
19. Hypotension often occurs after the laboring client receives a regional block. What is one of the first signs the nurse might observe?
20. How is the fourth stage of labor defined?
21. What actions can the nurse take to assist in preventing postpartum hemorrhage?
22. To promote comfort, what nursing interventions are used for a third-degree episiotomy that extends into the anal sphincter?
23. What nursing interventions are used to enhance maternal-infant bonding during the fourth stage of labor?
24. List three nursing interventions to ease the discomfort of afterpains.
25. List symptoms of a full bladder, which might occur in the fourth stage of labor.
26. What action should the nurse take first when a soft, boggy uterus is palpated?
27. How often should the nurse check the fundus during the fourth stage of labor?

Answers to Review

1. Lightening, Braxton Hicks contractions, increased bloody show, loss of mucus plug, burst of energy, and nesting behaviors.
2. True labor: regular, rhythmic contractions that intensify with ambulation; pain in the abdomen sweeping around from the back; and cervical changes. False labor: irregular rhythm, abdominal pain (not in back) that decreases with ambulation.
3. Nitrazine testing: paper turns dark blue or black. Demonstration of fluid "ferning" under microscope.
4. No, clients should use these techniques according to their discomfort level and change techniques when one is no longer working for relaxation.
5. Irritability, unwillingness to be touched but does not want to be left alone, nausea and vomiting, and hiccupping.
6. Vaginal exams should be done before analgesia/anesthesia to rule out cord prolapse, determine labor progress if it is questioned, and determine when pushing can begin.
7. The taking up of the lower cervical segment into the upper segment; shortening of the cervix expressed in percent from 0% to 100% or complete effacement.
8. Through the fetal back in vertex, OA positions.
9. 110 to 160 bpm. <140/90. <100 bpm. <100.4° F.
10. Gush of blood, lengthening of cord, and globular shape of uterus.

11. Oxytocin is given immediately after placenta is delivered to prevent postpartum hemorrhage/atony.
12. Tachypnea, dusky color, flaring nares, retractions, and grunting.
13. Arrange equipment for possible endotracheal tube placement to maintain airway.
14. 7 to 10.
15. Prevent ophthalmia neonatorum, which results from exposure to gonorrhea in vagina.
16. Hypotension resulting from vasodilation below the block, which pools blood in periphery, thereby reducing venous return.
17. Aspiration of gastric contents.
18. Gastric activity slows or stops in labor, decreasing absorption from oral route; may cause vomiting.
19. Nausea.
20. The first 1 to 4 hours after delivery of placenta.
21. Massage the fundus (gently) and keep the bladder emptied.
22. Ice pack, witch hazel compresses, and no rectal manipulation.
23. Withhold eye prophylaxis for up to 2 hours. Perform newborn admission/routine procedures in room with parents. Encourage early initiation of breastfeeding. Darken room to encourage newborn to open eyes.
24. Keep bladder empty. Provide a warm blanket for abdomen. Administer analgesics prescribed by health care provider.
25. Fundus above umbilicus, dextroverted (to the right side of abdomen), increased bleeding (uterine atony).
26. Perform fundal massage.
27. Every 15 min × 4 (1 hr), every 30 min × 2 hr if normal.

Normal Postpartum Period (Puerperium)

Description: Period after pregnancy and delivery (usually 6 weeks) when the body returns to the nonpregnant state.
A. Care in this period is focused on wellness and family integrity.
B. The teaching plan must be initiated early to cover the physical self-care needs and emotional needs of the mother, infant, and family.

Normal Postpartum (Puerperium) Changes

A. Reproductive system:
 1. Uterus:
  a. Myometrial contractions occur for 12 to 24 hr post-delivery because of high oxytocin levels (prominent in multiparas, breastfeeding clients, and women who experienced overdistention of the uterus).
   (1) First day: at 1 to 2 cm above umbilicus.
   (2) 7 to 10 days: decreases to 12-week size, slides back under symphysis pubis.
  b. Placenta site contracts and heals without scarring.
 2. Cervix:
  a. Becomes parous with a transverse slit.
  b. Heals within 6 weeks.
 3. Vagina:
  a. Rugae (folds) reappear within 3 weeks.
  b. Walls thin and dry.
 4. Breasts:
  a. Nonlactating:
   (1) Nodules palpable.
   (2) Engorgement may occur 2 to 3 days postpartum.
  b. Lactating:
   (1) Milk sinuses (lumps) palpable.
   (2) Colostrum (yellowish fluid) expressed first, and then milk (bluish-white).
   (3) May feel warm, firm, tender for 48 hours.
B. Cardiovascular system:
 1. At delivery:
  a. Maternal vascular bed reduced by 15%.
  b. Pulse may decrease to 50 (normal puerperal bradycardia).
  c. These changes are hypothesized to result in client "shivering."
  d. BP and pulse should quickly return to prepregnant levels.
 2. First 72 hours:
  a. 24 to 48 hours postpartum, cardiac output remains elevated (returns to nonpregnant levels in 2 to 3 weeks).
  b. Plasma loss greater than red blood cell (RBC) loss; reverses hemodilution of pregnancy (Hct rises).
  c. Diaphoresis (especially at night) helps restore normal plasma volume.
C. Hematologic system:
 1. Hct rises.
 2. WBC count elevated (12,000 up to 25,000).
 3. Difficult to use white count for determination of infection.
 4. Blood-clotting factors elevated; increases risk of thromboembolism.
D. Urinary system:
 1. Diuresis occurs; excretes up to 3000 mL/day of urine.
 2. Bladder distention and incomplete emptying common.

3. Persistent dilation of ureter/renal pelvis increase risk of urinary tract infection (UTI).
4. Urine glucose, creatinine, and BUN levels normal after 7 days.

E. Gastrointestinal system:
1. Excess analgesia/anesthesia may decrease peristalsis.
2. No bowel movements expected for 2 to 3 days.

F. Integumentary system:
1. Chloasma and hyperpigmentation areas (linea nigra, areolae) regress; some areas may remain permanently darker.
2. Palmar erythema declines quickly.
3. Spider nevi fade, some in legs may remain.

G. Musculoskeletal system:
1. Pelvic muscles regain tone in 3 to 6 weeks.
2. Abdominal muscles regain tone in 6 weeks unless diastasis recti (separation of rectus abdominis muscles) occurs.

HESI Hint • Normal leukocytosis of pregnancy averages 12,000 to 15,000 mm³. The first 10 to 12 days postdelivery, values of 25,000 mm³ are common. Elevated WBC and the normal elevated erythrocyte sedimentation rate may confuse interpretation of acute postpartal infections. For example, if the nurse assesses a client's temperature to be 101° F on the client's second postpartum day, what assessments should be made before notifying the physician? Obtain fundal height and firmness, perineal integrity; check for pain, warmth, redness, or swelling in calves and other symptoms of thromboembolism: pulse, respirations, and blood pressure; client's subjective description of symptoms—burning on urination, pain in leg, excessive tenderness of uterus.

HESI Hint • Reinforcement of client/family teaching is a common area for NCLEX-PN questions. Remember, when teaching, the first step is to assess the client's (parents') level of knowledge and identify their readiness to learn. Client teaching regarding lochia changes, perineal care, breastfeeding, and sore nipples is commonly tested content.

Nursing Assessment (Data Collection)

A. Review prenatal, antepartum, L&D (labor and delivery), and early postpartum records for status, estimated blood loss, lab data, and possible complications.
B. Review newborn record for Apgar scores, sex, possible complications, and relevant psychosocial information (adoption, single parent, etc.).
C. Obtain postpartum status: vital signs (Table 6-7, *Normal Postpartal Vital Signs*), fundal height and firmness, lochia, urination, perineum, bowel sounds, presence of thrombophlebitis.

D. Observe maternal/infant bonding and identify teaching needs of mother/family.

Analysis (Nursing Diagnoses)

A. Pain related to …
B. Risk for infection related to …
C. Urinary retention related to …
D. Deficient knowledge (specify) related to …
E. Situational low self-esteem related to …

Nursing Plans and Interventions

A. Monitor vital signs every 4 hours × 24 hours, then every 8 hours.
B. Check fundal height and firmness:
1. On the first postpartum day (first day following birth), the top of the fundus is located approximately 1 cm below the umbilicus (Figure 6-12, *Involution of the Uterus*).

TABLE 6-7 Normal Postpartal Vital Signs

Vital Sign	Description
Temperature	May rise to 100.4° F because of dehydrating effects of labor: *any* higher elevation may be caused by infection and must be reported.
Pulse	May decrease to 50 (normal puerperal bradycardia); pulse >100 may indicate excessive blood loss or infection.
Blood pressure	Should be normal; suspect hypovolemia if it decreases, preeclampsia if it increases.
Respirations	Rarely change: if respiration increases significantly, suspect pulmonary embolism, uterine atony, and/or hemorrhage.

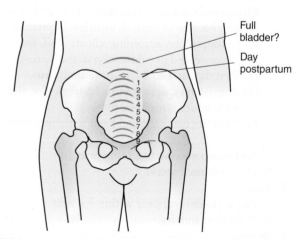

FIGURE 6-12 Involution of the Uterus. The height of the uterine fundus decreases approximately 1 cm per day until it is no longer palpable at 10 days postpartum. (From Perry S, Hockenberry MJ, Lowdermilk DL, Wilson D: *Maternal child nursing care*, ed 4, St. Louis, 2010, Mosby.)

2. Should be midline and firm immediately after delivery.
3. Massage if soft and/or boggy by stabilizing bottom of the uterus before applying pressure; teach mother procedure, but advise against overstimulation, which can lead to atony.
4. Have client void if not midline—full bladder may displace.
5. Reinforce teaching about normalcy of afterpains.

C. Observe and document lochia:
1. Lochia rubra: blood-tinged discharge, including shreds of tissue and decidua; lochia rubra lasts 2 to 3 days postpartum.
2. Lochia serosa: pale pinkish to brownish discharge lasting 1 week postpartum.
3. Lochia alba: thicker, whitish-yellowish discharge with leukocytes and degenerated cells; lochia alba lasts up to 4 weeks postpartum.

> **HESI Hint** • After the first postpartum day, the most common cause of uterine atony is retained placental fragments. The nurse must check for presence of fragments in lochial tissue.

4. Subinvolution: placental site does not heal, lochia persists with brisk periods of lochia rubra, and a D&C may be necessary.
5. Document amount:
   a. Scant: less than 1-inch stain on pad.
   b. Small: less than 4-inch stain on pad.
   c. Moderate: less than 6-inch stain on pad.
   d. Heavy: saturated pad within 1 hour.
   e. Clots should be less than 2 to 3 cm.
   f. Odor: fleshy, not foul.
6. Collaborate with RN to enhance and reinforce a teaching plan about normal lochia changes.
   a. Flow increases with ambulation and breastfeeding.
   b. Report if saturating 1 pad per hour.
   c. Expect color changes.

> **HESI Hint** • Women can tolerate blood loss, even slightly excessive blood loss, in the postpartal period because of the 40% increase in plasma volume during pregnancy. In the postpartum period, women may void up to 3000 mL/day to reduce this volume increase that occurred during pregnancy.

D. Observe perineum/episiotomy site:
1. Place in lateral Sims position, don gloves, and use flashlight to increase visualization.
2. Check for redness, edema, intactness, and presence of hematomas; show client technique of self-inspection with mirror.

3. Reinforce hygiene and comfort and healing measures:
   a. Change pad as needed and with every voiding/defecation.
   b. Use peri-bottle to cleanse perineum front to back.
   c. Use good handwashing technique.
   d. Use ice packs, sitz baths, peri-bottle lavage, and topical application of anesthetic spray or pads (Box 6-2, *Postpartum Teaching*).

E. Observe breasts:
1. Observe nipples for cracks, fissures, redness, and/or tenderness.
2. Observe breasts for engorgement.
3. Palpate breasts for lumps/nodules.
4. Determine motivation to breast- or bottle-feed.
5. If not breastfeeding, reinforce nonpharmacologic measures for milk suppression: wear supportive bra or binder, use ice packs, and avoid breast stimulation.
6. Reinforce teaching about breast self-exam (see Box 6-2).

> **HESI Hint** • Client should void within 4 hours of delivery. Monitor closely for urine retention. Suspect retention if voiding is frequent and less than 100 mL per voiding.

BOX 6-2   *Postpartum Teaching*

Breast Self-Exam
- Begin with inspection in a mirror. Place both hands at sides and observe; then look again with hands overhead, then hands on hips, and bending forward. Assess for:
  - Change in size and shape.
  - Dimpling, puckering, scaling, redness, swelling of any part of breast or deviations with a nipple pointing toward one side.
- Lie flat with right hand under head and pillow or towel under right shoulder.
  - Use left hand to palpate, using concentric circles around right breast all the way up to the underarm, feeling for lumps, nodules, or thickening.
  - Repeat with left breast.
- Squeeze nipples between thumb and forefinger to determine if there is any discharge (clear, bloody, milky, etc.). Remember to tell clients this is to be done after no longer breastfeeding.

Episiotomy Care
- Perineal care.
- Fill bottle with warm water, and if prescribed, an ounce of povidone/iodine solution.
- Lavage perineum with several squirts and blot dry instead of rubbing; avoid anal area.

> **HESI Hint** Women often have a syncopal spell (faint) on the first ambulation after delivery (usually related to vasomotor changes, orthostatic hypotension). The astute nurse will check client's Hgb and Hct for anemia and blood pressure, sitting and lying, for orthostatic hypotension.

F. Assist mother/infant with breastfeeding (Table 6-8, *Teaching Breastfeeding*).

G. Observe bladder and urine output:
   1. Palpate for spongy, full feeling over symphysis.
   2. Determine urge to void when bladder is palpated.
   3. Assist to ambulate for first void (possible orthostatic hypotension); measure if possible.
   4. Run warm water over perineum or place spirit of peppermint in bedpan to relax urethra if necessary.
   5. Catheterize *only* if necessary.
   6. Reinforce teaching about symptoms of UTI: dysuria, frequency, and urgency.
   7. Promote retoning of perineal muscles with Kegel exercises.

> **HESI Hint** Kegel exercises: increase integrity of introitus and improve urine retention. Teach client to alternate contraction and relaxation of the pubococcygeal muscles.

TABLE 6-8 Teaching Breastfeeding

Topics to Include	Data Related to Topics
Advantages of breastfeeding	• Low cost • Distinct immunologic advantages for newborn
Milk production	• Stimulated by the decrease in postpartum estrogen production, which allows release of prolactin from the pituitary • Prolactin responsible for milk production
Let-down reflex (milk ejection)	• Caused by action of oxytocin released from posterior pituitary, which stimulates myoepithelial cells around milk ducts/sinuses • Initiated by breast stimuli or even the mere presence or cry of the neonate
Breast size	• Has no relationship to successful breastfeeding
Inverted and retracted nipples	• Women with inverted or retracted nipples can wear shields, which may help the infant latch onto the nipple.
Diet during breastfeeding/lactation	• Avoid dieting. • Add 500 calories to prepregnant intake. • Drink 2 quarts (8 glasses) of noncaffeinated beverages daily.
Avoid	• Smoking and the intake of drugs, alcohol, and caffeine • Stress, most common reason for decreased milk supply
Encourage	• Rest
Care of breast and nipples	• Newborn should remain on first breast 10 minutes, switch to second breast and suckle until satisfied. (No longer recommended to limit breastfeeding time to 2 to 3 minutes first day, 5 minutes second, etc.). At the next feeding time, start with the last breast used for nursing. • Use warm water, not drying soap on nipples. • Let nipples air dry for 15 minutes two to three times daily. • Breast creams should not be routinely used; colostrum may be expressed and rubbed on nipples.
Engorgement	• Nurse more frequently and manually express milk to soften areola before feeding. • Wear supportive bra. • Take warm/hot showers (water over breasts promotes milk flow). • Watch for symptoms of mastitis (commonly occurs when breasts are not emptied). • If desired to wean, give up one feeding every week.
Incorrect positioning	• Incorrect positioning of baby on breast is most common reason for sore nipples. • Position so that baby is directly facing breast and be sure ear, shoulder, and hip are evenly aligned. • Make sure baby has as much of areola as possible in mouth. • Break suction with insertion of little finger into baby's mouth.

H. Observe bowel/anal area:
   1. Inspect for hemorrhoids; describe size and number.
   2. Administer antihemorrhoidal cream, ointment, or suppositories as prescribed.
   3. Auscultate bowel sounds; monitor for abdominal distention.
   4. Document flatus and/or bowel movement.
   5. Encourage early ambulation.
   6. Encourage increased fluids and use of roughage/bulk in diet.
   7. Administer stool softeners (Colace), enemas, or suppositories (Dulcolax) as prescribed (Table 6-9, *Postpartum Drugs*).
   8. Avoid rectal manipulation if third- or fourth-degree episiotomy was performed.
I. Prevent thrombophlebitis:
   1. Encourage early ambulation.
   2. Encourage foot paddling and ankle rolling after general anesthesia.

TABLE 6-9 Postpartum Drugs

Drugs	Indications	Adverse Reactions	Nursing Implications
Bisacodyl (Dulcolax suppository)	Constipation	Abdominal cramping	• Insert suppository into anus past internal rectal sphincter. • Because it is a contact laxative, stimulating rectal mucosa directly, there may be some burning. • Usually effective in 15 min to 1 hour. • Contraindicated with fourth-degree tear or episiotomy.
Docusate sodium (Colace)	Constipation Painful defecation because of fourth-degree tear	Abdominal cramping	• Encourage increased fluid intake. • Results usually occur within 1 to 3 days of continual use.
RhoGAM (Rh$_o$[D] immune globulin)	Prevention of Rh isoimmunization with next pregnancy	None known	• Given to Rh-negative women after miscarriage, abortion, or any procedure or complication that increases the risk of maternal-fetal blood exchange (amniocentesis, PUBs, abdominal trauma). • Routinely given at 28 weeks' gestation to Rh-negative mothers with a negative antibody titer. • Given postpartally to Rh-negative mother after delivery or abortion when fetus is Rh positive. • It is never given to an infant or the father. • Must be given within 72 hours of delivery. • Always given IM. • Is a blood product: → Must be checked by two nurses. → Return syringe to lab with label. → Not given to a mother with positive indirect Coombs or if baby has positive Coombs; she is already sensitized to fetal cells and has developed antibodies.
Rubella vaccine	Low rubella titer	Transient benign arthralgia Transient rash Hypersensitivity if allergic to duck eggs	• Given subcutaneously before hospital discharge to non-immune women. • May breastfeed. • Do not give if woman or other family members are immunocompromised. • Requires informed consent. • Reinforce teaching about contraception; women should avoid pregnancy for 3 months after immunization.

HESI Hint • Remember, if the Rh-negative mother delivers an Rh-positive infant, you do not give RhoGAM if the indirect Coombs on the mother is positive or the direct Coombs on the baby is positive. These results indicate the mother is already sensitized.

HESI Hint • Because Rh immune globulins suppress the immune system, the client who receives both RhoGAM and the rubella vaccine should be tested for rubella immunity at 3 months.

3. Monitor for pain, warmth, redness, or swelling in calves per institutional policy.
J. Administer RhoGAM (see Table 6-9) if prescribed by health care provider.
K. Administer rubella vaccine if prescribed by health care provider.
L. Observe maternal psychologic adaptation (Reva Rubin identified three distinct emotional stages after delivery):
   1. **Taking-in:** dependency behaviors for 24 to 48 hours; asking for help with simplest of tasks.
   2. **Taking-hold:** less focus on physical discomforts, beginning confidence with infant care taking. Not uncommon for mother to feel inadequate in caring for infant; the astute nurse will not "take over" but will praise efforts of parents. At this time new parents are usually most receptive to teaching about infant care.
   3. **Letting-go:** total separation of newborn from self; confident in care-taking activities for self and newborn.
M. Observe maternal/infant-bonding behaviors:
   1. Eye contact between mother/neonate.
   2. Exploration of infant from head to toe.
   3. Stroking, kissing, and fondling the neonate.
   4. Smiling, talking, singing to the neonate.
   5. Use of claiming expressions—for example, "He's got my feet."
   6. Absence of negative statements such as "She just doesn't like me."
   7. Naming the newborn quickly.
N. Promote maternal/infant-bonding:
   1. Ensure mother is comfortable: provide pain relief, hygiene, and adequate rest.
   2. If possible, have baby room-in; include family in teaching; praise and reinforce all positive parenting behaviors.
   3. Reinforce teaching about neonatal behavioral traits.
   4. Assure normalcy of comparing idealized child to looks/sex of real child but prevent long-term disappointment by encouraging verbalization of those feelings now.
   5. Reinforce teaching about responses to come from the baby:
      a. Pick baby up when crying (reciprocity).
      b. Soothe with calm, interactive responses until baby returns to quiet, active state (synchrony).
   6. Encourage verbalization of feelings; offer support in nonjudgmental manner.

> **HESI Hint** • "Postpartum blues" are usually normal, especially 5 to 7 days after delivery (unexplained tearfulness, feeling "down," and decreased appetite). Encourage use of support persons to help with housework for first 2 postpartum weeks. Refer to community resources. Instruct to inform health care provider if postpartum blues last 2 weeks or more or if severe with feelings of wanting to hurt self/baby.

O. Notify RN and/or health care provider or clinic promptly of:
   1. Heavy, vaginal bleeding with clots. Foul-smelling lochia.
   2. Temperature of 100.4° F or higher lasting 24 hours or longer.
   3. A red, warm lump in breast.
   4. Pain on urination.
   5. Tenderness in calf.
P. Collaborate with RN to enhance and reinforce a teaching plan about self-care for discharge:
   1. Continue perineal care and pad changes.
   2. Encourage balanced diet and fluid intake.
   3. Rest/nap when newborn does.
   4. Reinforce education about abstaining from sexual intercourse until lochia has ceased.
   5. Reinforce education to the client that the first sexual experience may not be pleasant because of vaginal dryness.
Q. Reinforce education about sibling rivalry, especially if a toddler is at home (age 18 months to 3 years):
   1. Alert parents that sibling may regress.
   2. Bring "present" to toddler from the newborn, and encourage mother to hug toddler.
   3. Plan time alone with sibling(s).
R. Assist RN with client education of contraceptive methods. Reinforce teaching about use, risks, and technique before discharge (Table 6-10, *Methods of Contraception*).

TABLE 6-10 Methods of Contraception

Method	Use, Risk, and Technique
Diaphragm	• Use with spermicide • Must be fitted by a nurse practitioner/physician • Must be left in place 6 hours after intercourse • Refit if excessive weight gain or loss (needs to be refitted after each pregnancy)
Cervical cap	• Use with spermicide • Contraindicated if cervical anomalies exist • Associated with cervical changes • Pap smear recommended 3 months after use

TABLE 6-10 Methods of Contraception—cont'd

Method	Use, Risk, and Technique
Condom (with spermicide)	• Use condom with spermicide to increase effectiveness • Recommended if any suspicion of STD • Withdraw penis while erect, or condom may fall off • Petroleum jelly can deteriorate rubber; use water-soluble jelly
symptothermal Pto-Thermal or fertility awareness	• Teach signs of ovulation: • Cervical mucus assessment • Basal body temperature assessment • Mittelschmerz (abdominal pain in the region of an ovary during ovulation)
IUD (intrauterine device)	• Contraindications: diabetes, anemia, abnormal pap, history of pelvic infections, smoking • High association with dysmenorrhea and infection
Oral contraceptives	• Estrogen in pills prevents pituitary secretion of FSH, preventing ovulation • Woman still menstruates • Lowest failure rate of methods • Contraindications: history of coagulation problems, thromboembolism, liver disease, reproductive cancer, coronary artery disease, smoking • Compliance is a problem because a pill has to be taken every day • What a woman should do if she misses taking a pill depends on the type of prescription. Consequently, reinforce the unique dose and missed pill regimen with each client
Transdermal contraceptive patch	• Mechanism of action, efficacy, contraindications, and side effects are similar to those of oral contraceptives • Delivers continuous levels of progesterone and estradiol • Can be applied to lower abdomen, upper outer arm, buttock, or upper torso (except the breasts) • Apply on the same day once a week for 3 weeks, followed by 1 week without patch
Norplant (Levonorgestrel implant)	• Sustained-release subdermal progestin-only contraceptive • Consists of six thin, flexible capsules made of soft Silastic tubing • Placed in a fanlike pattern just beneath the skin of the upper arm • Effective within 24 hours after insertion; effective for approximately 5 years • Efficacy is not dependent on client compliance once inserted • Reversible with return to previous level of fertility after removal • Side effects include menstrual pattern changes, headache, nervousness, weight gain, irregular bleeding or amenorrhea, headaches, depression • Works by suppression of ovulation as well as by thickening cervical mucus • Efficacy challenged—not available in United States; two-rod implant approved by FDA
Depo-Provera	• IM injection of 100 mg every 3 months for contraception • Administered during the first 5 days of menstrual cycle • New mothers may be given the injection during the postpartum period; before discharge • Efficacy of 99% • Protection from pregnancy is immediate after injection • Most women experience weight gain and irregular or unpredictable menstrual bleeding (after 1 year's use, many women stop having menstrual periods altogether) • Monitor for signs and symptoms of thrombophlebitis • Contraindications: history of breast cancer, stroke, blood clots, liver disease, smoking • Side effects include nervousness, dizziness, GI disturbances, headaches, and fatigue; may also increase risk of osteoporosis

Review of Normal Puerperium (Postpartum)

1. A nurse discovers a postpartum client with a boggy uterus, displaced above and to the right of the umbilicus. What nursing action is indicated?
2. Which women experience afterpains more than others?
3. Upon admission to the postpartum room, 3 hours after delivery, a client has a temperature of 99.5° F. What nursing actions are indicated?
4. A client feels faint on the way to the bathroom. What nursing assessments should be made?
5. What factor places the postpartum client at risk for thromboembolism?
6. A breastfeeding mother complains of very tender nipples. What nursing actions should be taken?
7. Three days postpartum, a lactating mother has full, warm, taut, tender breasts. What nursing actions should be taken?
8. What information should be given to a client regarding resumption of sexual intercourse after delivery?
9. A woman's white blood count returns to 17,000; she is afebrile and has no symptoms of infection. What nursing action is indicated?
10. What is the most common cause of uterine atony in the first 24 hours postpartum?
11. What is the purpose of giving docusate sodium (Colace) to the postpartum client?
12. What should the fundal height be at 3 days postpartum for a woman who has had a vaginal delivery?
13. List three signs of positive bonding between parents and newborn.

Answers to Review

1. Perform immediate fundal massage. Ambulate to the bathroom or use bedpan to empty bladder because cardinal signs of bladder distention are present.
2. Breastfeeding women, multiparas, and women who experienced overdistention of the uterus.
3. Probably elevated because of dehydration and work of labor; force fluids and retake temperature in an hour; notify health care provider if above 100.4° F.
4. Observe BP sitting and lying; assess Hgb and Hct for anemia.
5. Increased clotting factors.
6. Have her demonstrate infant position on breast (incorrect positioning often causes tenderness). Leave bra open to air-dry nipples for 15 minutes 3× daily. Express colostrums and rub on nipples.
7. She is engorged; have newborn suckle frequently; use measures to increase milk flow; warm water, breast massage, and supportive bra.
8. Avoid until postpartum exam. Use water-soluble jelly. Expect slight discomfort because of vaginal changes.
9. Continue routine observations; normal leukocytosis occurs during postpartum period because of placental site healing.
10. A full bladder.
11. To soften the stool in mothers with third- or fourth-degree episiotomies, hemorrhoids, or cesarean section delivery.
12. Three fingerbreadths/cm below the umbilicus.
13. Calling infant by name, exploration of newborn head-to-toe, in face position.

The Normal Newborn

During the immediate transitional period (first 6 to 8 hours of life) and early newborn period (first few days of life), the RN assesses, plans, and provides nursing interventions based on the outcomes of the individual newborn exam.

Nursing Assessment (Data Collection)

A. Review L&D report of neonatal history and newborn transition record:
   1. Cesarean delivery missing vaginal squeeze
   2. Prematurity or postmaturity
   3. Diabetic mother
   4. Prolonged rupture of membranes (ROM), more than 24 hours: sepsis workup
   5. Rh+ isoimmunization (+ direct Coombs)
   6. Traumatic/forceps vacuum suction delivery
B. Review L&D report of neonatal history and newborn transition record to determine risks caused by drugs/anesthesia in labor/delivery:
   1. Magnesium sulfate in labor: hypermagnesemia in neonate causes depressed respirations, hypocalcemia, and hypotonia.
   2. Narcosis (late administration of narcotic analgesics); causes decreased respirations and hypotonia.

C. Review L&D report of neonatal history and newborn transition record to determine risks caused by degree of birth asphyxia:
 1. Asphyxia in labor: documented late decelerations, decreased variability, severe variable decelerations.
 2. Apgar scores at 1 and 5 minutes.
D. Review significant labs: maternal Rh, Hep B, Group B strep.
E. Review significant social history: mother with STIs, single parent, language barrier, substance abuse, and lack of support system.

F. Obtain vital signs every 30 minutes × 2 hours, then every hour × 4 hours or until stabilized (Table 6-11, *Newborn Vital Sign Norms*).
G. Measure the neonate (Table 6-12, *Physical Measurements*).
H. Assist with initial physical examination of the newborn (Table 6-13, *Physical Exam of the Newborn*).
I. Assist with neuromuscular assessment. The absence of expected reflexes requires investigation into birth trauma/asphyxia or CNS anomaly (Table 6-14, *Neuromuscular Assessment*).

TABLE 6-11 Newborn Vital Sign Norms

Vital Sign	Normal	Nursing Implications
Respirations	Rate: 30 to 60 breaths per minute	• Remember the ABCs (airway, breathing, circulation) • Count 1 full minute by observing abdomen or auscultating breath sounds • Note five symptoms of respiratory distress: →Tachypnea →Cyanosis →Flaring nares →Expiratory grunt →Retractions
Heart rate	110 to 160 bpm; may fall as low as 100 during sleep, may rise as high as 180 during crying	• Auscultate for 1 full minute at the PMI (point of maximal impulse): third to fourth intercostal space
Temperature	Range 97.7 to 99.4° F, 36.5 to 37.5° C	• Measure axillary for 5 minutes • Rectal temps may perforate rectum; if taken rectally, insert only ¼ to ½ inch for 5 minutes and hold legs firmly to prevent trauma
Blood pressure	Average 80/50	• *Not* usually measured unless problems in circulation assessed

TABLE 6-12 Physical Measurements

Assessment	Normal	Nursing Implications
Weight	Average 7 lb, 8 oz (majority weigh between 2700 g and 4000 g; 6 to 9 lb)	• Weigh at birth and daily with neonate completely naked • Normally lose 5% to 15% (average, 10%) of birth weight in first week of life; document weight carefully
Length	Average range: 18 to 21 inches, 46 to 52.5 cm	• Measured from crown to rump and rump to heel, or from crown to heel at birth
Head circumference	Average range: 33 to 35 cm (normally, 2 cm larger than chest circumference)	• Place tape measure above eyebrows and stretch around fullest part of occiput, at posterior fontanel (FOC is designation for frontal-occipital circumference)
Chest circumference	Average range: 31 to 33 cm	• Stretch tape measure around scapulae and over nipple line

HESI Hint • PHYSICAL ASSESSMENT
The practical nurse should do a daily head-to-toe assessment. An initial detailed physical assessment is performed by the registered nurse or health care provider. Regardless of who performs the physical assessment, the nurse must know normal versus abnormal variations of the newborn. Observations must be recorded and the health care provider notified regarding abnormalities.

TABLE 6-13 Physical Exam of the Newborn

Normal	Abnormal	Rationale
General Appearance		
• Awake • Flexed extremities • Moves all extremities • Strong, lusty cry • Obvious presence of subcutaneous fat • No obvious anomalies	• Little subcutaneous fat	• Intrauterine growth problems • Fetal stress
	• Frog position	• Prematurity
	• Flaccid	• Asphyxia • Prematurity
	• Hard to arouse	• Sepsis • CNS problems • Asphyxia
	• High-pitched cry • Not moving arm on one side	• CNS damage/anomalies • Hypoglycemia • Drug withdrawal • Fractured clavicle or brachial plexus injury
Integument		
• Smooth, elastic turgor and subcutaneous fat, superficial peeling after 24 hours; rarely are veins visible • Milia, vernix in creases • Lanugo, mottling • Harlequin sign (pink/red skin on one side of body) • Erythema toxicum (pink papular rash is normal) • Mongolian spots (dark areas) • Telangiectatic nevi (stork bites)	• Extreme desquamation	• Postmaturity
	• Many visible veins	• Prematurity
	• Meconium staining	• Fetal distress
	• Cyanosis	• Heart disease • Asphyxia
	• Pathologic jaundice (within 24 hr) • Physiologic jaundice (at 24 degrees)	• Blood incompatibilities • Sepsis • Drug reactions
	• Vesicles	• Herpes, syphilis
	• Café-au-lait spots	• Neurofibromatosis
Head		
• Round or slightly molded • Caput succedaneum (edema over occiput) • Open, flat anterior and posterior fontanels, slightly separated sutures or overlapping because of molding	• Bulging fontanel	• Increased ICP
	• Sunken fontanel	• Dehydration
	• Widely separated sutures	• Hydrocephalus
	• Premature suture closure	• Genetic disorders
	• Cephalohematoma	• Blood under periosteum owing to trauma
Eyes		
• Symmetrically placed • Pseudo-strabismus • Chemical conjunctivitis (from eye prophylaxis) • Clear cornea • White-blue sclera • Subconjunctival hemorrhage from pressure • Absence of tears • Doll's eye movement (slight nystagmus)	• Purulent discharge	• Gonorrhea/chlamydia
	• Brushfield spots in iris	• Down syndrome
	• Absence of red reflex	• Congenital cataracts
	• Epicanthal folds	• Down syndrome
	• Setting sun sign	• CNS disorders
	• Absent glabellar reflex (blink)	• CNS or neuromuscular problem

TABLE 6-13 Physical Exam of the Newborn—cont'd

Normal	Abnormal	Rationale
Ears		
• Pinna at or above level of line drawn from outer canthus of eye • Well-formed and firm with instant recoil if folded against head	• Low set	• Down syndrome
	• Unformed, soft	• Prematurity
	• Preauricular sinus	• Possible renal anomaly
	• Short, upturned small philtrum (creases under nose)	• Fetal alcohol syndrome
	• Nasal flaring	• Respiratory distress
	• Grunting	• Respiratory distress • Choanal atresia (obstruction between nares and pharynx)
Nose		
• In midline • Appears flattened • Nose breather • Occasional sneezing	• Snuffles	• Syphilis
	• Excessive sneezing	• Drug withdrawal
Mouth and Chin		
• Symmetric movement • Intact lip/palate • Epstein pearls • Mobile tongue • Sucking pads in cheeks • Presence of rooting, sucking, swallowing, and gagging reflexes	• Asymmetry	• Facial nerve injury (Bell palsy)
	• Cleft lip	• Genetic disorder
	• White plaques on cheeks, tongue	• Monilial infection/thrush
	• Absence of protective reflexes	• Prematurity • CNS disorders
	• Excessive drooling	• Esophageal atresia
Neck		
• Short • ROM • Nonpalpable thyroid • Ability to lift head momentarily	• Limited range of motion	• Torticollis (wry neck)
	• Nuchal rigidity	• Meningitis
	• Enlarged thyroid	• Hyperthyroidism
	• Crepitus over clavicle	• Fractured clavicle
Chest		
• Symmetric excursion • Breath sounds clear and equal • Transient rales at birth • Round • Breast engorgement (hormonal) • Transient murmurs	• Persistent murmur	• Patent ductus arteriosus
	• Visible activity over precordium	• Congenital heart anomaly • Heart failure
	• Retractions	• Respiratory distress
	• Asymmetric chest	• Pneumothorax
Back, Hips, Buttocks, and Anus		
• Spine intact • Symmetric gluteal folds • Equal limb lengths • Patent anus	• Pilonidal dimple or sinus (at base of sacrum)	• CNS anomaly • Covert spina bifida
	• Hip click • Unequal limb lengths • Asymmetric gluteal folds	• Congenital hip dislocation
	• Absence of stools after 24 hours	• Imperforate anus • GI obstruction

Continued

TABLE 6-13 Physical Exam of the Newborn—cont'd

Normal	Abnormal	Rationale
Abdomen		
• Full, rounded, soft • Present bowel sounds • Palpable liver 1 to 2 cm below right costal margin • Two arteries, one vein in cord; white cord with Wharton jelly	• Scaphoid	• Diaphragmatic hernia
	• Distention	• Meconium ileus • GI obstruction • Hirschsprung disease
	• Hepatosplenomegaly	• Sepsis
	• Purulent discharge at base of cord, foul odor	• Omphalitis (cord infection)
	• One artery	• Renal/heart anomalies
	• Omphalocele	• Abdominal contents in umbilicus (anomaly)
	• Gastroschisis	• Abdominal contents outside of abdomen (anomaly)
Genitals		
Female		
• Slightly edematous labia covering clitoris and labia minora • Pseudomenstruation • Visible hymenal tag • Rugae on scrotum	• Labia minora and clitoris visible	• Prematurity
Male		
• Penis with foreskin intact • Meatus in middle at tip of penis • Descended testes • Slight edema of scrotum • Rugae on scrotum	• Undescended testes	• Prematurity
	• Meatus on dorsal surface penis	• Epispadias
	• Meatus on ventral surface penis	• Hypospadias
	• Fluid in testes	• Hydrocele
	• Intestine in inguinal canal	• Inguinal hernia
Extremities		
• Arms, hands, fingers, legs, feet, toes • Flexion • Symmetric movement • Palpable brachial and radial pulses • Strong grasp reflex • Multiple palmar and plantar creases • Slightly bowed legs • Femoral pulses present • Positive Babinski reflex	• Incurving little finger • Simian crease • Flapping tremors • Polydactyly • Syndactyly • Difference in pulses between upper and lower extremities • Absence of plantar creases • Rigid fixation of ankle • Absent Babinski reflex	• Down syndrome • Drug withdrawal • Extra digit (family trait) • Webbed digit (family trait) • Coarctation of aorta • Prematurity • Club feet (talipes) • CNS injury

HESI Hint • It is difficult to differentiate between caput succedaneum (edema under the scalp) and cephalohematoma (blood under the periosteum). The caput crosses suture lines and is usually present at birth, whereas the cephalohematoma does *not* cross suture lines and manifests a few hours after birth. The danger of cephalohematoma is increased hyperbilirubinemia because of excess RBC breakdown.

HESI Hint • The umbilical cord should always be checked at birth. It should contain three vessels: one vein that carries oxygenated blood to the fetus and two arteries that carry unoxygenated blood back to the placenta. This is the opposite of normal circulation in the adult. Cord abnormalities usually indicate cardiovascular or renal anomalies.

Postnatally, the fetal structures of foramen ovale, ductus arteriosus, and ductus venosus should close. If they do not, cardiac and pulmonary compromise will develop.

TABLE 6-14 **Neuromuscular Assessment**

Reflex	Normal Response	Lasts Until
Rooting	Turns toward stimuli when cheek or corner of lip is touched.	3 to 4 months (possibly 1 year)
Moro	When startled, baby symmetrically extends and abducts all extremities. Forefingers form a C.	3 to 4 months
Tonic neck	When neck is turned to side, baby assumes fencing posture.	3 to 4 months
Stepping	Infant is held in upright position with feet touching a hard surface, then makes walking motions.	3 to 4 months
Babinski	Stroke sole of foot from heel to ball and toes will hyperextend and fan apart from big toe.	1 year to 18 months
Palmar grasp	When examiner's finger is placed in the infant's palm, the newborn will curl his or her fingers around the examiner's finger.	Lessens by 3 to 4 months
Plantar	Finger in base of toes causes curling downward.	8 months

HESI Hint • These neurologic reflexes are transient and, as such, disappear usually within the first year of life. In the pediatric client, prolonged presence of these reflexes can indicate CNS defects. Anticipate NCLEX-PN questions regarding normal newborn reflexes. Physical assessment questions focus on normal characteristics of the newborn and the differentiation of conditions such as caput succedaneum and cephalohematoma.

TABLE 6-15 **Gestational Age Assessment**

By Date	By Weight
Preterm: 20 to 37 weeks' gestation	Small for gestational age (SGA): weight below the 10th percentile for estimated weeks of gestation
Term infant: 38 to 42 weeks' gestation	Average for gestational age (AGA): weight between the 10th and 90th percentiles for estimated weeks of gestation
Postterm: Over 42 weeks' gestation	Large for gestational age (LGA): weight above the 90th percentile for estimated weeks of gestation

J. Assist RN with a systematic gestational age assessment (Table 6-15, *Gestational Age Assessment*, and Figure 6-13, *Estimation of Gestational Age*). Plot measurements on percentile scale to determine if small, average, or large for gestational age.

K. Assist RN with a behavioral assessment using the Braselton Neonatal Behavioral Assessment Scale to evaluate newborn's behavioral uniqueness:
1. Waiting 2 to 3 days to perform test gives neonate a chance to rid body of effects of analgesia/anesthesia/trauma of birth.
2. Measures six categories: habituation, orientation, motor activity, self-quieting ability, social behaviors, sleep/awake states.
3. Performing test with parents present familiarizes them with their newborn's uniqueness and may provide them cues on the best ways to respond to the newborn.

Nursing Care of the Newborn

A. Aspirations:
1. Keep bulb syringe or suction immediately available: suction mouth and then nose.
2. Turn on side or stomach and pat firmly on the back, holding head 10 to 15 degrees lower than feet.

HESI Hint • Suction the mouth first and then the nose. Stimulating the nares can initiate inspiration that could cause aspiration of mucus in oral pharynx.

B. Infection:
1. HANDWASHING!! This is the most effective preventive measure.
2. Cord care performed per institutional policy.
3. Cover circumcision with petrolatum gauze; change gauze at each diaper change.
4. Do not allow visitors or personnel to attend to newborn if active infection, diarrhea, open wounds, infectious skin rash, and/or herpes virus are present.
5. Encourage breastfeeding for immunologic factors.
6. Keep diaper folded below level of cord.
7. Instruct parents to keep cord dry until it falls off (sponge bath only).

HESI Hint • Circumcision has become controversial because there is no real medical indication for the procedure, and it does cause trauma and pain to the newborn. It was once thought to decrease the incidence of penile and cervical cancer, but some researchers say this is unfounded.

MATURATIONAL ASSESSMENT OF GESTATIONAL AGE (New Ballard Score)

NAME _____   DATE/TIME OF BIRTH _____   SEX _____

HOSPITAL NO. _____   DATE/TIME OF EXAM _____   BIRTH WEIGHT _____

RACE _____   AGE WHEN EXAMINED _____   LENGTH _____

APGAR SCORE: 1 MINUTE _____ 5 MINUTES _____ 10 MINUTES _____   HEAD CIRC. _____

EXAMINER _____

NEUROMUSCULAR MATURITY

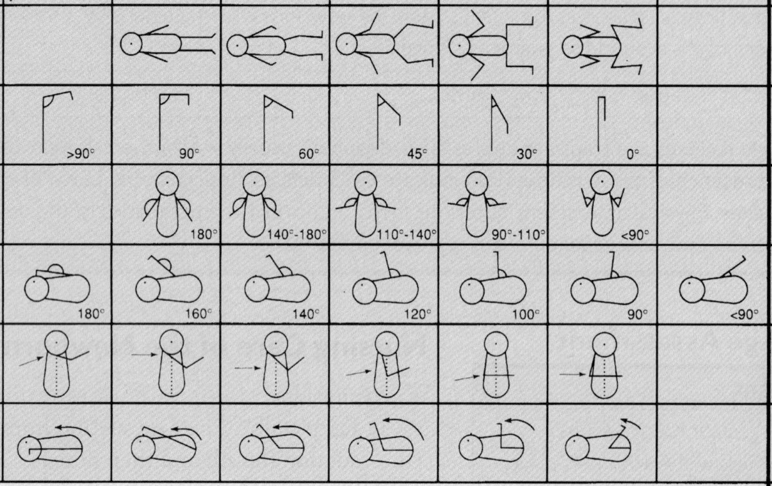

NEUROMUSCULAR MATURITY SIGN	SCORE							RECORD SCORE HERE
	-1	0	1	2	3	4	5	
POSTURE								
SQUARE WINDOW (Wrist)	>90°	90°	60°	45°	30°	0°		
ARM RECOIL		180°	140°-180°	110°-140°	90°-110°	<90°		
POPLITEAL ANGLE	180°	160°	140°	120°	100°	90°	<90°	
SCARF SIGN								
HEEL TO EAR								

TOTAL NEUROMUSCULAR MATURITY SCORE

PHYSICAL MATURITY

PHYSICAL MATURITY SIGN	SCORE							RECORD SCORE HERE
	-1	0	1	2	3	4	5	
SKIN	sticky friable transparent	gelatinous red translucent	smooth pink visible veins	superficial peeling &/or rash, few veins	cracking pale areas rare veins	parchment deep cracking no vessels	leathery cracked wrinkled	
LANUGO	none	sparse	abundant	thinning	bald areas	mostly bald		
PLANTAR SURFACE	heel-toe 40-50 mm:-1 <40 mm:-2	>50 mm no crease	faint red marks	anterior transverse crease only	creases ant. 2/3	creases over entire sole		
BREAST	imperceptible	barely perceptible	flat areola no bud	stippled areola 1-2 mm bud	raised areola 3-4 mm bud	full areola 5-10 mm bud		
EYE/EAR	lids fused loosely: -1 tightly: -2	lids open pinna flat stays folded	sl. curved pinna; soft; slow recoil	well-curved pinna; soft but ready recoil	formed & firm instant recoil	thick cartilage ear stiff		
GENITALS (Male)	scrotum flat, smooth	scrotum empty faint rugae	testes in upper canal rare rugae	testes descending few rugae	testes down good rugae	testes pendulous deep rugae		
GENITALS (Female)	clitoris prominent & labia flat	prominent clitoris & small labia minora	prominent clitoris & enlarging minora	majora & minora equally prominent	majora large minora small	majora cover clitoris & minora		

TOTAL PHYSICAL MATURITY SCORE

SCORE

Neuromuscular _____

Physical _____

Total _____

MATURITY RATING

score	weeks
-10	20
-5	22
0	24
5	26
10	28
15	30
20	32
25	34
30	36
35	38
40	40
45	42
50	44

GESTATIONAL AGE (weeks)

By dates _____

By ultrasound _____

By exam _____

Reference
Ballard JL, Khoury JC, Wedig K, et al: New Ballard Score, expanded to include extremely premature infants. *J Pediatr* 1991; 119:417-423. Reprinted by permission of Dr Ballard and Mosby · Year Book, Inc.

FIGURE 6-13 The new Ballard scale estimates gestational age based on the neonate's neuromuscular maturity **(A)** and physical maturity **(B).** A newborn will score 45 for a 42-week gestation or only 20 for a 32-week gestation **(C).** (Modified from Klaus MH, Fanaroff AA: *Care of the high-risk neonate,* ed 5, Philadelphia, 2001, Saunders.)

C. Hypothermia:
1. Keep dry and warm. Most important initial action in delivery room to prevent heat loss is to dry baby immediately.
2. Place stockinette cap on head (greatest heat loss is through scalp).
3. Take temperature at admission and every 4 to 6 hours; take every hour if temperature not stabilized.
4. If temperature falls below 97° F (36.4° C), place in radiant warmer and apply skin temperature probe to regulate isolette temperature if available. If not, double wrap or put skin to skin with mother. Monitor temperature closely for response. Report to RN and/or health care provider.

HESI Hint • Hypothermia (heat loss) leads to depletion of glucose and, therefore, the use of brown fat (special fat deposits fetus puts on in last trimester, which are important to thermoregulation) for energy, resulting in ketoacidosis and possible shock. Prevent by keeping neonate warm!

D. Hypoglycemia:
1. Perform a heel-stick blood glucose assessment on all small for gestational age or large for gestational age babies, infants of diabetic mothers, jittery babies, and babies with high-pitched cry (Box 6-3, *Heel-Stick for Newborns*).

BOX 6-3 *Heel-Stick for Newborns*

Procedure
• Wash hands and put on gloves.
• Clean heel with alcohol and dry with a gauze pad.
• Choose a site for puncture that avoids the plantar artery in the middle of the heel.
• Use only the lateral surfaces of the heel.
• Puncture deep enough to trigger a free flow of blood. Wipe away first drop with sterile gauze pad.
• Collect blood in appropriate tube, on card, or glucose "stick."

2. Report any blood glucose levels under 40 mg/dL in the full-term infant, under 30 mg/dL in the preterm infant. Normal serum glucose is 40 to 80 mg/dL.
3. Feed the baby early (5% dextrose water, breast milk, or formula) if a low glucose level is detected.
4. Prevent cold stress, which leads to hypoglycemia.
E. Hemorrhagic disorders: administer vitamin K to prevent hemorrhagic disorders (Table 6-16, *Vitamin K*).
F. Hyperbilirubinemia:
1. Bilirubin (byproduct of RBC destruction) binds to protein for excretion or metabolism.
2. Promote stooling by early feedings (protein binds bilirubin for excretion, and feedings increase peristalsis).
3. Observe daily for presence of jaundice:
   a. Yellowish skin color, sclera, and mucous membranes.
   b. Proceeds cephalocaudally (relationship between the head and the base of the spine).
4. Give adequate fluids.
5. Monitor bilirubin levels.
6. Assist with phototherapy if more than 12 mg/dL (varies by health care provider).

HESI Hint • Physiologic jaundice is caused by unconjugated bilirubin (inability of the immature liver to keep up with normal RBC destruction and bind bilirubin) and occurs on the second to third day of life. This is most common. Pathologic jaundice occurs before 24 hours or persists beyond 7 days and can lead to kernicterus (encephalopathy) and death. Typically, NCLEX-PN® questions ask about the normal problem of physiologic jaundice. Remember, unconjugated bilirubin is the culprit.

Nursing Plans and Interventions

A. The PN is responsible for monitoring the newborn whether infant is rooming-in or in the nursery.
B. Facilitate parent/infant attachment.
C. Document the elimination patterns daily:
1. Stool progression: meconium (black, tarry, sticky) stool within the first 24 hours to transitional (yellowish-green) to milk stool (yellow). Report if no stool within 24 hours.

TABLE 6-16 Vitamin K

Drugs	Indications	Adverse Reactions	Nursing Implications
Vitamin K (phytonadione) (Aquamephyton)	• Prevention of hemorrhagic disorder in newborn • Infants are born with sterile gut, and have no enteric bacteria present for synthesis of vitamin K	• Inflammation at the injection site	• Usual order is 0.5 to 1 mg of vitamin K given IM in the first hour after birth • Use the vastus lateralis muscle of the thigh (never the gluteus until walking for at least 1 year) • Hold knee secure during procedure, as neonate will try to move during injection

2. Monitor newborn for initial void. Report if no urination within 24 hours. To evaluate exact urine output, weigh dry diaper before and after voiding.

D. Screen for PKU (phenylketonuria) right before discharge and at first visit to health care provider. State laws differ regarding newborn screening. Some states also screen for hypothyroidism, sickle cell, and galactosemia.

E. Document nutritional intake and calculate nutritional needs:

> **HESI Hint** • Do not feed a newborn when the respiratory rate is over 60. Inform the RN and/or health care provider of respiratory status.

1. Demand feeding (bottle or breast) is preferred.
2. Most bottle-fed newborns eat every 3 to 4 hours; breastfed infants eat every 2 to 3 hours (breast milk is digested more quickly).
3. After initial weight loss period, infant should gain approximately 1 ounce (30 grams) per day.
4. Needs about 50 calories/lb or 108 calories/kg of body weight for the first 6 months.
5. Observe suck response and nutritional adequacy. The suck reflex should be strong, with coordinate suck/swallow. It should take less than 20 minutes to feed, and the newborn should gain 20 to 30 g per day.

> **HESI Hint** • A 7 lb, 8 oz baby would need 50 calories × 7 pounds = 350 calories plus 25 calories (½ pound or 8 ounces) = 375 calories per day. Most infant formulas contain 20 calories/ounce. Dividing 375 by 20 = 18.75 ounces of formula needed per day.

F. Monitor lab values for anemia, infection, and polycythemia (see Appendix A, *Normal Values*, p. 338):
1. Hct
2. Hgb
3. Platelets
4. WBC

G. Collaborate with RN to enhance and reinforce teaching for client/family about newborn care:
1. Bathing: *do not* submerge in water until cord falls off (7 to 10 days); continue cord care, and keep diaper off cord.
2. Diapering: use warm water to clean after voiding; soap and water with stools. (Remember, cleanse female perineum front to back; may use A&D cream for rashes.)
3. Crying: infant may cry 2 hours per day when hungry, wet, or bored. Pick up the baby; it is difficult to "spoil" the baby in the first year of life. Identify "fussy" periods and change environment when they occur.
4. Comfort: infant should enjoy "swaddling"; avoid startling infant when picking up; try to burp when "fussy" or crying (may be a gas bubble).

H. Recognize signs and symptoms of a sick newborn who needs medical attention:
1. Lethargy or difficulty waking
2. Temp above 100° F (32.2° C)
3. Vomiting (large emesis, *not* spitting up)
4. Green, liquid stools
5. Refusal of two feedings in a row or poor suck

> **HESI Hint** • Explain to parents how to take infant's temperature—*both* axillary and rectal. While axillary is recommended, some pediatricians will request a rectal temperature (core).
> **Axillary:** Place thermometer under arm, and hold thermometer in place for 5 minutes.
> **Rectally:** Use thermometer with *blunt* end. Insert thermometer ¼ to ½ inch, and hold in place for 5 minutes. Hold feet and legs firmly.

Review of the Normal Newborn

1. The newborn transitional period consists of the first _____ of life.
2. The nurse anticipates which newborn will be more at risk for problems in the transitional period. State three predisposing factors to respiratory depression in the newborn.
3. What is the danger of heat loss to the newborn in the first few hours of life?
4. Normal newborn temperature is _____. Normal newborn heart rate is _____. Normal newborn respiratory rate is _____. Normal newborn blood pressure is _____.
5. The nurse records a temperature below 97° F on admission of the newborn. What nursing actions should be taken?
6. True or False: The newborn's head is usually smaller than the chest.
7. During the physical exam of the newborn, the nurse notes the cry is shrill, high-pitched, and weak. What are the possible causes?
8. The nurse notes a swelling over the back part of the newborn's head. Is this a normal newborn variation?

9. Identify three ways to determine the presence of congenital hip dislocation in the newborn.
10. Should the normal newborn have a positive or negative Babinski reflex?
11. A small for gestational age newborn is identified as one who _____.
12. When the newborn is suctioned with a bulb syringe, which should be suctioned first—the mouth or the nose?
13. Normal blood glucose in the term neonate is _____.
14. Why does the newborn need vitamin K in the first hour after birth?
15. Physiologic jaundice in the newborn occurs _____. It is caused by _____.
16. When is the screening test for phenylketonuria done?
17. What factor should the nurse look for in evaluating the newborn's ability to suck and take in adequate nutrition?
18. A term newborn needs to take in _____ calories per pound per day. After the initial weight loss is sustained, the newborn should gain _____ per day.
19. List five signs and symptoms new parents should be taught to report immediately to a doctor or clinic.

Answers to Review

1. 6 to 8 hours.
2. Cesarean section delivery; magnesium sulfate given to mother in labor; asphyxia/fetal distress in labor.
3. Leads to depletion of glucose (very little glycogen storage in immature liver).
4. 97.7° F to 99.4° F; 110 to 160 bpm; pulse: 30 to 60; BP 80/50.
5. Place newborn in isolette or under radiant warmer and attach a temperature skin probe to regulate isolette or radiant warmer temperature. Wrap newborn double if no isolette or warmer available, and put cap on head. Watch for signs of hypothermia and hypoglycemia.
6. False: Head is usually 2 cm larger unless severe molding occurred.
7. CNS anomalies, brain damage, hypoglycemia, and drug withdrawal.
8. It depends on the exam. If it crosses suture lines and is a caput (edema), it is normal. If it does not cross suture lines, it is a cephalohematoma with bleeding between the skull and periosteum. This could cause hyperbilirubinemia. This is an abnormal variation.
9. Hip click determination, asymmetric gluteal folds, and unequal limb lengths.
10. Positive. The transient reflex is present until 12 to 18 months of age.
11. Has a weight below the tenth percentile for estimated weeks of gestation.
12. Mouth; stimulating the nares can initiate inspiration that could cause aspiration of mucus in oral pharynx.
13. 40 to 80 mg/dL.
14. Sterile gut at delivery lacks intestinal bacteria necessary for the synthesis of vitamin K; vitamin K is needed in the clotting cascade to prevent hemorrhagic disorders.
15. Jaundice occurs at 2 to 3 days of life and is caused by immature liver's inability to keep up with bilirubin production of normal RBC destruction.
16. At 2 to 3 days of life or after enough milk ingestion to determine body's ability to metabolize amino acid phenylalanine.
17. Good suck, coordinated suck-swallow takes less than 20 minutes to feed, and gains 20 to 30 g/day.
18. 50; 1 ounce or 30 grams.
19. Lethargy, temperature greater than 100° F, vomiting, green stools, and refusal of two feeds in a row or poor suck.

Complications of Pregnancy

A. The PN should anticipate and recognize complications of pregnancy, labor, delivery, and the puerperal period of involution.
B. The PN should assist the RN and/or health care provider with interventions as defined by local and state practice.

Antepartum Hemorrhage: Spontaneous Abortion

A. Bleeding from conception to 20 weeks' gestation.
B. Seventy-five percent of spontaneous abortions occur between 8 and 13 weeks and are usually related to chromosomal defects.
C. Considered a medical emergency.

Nursing Assessment (Data Collection)

A. Gestational age 20 weeks or less, fetal viability absent
B. Uterine cramping, backache, and pelvic pressure
C. Vaginal, bright red bleeding
  1. Note number of perineal pads/hour.
  2. Note symptoms of shock:
    a. Rapid, thready pulse
    b. Pallor
    c. Hypotension
    d. Cool, clammy skin
  3. Assess client/family emotional status, needs, and support system.

Analysis (Nursing Diagnoses)

A. Fluid volume deficit related to …
B. Anxiety related to …

Nursing Plans and Interventions

A. Monitor vital signs, level of consciousness every hour until stable.
B. Save all peripads, linens.
C. Observe IV site.
D. Assist in preparation for RhoGAM if indicated (Rh-negative mother).
E. Reinforce instruction to client to notify nurse if the following occurs:
  1. Temperature above 100.4° F
  2. Foul-smelling vaginal discharge
  3. Bright-red bleeding with any tissue larger than a dime
F. Implement grief protocol if fetus loss occurs:
  1. Provide a memory packet (footprints, bracelet).
  2. Give client/family opportunity to see fetus.
  3. Allow client/family to express their grief and loss and coordinate community resources for grief/loss.

Type and Treatment of Spontaneous Abortion

A. Threatened:
  1. Description: spotting without cervical changes.
  2. Treatment: bed rest for 24 to 48 hours; no sexual intercourse for 2 weeks.
B. Inevitable or incomplete:
  1. Description: moderate/heavy bleeding with tissue/products of conception present; open cervical os.
  2. Treatment: hospitalization; dilatation and curettage (D&C).
C. Complete:
  1. Description: all products of conception passed; cervix closed.
  2. Treatment: no need for treatment.
D. Septic:
  1. Description: fever, abdominal pain and tenderness; foul-smelling vaginal discharge/bleeding from scant to heavy.
  2. Treatment: termination of pregnancy; antibiotic therapy; monitor for septic shock.

E. Missed:
  1. Description: fetus has died/placenta atrophied, but passage of products of conception has not occurred; cervix closed.
  2. Treatment: watchful waiting; check clotting factors and possibly terminate pregnancy if disseminated intravascular coagulation (DIC) prevention considered necessary.
F. Recurrent/habitual:
  1. Description: loss of three or more previable pregnancies.
  2. Treatment: varies based on etiology; if premature cervical dilation (incompetent cervix) is cause, prophylactic cerclage may be done.

> **HESI Hint** • Clients with prior traumatic delivery, history of D&C, multiple abortions (spontaneous or induced), or daughters of DES mothers may experience miscarriage or preterm labor related to an incompetent cervix. The cervix may be surgically repaired prior to pregnancy or during gestation. A cerclage (McDonald suture) is placed around the cervix to constrict the internal os. The cerclage may be removed before labor if labor is planned or left in place if cesarean birth is planned.

Gestational Trophoblastic Disease (Hydatidiform Mole)

A. Chorionic villi degenerate into a bunch of clear vesicle, grapelike clusters.
B. Hydatidiform mole is a developmental anomaly.
C. An embryo is rarely present.
D. Predisposes the client to choriocarcinoma.

Nursing Assessment (Data Collection)

A. Vaginal bleeding usually in first trimester.
B. Size/date discrepancy (uterus larger than expected for gestational age).
C. Other common findings include:
  1. Anemia
  2. Excessive nausea and vomiting
  3. Abdominal cramping
  4. Early symptoms of preeclampsia

Analysis (Nursing Diagnoses)

A. Grieving related to …
B. Deficient knowledge (specify) related to …
C. Anxiety related to …

Nursing Plans and Interventions

A. Provide preoperative and postoperative D&C care.
B. Monitor:
  1. Vital signs
  2. Vaginal discharge
  3. Uterine cramping

C. Reinforce discharge instructions:
  1. Prevent pregnancy for 1 year.
  2. Obtain monthly serum human chorionic gonadotropin (HCG) levels for 1 year.
D. Review signs of complications with the client that need to be reported immediately to health care provider/clinic:
  1. Bright-red, frank vaginal bleeding
  2. Temperature spike over 100.4° F
  3. Foul-smelling vaginal discharge
E. Assist with referrals to community resource for grief/loss.

Ectopic Pregnancy

A. Fertilized ovum is implanted outside the uterine cavity, usually in the fallopian tube.
B. Occurs in 1 out of 200 pregnancies.
C. Often occurs as result of tubular obstruction or blockage that prevents normal transit of the fertilized ovum.
D. Considered a medical emergency.

Nursing Assessment (Data Collection)

A. Early symptoms of pregnancy may be absent.
B. Missed period; full feeling in lower abdomen, lower quadrant tenderness.
C. Positive pregnancy test.
D. Signs of acute rupture include:
  1. Vaginal bleeding
  2. Adnexal or abdominal mass
  3. Sharp, unilateral or bilateral pelvic pain; abdominal pain
  4. Referred shoulder pain
  5. Syncope; shock

Analysis (Nursing Diagnoses)

A. Acute pain related to …
B. Grieving related to …
C. Risk for deficient fluid volume related to …

Nursing Plans and Interventions

A. Assist with admission care:
  1. Assess vital signs STAT.
  2. Check for vaginal bleeding.
  3. Monitor IV fluids.
  4. Notify RN or health care provider immediately.
B. Reinforce explanation of procedures as interventions continue; allow family member to be present if possible.
C. Prepare client for abdominal ultrasound.
D. Prepare client for possible laparotomy.
E. Verify availability of two units packed red blood cells.

> **HESI Hint** • Suspect ectopic pregnancy in any woman of childbearing age who presents at an emergency room, clinic, or office with unilateral or bilateral abdominal pain. Most are misdiagnosed as appendicitis.

Abruptio Placentae and Placenta Previa

> **HESI Hint** • A client who is 32 weeks' gestation calls the health care provider because she is experiencing dark-red vaginal bleeding. She is admitted to the emergency room, where the nurse determines the FHR to be 100 bpm. The client's abdomen is rigid and boardlike, and she is complaining of severe pain. What action should the nurse take first? First the nurse must use his or her knowledge base to differentiate between abruptio placentae (this client) and placenta previa (painless bright-red bleeding occurring in the third trimester). The nurse should immediately notify the health care provider, and no abdominal or vaginal manipulation or exams should be done. Administer O_2 per face mask. Monitor for bleeding at IV sites and gums because of the increased risk for DIC. Emergency cesarean section is required because uteroplacental perfusion to the fetus is being compromised by early separation of the placenta from the uterus.

Comparison of Abruptio Placentae and Placenta Previa

Description: Abruptio placentae: partial or complete premature detachment of the placenta from its site of implantation in the uterus.
A. Occurs in 1 out of 200 pregnancies.
B. Usually occurs in late third trimester or in labor.
C. Is the cause of 15% of maternal deaths.
D. One third of infants born to mothers with abruptio placentae die.
E. A medical emergency.
F. Cause unknown but is related to:
  1. Hypertensive disorders
  2. High gravidity
  3. Abdominal trauma (uncommon)
  4. Short umbilical cord
  5. Cocaine abuse

Description: Placenta previa: abnormal implantation of placenta in lower uterine segment.
A. Occurs in 1 out of 250 pregnancies.
B. Bleeding usually begins in the third trimester.
C. Degrees of previa described as:
  1. Partial: placenta lies over part of cervical os.
  2. Complete: placenta lies over entire cervical os.
  3. Marginal: edge of placenta meets the rim of the cervical os.
  4. Low-lying: placenta implants in lower uterine segment with a placental edge lying near the cervical os.
D. Associated with previous uterine scars, surgery, or fibroid tumors.
E. Considered a medical emergency.

Nursing Assessment (Data Collection)

Abruptio Placentae

A. Bleeding can be concealed or overt (if overt, is dark red)
B. Uterine tenderness
C. Persistent abdominal pain
D. Rigid, boardlike abdomen
E. Fetal heart rate abnormalities

Placenta Previa

A. Painless, bright-red vaginal bleeding in third trimester
B. Soft uterus
C. Possible signs of shock
D. Placenta in lower uterine segment (indicated by ultrasound)
E. Fetal heart rate is usually normal

Nursing Plans and Interventions

Abruptio Placentae

A. Institute bed rest with *no* vaginal or rectal manipulation, and notify health care provider immediately.
B. Monitor BP and pulse every 15 minutes; apply electric BP monitor if available.
C. Apply external uterine and fetal monitor.
D. Place client in side-lying position to increase uterine perfusion.
E. Closely monitor contractions and FHR.
F. Monitor IV infusion.
G. Review results for CBC, clotting studies, Rh factor, and type/crossmatch STAT.
H. Watch for signs of developing DIC:
   1. Bleeding gums/nose
   2. Reduced lab values for platelets, fibrinogen, and prothrombin
   3. Bleeding from injection sites, IV sites
   4. Ecchymosis
I. Prepare for immediate emergency cesarean section.
J. Monitor blood loss; save pads, linens.
K. Provide constant nurse surveillance and allow presence of family if available.
L. Provide emotional support, and reinforce teaching regarding usual management and expected outcomes of abruption.

Placenta Previa

A. Manage with bed rest to extend the period of gestation until fetal lung maturity is achieved (determined by an L/S ratio of at least 2:1), and then delivery is accomplished.
B. If determined during labor, institute bed rest immediately and notify physician.
C. Monitor BP and pulse every 15 minutes.
D. Monitor IV.
E. Obtain blood specimen for CBC, clotting studies, Rh factor, and type/crossmatch.
F. Monitor contractions and fetal heart rate; place external monitor on client immediately.
G. Position side-lying.
H. Continue monitoring blood loss; save pads/linen.
I. Prepare client for ultrasound diagnosis.
J. Prepare client/family for possible cesarean birth if placenta previa is complete.
K. Provide emotional support and reinforce appropriate teaching regarding usual management and outcomes of placenta previa.

> **HESI Hint** • Disseminated intravascular coagulation (DIC) is a syndrome of abnormal clotting that is systematic and pathologic. Large amounts of clotting factors, especially fibrinogen, are depleted, causing widespread external and/or internal bleeding. DIC is related to fetal demise, infection/sepsis, pregnancy-induced hypertension (preeclampsia), and abruptio placentae. (DIC is discussed in more detail in Chapter 3, *Advanced Clinical Concepts*, p. 30.)

> **HESI Hint** • Clients with abruptio placentae or placenta previa (actual or suspected) should have *no* abdominal or vaginal manipulation.
> • *No* Leopold's maneuvers.
> • *No* vaginal exam.
> • *No* rectal exams, enemas, or suppositories.
> • *No* internal monitoring.

Anemia

Description: Anemia is a decrease in the oxygen-carrying capacity of blood; often related to iron deficiency and reduced dietary intake.

A. Occurs in 20% of pregnant women.
B. Associated with increased incidence of abortion, preterm labor, preeclampsia, infection, postpartum hemorrhage, and intrauterine growth retardation.

Nursing Assessment (Data Collection)

A. Fatigue, pallor
B. Hgb and Hct signs of anemia:
   1. Hgb <11 g/dL, Hct <37% in FIRST trimester
   2. Hgb <10.5 g/dL, Hct <35% in SECOND trimester
   3. Hgb <10 g/dL, Hct <32% in THIRD trimester
C. See Chapter 5, *Pediatric Nursing*, p. 203, for description of sickle cell anemia
D. Poor nutritional intake
E. Noncompliance with prenatal vitamin/iron supplement

Analysis (Nursing Diagnoses)

A. Ineffective peripheral tissue perfusion (specify) related to …
B. Imbalanced nutrition: less than body requirements related to …

TABLE 6-17 **Iron**

Drug	Indications	Adverse Reactions	Nursing Implications
Ferrous sulfate (Feosol)	Iron deficiency anemia	• Constipation • Diarrhea • Gastric irritation • Nausea or vomiting	• Iron is best absorbed on an empty stomach. • Take with vitamin C source such as orange juice to increase absorption. • Avoid taking with cereal, eggs, or milk, which decrease absorption. • Take in the evening if problem exists with morning sickness. • Stools will turn dark green to black. • Check lab values for increased reticulocytes and rising Hgb and Hct.

Nursing Plans and Interventions

A. Obtain 24-hour dietary recall.

B. Review and reinforce nutritional requirements for pregnancy (see Appendix A, *Normal Values,* p. 338).

C. Reinforce teaching about oral administration of iron (Table 6-17, *Iron*).

Infections

A. Sexually transmitted infections (STIs) and general infections.

B. Infections can be harmful to mother and fetus during the antepartum period (Table 6-18, *Infections, Maternal/Fetal Effects*).

C. Simple viral infections in the first trimester can cause serious fetal teratogenic effects.

D. STIs have a predilection for genital and perigenital site manifestations.

Nursing Assessment (Data Collection)

A. History of multiple sex partners

B. Previous history of STI or vaginal infections

C. Employment with high exposure to infection—for example, child care worker, health care worker

D. Nonspecific symptoms: fever, malaise

E. General symptoms of STIs: vaginal discharge, genital lesions, dysuria, and dyspareunia

F. Specific symptoms—for example, herpes simplex blisters

G. Laboratory studies: antibody titers, TORCH, VDRL (may be negative if drawn too early), RPR, gonorrhea screen, vaginal wet-mount

> **HESI Hint** • Some maternal infections that harm the embryo or fetus (teratogenic) are known as TORCH infections: Toxoplasmosis, Other infections, Rubella, Cytomegalovirus, and Herpes virus type 2.

Analysis (Nursing Diagnoses)

A. Risk for injury (mother/fetus) related to …

B. Deficient knowledge (specify) related to …

Nursing Plans and Interventions

A. See Nursing Plans and Interventions for STIs in Chapter 4, *Medical-Surgical Nursing,* p. 157.

B. Reinforce teaching about immunity to rubella; if client lacks immunity, advise against working with children in terms of risk for exposure.

C. If diagnosed with infection, reinforce instructions regarding maternal/fetal effects and how/why to follow the prescribed medical regimen.

Psychosocial Concerns: Teenage (Adolescent) Pregnancy

Definition: Pregnancy occurring at age 19 or younger.

A. Teen pregnancy remains a problem and is addressed in *Healthy People 2020.*

B. Teen pregnancy is associated with anemia, preeclampsia, cephalopelvic disproportion, sexually transmitted infections, intrauterine growth restriction, and ineffective parenting.

Nursing Assessment (Data Collection)

A. Age 12 to 19

B. Inquire about factors that influence the outcome of pregnancy:
  1. Previous history of menstrual or obstetric complications
  2. Nutritional status: 24-hour diet recall and analysis
  3. Attitude toward pregnancy and becoming a mother
  4. Social support system—that is, family, spouse/boyfriend, friends, classmates
  5. Exposure to battering from boyfriend, spouse, father, or other male
  6. Peer activities regarding smoking, drugs, and unsafe behaviors
  7. Client's activities regarding smoking, drugs, and unsafe behaviors
  8. Economic status
  9. Educational level; knowledge of pregnancy, childbearing, and child rearing
  10. Access to prenatal care

TABLE 6-18 Infections, Maternal/Fetal Effects

Infection	Maternal Effect	Fetal Effects	Treatment
Chlamydia trachomatis	• Mucopurulent vaginal discharge • Dysuria • Acute salpingitis • Pelvic inflammatory disease (PID) • Sterility or infertility	• Stillbirth/neonatal death • Preterm birth • Ophthalmia neonatorum • Pneumonia	• Treat with erythromycin; may need to treat partner • Azithromycin (Zithromax)
Human papillomavirus (HPV)	• Small or large, dry, wart-like growth on vulva, vagina, cervix, and/or rectum (condylomata acuminata)	• Possible chronic respiratory papillomatosis	• Laser ablation or cryotherapy • When pregnant, lesions usually left alone, unless mild laser treatment needed • Explain need for possible abdominal delivery because of fetal effect
Gonorrhea	• Dysuria • Purulent vaginal discharge • PID	• Ophthalmia neonatorum • Sepsis	• Includes both partners: penicillin and/or erythromycin and Ceftriaxone used in pregnancy • Have partner(s) use condoms until cultures negative two times
Syphilis	• Chancre • Late abortion (syphilis is most common cause) • Positive antibody screen; will not show positive if tested too soon after exposure (usually positive 6 weeks after exposure) • Positive tests for *Treponema pallidum* (FTA-ABS)	• Stillbirth • Congenital syphilis, characterized by snuffles (rhinitis) if mother has latent or tertiary syphilis • Hydrocephaly • Congenital cataracts • Copper-colored rash • Cracks around the mouth • Hypothermia (neonate may have difficulty with thermoregulation)	• Treatment before 16 weeks prevents placental transmission to fetus • Penicillin G • Erythromycin
Toxoplasmosis (TORCH disease)	• Effects are absent or manifest as flulike symptoms	• Stillbirth • Microcephaly • Hydrocephalus • Blindness • Deafness	• Treatment during pregnancy by sulfa drugs • May consider therapeutic abortion if discovered before 20 weeks
Hepatitis	• May result in preterm birth	• Baby is HBsAg positive, IgM positive	• Carriers of hepatitis B are given a series of hepatitis immunizations that may prevent carrier status and chronic liver disease in newborn
Rubella (TORCH disease)	• Most severe if contracted in *first* trimester • Therapeutic abortion offered	• Congenital heart defects • IUGR • Congenital cataracts • Hearing or vision problems may arise in later childhood	• No maternal treatment for the virus is available
Cytomegalovirus (CMV) or cytomegalic inclusion disease (CID) (TORCH disease)	• Maternal effects are absent or mononucleosis-like	• Stillbirth • Congenital CMV • Microcephaly • IUGR • Cerebral palsy • Mental retardation • Rash, jaundice, hepatosplenomegaly	• No treatment is available for mother or infant

TABLE 6-18 Infections, Maternal/Fetal Effects—cont'd

Infection	Maternal Effect	Fetal Effects	Treatment
Herpes virus type 2 (HSV) (TORCH disease)	• A primary or recurrent infection • Painful vesicular genital lesions • Cesarean delivery recommended during active lesion breakout	• Disseminated or localized skin infection • CNS abnormalities	• Safety of systematic acyclovir (Zovirax) in pregnant clients has not been established; should be used only in pregnant clients with life-threatening infection
Human immunodeficiency virus (HIV) Acquired immune deficiency syndrome (AIDS)	• Usually asymptomatic • Chronic vaginitis • Susceptible to opportunistic diseases and immunologic suppression	• Affects fetus through transplacental transfer, exposure to maternal blood/body fluids, or through breast milk	• See HIV Infection in Chapter 3, *Advanced Clinical Concepts*, p. 55, for further discussion
Bacterial vaginosis (vaginal infection)	• Milk-like discharge with fishlike odor • Itching, burning pain • Can cause premature rupture of membranes • Postpartum endometritis	• Neonatal sepsis and death	• Treated with clindamycin or ampicillin or metronidazole (Flagyl)
Monilial vaginitis (*Candida albicans*, yeast; vaginal infection)	• Common in diabetes and clients on long-term antibiotic therapy • Odorless, thick, cheesy vaginal discharge • Severe vaginal itching • Dyspareunia	• Oral thrush or perineal rash	• Treated with miconazole nitrate cream or nystatin cream in pregnancy • Teach client to wear cotton undergarments and abstain from intercourse until cured
Trichomoniasis vaginitis (Trichomonas protozoa)	• Profuse, frothy, yellowish discharge • Irritation, itching • Dysuria • Dyspareunia	• Usually no fetal effects	• Treat with vagina suppositories to reduce symptoms during the first and second trimesters of pregnancy

HESI Hint • Tetracycline is contraindicated in pregnancy because it darkens the teeth of the newborn.

HESI Hint • Podophyllin, which is usually used to treat HPV, is contraindicated in pregnancy because it is associated with fetal death, preterm labor, and cervical carcinoma.
Quadrivalent human papillomavirus (types 6, 11, 16, and 18) recombinant vaccine (Gardasil) is available to nonpregnant females age 9 years and older to prevent HPV.

HESI Hint • Toxoplasmosis is usually related to exposure to cats, gardening (where cat feces may be found), or eating raw meat.

HESI Hint • Acyclovir (used to treat herpes simplex) is *not recommended* during pregnancy.

HESI Hint • Rubella is teratogenic to the fetus during the *first* trimester, causing congenital heart disease and/or congenital cataracts. All women should have their titers checked during pregnancy. If a woman's titers are low, she should receive the vaccine *after* delivery and be instructed not to get pregnant within 3 months. Breastfeeding mothers may take the vaccine.

HESI Hint • Although metronidazole (Flagyl) is the treatment of choice for some vaginal infections, its use is contraindicated in the first trimester of pregnancy, and its use during the second trimester is controversial.

HESI Hint • Medications usually recommended for the nonpregnant client with STDs may be contraindicated for the pregnant client because of the effects on the fetus.

Analysis (Nursing Diagnoses)

A. Deficient knowledge (specify) related to …

B. Imbalanced nutrition: less than/more than body requirements related to …

Nursing Plans and Interventions

A. Establish trust and rapport through interview first, and then proceed to therapeutic relationship.

B. Avoid authoritative, punitive approach to counseling; use an information-sharing approach.

C. Reinforce information in private regarding options of pregnancy termination, adoption, and local agencies supporting pregnant adolescents.

D. Praise adolescent for all health-maintenance activities—that is, coming for pregnancy testing, making prenatal visits, and asking well-thought-out questions.

E. Allow support person to attend prenatal visits.

F. Relate nutritional information to resumption of figure postpartum, skin health, hair integrity, and other normal adolescent concerns.

G. Reinforce dangers related to substance abuse in pregnancy:
1. Smoking: low-birth-weight infant
2. Alcohol: fetal alcohol syndrome
3. Cocaine: preterm labor and abruption placentae; subtle neurologic changes in the neonate

H. Teratogenic fetal effects highest in first trimester.

I. Encourage normal activities to achieve early developmental task of identity versus role-confusion; late adolescent developmental task of intimacy versus isolation.

J. Encourage adolescent to stay in school, continue identity as student.

K. Prevent social isolation by encouraging adolescent to continue normal activities, such as attendance at school functions, games, and family activities.

L. Reinforce information regarding childbirth classes, peer support groups.

M. Reinforce information on major milestones in fetal development (major fetal growth in third trimester).

N. Monitor carefully for development of preeclampsia, nutritional disorders (anemia, IUGR).

HESI Hint • The outcome of adolescent pregnancy depends on prenatal care. Nutrition is a key factor because the adolescent's physiologic needs for growth are already higher, and the additional stress of pregnancy only increases these needs.

Preterm Labor

Description: Onset of labor between 20 and 37 weeks' gestation.

A. Predisposing factors to preterm labor include:
1. Diabetes, cardiac disease, preeclampsia, and placenta previa.
2. Infection, especially urinary tract.
3. Overdistention of uterus resulting from multiple pregnancies, hydramnios, large for gestational age baby.

B. Psychosocial factors:
1. Working outside home, if job is stressful
2. Having two or more children under age 5
3. Financial stress
4. No social support system
5. Smoking more than 10 cigarettes/day

C. Preterm labor is responsible for two out of three neonatal deaths.

D. Neonates weighing over 2000 g (4.5 lb) or 32 weeks' gestation have best chance of survival.

Nursing Assessment (Data Collection)

A. True labor present—that is, contractions with cervical change are occurring.

B. FHR 110 to 160 bpm with no distress.

C. No medical or obstetric disorder contraindicating continuance of pregnancy.

D. Fetal fibronectin test is obtained with a cervical swab detecting that preterm labor has begun.

Analysis (Nursing Diagnoses)

A. Anxiety related to …

B. Deficient knowledge (specify) related to …

C. Risk for injury (mother/fetus) related to …

Nursing Plans and Interventions

Antepartum

A. Use fetal development chart to show client when baby has mature lungs (36 weeks).

B. Reinforce instructions of preterm labor:
1. Uterine contractions every 10 minutes or more often
2. Menstrual-like cramps: low, dull backache and pelvic pressure
3. Increase or change in vaginal discharge.
4. Rupture of membranes

C. Reinforce instructions for self-assessment of uterine contractions:
1. Lying on left side, place fingers on top of uterus.
2. Note a periodic hardening or tightening with or without pain (contraction).
3. More than five contractions in an hour should be reported immediately to health care provider or clinic.

D. Follow up teaching with written instructions about signs of impending labor.

Intrapartum

A. Home management:
1. Reinforce teaching about the need for bed rest with fetus off of the cervix—that is, no sitting or kneeling.

2. Reinforce teaching about the side-lying position and elevation of foot of bed to increase uterine perfusion and decrease uterine irritability.
3. Reinforce teaching about side effects and warning signs of medications. (May be taking oral tocolytic drugs [terbutaline]; Table 6-19, *Medications for Intrapartal Complications*.)
4. Avoid sexual stimulation: no sexual intercourse, nipple stimulation, or orgasm.
5. Increase oral fluid (2 to 3 liters/day).
6. Empty bladder every 2 hours.
7. Review what to do if membranes rupture or if signs of infection occur (fever, foul-smelling vaginal discharge).
B. Hospital management:
   1. Place on bed rest in side-lying position with continuous fetal monitoring (external).
   2. Notify health care provider immediately.
   3. Assist RN and/or health care provider with medication administration as prescribed:
      a. Magnesium sulfate: decreases uterine activity.
      b. Terbutaline (Brethine): causes uterine muscle relaxation.
      c. Tocolytics: reduce uterine contractions (see Table 6-19).
      d. Glucocorticoids (betamethasone): enhance fetal lung maturation if fetus is less than 35 weeks' gestation.
   5. Prepare for birth of low-birth-weight infant if preterm labor is not arrested.
   6. Continuously monitor fetal heart rate.

Dystocia

Description: Dystocia is a difficult birth resulting from any cause.
A. Can result from any one or all of the "5 Ps":
   1. Powers: primary uterine contractions and secondary abdominal bearing down efforts
   2. Passage: maternal pelvis, uterus, cervix, vagina, perineum
   3. Passenger: fetus and placenta
   4. Psyche: response to labor by woman
   5. Position: of the laboring woman
B. Dystocia is suspected when there is:
   1. A lack of progress in cervical dilation.
   2. A lack of fetal descent.
   3. A lack of change in uterine contraction characteristics (frequency, strength, and duration).
C. Dystocia, dysfunctional labor, and uterine inertia are terms used interchangeably.

Nursing Assessment (Data Collection)

A. Hypertonic or hypotonic uterine contractions
B. Inability to bear down or push efficiently
C. Prolonged labor patterns (Table 6-20, *Prolonged Labor Patterns*)

Analysis (Nursing Diagnoses)

A. Pain related to …
B. Anxiety related to …
C. Risk for injury (mother/fetus) related to …

Nursing Plans and Interventions

A. Assist with diagnostic procedures (ultrasound, pelvimetry, vaginal exam) to rule out cephalopelvic disproportion (CPD).
B. Assist with amniotomy performed by health care provider: artificial rupture of membranes (AROM) may enhance labor forces.
   1. Explain procedure (it is painless).
   2. FHR assessed immediately after rupture to determine cord prolapse.
   3. Assess fluid for color, odor, and consistency (blood, meconium, or vernix particles).
C. Assist with IV oxytocin infusion for induction (initiation) or augmentation (stimulation) of labor and manage infusion delivery (Box 6-4, *Nursing Protocol for Administration of Oxytocin*).

Hypertensive Disorders of Pregnancy

A. Gestational hypertension:
   1. BP elevation occurs for the first time after midpregnancy.
   2. No proteinuria.
B. Transient hypertension:
   1. Gestational hypertension with no other signs of preeclampsia present at time of birth.
   2. Resolves by 12 weeks' gestation.
C. Preeclampsia:
   1. Pregnancy-specific syndrome that usually occurs after 20 weeks' gestation (except with gestational trophoblastic disease [hydatidiform mole]).
   2. Characterized by an increase in BP of 30 mm Hg systolic and/or 15 mm Hg diastolic or a BP of 140/90 mm or higher.
   3. Gestational hypertension plus proteinuria.
D. HELLP syndrome:
   1. Although not technically classified as a separate hypertensive disorder of pregnancy, HELLP syndrome is a variant of severe preeclampsia with often very different risk factors and signs/symptoms.
   2. HELLP is an acronym for Hemolysis, Elevated Liver enzymes, Low Platelets.
E. Eclampsia: seizures (with no known etiology, like epilepsy) in a woman with preeclampsia.
F. Chronic hypertension: hypertension that is observable before pregnancy or that is diagnosed before the twentieth week of gestation (with the exception of hydatidiform mole).
G. Preeclampsia superimposed on chronic hypertension: chronic hypertension with new onset proteinuria and/or a worsening of the already present hypertension, thrombocytopenia, or increased liver enzyme values.

TABLE 6-19 Medications for Intrapartal Complications

Drug	Indications	Adverse Reactions	Nursing Implications
Terbutaline sulfate (Brethine) beta-sympathomimetic agent, bronchodilator	Stops preterm labor contractions	• CNS effects: →Severe nervousness →Tremulousness →Headache • CV effects: →Severe palpitations →Tachycardia →Chest pain →Pulmonary edema • GI effects: →Nausea →Vomiting →Diarrhea →Epigastric pain • Lab value distortions →Low K+ →Hyperglycemia	• Administer IV • Increase infusion rate every 15 min, depending on uterine response and maternal side effects • Get maternal EKG and lab values before beginning infusion • Place mother on bedside cardiac monitor • Monitor fetus continuously • Monitor vital signs every 15 min • Maternal pulse should not exceed 140 bpm • FHR should not exceed 180 bpm • I&O; weigh daily • Prepare woman for side effects, especially to expect jitteriness • Notify health care provider of: →High pulse, FHR changes, abnormal lab values →Signs of HF: dyspnea, jugular vein distention, dry cough, rales in lung bases →Have antidote available—that is, a beta-blocking agent such as propranolol (Inderal)
Magnesium sulfate	• Central nervous system depressant administered to preeclamptic client to prevent seizures • May be used as a tocolytic to stop preterm labor contractions	• CNS depression manifested by: →Depressed respirations →Depressed DTRs • Decreased urine output • Pulmonary edema	• Hold if respiration <12/min, urine output <100 mL/4 hr • DTRs absent (check hourly) • Monitor magnesium levels as prescribed and report values outside therapeutic range (5 to 8 mg/dL) • Remind client of warm, flushed feeling with IV administration • Keep calcium gluconate at bedside (antidote)

HESI Hint • Although the toxic side effects of magnesium sulfate are well known and watched for, it is just as important to get serum blood levels of magnesium sulfate above 4 mg/dL to prevent convulsions and reach therapeutic range.

HESI Hint • Hold next dose of magnesium sulfate and notify health care provider if any toxic symptoms occur (<12 respirations/min, urine output <100 mL/4 hr, absent DTRs, magnesium sulfate >8 mg/dL).

HESI Hint • When administering magnesium sulfate, *always* have the antidote available (calcium gluconate, 10 mL vial of a 10% solution).

HESI Hint • Tachycardia is the major side effect of tocolytic drugs, which are beta-adrenergic agents such as terbutaline (Brethine) used to stop preterm labor. Teach the client to take her pulse before administration, and withhold medication if pulse is not within the prescribed parameters (usually withheld if pulse is higher than 120 to 140). If administration is via a continuous pump, teach client to monitor pulse periodically.

TABLE 6-20 Prolonged Labor Patterns

Pattern	Nullipara	Multipara
Prolonged latent phase	>20 hr	>14 hr
Prolonged active phase	<1.2 cm/hr	<1.5 cm/hr
Secondary arrest	No change for >2 hr	No change for >2 hr
Prolonged deceleration phase	>3 hr	>1 hr
Protracted descent	Descent of fetus <1 cm/hr	Descent of fetus <2 cm/hr
Arrest of descent	>1 hr	>½ hr

BOX 6-4 *Nursing Protocol for Administration of Oxytocin (Pitocin)*

- Determine any contraindications to use of oxytocin:
  - → Known cephalopelvic disproportion (CPD)
  - → Fetal stress
  - → Placenta previa
  - → Prior classical incision into uterus
  - → Active genital herpes infection
  - → Floating fetus
  - → Unripe cervix
- Monitor IV infusion per protocol.
  - → Piggyback at the lowest port on the primary IV line
- Using external or internal fetal monitoring, continuously monitor the following:
  - → FHR
  - → Uterine resting tone
  - → Contraction frequency, duration, and strength

HESI Hint   Dystocia frequently requires the use of oxytocin for augmentation or induction of labor. Uterine tetany is a harmful complication, and careful monitoring is required. The desired effect is contractions every 2 to 3 minutes, with duration of contractions no longer than 90 seconds. Continuously monitor FHR and uterine resting tone. If tetany occurs, turn off Pitocin, turn client to a side-lying position, and administer O₂ by face mask. Check output (should be at least 100 mL/4 hours). Oxytocin's most important side effect is its antidiuretic (ADH) effect, which can cause water intoxication and can lead to pulmonary edema. Using IV fluids containing electrolytes decreases the risk of water intoxication.

HESI Hint   The uterus is most sensitive to becoming tetanic at the beginning of the infusion. The client must *always* be attended and contractions monitored. Contractions should last *no* longer than 90 seconds to prevent fetal hypoxia.

HESI Hint   Women with previous uterine scars are prone to uterine rupture, especially if oxytocin or forceps are used. If a woman complains of a sharp pain accompanied by the abrupt cessation of contractions, suspect uterine rupture—*a medical emergency*. Immediate surgical delivery is indicated to save the fetus and the mother.

Preeclampsia/Eclampsia, also Called Pregnancy-Induced Hypertension

Definition: Most common hypertensive disorder that develops during pregnancy, characterized by elevated blood pressure, edema, and proteinuria.

A. Preeclampsia is characterized by an increase in BP of 30 mm Hg systolic and/or 15 mm Hg diastolic over previous/usual baseline, with concomitant evidence of preeclampsia by a BP of over 140/90 mm Hg.

B. Usually develops during last 10 weeks of gestation or up to 48 hours after delivery.

C. Occurs in 6% to 7% of all pregnancies.

D. Occurs predominately in primigravidas.

E. Preeclampsia is a major cause of maternal death and fetal hypoxia/death.

F. Differentiated into three types:
  1. Preeclampsia
  2. Eclampsia: preeclampsia with seizures/coma
  3. HELLP syndrome

G. There is *no* known cause of preeclampsia. Pathophysiology is characterized by:
  1. Generalized vasospasm and vasoconstriction leading to vascular damage over time.
  2. Loss of plasma protein into the interstitial space (fluid is drawn into the extravascular spaces, which results in hypovolemia).

3. Hypovolemia results in decreased perfusion to major organs, including the uterus.

Nursing Assessment (Data Collection)

A. Obtain baseline BP at first prenatal visit.
B. Risk factors associated with preeclampsia:
   1. Age less than 17 years or greater than 35 years
   2. Low socioeconomic status
   3. Poor protein intake
   4. Previous hypertension
   5. Diabetes (gestational or preexisting)
   6. Multiple gestation
   7. Hydatidiform mole
   8. Family history (mothers or sisters with preeclampsia)
C. Mild preeclampsia:
   1. BP rises 30 mm Hg systolic/15 mm Hg diastolic over previous baseline or 140/90 or greater
   2. Presence of associated conditions (outlined above)
   3. Weight gain of more than 2 lb/week
   4. Proteinuria of 1+ or greater
   5. Edema, especially around eyes, face, and fingers
   6. Hyperreflexia of 3+
   7. CNS symptoms: possible mild headache, slight irritability
   8. Intrauterine growth retardation (IUGR), evidenced by size/date discrepancy
D. *Severe* preeclampsia consists of all of the above symptoms *plus* any two of the following:
   1. BP rises to 160 mm Hg/110 mm Hg on two or more occasions
   2. Proteinuria of 2+ to 4+
   3. Generalized edema (very puffy face and/or hands)
   4. Deep tendon reflexes (DTRs) 3+ or greater, plus clonus
   5. Oliguria (less than 100 mL/4 hr)
   6. CNS symptoms: severe headache, visual disturbances (blurred vision, photophobia, blind spots), and possibly epigastric pain
   7. Elevated serum creatinine, thrombocytopenia, and marked liver enzyme elevation with epigastric pain related to liver spasms
   8. Severe IUGR; late decelerations of the FHR
E. Eclampsia:
   1. Presence of seizure in the woman with preeclampsia
   2. Tonic-clonic type seizures
F. HELLP syndrome:
   1. Characterized by hemolysis (H), elevated liver enzymes (EL), and low platelets (LP).
   2. Increased risk for abruption, acute renal failure, hepatic rupture, preterm birth, and fetal and/or maternal death.
   3. Etiology arises out of changes that occur with preeclampsia.
   4. More commonly seen in older, white, multiparous women.
   5. Signs and symptoms include history of malaise, epigastric or right upper quadrant pain, nausea and vomiting.

6. Many women are normotensive and do not have proteinuria.
7. Should still be treated prophylactically with magnesium sulfate (because of increased CNS irritability that is part of the disease), even if hypertension is not present.
8. Women with HELLP syndrome are at high risk for developing the syndrome again in future pregnancies as well as for developing preeclampsia in other pregnancies not complicated by HELLP syndrome.
9. Women with HELLP syndrome may develop DIC.

Nursing Analysis (Nursing Diagnoses)

A. Risk for injury (fetus/mother) related to …
B. Deficient knowledge (specify) related to …

Nursing Care for Client with Preeclampsia Antepartum

A. Home management:
   1. Reinforce to client that absolute bed rest with bathroom privileges is necessary (except for regularly scheduled prenatal visits).
   2. Have client weigh daily and report greater than 2 lb/week gain.
   3. Reinforce teaching that client test urine daily for protein.
   4. Provide client with list of signs to report immediately to caregiver.
      a. CNS symptoms: visual disturbances, headache, nausea and vomiting, hyperreflexia, convulsions
      b. Hepatic sign: epigastric pain
      c. Renal signs: oliguria, proteinuria
      d. Fetal distress signs: decreased or absent fetal activity, unusual or extremely active fetus
      e. Signs of abruptio placentae: vaginal bleeding, abdominal pain
   5. Collaborate with RN to enhance and reinforce a teaching plan about the prescribed diet:
      a. High-protein diet
      b. Limit salt intake (no longer completely restricted)
      c. Maintain minimum of 35 cal/kg of body weight
   6. Reinforce client teaching about therapeutic rationale of bed rest in left side-lying position (to increase uterine perfusion and prevent fetal distress).
   7. Reinforce need for stress reduction and home help in order to prevent further vascular constriction from circulating stress hormones/catecholamines.
B. Hospital management:
   1. If mild preeclampsia progresses to severe preeclampsia, hospitalization will be necessary.
   2. Monitor level of consciousness, BP, and vital signs every 4 hours or more often if elevated/abnormal.
   3. Obtain fetal assessment continuously; apply external fetal monitor.
   4. Observe for vaginal bleeding/abdominal pain and report to RN and health care provider.

5. Provide bed rest in left side-lying position.
6. Assist with and monitor intravenous infusion for fluid and medication access.
7. Insert indwelling urinary catheter with urine meter.
8. Monitor I&O hourly.
9. Maintain quiet, slightly darkened environment with limited visitors.
10. Assist with administration of magnesium sulfate and antihypertensive drugs (rare unless diastolic BP consistently over 110), and possibly oxytocin (Pitocin) for initiation/augmentation of labor (see Table 6-19).
11. Observe daily for signs of coagulopathy:
    a. Petechiae under BP cuff
    b. Platelet decrease or increase
    c. Fibrinogen increase or decrease
12. Assist with assessment of deep tendon reflexes (DTR) and assess for clonus once each shift or more often if prescribed or abnormal.
13. Assist with transfer to labor/delivery if necessary:
    a. Signs of pulmonary edema occur.
    b. HELLP syndrome occurs.
    c. Late decelerations of the fetal heart rate occur.
    d. Preterm labor begins.

> **HESI Hint** • Rarely are antihypertensive drugs used in the preeclamptic client. They are given only in the event of diastolic blood pressure over 110 mm Hg (cerebrovascular accident [CVA] danger). Drug of choice is hydralazine HCl (Apresoline).

> **HESI Hint** • Although delivery is often described as the "cure" for preeclampsia, the client can convulse up to 48 hours after delivery.

> **HESI Hint** • DTRs are important to check hourly if client is on magnesium sulfate. Loss of DTRs always proceeds to respiratory depression.

> **HESI Hint** • Remember magnesium sulfate is given for preeclampsia to help prevent seizures, not to lower BP.

Nursing Care for the Client with Preeclampsia Intrapartum

A. When the client with preeclampsia begins labor, control the amount of stimulation in the labor room:
   1. Keep nurse/client ratio at 1:1.
   2. If possible, put client in darkened, quiet, private room.
   3. Keep client on absolute bed rest, side-lying, with bed rails up.
   4. Disturb client as little as possible with nursing interventions.

B. Have client choose support person to stay with her and limit other visitors.
C. Constantly reinforce rationale for procedures and care.
D. Monitor intravenous line to maintain fluid and medication access.
E. Monitor blood pressure every 15 to 30 minutes, keeping blood pressure cuff on or using electronic blood pressure monitor if available.
F. Check urine for protein every hour and report increase.
G. Determine deep tendon reflexes every hour and report increases or decreases.
H. Support the RN in the administration of magnesium sulfate (see Table 6-19).
   1. Usually given IV with a loading dose of 4 g in 100 mL to 250 mL of solution. Give over 20 to 30 minutes to get the blood level up to therapeutic serum levels (5 to 8 mg/dL).
   2. Serum blood levels are usually maintained by infusing 2 g/hr after loading dose.
I. Monitor for toxicity during magnesium sulfate administration:
   1. Urinary output less than 33 mL/hr.
   2. Respirations less than 12/min.
   3. DTRs absent.
   4. Deceleration of the FHR, bradycardia.
J. When magnesium sulfate is prescribed to be given IM:
   1. Give 10 g (5 g in each buttock) with 1 mL 1% lidocaine to decrease pain.
   2. Give deep in dorsal gluteal site with 3-inch, 20-gauge needle; give z-track or with rotation method.
   3. Expect onset within 30 min/1 hr, lasting 3 to 4 hr.
K. If convulsions/seizures do occur:
   1. Stay with client and use call button to summon help. Have someone get health care provider STAT!
   2. Turn client on side to prevent aspiration.
   3. Do not attempt to put objects or fingers in the client's mouth.
   4. Administer O_2 at 10 L/min by face mask and have suction available.
   5. Give magnesium sulfate as prescribed (see Table 6-19).
   6. Monitor labor/delivery status.
L. During the postdelivery period:
   1. Continue magnesium sulfate as prescribed (usually given first 24 hours after delivery) or more often per institutional policy.
   2. Monitor blood pressure, respirations, DTRs, and urine output every 4 hours for 48 hours. (If still on magnesium sulfate, may be every hour.)
   3. Carefully obtain uterine tone/fundal height for uterine atony resulting from magnesium sulfate administration.
   4. Monitor for blood loss: preexisting hypovolemia makes these women sensitive to even normal blood loss.
   5. Reinforce client instructions to report headache, visual disturbances, or epigastric pain.

6. Check with the registered nurse before administration of *any ergot* derivatives.
7. Complete bed rest while on magnesium sulfate.

HESI Hint • The major goal of nursing care for a client with preeclampsia is to maintain uteroplacental perfusion and prevent seizures. This requires the administration of magnesium sulfate. Withhold administration of magnesium sulfate if signs of toxicity exist: respirations less than 12/min, absence of DTRs, and/ or urine output less than 30 mL/hr.

HESI Hint • Increased DTRs indicates worsening preeclampsia, and decreased DTRs may indicate magnesium sulfate toxicity.

Maternal/Infant Cardiac Disease

A. Impaired cardiac function usually results from a congenital defect or a history of rheumatic heart disease with valve prolapse or stenosis.
B. More commonly seen in women today because of surgical correction techniques in infancy enabling them to live to childbearing age.
C. Dangerous because of plasma volume increase that accompanies pregnancy.
D. Type and extent of disease:
  1. Class I: ordinary physical activity does not cause cardiac symptomatology. Unrestricted physical activity.
  2. Class II: ordinary activity causes fatigue, palpitations, dyspnea, and angina. Physical activity limited.
  3. Class III: with less than ordinary activity, cardiac decompensation symptoms ensue. Moderate to marked limitation of activity.
  4. Class IV: symptoms of cardiac insufficiency occur even at rest. No activity allowed.

Nursing Assessment (Data Collection)

A. History of preexisting cardiac disease
B. Cardiac decompensation:
  1. Subjective symptoms determined by client:
    a. Increasing fatigue
    b. Dyspnea
    c. Feeling of smothering
    d. Dry, hacky cough
    e. "Racing" heart
    f. Swelling of feet, legs, and fingers
  2. Objective symptoms determined by health professional:
    a. Pulse greater than 100 bpm
    b. Crackles at lung bases even after deep breathing
    c. Orthopnea/dyspnea
    d. Respirations greater than 25/min
C. Anemia possible (Hct <32%, Hgb <10 mg/dL)

Analysis (Nursing Diagnoses)

A. Deficient knowledge related to …
B. Anxiety related to …
C. Ineffective family coping related to …
D. Ineffective peripheral tissue perfusion (specify) related to …

Nursing Care for the Cardiac Maternity Client

A. Antepartum:
  1. Reinforce information related to cardiac disease and for client to report any symptoms of cardiac decompensation
  2. Encourage 8 to 10 hours' sleep each night with daily rest periods.
  3. Reinforce teaching of self-administration of heparin if prescribed.
  4. Give diet plan, which includes high iron, high protein, and adequate calorie intake.
  5. Inform client of anticipated difficult period for control at 28 to 32 weeks when plasma volume peaks in pregnancy.
  6. Reinforce client teaching to notify health care provider at first sign of infection.
B. Intrapartum:
  1. Maintain a calm atmosphere, allowing presence of support persons, and keep family informed at all times.
  2. Maintain cardiac perfusion.
    a. Put client in semi-Fowler side-lying position.
    b. Prevent Valsalva maneuvers even during second stage (obstructs left ventricular outflow).
    c. Avoid hypotension if epidural anesthesia used.
    d. Avoid use of stirrups in delivery room (can cause popliteal vein compression and decreased venous return).
  3. Provide pain relief and supportive measures because pain can contribute to cardiac distress.
  4. Monitor during forceps delivery and episiotomy (will likely be performed to decrease the time of the second stage).
B. Postpartum:
  1. Tailor care to the woman's functional classification.
  2. Continue semi- or high-Fowler position (head of bed raised) with side-lying maintained.
  3. Progress ambulation: dangling, sitting, standing, short to long ambulation, according to tolerance and no symptoms of cardiac decompensation.
  4. Administer stool softeners as prescribed to prevent straining during bowel movement.
  5. Watch for symptoms of urinary infection: dysuria, white cells in urine, and pus in urine.
  6. Report *any* symptoms of cardiac decompensation to health care provider immediately:
    a. Tachycardia (pulse >100)
    b. Tachypnea (respirations >25)
    c. Dry cough
    d. Rales in the lung bases

7. Report immediately any temperature spike over 100.4° F.
8. Coordinate with the mother and family for support when returning home. If necessary, refer to community resource for homemaking services.

> **HESI Hint** • Nursing care during labor and delivery for the client with cardiac disease is focused on prevention of cardiac embarrassment, maintenance of uterine perfusion, and alleviation of anxiety.

> **HESI Hint** • Should these clients experience preterm labor, the use of beta-adrenergic agents such as terbutaline (Brethine) are contraindicated because of the chance of myocardial ischemia.

> **HESI Hint** • Normal diuresis, which occurs in the postpartum period, can pose serious problems to the new mother with cardiac disease because of the increased cardiac output.

Congenital Heart Disease in the Newborn

Nursing Assessment (Data Collection)
A. Weak cry, cyanosis worsening with crying
B. Lethargy, hypotonia, and flaccidity
C. Persistent bradycardia or tachycardia
D. Tachypnea or other signs of respiratory distress
E. Decreased/absent femoral or pedal pulses

Nursing Plans and Interventions
A. Decrease energy use immediately:
   1. No nippling (no pacifiers, no excessive stimulation).
B. Notify health care provider STAT of findings.
C. Transfer neonate to NICU for diagnostic workup.

> **HESI Hint** • Coumadin may not be taken during pregnancy because of its ability to cross the placenta and affect the fetus. HEPARIN is the drug of choice; it does not cross the placental membrane.

Hyperemesis Gravidarum

A. Inability to control nausea and vomiting during pregnancy.
B. Hyperemesis gravidarum is characterized by the inability to keep down solid food/fluids for 24 hours.
C. It is linked to maternal hormones and possible psychologic reaction to pregnancy.

Nursing Assessment (Data Collection)
A. Weight loss in pregnancy.
B. Signs of dehydration:
   1. Increased urine-specific gravity
   2. Oliguria
C. Psychologic distress (different from normal ambivalence in pregnancy).
D. Fluid and electrolyte imbalance; potential metabolic acidosis.

Analysis (Nursing Diagnoses)
A. Risk for deficient fluid volume related to …
B. Anxiety related to …
C. Imbalanced nutrition: less than bodily requirements related to …

Nursing Plans and Interventions
A. Weigh daily at same time with like clothing.
B. Check urine 3× daily for ketones.
C. Monitor electrolytes, serum albumin levels, and hydration status. Report abnormal lab values STAT to health care provider.
D. Progress diet from clear liquids to full liquids to bland to full diet.
E. Check fetal heart rate (if possible, auscultate by Doppler) every 8 hours.
F. Provide psychologic support to offset client's concerns.
G. Assist with administration of total parenteral nutrition (TPN) as prescribed.
H. Administer antiemetics as prescribed.

> **HESI Hint** • Recent research has found that *Helicobacter pylori* (the bacterium that causes stomach ulcers) infection is another possible causative factor in hyperemesis. Other pregnancy and nonpregnancy risk factors for hyperemesis gravidarum include first pregnancy, multiple fetuses, age under 24, history of this condition in other pregnancies, obesity, and high-fat diets.

> **HESI Hint** • In severe cases of hyperemesis gravidarum, the health care provider may prescribe antihistamines, vitamin B_6, or phenothiazines to relieve nausea. The provider may also prescribe metoclopramide (Reglan) to increase the rate at which the stomach moves food into the intestines or antacids to absorb stomach acid and help prevent acid reflux.

> **HESI Hint** • Women who suffer from hyperemesis gravidarum are often deficient in thiamin, riboflavin, vitamin B_6, vitamin A, and retinol-binding proteins.

Diabetes Mellitus

A. May manifest for the first time in pregnancy as the diabetogenic effects of pregnancy increase.
B. Hormonal changes during pregnancy act to increase maternal cell resistance to insulin so that an abundant supply of glucose is available to the fetus.
C. A preexisting reduction in insulin and the glucose-sparing effects of pregnancy compromise health of the mother/fetus.
D. If insulin cannot move glucose into maternal cells, the mother will begin to metabolize fat and protein for energy-producing ketones and fatty acids that result in ketoacidosis.

Nursing Assessment (Data Collection)

A. Predisposing factors include the following:
1. Family history of diabetes
2. History of more than two spontaneous abortions
3. Hydramnios
4. Previous baby with a weight over 4000 g (8 lb, 13.5 oz)
5. Previous baby with congenital anomalies
6. High parity
7. Obesity
8. Recurrent monilial vaginitis
9. Glycosuria
B. Abnormal glucose screen. A 1-hour glucose screen is routinely done on all pregnant women between 24 and 26 weeks' gestation.
C. Elevated glycosylated hemoglobin (used to evaluate diabetic control by reflecting blood glucose level during the previous 6 to 8 weeks) indicates uncontrolled diabetes.
D. Types of diabetes mellitus include:
1. Type 1 (insulin dependent): schedule for hemoglobin A1C test (glycosylated hemoglobin reflects glucose control for the lifespan of the red blood cell, 120 days). Prone to ketosis.
2. Type 2 (noninsulin dependent): in pregnancy, insulin is required to control maternal blood glucose levels.
3. Type 3 (gestational diabetes): onset during pregnancy with return to normal glucose tolerance after delivery.
E. Symptoms include the "three Ps": polyphagia, polydipsia, and polyuria.
F. Hypoglycemia (usually first trimester); insulin need may decrease.
G. Hyperglycemia (second and third trimesters); amount of insulin needed increases.
H. Increased incidence of preeclampsia, infection, and hydramnios.

Analysis (Nursing Diagnoses)

A. Deficient knowledge (diabetes mellitus during pregnancy) related to ...
B. Risk for injury (fetus/mother) related to ...

Nursing Plans and Interventions

A. At diagnosis, implement the following:
1. Review pathophysiology of disease.
2. Reinforce teaching of home glucose monitoring (urine and blood).
3. Demonstrate insulin administration (oral hypoglycemics are contraindicated during pregnancy).
4. Identify signs of hypo- and hyperglycemia and the immediate actions to be taken if signs are noted (see Diabetes Mellitus in Chapter 4, *Medical-Surgical Nursing*, p. 117).
5. Stress importance of regular prenatal visits.
6. Encourage verbalization of concerns regarding diagnosis.
B. Coordinate referral with dietitian for individualized diet management:
1. Calories: 35 to 50 cal/kg of ideal body weight
2. Complex carbohydrates: 50% of diet
3. Proteins: 20% of diet
4. Fat: Less than 30% of diet
5. Distribute calories among three meals and four snacks
6. Review relationship between exercise and diet. Hyperglycemia can be prevented by consistent use of calories through exercise.
C. Remind client of expected increased insulin needs in second and third trimesters related to increasing diabetogenic effects of pregnancy.
D. Review situations that will complicate diabetic control: illness, diarrhea, and vomiting.
E. Reinforce client teaching to drink orange juice followed by glass of low-fat milk for hypoglycemic reaction or insulin reaction.
F. Reinforce teaching about signs and symptoms of ketoacidosis (fruity odor to breath, nausea and vomiting, exaggerated respiratory effort, altered mental state) and to come to hospital immediately if any of these symptoms occur.
G. Remind client of need for scheduled delivery date, usually around 37 to 38 weeks' gestation, when control becomes more difficult.
H. See Nursing Care for the Maternity Client with Diabetes.
I. Provide care for the infant (see Nursing Care for Infant of Mother with Diabetes).

HESI Hint • GLUCOSE SCREEN
Client does not have to fast for this test: 50 g of glucose is given and blood is drawn after 1 hour. If the blood glucose is greater than 135 mg/dL, then a 3-hour glucose tolerance test is done.

HESI Hint • A high incidence of fetal anomalies occurs in pregnant women with diabetes. Therefore, fetal surveillance is very important.
• Ultrasound exam
• Alpha-fetoprotein (to determine neural tube anomalies)
• Nonstress and contraction stress tests

HESI Hint • Oral hypoglycemics are not taken in pregnancy because of potential teratogenic effects on the fetus. Insulin is used for therapeutic management.

HESI Hint • When a woman with a diagnosis of diabetes mellitus is admitted in labor:
- She is more prone to preeclampsia, hemorrhage, and infection.
- Delivery is often scheduled between 37 to 38 weeks' gestation to avoid the end of the third trimester of pregnancy because this is a *very* difficult time to maintain diabetic control.

Nursing Care for the Maternity Client with Diabetes

A. Predelivery period:
1. On the day of delivery, carefully assess client for insulin administration.
2. Monitor infusion of insulin/glucose to maintain blood glucose levels between 60 and 80 mg/dL in labor.
3. Hourly determinations of blood glucose are done by finger stick.
4. Position on left side to avoid pressure on vena cava from large fetus or hydramnios.
5. Check urine for ketones hourly. Report any over 2+.
6. Monitor fetus continuously using electronic fetal monitoring system.
B. Postdelivery period:
1. Use a sliding-scale approach to insulin administration because of the precipitous fall in insulin requirements postdelivery.
2. Continue monitoring a 5% glucose infusion at 100 to 125 mL/hr as prescribed.
3. Check urine each shift for ketones (sign of hyperglycemia, use of fat/protein for energy).
4. Monitor for complications:
   a. Preeclampsia
   b. Postpartum uterine atony associated with uterine overdistention
   c. Infection
5. Encourage breastfeeding, which decreases insulin requirements. Insulin *does not* cross into breast milk.
6. Contraception: diaphragm with spermicide.

HESI Hint • It is useful to discontinue long-acting insulin administration on the day before delivery is planned because insulin requirements are less in labor and drop precipitously after delivery.

HESI Hint • Estrogen-containing birth control pills affect glucose metabolism by increasing resistance to insulin. The intrauterine device may be associated with an increased risk of infection in these already vulnerable women.

Nursing Care for Infant of Mother with Diabetes
Nursing Assessment (Data Collection)

A. Macrosomia
B. IUGR
C. Hypoglycemia, hypocalcemia
D. Hyperbilirubinemia, polycythemia
E. Congenital anomalies
F. Infection
G. Prematurity

Nursing Plans and Interventions

A. Observe for birth trauma: clavicle fracture or cerebral trauma.
B. Perform heel sticks for glucose assessment at 30 minutes of age, 1 hour, and as prescribed.
C. Observe for hypoglycemia: jitteriness.
D. Observe for hypocalcemia: jitteriness.
E. Begin small, frequent feedings at 1 hour of age.

Emergency Delivery

Description: Emergency delivery (rapid, uncontrolled delivery) is an unsterile or an unassisted delivery that can be managed without complications to mother or fetus.

Nursing Assessment (Data Collection)

A. Bulging perineum.
B. Woman screaming that the baby is coming.
C. Presenting part visible at introitus.

Analysis (Nursing Diagnoses)

A. Risk for injury (mother/fetus) related to …
B. Anxiety related to …

Nursing Plans and Interventions

A. Do not, at any time, leave the client alone.
B. If possible, summon RN and health care provider if occurring in labor room (precip basin includes towels, scissors, cord clamps, bulb syringe, and placenta basin).
C. Place clean towel under mother's buttocks.
D. Have client use hee-blow or blow-blow breathing technique to slow expulsion of head over perineum.
E. If amnion is still present, rupture with fingers or clean implement when head crowns.
F. Apply gentle counter pressure against presenting part (vertex) to prevent the fetus from "popping" over the

perineum, which can lacerate tissue and cause fetal cerebral trauma.
G. Check for cord around neck and remove if loose; cut if tight.
H. Deliver anterior shoulder first by gently pressing downward under symphysis.
I. Apply upward pressure over perineum to deliver posterior shoulder.
J. Deliver entire body, holding baby in slightly head down position to facilitate mucus drainage.
K. Suction baby with bulb syringe quickly (mouth and nares). If meconium is present, this must be done before delivery of the body.
L. Dry infant and cover with blanket or towel.
M. If equipment is available, clamp cord in two places and cut in between. If sterile supplies are not available, leave cord intact.
N. Do not milk the cord.
O. When signs of placental separation are seen (gush of blood, lengthening of cord), ask woman to gently push placenta out.
P. Put baby to mother's breast to contract uterus.

Cesarean Birth

Description: Delivery of a fetus or fetuses through the abdomen.
A. Whether planned (elective) or unplanned (emergency), such a client is prone to complications:
  1. Anesthesia complications
  2. Usual abdominal surgery complications
  3. Sepsis
  4. Thromboembolism
  5. Injury to the urinary tract
B. The rate of cesarean section births is more than 30% in the United States and is increasing.
C. Vaginal birth after cesarean (VBAC) rate is decreasing due to the complications associated with the procedure.

Nursing Assessment (Data Collection)

A. Elective or repeat cesarean birth scheduled.
B. Emergency cesarean birth performed to prevent harm to mother/fetus.

Analysis (Nursing Diagnoses)

A. Anxiety related to …
B. Risk for injury (mother) related to …
C. Risk for impaired urinary elimination related to …

Nursing Care for the Client with Cesarean Birth

A. Before cesarean birth:
  1. If surgery is planned, encourage couple to attend cesarean birth class:
    a. Tour of surgical area is usually provided.
    b. Film of cesarean birth is shown.
    c. Discussion is led by staff member.
  2. If emergency cesarean is necessary, check for informed consent, including health care provider's explanation of risks, benefits, and alternatives to surgery.
  3. Inform anesthesiologist of need for preoperative assessment.
  4. Assist health care provider with anesthesia—that is, epidural.
  5. Administer preoperative medications if prescribed.
    a. Usually, because of fetus in utero, no analgesia or sedative is prescribed preoperative.
    b. May receive antacid to alkalize stomach contents (if aspiration occurs, less damage will be done to lung tissue) or drug such as a histamine receptor antagonist, which is a gastric antisecretory drug, to reduce production of gastric secretions.
  6. Shave abdomen from xiphoid to ¼ way down thigh, including pubic area (varies by institution).
  7. Insert Foley catheter.
  8. Preview lab studies: Type and cross-match for 2 units packed red blood cells, CBC, and chemistry urinalysis.
  9. Remove dentures, contact lenses, rings, and fingernail polish and give to support person.
  10. Notify registered nurse, nursery, neonatologist, and/or pediatrician of impending cesarean birth.
  11. Allow presence of support person in operative suite unless hospital policy contraindicates.
  12. Maintain safety during transfer to operative suite.
B. Intraoperative care:
  1. Before abdominal prep:
    a. Place wedge under one hip to displace uterus laterally.
    b. Keep client warm via warm blankets.
    c. Monitor and document fetal heart tones continually.
  2. Apply grounding pad to leg.
  3. Perform abdominal scrub (prep).
  4. Assist circulating nurse per institutional protocol.
  5. If client is awake, assess and meet psychosocial needs.
C. Post cesarean birth:
  1. Receive complete report, including the type of uterine incision performed, and assist RN with initial assessment.
  2. Obtaining fundal height and consistency may be difficult because of abdominal bandage and pain. Note on chart if unable to determine, but gentle attempts should be made.
  3. Monitor temperature every hour in recovery room, then every 4 hours × 24 hours, every 8 hours thereafter if within normal limits.
  4. Monitor heart rate, respirations, breath sounds, bowel sounds, and SaO_2 per unit protocol.
  5. Begin I&O assessment every 8 hours.

TABLE 6-21 **Narcotic Analgesics**

Drug	Indications	Adverse Reactions	Nursing Implications
Fentanyl citrate (Sublimaze)	Used as an adjunct to anesthesia	• Respiratory depression, apnea • Bradycardia, hypotension	• Have resuscitation equipment readily available • Do not mix with IV barbiturates
Morphine sulfate (Astramorph Pf, Duramorph, MS Contin) (see Table 3-16, *Onset of Commonly Administered Narcotics*, p. 64, for more narcotic information)	Often first choice for severe pain	• Nausea, vomiting, constipation • Respiratory depression, depression of cough reflexes • Hypotension	• Check respirations and BP before administration; hold administration if respirations <12 or if hypotension exists • Have antagonist, naloxone HCl (Narcan), available in case of respiratory depression

6. Administer pain medication as prescribed. Instruct client to use patient-controlled analgesia (PCA pumps) (Table 6-21, *Narcotic Analgesics*).
7. Encourage participation in infant care ASAP, and take mother/couple to nursery often.
8. Demonstrate splinting of abdomen, coughing, deep breathing, and incentive spirometer use to prevent respiratory complications from stasis of lung secretions.
9. Maintain aseptic technique to prevent sepsis:
   a. Reinforce teaching about handwashing technique.
   b. Assess incisional healing every 8 hours.
   c. Perform scrupulous peri care/pad changes.
   d. Assess lochia for foul odor (indicative of infection).

HESI Hint • If a woman is medicated, the responsible adult accompanying her must sign the necessary consent forms. State laws differ as to the acceptability of a friend signing the consent form rather than a relative.

HESI Hint • Babies delivered abdominally miss out on the vaginal squeeze and are born with more fluid in the lungs, predisposing the newborn to transient tachypnea and respiratory distress.

HESI Hint • The preferable low-transverse uterine incision usually results in less postoperative pain, less bleeding, and fewer incidents of ruptured uterus. The classical, vertical incision on the uterus may involve part of the fundus, resulting in more postoperative pain, more bleeding, and an increased chance of uterine rupture.

HESI Hint • Because of the exploration and cleansing of the uterus just after delivery of the placenta, the amount of lochia may be scant in the recovery room. However, pooling in the vagina and uterus while the client is on bed rest may result in blood running down the client's leg when she first ambulates. Cesarean birth clients have the same lochial changes, placental site healing, and aseptic needs as do vaginal birth clients.

HESI Hint • A laparotomy of any kind, including cesarean birth, predisposes the client to postoperative paralytic ileus. When the bowel is manipulated in surgery, it ceases peristalsis, which may persist. Symptoms include absent bowel sounds, abdominal distention, tympany on percussion, nausea and vomiting, and, of course, obstipation (intractable constipation). Early ambulation is an effective nursing intervention.

Review of Complications of Pregnancy

1. What instructions should the nurse give the woman with a threatened abortion?
2. What condition should the nurse suspect if a woman of childbearing age presents to an emergency room with bilateral or unilateral abdominal pain with or without bleeding?
3. List three symptoms of abruptio placentae and three symptoms of placenta previa.
4. State three principles pertinent to counseling and/or teaching a pregnant adolescent.
5. What complications are pregnant adolescents more prone to develop?

6. All pregnant women should be taught preterm labor recognition. Describe the warning symptoms of preterm labor.
7. List the predisposing factors to preterm labor.
8. When is preterm labor able to be arrested?
9. What is the major side effect of beta-adrenergic (Terbutaline) tocolytic drugs?
10. What are the major goals of nursing care related to pregnancy-induced hypertension with preeclampsia?
11. Magnesium sulfate is used to treat preeclampsia.
    A. What is the purpose for administration of magnesium sulfate?
    B. What is the main action of magnesium sulfate?
    C. What is the antidote for magnesium sulfate?
    D. List the three main assessment findings indicating toxic effects of magnesium sulfate.
12. What are the major symptoms of preeclampsia?
13. What is the priority nursing action after spontaneous or artificial rupture of membranes?
14. What is the most common complication of oxytocin augmentation or induction of labor? List three actions the nurse should take if such a complication occurs.
15. State three nursing interventions during forceps delivery.
16. What is the cause of preeclampsia?
17. What interventions should the nurse implement to prevent further CNS irritability in the preeclampsia client?
18. A woman on tolbutamide (Orinase) (oral hypoglycemic) asks the nurse if she can continue this medication in pregnancy. How should the nurse respond?
19. Name three maternal and three fetal complications of gestational diabetes.
20. State three priority nursing actions in the postdelivery period for the client with preeclampsia.
21. Why is regular insulin used in labor?
22. List three conditions clients with diabetes mellitus are more prone to develop.
23. Does insulin cross the placental/breast barrier?
24. The goal for diabetic management during labor is euglycemia. How is it defined?
25. What contraceptive technique is recommended for diabetic women?
26. What interventions can the nurse implement to maintain cardiac perfusion in a laboring cardiac client?
27. Gentle counter pressure against the perineum during an emergency delivery prevents _____ and _____.
28. When may a vaginal birth after cesarean be considered by a woman with a previous cesarean section?
29. Clients who have had a cesarean section are prone to what postoperative complications?

Answers to Review

1. Maintain strict bed rest for 24 to 48 hours. Avoid sexual intercourse for 2 weeks.
2. Ectopic pregnancy.
3. Abruption: fetal distress; rigid, boardlike abdomen; pain; dark-red or absent bleeding. Previa: painless, bright-red vaginal bleeding; fetal heart rate normal; soft uterus.
4. Nurse must establish trust/rapport before counseling/teaching begins. Adolescents do not respond to an authoritarian approach. Consider the developmental tasks of identity and social/individual intimacy.
5. Preeclampsia, IUGR, CPD, STIs, anemia.
6. More than 5 contractions/hour; cramps, low, dull backache; pelvic pressure; change in vaginal discharge.
7. Urinary tract infection; overdistention of uterus; diabetes; preeclampsia; cardiac disease; placenta previa; psychosocial factors, such as stress.
8. Cervix is less than 4 cm dilated, less than 50% effacement, and membranes intact and not bulging out of the cervical os.
9. Tachycardia.
10. Maintenance of uteroplacental perfusion; prevention of seizures; prevention of complications such as HELLP syndrome, DIC, and abruption.
11. Answers are as follows:
    A. Prevent seizures by decreasing CNS irritability.
    B. CNS depression (seizure prevention).
    C. Calcium gluconate.
    D. Reduced urinary output, reduced respiratory rate, and decreased reflexes.

12. Increase in BP of 30 mm Hg systolic and 15 mm Hg diastolic over previous baseline; hyperreflexia; proteinuria (albuminuria); CNS disturbances; headache and visual disturbances; epigastric pain.
13. Assessment of the fetal heart rate.
14. Tetany. Turn off Pitocin. Turn pregnant woman to side. Administer O_2 by mask.
15. Ensure empty bladder. Auscultate FHR before application, during application, and between traction periods. Observe for maternal lacerations and newborn cerebral/facial trauma.
16. The exact cause of preeclampsia is unknown, but the underlying pathophysiology appears to be generalized vasospasm with increased peripheral resistance and vascular damage. This decreased perfusion results in damage to numerous organs.
17. Darken room, limit visitors, maintain close 1:1 nurse/client ratio, place in private room, plan nursing interventions all together so client is disturbed as little as possible.
18. No, oral hypoglycemic medications are teratogenic to the fetus. Insulin will be used.
19. *Maternal:* hypoglycemia, hyperglycemia, ketoacidosis. *Fetal:* macrosomia, hypoglycemia at birth, fetal anomalies.
20. Monitor for signs of blood loss. Continue to assess BP and DTRs every 4 hours. Monitor for uterine atony.
21. It is short-acting, predictable, can be infused intravenously, and can be discontinued quickly if necessary.
22. Preeclampsia, hydramnios, and infection.
23. No, therefore insulin-dependent women may breastfeed.
24. 60 to 100 mg/dL.
25. Diaphragm with spermicide. Avoid birth control pills that contain estrogen and IUDs, which are an infection risk.
26. Position client in a semi- or high-Fowler position. Prevent Valsalva maneuvers. Position client in a supine position or R/T for regional anesthesia. Avoid stirrups because of possible popliteal vein compression and decreased venous return.
27. Maternal lacerations, fetal cerebral trauma.
28. If a low uterine transverse incision was performed and can be documented *and* if the original complication does not recur—that is, CPD.
29. Paralytic ileus, infection, thromboembolism, respiratory complications, and impaired maternal infant bonding.

Postpartum Complications

Postpartum Infections

Description: Any clinical infection of the genital canal that occurs within 28 days of delivery.

Nursing Assessment (Data Collection)

A. Women predisposed to infection include those with:
1. Rupture of membranes more than 24 hours before delivery.
2. Any lacerations or operative incisions (forceps, episiotomy, or cesarean section).
3. Hemorrhage.
4. Hematomas.
5. Lapses in aseptic technique before or after delivery—for example, faulty perineal care.
6. Anemia or poor physical health before delivery.
7. Intrauterine manipulation, manual removal of placenta, retained placental fragments.
B. Puerperal morbidity:
1. Temperature of 100.4° F or higher
2. Occurs within the first 24 hours after delivery
3. Temperature elevation on two successive days or two successive 4-hour assessments
C. Signs of infection (see Assessment Data for Puerperal Infection, below).
D. Most common organisms are streptococcal and anaerobic organisms; least common organism is staphylococcus.

Assessment Data for Puerperal Infection

A. Perineal infection:
1. Temperature 101° to 104° F (38.3° to 40° C)
2. Red, swollen, very tender perineum (episiotomy site)
3. Purulent drainage, induration
B. Endometritis (infection of lining of uterus):
1. Temperature 101° to 102° F (38.3° to 39.9° C)
2. Pulse greater than 100
3. Malaise, anorexia
4. Excess fundal tenderness long after expected
5. Uterine subinvolution
6. Lochia return to rubra from serosa
7. Foul-smelling lochia
C. Parametritis (pelvic cellulites):
1. Temperature 103° to 104° F (39.4° to 40° C).
2. Tachycardia, tachypnea
3. Severe uterine and cervical tenderness
4. WBC >25,000
5. Palpable pelvic abscess
D. Peritonitis:
1. Chills and temperature to 105° F
2. Rapid, thready pulse to 140 bpm
3. Decreased urinary output
4. Paralytic ileus, abdominal distention, absence of bowel sounds
E. Thrombophlebitis (deep vein):
1. Minimal, if any, fever
2. Positive Homan sign
3. Pain in calf or dull ache in leg
4. Swelling in extremity below pain

F. Urinary tract infection/cystitis (bladder):
   1. Slight or no fever
   2. Dysuria, frequency, urgency, suprapubic tenderness
   3. Hematuria, bacteriuria
   4. Cloudy urine
G. Pyelonephritis (kidney):
   1. Temperature 102° F and higher, chills
   2. Flank pain and costovertebral angle tenderness
   3. Nausea and vomiting.
   4. Dysuria, urgency, cloudy urine, hematuria, bacteriuria
H. Mastitis (breast):
   1. Sore, cracked nipple
   2. Flulike symptoms: malaise, chills, and fever
   3. Red, warm lump in breast

Analysis (Nursing Diagnoses)

A. Risk for injury related to …
B. Deficient knowledge (specify) related to …
C. Pain related to …

Nursing Plans and Interventions

A. Implement general care pertinent to any client with a diagnosed infection:
   1. Use and reinforce teaching about good handwashing technique (HWT).
   2. Observe and record vital signs, especially temperature, every 4 hours or more often if indicated.
   3. Manage fever by increasing fluids, giving cool baths, administration of acetaminophen (Tylenol) orally or by suppository.
   4. Observe for signs of dehydration: inelastic skin turgor, dry mucous membranes, increased urine specific gravity.
   5. Maintain hydration: increase fluid intake to 2 to 3 L/day.
   6. Promote nutrition: basic four food groups and increase intake of vitamin C foods (for healing) and protein (for tissue repair).
   7. Emphasize need for adherence to medication regimen (take entire antibiotic series).
   8. Maintain cleanliness, personal hygiene.
   9. Implement medical and nursing interventions for specific diagnosed infections.
B. Perineal infection:
   1. Keep warm; may use hot water bottle in bed if chilled.
   2. Observe site daily for decrease in redness, pain, and discharge.
   3. Assist with sitz bath and peri lamp two to three times daily; encourage meticulous peri care.
   4. Administer antibiotics and analgesics as prescribed.
C. Endometritis:
   1. Usually maintain bed rest with bathroom privileges (Fowler or semi-Fowler position).
   2. Palpate fundus and abdomen every 8 hours to assess pain and involution.
   3. Assist with IV antibiotic administration, often using a heparin lock (Table 6-22, Antibiotics).
D. Parametritis:
   1. Promote lochial/uterine drainage by semi-Fowler position.
   2. Observe amount and odor of lochia (heavy, foul-smelling usually indicates anaerobic bacteria).
   3. Monitor for development of pelvic thrombophlebitis: clot in ovarian vein will cause acute abdominal pain.
   4. Assist with administration of IV antibiotics.

TABLE 6-22 Antibiotics

Drug	Indications	Adverse Reactions	Nursing Implications
Clindamycin	Broad-spectrum antibiotic used to treat postpartum endometritis	• Nausea, vomiting • GI irritation • Diarrhea	• Must be used in combination with gentamicin
Ampicillin-sulbactam (Unasyn)	Broad-spectrum antibiotic used to treat postpartum endometritis	• Rash, dermatitis • Nausea, vomiting • GI irritation	• Do not administer to clients with penicillin sensitivity • Alternative to clindamycin and gentamicin combination
Gentamicin sulfate (Garamycin)	Aminoglycoside antibiotic used for serious puerperal infections	• GI irritation • Nephrotoxicity • Ototoxicity • Neurotoxicity • Possible hypersensitivity	• Do not mix with any other drug • Observe for ototoxicity: ataxia, tinnitus, headache • Observe for nephrotoxicity: elevated BUN and creatinine • Observe for neurotoxicity: paresthesia, muscle weakness • Monitor I&O closely
Dicloxicillin Cephalexin (Keflex)	Broad-spectrum antibiotic used to treat lactational mastitis	• Rash, dermatitis • Nausea, vomiting	• Do not administer to clients with penicillin allergy

E. Peritonitis:
1. Client usually transferred to intensive care: medical emergency.
2. O$_2$ by mask.
3. Prepare client for IV antibiotics.
4. Insertion of nasogastric tube for gastric decompression, prevention of vomiting from paralytic ileus.
5. Observe abdomen three times daily for tympany, distention, and bowel sounds.
6. Monitor and document I&O.

F. Mastitis:
1. Obtain culture and sensitivity on breast milk.
2. Breastfeed every 2 to 3 hours and make sure breasts are emptied with each feed.
3. Do not abruptly cease breastfeeding unless health care provider prescribes.
4. May have to discontinue breastfeeding if pus is in breast milk or if antibiotic is contraindicated in breastfeeding. Mother should manually empty the breasts and discard the milk to maintain milk production and reduce congestion.
5. If newborn develops diarrhea, contact health care provider regarding changing antibiotic.
6. Usually treated at home by oral antibiotics.
7. Bed rest for 48 hours.
8. Monitor for abscess formation, need for incision and drainage.

G. Deep vein thrombophlebitis:
1. See Chapter 4, *Medical-Surgical Nursing*, p. 91, for interventions.
2. Administer anticoagulant therapy (heparin for 6 weeks) (see Table 4-15, *Anticoagulants*, p. 92).

H. Cystitis and pyelonephritis:
1. Collect urine for analysis and culture.
2. Avoid catheterization if at all possible.

I. Sexually transmitted infections (STIs):
1. See Chapter 4, *Medical-Surgical Nursing*, p. 157, for interventions.
2. Breastfeeding and rooming-in are affected when the mother has an STI (Table 6-23, *Breastfeeding/Rooming-In Procedures for Mothers with STIs*).

> **HESI Hint** • Clients taking anticoagulants can usually expect to have heavy menstrual periods.

> **HESI Hint** • Nurse must be especially supportive of postpartum client with infection because it usually implies isolation from newborn until organism is identified and treatment is begun. Arrange phone calls to nursery and window viewing. Involve family, spouse, and significant others in teaching, and encourage other family members to continue neonatal attachment activities.

> **HESI Hint** • Most common iatrogenic cause of UTI is urinary catheterization.
> • Encourage clients to void frequently and to not ignore the urge.
> • IV antibiotics are usually administered to clients with pyelonephritis.

> **HESI Hint** • Remember, the risk of postpartum infections increases for clients who experienced problems during pregnancy (e.g., anemia, diabetes) or who experienced trauma during labor and delivery.

Postpartum Hemorrhage

Description: A leading cause of maternal mortality that demands prompt recognition and intervention.

A. Hemorrhage can be caused by:
1. Uterine atony (poor muscle tone).
2. Lacerations of the vagina.
3. Cervix, perineum, or labia hematoma development.
4. Retained placental fragments.
5. Full bladder.

TABLE 6-23 Breastfeeding/Rooming-In Procedures for Mothers with STIs

STI	Rooming-In	Breastfeeding
AIDS/HIV positive	Yes	No
Cytomegalovirus (CMV)	Yes	No
Chlamydia	Yes	Yes
Gonorrhea (untreated)	No	No
Medication × 24 hr	Yes	Yes
Hepatitis	Yes	Yes
Herpes	Yes	Yes
Syphilis (untreated)	No	No
Medication × 24 hours	Yes	Yes
Trichomoniasis	Yes	Yes

> **HESI Hint** • In most cases, a mother who is on antibiotic therapy can continue to breastfeed unless the health care provider thinks the neonate is at risk for sepsis by maternal contact. Sulfa drugs are used cautiously in lactating mothers because they can be transferred to the infant in breast milk.

> **HESI Hint** • Many times mastitis can be confused with a blocked milk sinus, which is treated by nursing closer to the lump and by rotating the baby on the breast. Breastfeeding is not contraindicated for women with mastitis unless pus is in the breast milk or the antibiotic of choice is harmful to the infant. If either of these occurs, milk production can still be fostered by manual expression.

B. Predisposing factors include:
1. High parity.
2. Dystocia, prolonged labor.
3. Operative delivery: cesarean or forceps delivery; intrauterine manipulation.
4. Overdistention of the uterus: polyhydramnios, multiple gestations, large neonate.
5. Abruptio placentae.
6. Previous history of postpartum hemorrhage.
7. Infection.
8. Placenta previa.

Nursing Assessment (Data Collection)

A. Excessive uterine bleeding during the first hour following delivery (more than one saturated pad/15 min).
B. Excessive uterine bleeding during the postpartum period (more than one saturated pad/hour).
C. Blood loss of more than 500 mL during vaginal delivery, or loss of 1% or more of body weight (1 mL = 1 g).
D. Signs of hypovolemic shock:
1. Decreased blood pressure
2. Weak, rapid pulse
3. Cool, clammy skin, color ashen or gray
E. Signs of hematomas developing in perineum:
1. Intense perineal pain
2. Swelling and blue-black discoloration on perineum
3. Pallor, tachycardia, and hypotension (great blood loss); feeling of pressure in vagina, urethra, and bladder.
4. Possible urinary retention, uterine displacement
F. Signs of bleeding from unrepaired laceration:
1. Continuous trickle from vagina
2. Bleeding in spurts
3. Bleeding in presence of contracted fundus
G. Signs of bleeding from uterine atony:
1. Soft, boggy uterus, usually above umbilicus
2. Fundus does not firm up with massage

Analysis (Nursing Diagnoses)

A. Deficient fluid volume related to …
B. Anxiety related to …
C. Risk for infection related to …

Nursing Plans and Interventions

A. Early postpartum:
1. Review chart for predisposing factors.
2. Monitor vital signs, fundus, lochia every 15 min × 1 hour, every 30 min × 10 hours, every 1 hour × 2 hours per institutional policy.
3. Monitor level of consciousness.
4. Keep the bladder empty.
5. Call health care provider if atony/bleeding continues despite massage.
6. Anticipate an increase in Pitocin (oxytocin) IV infusion and/or administering ergot preparation IM.
7. Count pads saturated and time required to saturate.
8. Monitor I&O (at least 30 mL/hr output); be sure to maintain fluid replacement.
B. Late postpartum:
1. Anticipate quick hospitalization and determination of cause of bleeding.
2. Type and cross-match for possible blood transfusion.
3. Prepare for administration of oxytocic drugs and possibly ergot preparations as prescribed.
4. Administer antibiotics as prescribed.
5. Keep the client warm, and be alert to symptoms of shock.
6. Prepare the client for possible surgical repair of laceration, evacuation of hematomas, or curettage for removal of placental fragments (most common reason for late postpartum hemorrhage).
B. Hematoma development:
1. Apply ice pack to perineum to decrease swelling and pain.
2. Prepare client for surgical incision if hematoma is large.
3. Monitor vital signs closely.
4. Administer analgesics and antibiotics as prescribed.
5. If severe hemorrhage and hypovolemic shock occur, notify health care provider immediately and:
a. Monitor IV infusion.
b. Give O_2 by mask at 10 liters.
c. Monitor vital signs every 5 to 15 min.
d. Lower head of bed, position client supine.
e. Insert Foley catheter.
f. Prepare for vascular access and monitoring devices.

HESI Hint • During medical emergencies such as bleeding episodes, clients need calm, direct explanations and assurance that all is being done that can be done. If possible, allow support person at bedside. Risk-management principles state that the suit-prone client is one who feels that things are being hidden from her or that adequate attention is *not* being given to *her* problem.

HESI Hint • Risk factors for hemorrhage include dystocia, prolonged labor, overdistended uterus, abruptio placentae, and infection.

HESI Hint • What immediate nursing action should be taken when a postpartum hemorrhage is detected?
• Perform fundal massage.
• Notify the health care provider if the fundus does not become firm with massage.
• Count pads to estimate blood loss.
• Assess and record vital signs.
• Increase IV fluids (additional IV fluids may be indicated).
• Administer oxytocin infusion as prescribed.
• Initiate breastfeeding to allow natural oxytocin to be initiated.

Review of Postpartum Complications

1. May women with a positive HIV antibody try to test breastfeed?
2. What are the common side effects of antibiotics used to treat puerperal infection?
3. How does the nurse differentiate symptomatology of cystitis from pyelonephritis?
4. What are the signs of endometritis?
5. What are the nursing actions for endometritis and parametritis?
6. State four risk factors or predisposing factors to postpartum infection.
7. State four risk factors or predisposing factors to postpartum hemorrhage.
8. What immediate nursing actions should be taken when a postpartum hemorrhage is detected?
9. Must women diagnosed with mastitis stop breastfeeding?

Answers to Review

1. No, HIV has been found in breast milk (*New England Journal of Medicine*, August 1991).
2. GI adverse reactions: nausea, vomiting, diarrhea, and cramping. Hypersensitivity reactions: rashes, urticaria, and hives.
3. Pyelonephritis has the same symptoms as cystitis (dysuria, frequency, and urgency), with the addition of flank pain, fever, and pain at costovertebral angle.
4. Subinvolution (boggy, high uterus), lochia returns to rubra with possible foul smell, temperature 100.4° F or higher, and unusual fundal tenderness.
5. Measures to promote lochial drainage; antipyretic measures (acetaminophen, cool baths); administration of analgesics and antibiotics as prescribed; increase fluids with attention to high-protein/high–vitamin C diet.
6. Operative delivery, intrauterine manipulation, anemia or poor physical health, traumatic delivery, and hemorrhage.
7. Dystocia or prolonged labor, overdistention of the uterus, abruptio placentae, and infection.
8. Fundal massage. Notify health care provider if massage does *not* firm fundus. Count pads to estimate blood loss. Assess/record vital signs. Increase IV fluids and administer oxytocin infusion as prescribed.
9. No, women who abruptly stop breastfeeding may make the situation worse by increasing congestion/engorgement and providing further media for bacterial growth. Client may *have* to discontinue breastfeeding if pus is present or antibiotics are contraindicated for neonate.

Complications of the Newborn

Major Danger Signals in the Newborn

A. Sixty percent of neonates requiring special care at birth can be identified through the prenatal history and another 20% through a review of intrapartal risk factors.
B. Infants with Apgar scores of 7 to 10 rarely need resuscitative efforts, scores of 4 to 6 indicate mild to moderate asphyxia, and scores of 0 to 3 indicate severe asphyxia.
C. The family experiences extreme challenges in adapting to the crisis of a sick baby.

Danger Signs by System

A. Central nervous system: lethargy, high-pitched cry, jitteriness, seizures, and bulging fontanels.
B. Respiratory system: apnea (lack of breathing for 15 to 20 seconds), tachypnea, flaring nares, retractions, seesaw breathing, grunting, abnormal blood gases.
C. Cardiovascular system: abnormal rate and rhythm, persistent murmurs, differentials in pulse, dusky skin color, and circumoral cyanosis.

D. Gastrointestinal system: absent feeding reflexes, vomiting, abdominal distention, changes in stool patterns, and no stool.
E. Metabolic system: hypoglycemia, hypocalcemia, hyperbilirubinemia, labile temperature, infection.
F. Newborn weight is a major variable in determining survival:
  1. Low birth weight (LBW): 2500 g or less
  2. Very low birth weight (VLBW): 1500 g or less

HESI Hint "Jitteriness" is a clinical manifestation of hypoglycemia and hypocalcemia. Laboratory analysis is indicated to differentiate between the two etiologies.

HESI Hint To avoid metabolic problems brought on by cold stress, the first step—and number one priority—in management of the newborn is to prevent loss of body heat, followed by ABCs. Neonates produce heat by nonshivering thermogenesis, by burning brown fat. The neonate is easily stressed by hypothermia and develops acidosis from hypoxia. Prevent chilling (keep

Continued

under radiant warmer or in isolette). If cold, the first signs exhibited are prolonged acrocyanosis, skin mottling, tachycardia, and tachypnea. If cold stressed, warm slowly over 2 to 4 hours because rapid warming may produce apnea. The neonate needs glucose; he or she has little glycogen storage and needs to be fed.

Nursing Plans and Interventions for Management of Newborn Resuscitation

A. Assist with ventilations that are done over mouth and nose using a size 1 mask with a term neonate, size 0 for a preterm.

B. With neonates, initial ventilation with peak inflating pressures of 30 to 40 cm H_2O at a rate of 40 to 60/min is usually successful in unresponsive term infants.

C. If the heart rate is under 60, compressions are done with thumb side-by-side encircling the thorax and over the lower third of the sternum, to a depth of one third the A/P chest diameter with a compression to ventilation ratio of 3:1 to achieve 120 events per min (90 compressions plus 30 breaths).

D. Prepare for prescribed IV fluids (usually umbilical vein, may use peripheral vein).

E. Assist with administration of sodium bicarbonate and/or epinephrine as prescribed (Table 6-24, *Newborn Resuscitation*).

F. Assist with administration of glucose as prescribed (stress rapidly causes hypoglycemia).

G. Support parents during resuscitation.

H. Resuscitative efforts may be evaluated by the Silverman-Anderson Index of Respiratory Distress. Five criteria are graded, so observe and monitor respiration effort:
1. Upper chest synchronization
2. Lower chest retractions
3. Xiphoid retractions
4. Nares dilation (flaring)
5. Expiratory grunt

HESI Hint • The lower score on the Silverman-Anderson Index of Respiratory Distress, the better the respiratory status of the neonate. A score of 10 indicates

Continued

that a newborn is in severe respiratory distress. This is the exact *opposite* of the method used for Apgar scoring.

Oxygen Therapy for the Newborn

Nursing Plans and Interventions

A. Principle: always administer O_2 at the lowest concentration possible to correct hypoxia. Use an O_2 analyzer to determine exact O_2 concentration. Oxygen is a "drug." Hypoxia and hyperoxia are both dangerous.

B. O_2 toxicity results in:
1. Retinopathy of prematurity (retrolental fibroplasias).
2. Bronchopulmonary dysplasia.

C. Monitor O_2 administration to the newborn via:
1. Oxyhood: concentrations up to 100%.
2. Nasal prongs: low concentrations.

D. Closely monitor the partial pressure of O_2 in the newborn's arterial blood—that is, Po_2.

E. Monitor oxygenation saturation using pulse oximetry. It has a direct relationship to the partial pressure of O_2 in the arterial blood. Oxygen saturation should *not* fall below 90 mm Hg.

HESI Hint • *Watch* the newborn Hct. It is difficult to oxygenate either an anemic newborn (lack of oxygen-carrying capacity) or a newborn with polycythemia (Hct >80%, thick, sluggish circulation).

HESI Hint • The Po_2 should be maintained between 50 and 90 mm Hg. Po_2 less than 50 signifies hypoxia; Po_2 greater than 90 signifies oxygen toxicity problems.

Neonate with an Infection

Infections in the infant can be overwhelming because of the immaturity of the immune system.

TABLE 6-24 **Newborn Resuscitation**

Drug	Indications	Adverse Reactions	Nursing Implications
Sodium bicarbonate	Correction of severe metabolic acidosis in asphyxiated infants after adequate ventilation begun	• Fluid overload • Hypernatremia • Intracranial hemorrhage	• Do not mix with calcium solutions; causes precipitate • Use *pediatric* concentration of the drug • Infuse slowly and monitor I&O
Epinephrine	Asystole or severe bradycardia	• Tachydysrhythmias	• Make sure ventilation of newborn is adequate • Do not inject directly into artery • Monitor apical pulse or connect to ECG before use

Nursing Assessment (Data Collection)

A. Lethargy
B. Temperature instability
C. Difficulty feeding
D. Subtle color changes; mottling, duskiness
E. "Just acts funny;" subtle changes in behavior
F. Respiratory distress, apnea
G. Hyperbilirubinemia

Analysis (Nursing Diagnoses)

A. Ineffective thermoregulation related to …
B. Risk for injury related to …

Nursing Plans and Interventions

A. Prevent infection in the newborn by:
   1. Meticulous handwashing: 3 minutes before day begins, 1 minute in between each baby.
   2. Perform cord care according to institutional policy (triple-dye antimicrobial, alcohol, etc.).
   3. Maintain sterile technique during procedures.
   4. Avoid rings and other jewelry in nursery.
   5. Do not wear acrylic nails in nursery.
   6. During contact with body secretions, use universal precautions
   7. Document IV site appearance.
   8. Watch skin integrity: use little tape; use sheepskin, waterbed, and ROM.
   9. Staff member with *any* herpes lesion that has *not* reached the crusting stage should not be in the nursery.
   10. Maintain adequate nutrition: calculate calorie, protein, and fluid needs according to weight.
B. If neonate develops signs of sepsis:
   1. Prepare isolation room.
   2. Assist RN and health care provider with a sepsis workup: blood cultures, spinal tap, urine collection, chest x-ray, chemistry, and CBC with differential.

> **HESI Hint** • Antibiotic dosage is based on the neonate's weight in kilograms. Peak and trough drug levels are drawn to evaluate whether therapeutic drug levels have been achieved. Closely monitor the neonate for adverse effects of all drugs.

Hyperbilirubinemia

Definition: Hyperbilirubinemia is excessive accumulation of bilirubin (usually unconjugated) in the blood because of red blood cell hemolysis.

Nursing Assessment (Data Collection)

A. Predisposing risk factors:
   1. Rh incompatibility
   2. ABO incompatibility
   3. IUGR pitocin induction
   4. Prematurity
   5. Sepsis
   6. Perinatal asphyxia
   7. Maternal diabetes mellitus or intrauterine infections
   8. Cephalohematoma
B. Jaundice: sclera, skin (if whole body is yellow *or* palms are yellow, there is a danger of kernicterus, bilirubin encephalopathy, resulting from bilirubin deposition in brain).
C. Total bilirubin determinations:
   1. Level increases more than 5 mg/day.
   2. Term: level greater than 12 mg/dL.
   3. LBW: level 10 to 12 mg/dL or greater.
   4. Preterm: level greater than 5 mg (more sensitive to kernicterus at lower bilirubin concentrations).
D. Positive direct Coombs test: indicates presence of maternal antibody on the fetal RBC (an indication of sensitization). If greater than 1:64, an exchange transfusion is indicated.
E. Increased reticulocyte count usually indicates ABO incompatibility.
F. Anemia.
G. Urine/stools may be dark.

Analysis (Nursing Diagnoses)

A. Risk for injury related to …
B. Impaired gas exchange related to …
C. Anxiety (parental) related to …

Nursing Plans and Interventions

A. Notify registered nurse of any abnormal assessment factors present.
B. Assist RN with prescribed phototherapy. Phototherapy decomposes bilirubin in the skin through oxidation.
   1. Place unclothed neonate 18 inches below a bank of lights for several hours or days until bilirubin levels fall below 12 mg/dL.
   2. Place opaque mask over eyes to prevent retinal damage.
   3. Monitor skin temperature.
   4. Cover genitals with a small diaper or mask to catch urine/stool while leaving skin surface open to light.
   5. Turn every 2 hours to avoid skin breakdown.
   6. Turn off the lights for 5 to 15 minutes every 8 hours to assess for conjunctivitis.
   7. Monitor for signs of dehydration.
C. Maintain hydration: nipple, gavage feedings, and monitor IV fluids.
D. Assist with exchange transfusion.
E. Promote excretion of bilirubin through feeding and stools.
F. BiliBed or blanket are frequently used to allow rooming-in or home phototherapy (no need for eye patches).

HESI Hint • To assess for skin jaundice, apply pressure with thumb over bony prominences to blanch skin. After thumb is removed, the area will look yellow before normal skin color reappears. The best areas for assessment are the nose, forehead, and sternum. In dark-skinned infants, observe conjunctival sac and oral mucosa.

HESI Hint • Lab tests measure total and direct (conjugated, excretable, nonfat soluble) bilirubin levels. The dangerous bilirubin is the unconjugated, indirect (fat-soluble) bilirubin, which is measured by subtracting the direct from the total bilirubin.

HESI Hint • Maintenance of hydration is crucial for all infants. The preterm infant is already at risk for fluid and electrolyte imbalances because of increased body surface area from extended body positioning and larger body area in relation to body weight. Phototherapy treatment for hyperbilirubinemia (level greater than 12 mg/dL) increases the risk for dehydration.

Substance Abuse Effects on the Neonate

Effects on the neonate from maternal substance abuse are related to the substance as well as the amount of the substance abused.

Cigarette Smoking

Nursing Assessment (Data Collection)
A. Small neonate.
B. IUGR (increases with the number of cigarettes smoked).
C. Neonates of mothers who are exposed to smoke-filled environments are also at risk.

Nursing Plans and Interventions
A. Reinforce teaching for the antepartum client that IUGR can be minimized or eliminated when smoking is stopped early in pregnancy.
B. Consider the infant as a small-for-gestational-age infant.

Narcotic Use

Nursing Assessment (Data Collection)
A. Neonatal narcotic withdrawal syndrome:
  1. Irritability, hyperactivity
  2. High-pitched cry
  3. Coarse, flapping tremors
  4. Poor feeding, frantic sucking, vomiting/diarrhea
  5. Nasal stuffiness

Nursing Plans and Interventions
A. Swaddle and minimize handling.
B. Decreased environmental stimuli.
C. Provide pacifier.
D. Position on sheepskin.
E. Cover elbows, knees to prevent skin breakdown.
F. Keep bulb syringe close at hand.

Alcohol Intake

Nursing Assessment (Data Collection)
A. Fetal alcohol syndrome (FAS):
  1. Microcephaly
  2. Growth retardation
  3. Short palpebral fissures
  4. Maxillary hypoplasia
B. Long-term complications of FAS:
  1. Mental retardation
  2. Poor coordination
  3. Facial abnormalities
  4. Behavioral deviations (irritability)
  5. Cardiac and joint abnormalities
C. The combined effects of cigarette smoking and alcohol consumption during pregnancy cause greater fetal anomalies than the sum of their individual effects.

Nursing Plans and Interventions
A. Determine how much and how often the mother drank alcoholic beverages during pregnancy and/or while breastfeeding (alcohol intake has serious harmful effects on the fetus, especially when consumed during the 16th to 18th weeks of pregnancy).
B. Decrease environmental stimuli.
C. Assist with enteral feedings if neonate has incoordinate sucking and swallowing.

Review of Complications of the Newborn

1. List the major CNS danger signals that occur in the neonate.
2. A baby is delivered blue, limp, and with a heart rate less than 100. The nurse dries the infant, suctions the oropharynx, and gently stimulates the infant while blowing O_2 over the face. The infant still does not respond. What is the next nursing action?
3. What does the Silverman-Anderson Index measure?
4. What are the two major complications of O_2 toxicity?
5. Intraventricular hemorrhage is more common in _____ and results in symptoms of _____.
6. What conditions make oxygenation of the newborn more difficult?

7. What parameters can the nurse observe to prevent problems oxygenating the newborn?
8. What are the cardinal symptoms of an infection in a newborn?
9. List risk factors for hyperbilirubinemia.
10. List symptoms of hyperbilirubinemia in the neonate.
11. List three nursing interventions for the neonate undergoing phototherapy.
12. List the symptoms of neonatal narcotic withdrawal.
13. Neonates who are "sick" are prone to receive too much stimulation in the form of invasive procedures and handling, and too little developmentally appropriate stimulation and affection. How might such an infant respond?
14. What characteristics would the nurse expect to see in a neonate with fetal alcohol syndrome?

Answers to Review

1. Lethargy, high-pitched cry, jitteriness, seizures, and bulging fontanels.
2. Begin oxygenation by bag and mask at 30 breaths/min. If heart rate is less than 60, start cardiac massage at 120 events/min: 30 breaths and 90 compressions. Assist health care provider in setting up for intubation procedure.
3. Respiratory difficulty.
4. Retrolental fibroplasias and bronchopulmonary dysplasia.
5. Premature neonates and VLBW babies; increased intracranial pressure.
6. Respiratory distress syndrome: alveolar prematurity/lack of surfactant, anemia, and polycythemia.
7. Po_2 50 to 90, Sao_2 60 to 80 mm Hg.
8. Lethargy, temperature instability, difficulty feeding, subtle color changes, subtle behavioral changes, and hyperbilirubinemia.
9. Rh incompatibility, ABO incompatibility, prematurity, sepsis, and perinatal asphyxia.
10. Bilirubin levels rising 5 mg/day, jaundice, dark urine, anemia, high reticulocyte (RBC) count, and dark stools.
11. Apply opaque mask over eyes. Leave diaper loose so stools/urine can be monitored. Turn every 2 hours. Watch for dehydration.
12. Irritability, hyperactivity, high-pitched cry, frantic sucking, coarse flapping tremors, and poor feeding.
13. Failure to thrive, lack of crying.
14. Microcephaly, growth retardation, short palpebral fissures, and maxillary hypoplasia.

7

PSYCHIATRIC NURSING

Therapeutic Communication

Description: Therapeutic communication is the exchange of verbal and nonverbal interactions between health care providers and clients for a goal-directed purpose.

A. Communication is the primary tool used in the delivery of psychiatric nursing care and all nurse–client interactions (Table 7-1, *Helpful Techniques*).

B. The focus of therapeutic interaction is to assist the client with gaining insight into thoughts, feelings, and behaviors (Table 7-2, *Useful and Nontherapeutic Phrases*).

Coping Styles (Defense Mechanisms)

Description: Coping styles are automatic psychologic processes that protect the individual from anxiety and the awareness of internal and external dangers or stressors. The individual may or may not be aware of these processes (Table 7-3, *Coping Styles [Defense Mechanisms]*).

Treatment Modalities

Description: Treatment modalities are psychiatric/mental health treatment modalities used to promote mental health.

> **HESI Hint** · The nurse should be aware that all behavior has meaning.

Types of Treatment Modalities

A. Milieu therapy:
1. It is the planned use of people, resources, and activities in the environment to assist with improving interpersonal skills, social functioning, and activities of daily living, as well as safety and protection for all clients.
2. The focus is on the here and now (i.e., assisting the client to deal with the realities of today rather than focusing on situations and behaviors of the past).
3. It uses limit setting.

4. It involves the client in making decisions about his or her own care.
5. It uses activities that support group sharing, cooperation, and compromise (e.g., unit government groups).
6. Nursing interventions support client privacy and autonomy and give clear expectations.

B. Behavior modification:
1. It is a process used to change ineffective behavior patterns. It focuses on consequences for actions rather than peer pressure.
2. Positive reinforcement is used to strengthen desired behavior (e.g., a client is praised or given a token that can be exchanged for a treat or a desired activity).
3. Negative reinforcement is used to decrease or eliminate inappropriate behavior (e.g., ignoring undesirable behavior, removing a token or privilege, "time out").
4. Role modeling, teaching, and reinforcement of new behaviors are important interventions.

C. Family therapy:
1. It is a form of group therapy that identifies the entire family as the client.
2. It is based on the concept of the family as a system of interrelated parts forming a whole.
3. The focus is on the patterns of interaction within the family and not on any one individual member.
4. The therapist assists the family in identifying roles assigned to each member based on family rules.
5. Life scripts (living out parents' dreams) and self-fulfilling prophecies (unconsciously following what one thinks should happen, therefore setting it up to happen) are identified.
6. Congruent and incongruent communication patterns and behaviors are identified.
7. The goal is to decrease family conflict and anxiety and to develop appropriate role relationships.

D. Crisis intervention:
1. It is a form of therapy that is directed at the resolution of an immediate crisis that the individual is unable to handle alone.

TABLE 7-1 Helpful Techniques

Technique	Description
Acknowledgment	Recognizing the client's opinions and/or statements without imposing your own values and judgments
Clarifying	The process of making sure you understood the meaning of what was said
Confrontation	Calling attention to inconsistent behavior, information shared or not shared
Focusing	Assisting the client to explore a specific topic
Information-giving	Feedback about client's observed behavior
Open-ended questions	Questions that require more than a "Yes" or "No" response
Reflecting/restating	Paraphrasing/repeating what the client said. (Be careful not to overuse; client will feel as though you are not listening.)
Silence	Can be therapeutic or can be used to control interaction. Use carefully with paranoid client; may be misinterpreted or could be used to support paranoid ideation
Suggesting	Offering alternatives (e.g., "Have you ever considered … ?")

HESI Hint • The purpose of therapeutic interaction with clients is to allow them the autonomy to make choices when appropriate. Keep statements value free, advice free, and reassurance free. Remember, just the facts. No opinions.

HESI Hint • What action should the nurse take in a psychiatric situation when the client describes a physical problem? Monitor! If the client with paranoid schizophrenia on the psychiatric unit complains of chest pain, take his or her vital signs and report this to the RN or primary health care provider. If the OB client who has delivered a dead fetus complains of perineal pain, look at the perineal area (she may have a hematoma). Just because the focus of the client's situation is on his or her psychologic needs, it does not mean that the nurse can ignore physiologic needs.

TABLE 7-2 Useful and Nontherapeutic Phrases

Description	Examples
Useful Phrases	
• These are phrases that are useful in therapeutic interactions. • Keep the interaction open, genuine, and client-centered. • Keep the client as the focus. • Be aware of your own feelings and anxiety level.	• "Tell me about …" • "Go on …" • "I'd like to discuss what you're thinking …" • "What are your thoughts …" • "Are you saying that …" • "What are you feeling?" or "I'd be interested to know how you're feeling." • "It seems as if …"
Nontherapeutic Responses/Responses to Avoid	
• These are phrases that should not be used when interacting with clients. Avoid them at all costs (especially if they appear on an exam). • Avoid social interaction, clichés, and saying too much. • Avoid changing subjects. • Avoid words such as "good," "bad," "right," "wrong," and "nice."	• "You should …" • "You'll have to …" • "You can't …" • "If it were me, I'd …" • "Why don't you …" • "I think you …" • "It's the policy on this unit." • "Don't worry." • "Everyone …" • "Why … ?" • "Just a second …" • "I know …"

HESI Hint • Remember, nurses are nice people, but they are also therapeutic.

HESI Hint • Basic communication principles can be applied to all clients:
• Establish trust.
• Demonstrate a nonjudgmental attitude.
• Offer self; be empathetic, *not* sympathetic.
• Use active listening.
• Accept and support client's feelings.
• Clarify and validate client's statement.
• Use a matter-of-fact approach.
• Be aware of body language.

HESI Hint • Remember, a nurse's nonverbal communication may be more important than his or her verbal communication.

HESI Hint • A question concerning nurse-client confidentiality often appears on the NCLEX-PN. If the nurse tells a client that she or he will not tell anyone about their discussion, it puts the nurse in a difficult position. Some information *must* be shared with other team members for the client's safety (e.g., suicide plan) and optimal therapy.

2. A crisis may develop when previously learned coping mechanisms are ineffective in dealing with the current problem.
3. The individual is usually in a state of disequilibrium.
4. If the client is in a panic state as a result of the disorganization, be very directive.

TABLE 7-3 Coping Styles (Defense Mechanisms)

Style	Description	Example
Denial	Unconscious failure to acknowledge an event, thought, or feeling that is too painful for conscious awareness	A woman diagnosed with cancer tells her family all the tests were negative.
Displacement	The transference of feelings to another person or object	After being scolded by his supervisor at work, a man comes home and kicks the dog for barking.
Identification	Attempt to be like someone or emulate the personality, traits, or behaviors of another person	A teenage boy dresses and behaves like his favorite singer.
Intellectualization	Using reason to avoid emotional conflicts	A wife of a substance abuser describes, in detail, the dynamics of enabling behavior, yet continues to call her husband's place of work to report his Monday morning absence as an "illness."
Introjection	Incorporation of values or qualities of an admired person or group into one's own ego structure	A young man deals with a business client in the same fashion his father deals with business clients.
Isolation	Separation of an unacceptable feeling, idea, or impulse from one's thought process	A nurse working in an emergency room is able to care for the seriously injured by isolating or separating her feelings and emotions related to the clients' pain, injuries, or death.
Passive-aggression	Indirectly expressing aggression toward others; a facade of overt compliance masks covert resentment	An employee arrives late to a meeting and disrupts others after being reminded of the meeting earlier that day and promising to be on time.
Projection	Attributing one's own thoughts or impulses to another person	A student who has sexual feelings toward her teacher tells her friends the teacher is "coming on to her."
Rationalization	Offering an acceptable, logical explanation to make unacceptable feelings and behavior acceptable	A student who did not do well in a course says it was poorly taught and the course content was not important anyway.
Reaction formation	Development of conscious attitudes and behaviors that are opposite of what is really felt	A person who dislikes animals does volunteer work for the Humane Society.
Regression	Reverting to an earlier level of development when anxious or highly stressed	After moving to a new home, a 6-year-old starts wetting the bed.
Repression	The involuntary exclusion of a painful thought or memory from awareness	A young man whose mother died when he was 12 cannot tell you how old he was or the year she died.
Sublimation	Substitution of an unacceptable feeling with a more socially acceptable one	A student who feels too small to play football becomes a champion marathon swimmer.
Suppression	The intentional exclusion of feelings and ideas	When about to lose Tara, Scarlett O'Hara says, "I'll think about it tomorrow."
Undoing	Communication or behavior done to negate a previously unacceptable act	A young man who used to hunt wild animals now chairs a committee for the protection of animals.

5. Focus on the problem, not the cause.
6. Identify support systems.
7. Identify past-coping patterns used in other stressful situations.
8. The goal is to return the individual to precrisis level of functioning.
9. Crisis intervention is usually limited to 6 weeks.

E. Cognitive therapy:
   1. It is directed at replacing clients' irrational beliefs and distorted attitudes with more appropriate responses.
   2. It is focused, problem-solving therapy.
   3. The therapist and client work together to identify and solve problems and overcome difficulties.

4. It is short term, of 2 to 3 months' duration.
5. It involves cognitive restructuring.
F. Electroconvulsive therapy (ECT) and electroshock therapy (EST):
   1. **Description:** Use of electrically induced seizures for psychiatric purposes. Used with severely depressed clients who fail to respond to antidepressant medication and therapy. May be used with extremely suicidal clients because 2 weeks are needed for antidepressants to take effect.
   2. Most times ECT takes place in a treatment suite, and then the client is taken to a recovery area.
   3. Nursing care before ECT. (Practical nurses [PNs] assist with care as dictated by the practical nurse scope of practice and by the agency's policies and procedures.)
      a. An informed consent must have been signed by the client or a legally designated person if the client is unable to sign.
      b. Prepare client by reinforcing teaching regarding what the treatment involves.
      c. Avoid the word "shock" when discussing treatment with client and family.
      d. Anticholinergic (e.g., atropine sulfate) is usually given 30 minutes before treatment to dry oral secretions.
      e. A quick-acting muscle relaxant (e.g., Anectine) or a general anesthetic agent is usually given to client before the ECT. This helps prevent any bone or muscle damage.
      f. Have an emergency cart, suction equipment, and O_2 available in the room.
   4. Nursing care after ECT:
      a. Maintain patent airway; client is in an unconscious state immediately after ECT.
      b. Check vital signs every 15 minutes until client is alert.
      c. Reorient client after ECT. (Client is usually confused on awakening, and short-term memory impairment may occur.)
      d. Common complaints after ECT include:
         (1) Headache
         (2) Muscle soreness
         (3) Nausea
         (4) Confusion

HESI Hint • Nausea is a common complaint after ECT. Vomiting by the unconscious client can lead to aspiration. Because post-ECT clients are unconscious, the nurse must observe closely for the possibility of aspiration—that is, MAINTAIN A PATENT AIRWAY!

G. Group intervention:
   1. **Description:** Process involving two or more clients who will develop an interactive relationship and share at least one common issue or goal.
   2. Types of groups:
      a. The groups may be closed (set group) or open (new members may join).
      b. The groups may be small or large (more than 10 members).
      c. The specific purpose of the group may be psychoeducation, supportive therapy, psychotherapy, or self-help.
      d. Common nurse-led intervention groups include use of medication, symptom management, anger management, and self-care.
   3. Phases of group therapy:
      a. Initial/orientation phase characterized by:
         (1) High anxiety.
         (2) Superficial interactions.
         (3) Testing the therapist to see whether he or she can be trusted.
      b. Middle/working phase characterized by:
         (1) Problem identification.
         (2) Beginning of problem solving.
         (3) Beginning of the group sense of "we."
      c. Termination phase characterized by:
         (1) Evaluation of experience.
         (2) Expression of feelings ranging from anger to joy.
   4. Advantages:
      a. Develops socializing techniques.
      b. Provides the opportunity to try new behaviors.
      c. Promotes a feeling of universality (i.e., not being alone with problems).
      d. Provides an opportunity for feedback from the group, which may correct distorted perceptions.
      e. Provides clients alternate ways to analyze and deal with problems.

Review of Therapeutic Communication and Treatment Modalities

1. After the fourth group meeting, the informal leader makes a statement that she believes she can help the group more than the assigned facilitator and has better credentials. Identify the group dynamics and stage of development.
2. On an in-patient psychiatric unit, clients are expected to get up at a certain time, attend breakfast at a certain time, and come for their medication at the correct time. What form of therapy is incorporated into this unit?
3. The wife of a man killed in a motor vehicle accident has just arrived at the emergency room and is told of her husband's death. What nursing actions are appropriate for dealing with this crisis?

4. A 10-year-old boy is admitted to the children's unit of the psychiatric facility after stabbing his sister. His behavior is extremely aggressive with the other children on the unit. Using a behavior modification approach with positive reinforcement, design a treatment plan for this child.
5. The 10-year-old boy, his sister, his mother, and his mother's live-in boyfriend are asked to attend a therapy meeting. Who is the "client" who will be treated during this session?
6. A 66-year-old woman is admitted to the psychiatric unit with agitated depression. She has not responded to antidepressants in the past. What would be the medical treatment of choice for this client?
7. Describe the nursing interventions used to care for a client during and after electroconvulsive therapy.

Answers to Review

1. The informal leader is "testing," which is a behavior indicative of a new group trying to establish trust. This group is still in the orientation phase of development.
2. Milieu.
3. Take her to a quiet room, and ask her if there are family, friends, or clergy you can call for her. Stay with her, be firm and directive, and identify her previous successful coping strategies.
4. Assess what activities he enjoys. Set up a token system: When he displays nonaggressive behavior, he earns a token good toward participating in the activity selected. He loses a token when he becomes aggressive.
5. The entire family.
6. Electroconvulsive therapy (ECT).
7. Maintain patent airway. Check vital signs every 15 minutes until client is alert. Remain with client after treatment until client is conscious. Reorient if client is confused.

Anxiety

Description: Anxiety is unexplained discomfort, tension, apprehension, or uneasiness that occurs when a person feels a threat to self. The threat may be real or imagined and is a very subjective experience.

Levels of Anxiety

A. Mild anxiety:
1. Is associated with daily life; motivates learning.
2. Produces increased level of sensory awareness and alertness.
3. Allows for thoughts that are logical; client is able to concentrate and problem solve.
4. Permits client to appear calm and in control.
B. Moderate anxiety:
1. Continues to motivate learning with assistance from others.
2. Allows client to be attentive and able to focus and problem solve, but not at optimal level.
3. Dulls perceptions of sensory stimuli; client becomes hesitant.
4. Causes client's speech rate and volume to increase; client becomes wordy.
5. Produces restlessness in client (frequent body movements and gestures).
6. May be converted to physical symptoms such as headaches, nausea, diarrhea, and tachycardia.

C. Severe anxiety:
1. Stimulates "fight or flight" response.
2. Causes sensory stimuli input to be disorganized.
3. May cause perceptions to be distorted.
4. Impairs concentration and problem-solving ability.
5. Results in selective attention; focuses on only one detail.
6. Verbalizes emotional pain—for example, "I need help; I can't stand this."
7. May cause tremors, increased motor activity—for example, pacing, wringing hands.
D. Panic:
1. Causes perceptions to be grossly distorted, unable to differentiate between real and unreal.
2. Brings about client's inability to concentrate or problem solve; causes loss of rational, logical thinking.
3. Produces feelings of being overwhelmed, helpless.
4. Results in loss of control; inability to function.
5. Can elicit behaviors of anger, aggression, withdrawal, clinging, and crying.
6. Requires immediate intervention.

HESI Hint Common physiologic responses to anxiety include increased heart rate and blood pressure; rapid, shallow respirations; dry mouth, tight feeling in throat; tremors, muscle tension; anorexia; urinary frequency; and palmar sweating.

> **HESI Hint** · Anxiety is very contagious and is easily transferred from client to nurse *and* from nurse to client. *First,* the nurse must assess his or her own level of anxiety and remain calm. A calm nurse assists the client to gain control, decrease anxiety, and increase feelings of security.

Anxiety Disorders

Generalized Anxiety Disorders

Description: Unrealistic, excessive, and/or persistent (lasting 6 months or longer) anxiety and worry about two or more life circumstances. Previously learned coping mechanisms are inadequate to deal with this level of anxiety. Multiple etiologic theories exist, including but not limited to neurobiochemical and psychodynamic theories.

Nursing Assessment (Data Collection)

A. Severe anxiety
B. Motor tension:
   1. Restlessness
   2. Easily fatigued
   3. Feelings of shakiness
   4. Tension
C. Autonomic hyperactivity:
   1. Shortness of breath
   2. Heart palpitations
   3. Dizziness
   4. Diaphoresis
   5. Frequent urination
D. Vigilance and scanning:
   1. Difficulty concentrating
   2. Sleep disturbance
   3. Irritability, easily angered
E. "On edge," appearance of being nervous
F. Low self-esteem

Analysis (Nursing Diagnosis)

A. Anxiety related to …
B. Ineffective coping related to …
C. Disturbed sleep pattern related to …
D. Imbalanced nutrition: less than/more than body requirements related to …

Nursing Plans and Interventions

A. Observe client to recognize anxiety and label the feeling (e.g., "What are you feeling now?").
B. Help client identify the relationship between the stressor and the level of anxiety.
C. Provide opportunities to learn and test different adaptive coping responses.
D. Encourage exercise, deep-breathing techniques, visualization, relaxation techniques, and biofeedback.

E. Decrease environmental stimuli.
F. Remain with client until client is calmer.
G. Administer medications as ordered by the health care provider (Table 7-4, *Antianxiety Drugs*).

Panic Disorders/Phobias

A. These are discrete periods of intense fear or discomfort that are unexpected and may be incapacitating.
B. It is characterized by an irrational fear of an external object, activity, or situation and feelings of impending doom.
C. A chronic condition that has exacerbations and remissions.
D. The client transfers anxiety or fear from its source to a symbolic object, idea, or situation.
E. The client recognizes that the fear is excessive and unrealistic but "can't help it."

Common Phobias

A. Acrophobia: fear of heights
B. Agoraphobia: fear of crowds or open places
C. Claustrophobia: fear of closed-in places
D. Hydrophobia: fear of water
E. Nyctophobia: fear of the dark
F. Thanatophobia: fear of death

Nursing Assessment (Data Collection)

A. Coping styles used (see Table 7-3):
   1. Displacement
   2. Projection
   3. Repression
   4. Sublimation
   5. Additional coping styles listed (see Table 7-3)
B. Autonomic hyperactivity
C. Panic attacks usually peak at 10 minutes but can last up to 30 minutes with a gradual return to normal functioning.
D. Disruption in personal life as well as work life
E. Possible use of alcohol and drugs to decrease anxiety

Analysis (Nursing Diagnoses)

A. Ineffective coping related to …
B. Social isolation related to …

> **HESI Hint** · When a client describes a phobia or expresses an unreasonable fear, the nurse should acknowledge the feeling (fear) and refrain from exposing the client to the identified fear. After trust is established, a desensitization process may be prescribed.
> Desensitization is the nursing intervention for phobia disorders. The nurse should:
> • Assist client to recognize factors associated with feared stimuli that precipitate a phobic response.

Continued

- Collaborate with RN to reinforce teaching and practice with client alternative adaptive coping strategies, such as the use of thought substitution (replacing a fearful thought with a pleasant thought) and relaxation techniques. Role-playing is useful when the client is in a calm state.
- Expose client progressively to feared stimuli, offering support with the nurse's presence.
- Provide positive reinforcement whenever a decrease in phobic reaction occurs.
- NOTE: In all likelihood, the desensitization process will be overseen by a mental health practitioner (nurse practitioner [NP], psychiatric clinical nurse specialist [CNS], or psychologist).

HESI Hint • The nurse should place an anxious client where there are reduced environmental stimuli—a quiet area of the unit, away from the nurse's station.

Nursing Plans and Interventions

A. Establish trust; listen, use calm approach and direct, simple questions.
B. Provide safe environment.
C. Draw client's attention away from feared object/situation.
D. Remain with client; do not leave client alone.
E. Reinforce and encourage use of alternative coping strategies.
F. Suggest substitution of positive thoughts for negative ones.
G. Assist in desensitizing client.
H. Encourage sharing of fears and feelings with others.
I. Administer antianxiety medications as prescribed (see Table 7-4).
J. Administer selective serotonin reuptake inhibitors (SSRIs) or other medications as prescribed (see Table 7-6).
K. Encourage client to decrease intake of caffeine and nicotine.
L. Report client responses to the mental health practitioner directing care.

TABLE 7-4 Antianxiety Drugs

Drugs	Indications	Reactions	Nursing Implications
Benzodiazepines			
• Chlordiazepoxide HCl (Librium) • Diazepam (Valium) • Alprazolam (Xanax) • Clorazepate dipotassium (Tranxene) • Lorazepam (Ativan)	• Reduce anxiety • Induce sedation, relax muscles, inhibit convulsions • Treat alcohol and drug withdrawal symptoms • Safer than sedative-hypnotics	• Sedation • Drowsiness • Ataxia • Dizziness • Irritability • Blood dyscrasias • Habituation and increased tolerance	• Administer at bedtime to alleviate daytime sedation. • Greatest harm occurs when combined with alcohol or other CNS depressants. • Instruct to avoid driving or working around equipment. • Gradually taper drug therapy due to withdrawal effects; do not stop suddenly. • Used only as short-term drug and as supplement to other medications.
Nonbenzodiazepines			
• Buspirone (BuSpar)	• Reduces anxiety • Helps to control symptoms such as insomnia, sweating, and palpitations associated with anxiety	• Dizziness	• Takes several weeks for antianxiety effects to become apparent. • Intended for short-term use.
• Zolpidem (Ambien)	• Used for short-term treatment of insomnia	• Daytime drowsiness	• Give with food 1 to 1½ hours before bedtime.
• Ramelteon (Rozerem)	• Approved for long-term treatment of insomnia • Selectively binds to melatonin receptors	• Dizziness	• Appropriate for clients with delayed sleep onset.

Obsessive-Compulsive Disorder

Description: Anxiety associated with repetitive thoughts (obsession) or irresistible impulses (compulsion) to perform an action. Fear of losing control is a major symptom of this disorder.

Nursing Assessment (Data Collection)

A. Use of coping styles to control anxiety (see Table 7-3):
   1. Repression
   2. Isolation
   3. Undoing
B. Magical thinking (belief that one's thoughts or wishes can control other people or events).
C. Evidence of destructive, hostile, aggressive, and delusional thought content.
D. Difficulty with interpersonal relationships.
E. Interference with normal activities (e.g., a client who "must" wash her hands all morning and cannot take her children to school).
F. Safety issues involved in repetitive performance of the ritualistic activity (e.g., dermatitis may occur as a result of the continuous washing of hands).
G. Recurring intrusive thoughts.
H. Recurring, repetitive behaviors that interfere with normal functioning.

Analysis (Nursing Diagnoses)

A. Ineffective coping related to …
B. Social isolation related to …

Nursing Plans and Interventions

A. Provide for client's physical needs.
B. Allow performance of the compulsive activity with attention given to safety (e.g., skin integrity of a hand washer).
C. Explore meaning and purpose of the behavior with client.
D. Avoid punishment or criticism.
E. Establish routine to avoid anxiety-producing changes.
F. Assist client with learning alternative methods of dealing with stress.
G. Avoid reinforcing compulsive behavior.
H. Limit the amount of time for performance of ritual, and encourage client to gradually decrease the time.
I. Administer antianxiety medications as prescribed (see Table 7-4).
J. Administer SSRIs and tricyclic antidepressants as prescribed (see Table 7-6).
K. Observe client response, document, and report responses to the RN.

> **HESI Hint** • The best time for interaction with a client is at the completion of the performed ritual. The client's anxiety is lowest at this time; therefore, it is an optimal time for learning.

> **HESI Hint** • Compulsive acts are used in response to anxiety, which may or may not be related to the obsession. It is the nurse's responsibility to help alleviate anxiety.
> Interfering will increase anxiety. These acts should be allowed as long as the client's acts are free of violence. The nurse should:
> • Actively listen to the client's obsessive themes.
> • Acknowledge effects that ritualistic acts have on the client.
> • Demonstrate empathy.
> • Avoid being judgmental.

Posttraumatic Stress Disorder

Description: Severe anxiety, which results from a traumatic experience (war, earthquake, rape, incest) and can be a persistent reexperiencing of the trauma.

Nursing Assessment (Data Collection)

A. Anxiety; level is proportional to the perceived degree of threat experienced by the client.
B. Anxiety manifested in symptomatic behaviors:
   1. Intrusive thoughts
   2. Flashbacks of the experience
   3. Nightmares
   4. Emotional detachment
C. Responses to anxiety include:
   1. Shock
   2. Anger
   3. Panic
   4. Denial
D. Self-destructive behavior such as suicidal ideation and substance abuse.
E. Visible reminders of trauma (e.g., scars, physical disabilities).

Analysis (Nursing Diagnoses)

A. Posttrauma syndrome related to …
B. Ineffective coping related to …
C. Risk for other-directed/self-directed violence related to …

Nursing Plans and Interventions

A. Provide consistent, nonthreatening environment.
B. Implement suicidal/homicidal precautions if the client's behavior indicates risk, and report findings to the RN.
C. Listen to client's details of events to identify most troubling aspect of event.
D. Assist client to develop objectivity in perception of event and identify areas of no control.
E. Assist client to regain control by identifying past situations that have been handled successfully.
F. Administer antianxiety and antipsychotic medications, as prescribed, to decrease anxiety, manage behavior, and provide rest (see Table 7-3 and Table 7-8, *Antipsychotic Drugs*).
G. Observe client responses to the nursing care plan and report changes to the RN.

HESI Hint • For clients with posttraumatic stress disorder, the nurse should:
- Actively listen to client's stories of experiences surrounding the traumatic event.
- Monitor for suicide risk.
- Assist client to develop objectivity about the event and problem solve regarding possible means of controlling anxiety related to the event.
- Encourage group therapy with other clients who have experienced the same or related traumatic events.

Continued

Review of Anxiety Disorders

1. State five autonomic nervous system responses to anxiety.
2. Identify the coping style used by a person who feels guilty about masturbating as a child and develops a hand-washing compulsion as an adult.
3. Identify anxiety-reducing strategies the nurse can teach.
4. Which levels of anxiety facilitate learning?
5. A Vietnam veteran is plagued by nightmares and is found trying to strangle his roommate one night. List, in order of priority, the appropriate nursing interventions.
6. A client is in the middle of an extensive ritual, which focuses on food during lunch. However, the client is scheduled for group therapy, which is about to start. What action should the nurse take?

Answers to Review

1. Shortness of breath, heart palpitations, dizziness, diaphoresis, and frequent urination.
2. Undoing.
3. Deep breathing techniques, visualization, relaxation techniques, exercise, and biofeedback.
4. Mild to moderate.
5. Protect roommate from harm. Stay with client. If the client is agitated, administer antianxiety medications as prescribed. Arrange for private room. Place client on homicidal precautions at night.
6. Allow client to complete the ritual. Discuss with the group leader the possibility of allowing the client to enter the group late. Arrange for client to begin lunch earlier so that the ritual can be completed before scheduled activities.

Somatoform Disorders

A. A group of disorders characterized by the expression of unexplained physical symptoms that have no physical basis.
B. The physical symptom is thought to be an unconscious expression of an internal conflict.
C. Somatoform disorders occur more often in women and begin before 30 years of age.
D. Children may learn that physical complaints are an acceptable coping strategy and are rewarded by receiving attention for this behavior. This is referred to as a secondary gain.
E. These clients may abuse analgesics and yet receive no relief from pain and/or discomfort. Accumulate prescriptions from "doctor shopping" to relieve physical symptoms.

Types of Somatoform Disorders

A. Somatization disorder:
   1. Recurrent somatic complaints for which frequent medical attention is sought. No medical pathology is present.
   2. Example: a client who complains of chest pains but has a normal ECG and normal cardiac enzymes.
B. Hypochondriasis:
   1. The belief and fear of having a disease, which includes misinterpretation of physical signs as "proof" of the presence of the disease.
   2. Example: a client has a rash that is quite minor but insists that he has a serious disease such as lupus.
C. Conversion disorder:
   1. A disorder characterized by transferring a mental conflict into a physical symptom for which there is no organic cause.
   2. Example: blindness, paralysis, seizures, deafness, or pseudocyesis (false pregnancy).

Nursing Assessment (Data Collection)

A. Preoccupation with pain or bodily function for at least 6 months' duration
B. History of frequent "doctor shopping"
C. Absence of emotional concern regarding the physical impairment
D. May report excessive dysmenorrhea

E. Vital signs may be elevated, similar to a panic attack
F. Fear of having a serious disease
G. Excessive use of analgesics
H. Rumination about physical symptoms
I. Drug abuse; drug screening needed to determine presence of abuse and, if present, the level of abuse
J. Depression and presence of suicidal ideation
K. Social or occupational impairment
L. Presence of blindness, deafness, paralysis, or seizures suggestive of a neurologic disease

Analysis (Nursing Diagnoses)

A. Chronic pain related to …
B. Ineffective coping related to …
C. Disturbed personal identity related to …

Nursing Plans and Interventions

A. Convey a nonjudgmental attitude.
B. Record duration and intensity of pain with attention to factors that precipitate onset.
C. Encourage expression of angry feelings.
D. Implement suicide precautions if indicated and report to RN.
E. Focus interactions and activities away from self and pain.
F. Help client identify connection between pain and anxiety.
G. Increase time and attention given to client as reward for not focusing on self or physical symptoms.
H. Help client identify needs met by the sick role and secondary gains, e.g., attention and freedom from responsibility (Table 7-5, *Terms Associated with Somatoform Disorders*).

TABLE 7-5 Terms Associated with Somatoform Disorders

Term	Definition
La Belle indifference	Term used to describe the lack of concern over physical illness; seen in conversion reactions
Primary gain	A decrease in anxiety resulting from the ability to deal with a stressful situation
Secondary gain	The rewards obtained from the sick role (e.g., freedom from certain responsibilities, sympathy, attention)

I. Encourage use of anxiety-reducing techniques such as deep breathing, visualization, meditation, exercise, and relaxation.

> **HESI Hint** • Be aware of your own feelings when dealing with this type of client. It is a challenge to be nonjudgmental. The pain is real to the person experiencing it. These disorders cannot be explained medically; they result from internal conflict. The nurse should:
> • Acknowledge the symptom or complaint.
> • Reaffirm that diagnostic test results reveal no organic pathology.
> • Determine the secondary gains acquired by the client.

Review of Somatoform Disorders

1. Describe the difference between primary and secondary gains.
2. Explain the difference between somatization and hypochondriasis.
3. An air traffic controller suddenly develops blindness. All physical findings are negative. The client's history reveals an increased anxiety about job performance and fear about job security. What type of disorder is this? What purpose is the blindness serving? What nursing interventions are indicated?
4. A 29-year-old secretary has visited seven different doctors in the last year with a complaint of chest pain, heart palpitations, and shortness of breath. She is certain she is having a heart attack in spite of the health care provider's reassurance that all tests are normal. What type of disorder is this? What nursing actions are indicated?
5. Five years ago, a woman was involved in a motor vehicle accident that killed her friend who was a passenger in the car she was driving. Since that time, she has been unable to work because of severe back pain. The pain is unrelieved by prescribed medications. What type of disorder is this? What are the contributing causes? Describe the nursing care.

Answers to Review

1. Primary gain is a decrease in anxiety, which results from some effort made to deal with stress. Secondary gain is the advantage, other than reduced anxiety, which occurs from the sick role.
2. Somatization is used to describe a person who has many recurrent complaints with no organic basis as opposed to someone with hypochondriasis, who has unrealistic or exaggerated physical complaints. The concerns of those who are experiencing

somatization, as well as those who are hypochondriacal, are so exaggerated that they interfere with social and occupational functioning.

3. Conversion reaction; decreases the anxiety about job; assist with activities of daily living (ADL), encourage expression of anger, teach relaxation techniques, and assist with the identification of anxiety related to job security and performance.

4. Hypochondriacal disorder; decrease anxiety, teach relaxation techniques, explore relationship between the symptoms and past experiences with heart disease. Focus interactions away from bodily concerns.

5. Somatization disorder; unresolved grief, anxiety. Evaluate pain medication use and/or abuse. Document duration and intensity of pain. Assist client to identify precipitating factors related to request for medication.

Dissociative Disorders

Description: An alteration in the function of consciousness, personality, memory, or identity.

A. Dissociative disorders may be sudden and temporary or gradual and chronic.

B. Persons afflicted with these types of disorders handle stressful situations by "splitting" from the situation into a fantasy state.

Types of Dissociative Disorders

A. Psychogenic amnesia:
   1. It is the sudden temporary inability to recall extensive personal information.
   2. It usually occurs after a traumatic event such as a threat of death or injury, an intolerable life situation, or a natural disaster.
   3. It is the most common dissociative disorder.

B. Psychogenic fugue:
   1. It is characterized by a person suddenly leaving home or work with the inability to recall his or her identity.
   2. The behavior may even include the client assuming a new identity.
   3. This disorder rarely occurs.
   4. Excessive use of alcohol may contribute to a fugue state.

C. Dissociative identity disorder:
   1. Presence of two or more distinct personalities within an individual.
   2. The personalities emerge during stress; they emerge one at a time.

D. Depersonalization:
   1. Characterized by a temporary loss of one's reality and/or the ability to feel and express emotions.
   2. Client expresses a fear of "going crazy."
   3. Client describes a sense of "strangeness" in the surrounding environment.

Nursing Assessment (Data Collection)

A. Depression, mood swings, insomnia, potential for suicide

B. Varying degrees of orientation

C. Varying levels of anxiety

D. Impairment of social and occupational functioning

E. Alcohol and/or drug abuse (drug screening is necessary to determine presence and level of abuse)

Analysis (Nursing Diagnoses)

A. Ineffective coping related to …

B. Potential for self-directed/other-directed violence related to …

C. Disturbed personal identity related to…

Nursing Plans and Interventions

A. Reduce environmental stimulation to decrease anxiety.

B. Stay with client during periods of depersonalization (client is often fearful, and the nurse's presence will assist in providing support/comfort during fearful episode).

C. Demonstrate acceptance of client's behavior during various experiences and personalities.

D. Document emergence of different personalities if present.

E. Report to RN any behaviors that might indicate the need to implement suicide precautions.

F. Encourage client to identify stressful situations that cause a transition from one personality to another.

G. Help client identify effective coping patterns used in other stressful situations.

H. Assist client to use new alternative coping methods. Observe successes and report to RN.

HESI Hint • Avoid giving clients with dissociative disorders too much information about past events at one time. The various types of amnesia, which accompany dissociative disorders, provide protection from pain. Too much, too soon may cause decompensation.

Review of Dissociative Disorders

1. Describe the difference between psychogenic amnesia and a psychogenic fugue.
2. What is a dissociative identity disorder?
3. List three possible causes of psychogenic amnesia.
4. Describe depersonalization disorder.

Answers to Review

1. Psychogenic amnesia is the sudden inability to recall certain events in one's life. A psychogenic fugue state is characterized by the individual leaving home and being unable to recall his or her identity or past.
2. Presence of two or more distinct personalities within an individual. The personalities emerge one at a time during stress.
3. Traumatic event such as a threat of death or injury, an intolerable life situation, or a natural disaster.
4. A temporary loss of one's reality, a loss of the ability to feel and express emotions, or a sense of "strangeness" in the surrounding environment. These individuals express a fear of "going crazy."

Personality Disorders

Cluster A—Paranoid, Schizoid, Schizotypal

Description: Characterized by suspicious, strange behavior that may be odd or eccentric: may be precipitated by a stressful event; may manifest as intense hypochondriasis.

A. Paranoid personality:
1. Displays pervasive and long-standing suspiciousness.
2. Mistrusts others, suspicious, fearful.
3. Projects blame for own problems onto others.
4. Is in touch with reality.
5. Verbally: hostile, accusatory dialogue, which is reality based.
6. Nonverbally: appears suspicious, tense, distant, watchful, and angry.
7. Example: teacher always suspects students of cheating during an exam or obtaining test questions before the exam.

B. Schizoid personality:
1. Is socially detached, shy, introverted.
2. Avoids interpersonal relationships, lacks social skills.
3. Has few friends; emotionally detached, quiet, and aloof.
4. Is introverted, unresponsive, with autistic thinking.
5. Verbally: says little, appears withdrawn and reclusive.
6. Nonverbally: dull, humorless, with little expression.
7. Example: computer programmer who works day and night; his only "relationship" is with his computer.

C. Schizotypal personality:
1. Has interpersonal deficits; sensitive to being rejected.
2. Has eccentricities and odd beliefs.
3. Is socially isolated.
4. Example: a person who spends hours walking on the street, wears a hat with all kinds of things hanging from it, and all sorts of mismatched clothing.

Nursing Assessment (Data Collection)

A. Determine degree of suspiciousness and mistrust of others.
B. Observe and report to RN degree of anxiety.
C. Determine whether delusions are present and report to RN:
1. Reference or control
2. Persecution
3. Grandeur
4. Somatic
D. Observe and report to RN degree of insecurity.

Analysis (Nursing Diagnoses)

A. Risk for self-directed violence related to …
B. Risk for other-directed violence related to …
C. Social isolation related to …

Nursing Plans and Interventions

A. Establish trust.
B. Be truthful and honest; follow through on commitments.
C. Assist client to identify situations that provoke anxiety and aggressive behaviors.
D. Avoid confrontation with the client over delusions.
E. Help client to focus on feelings that cause the delusions.
F. Assist in identifying thoughts, perceptions, and own conclusions of reality.
G. Avoid talking and laughing where client can see but not hear you.
H. Engage in noncompetitive activities that require concentration.
I. Involve client in treatment plan.
J. Promote family involvement in therapy and medication compliance.
K. Avoid stepping into client's personal space or touching client.

Cluster B: Dramatic—Emotional

A. Antisocial personality:
1. Shows aggressive "acting out" behavior pattern without any remorse.
2. Is clever and manipulative in order to meet own self-centered needs.
3. Lacks social conscience and ability to feel remorse; is emotionally immature and impulsive.
4. Has ineffective interpersonal skills that impair ability to form close and lasting relationships.
5. Verbally: is disparaging, humiliating, belligerent toward those perceived as a threat.
6. Nonverbally: is cold, callous, and insensitive to others; can display socially gracious behaviors so as to meet own needs; can be charming, smooth talking, and reckless with behavior.
7. Example: a prison inmate tries to get special privileges by bribing the guards—that is, he acts out the role of a "con artist."

B. Borderline personality:
1. Has disturbances regarding self-image, sexual, social, and occupational roles.
2. Shows impulsive, self-damaging behavior, suicidal gestures, self-mutilation.
3. Is "other directed" and overly dependent on others.
4. Is unable to problem solve or learn from experiences; may blame others for their problems.
5. Tends to view others as either "all good" or "all bad" (e.g., "splitting" behavior).
6. Verbally: is self-critical, demanding, whiny, manipulative, argumentative, can become verbally abusive.
7. Nonverbally: has highly changeable and intense affect, impulsive behaviors.
8. Example: teenage girl who threatens to commit suicide when her boyfriend leaves, but in 6 weeks has new boyfriend and is "clinging" to him.

C. Histrionic personality:
1. Seeks attention by overreacting and exhibiting hyperexcitable emotions.
2. Is overly dramatic, seeks attention, and tends to exaggerate.
3. Has chaotic relationships, demonstrates angry outbursts or tantrums.
4. Verbally: is loud, excitable, overreactive, attempts to draw attention to self.
5. Nonverbally: is immature, self-centered, dependent on attention and care from others, seductive and flirty.
6. Uses physical appearance to draw attention to self.
7. Example: hostess at a party who is overly excited to see the guests and welcomes them in a loud, "showy" manner that draws attention to herself.

D. Narcissistic personality:
1. Perceives self as all-powerful and important, critical of others, arrogant.
2. Has exaggerated feeling of self-importance and self-love.
3. Needs attention and admiration.
4. Is preoccupied with power and appearance.
5. Exploits others.
6. Verbally: talks about self incessantly and does whatever necessary to draw attention to self.
7. Nonverbally: is inattentive and indifferent to others, appears only concerned with self.
8. Example: star football player whose success has "gone to his head."

Cluster C: Anxious—Fearful

A. Avoidant personality:
1. Is socially inhibited.
2. Feels inadequate; avoids situations where rejection is a possibility.
3. Is hypersensitive to negative criticism, rejection.
4. Longs for relationships.
5. Example: a man who refuses to play on the work softball team because he is afraid his teammates will make fun of him.

B. Dependent personality:
1. Has unreasonable wishes and wants; needs are expressed in a demanding, whining manner while professing independence and denying dependent behavior.
2. Is passive without accepting responsibility for consequences of his or her own behavior.
3. Has low self-esteem; sees self as stupid, unable to make decisions.
4. Is dependent on others to meet his or her needs.
5. Verbally: is self-depreciating, demanding others to meet needs.
6. Nonverbally: appears dull, uninterested in others, dissatisfied with self.
7. Example: adult who exhibits adolescent-type behavior; wants others to take care of him or her while at the same time declares independence.

C. Obsessive-compulsive personality:
1. Attempts to control self through the control of others or the environment.
2. Shows inattention to new facts or different viewpoints.
3. Is cold and rigid toward others.
4. Has perfectionistic, inflexible, and stubborn characteristics.
5. Acts with blind conformity and obedience toward rules.
6. Is excessively neat and clean.
7. Preoccupies self with work efficiency and productivity.
8. Verbally and nonverbally expresses disapproval of those whose behaviors/standards are different from theirs.

9. Example: a nurse who insists that all staff on his or her unit wear a freshly starched uniform every day and has no tolerance for those who are not as "professionally" dressed.

Nursing Assessment (Data Collection) of Personality Disorders, Clusters B and C

A. Observe and report to RN degree of social impairment.
B. Determine degree of manipulative behavior.
C. Observe and report to RN degree of anxiety.
D. Monitor for risk of self- or other-directed violence, then report to RN.

Analysis (Nursing Diagnoses)

A. Disturbed personal identity related to …
B. Ineffective coping related to …
C. Social isolation related to …
D. Risk for self-directed/other-directed violence related to …

Nursing Plans and Interventions

A. Establish trust; use straightforward approach.
B. Protect client from injury to self or others.
C. Assist client to recognize manipulative behavior.

D. Focus on client's strengths and accomplishments.
E. Set limits on manipulative behaviors when necessary.
F. Reinforce independent, responsible behaviors.
G. Assist client to recognize the need to respect the needs and rights of others.
H. Encourage socialization with others to improve skills.

HESI Hint Personality disorders are long-standing behavioral traits that are maladaptive responses to anxiety and cause difficulty in relating and working with other individuals. Questions on the NCLEX-PN® exam sometimes test personality disorder content by describing management situations.

HESI Hint People with personality disorders are usually comfortable with their disorder and believe they are right and the world is wrong. These individuals usually have very little motivation to change.

Review of Personality Disorders

Give an example of a behavior or a description of an individual who exhibits each of the following personality disorders:
1. Obsessive-compulsive:
2. Antisocial:
3. Borderline:
4. Dependent:
5. Narcissistic:
6. Histrionic:
7. Paranoid:
8. Schizoid:

Answers to Review

1. Orderliness, rigid.
2. Inability to conform to social norms.
3. Needy, always in a crisis, self-mutilating, unable to sustain relationships, splitting behavior.
4. Unable to make decisions for self, allows others to assume responsibility for his or her life.
5. Feelings of self-importance and entitlement; may exploit others to get own needs met.
6. Dramatic, flamboyant, needs to be the center of attention.
7. Suspicious, shows mistrust of others, is watchful and secretive.
8. Isolated and introverted, has no close friends.

Eating Disorders

Anorexia Nervosa

Description: A psychiatric disorder involving a voluntary refusal to eat and maintain minimal weight for height and age.

A. A distorted body image and fear of becoming obese drive the excessive dieting and exercise.
B. A reported 15% to 20% of those diagnosed die.
C. It is more common in females than males.
D. It occurs in adolescents and young adults.
E. It is often associated with parent-child conflicts about dependency issues. The child often feels as though his or her body and weight are the only areas of control.
F. Possible etiologic factors:
  1. A dysfunctional family system
  2. Unrealistic expectations of perfection
  3. Ambivalence about maturation and the assumption of independence
  4. Chemical imbalance

Nursing Assessment (Data Collection)

A. Weight loss of at least 15% of ideal/original body weight
B. Excessive exercise
C. Apathy about physical condition and inordinate pleasure in weight loss
D. Skeletal appearance (usually hidden by baggy clothes)
E. Distorted body image (usually sees self as fat)
F. Low self-esteem
G. Hair loss and dry skin
H. Irregular heartbeat, decreased pulse and BP resulting from decreased fluid volume and from electrolyte imbalance
I. Amenorrhea for at least 3 months (female)
J. Delayed psychosexual development (adolescents) or disinterest in sex (adults)
K. Dehydration and electrolyte imbalance (decreased potassium, sodium, and chloride) resulting from:
  1. Diet pill abuse.
  2. Enema and laxative abuse.
  3. Diuretic abuse.
  4. Self-induced vomiting.

Analysis (Nursing Diagnoses)

A. Imbalanced nutrition: less than body requirements related to …
B. Disturbed personal identity related to… .
C. Interrupted family process related to …

Nursing Plans and Interventions

A. Monitor weight, vital signs, and electrolytes (especially potassium, thyroid levels, and calcium/phosphorus for osteoporosis).
B. Provide a structured, supportive environment, especially during mealtimes.
C. Set a time limit for eating.
D. Carefully monitor food and fluid intake.
E. Provide snacks in between meals.
F. Be alert to client choosing low-calorie foods.
G. Be alert to possible discarding of food through others or in pockets, wastebaskets, or drawers.
H. Monitor client for 1 or 2 hours after meals for possible vomiting.
I. Monitor activity level to prevent excessive exercise.
J. Use positive reinforcement to build self-esteem and develop a realistic body image.
K. Implement a behavior modification treatment program if prescribed:
  1. Weigh on a regular schedule.
  2. Weigh in same clothes with back to scale; this prevents manipulation and arguing about exact weight.
  3. Praise weight gain versus food intake.
L. Focus interactions away from food and eating.
M. Administer antidepressant medications as prescribed (see Table 7-6).
N. Encourage family therapy.
O. Monitor activity and watch for weakness, fatigue, and pathologic fractures.
P. Provide safe environment and identify suicide ideation; implement suicide precaution if necessary and immediately report to RN.
Q. Use the nursing process to add to the established client plan of care and report significant changes to the RN.
R. Watch for "water loading" before weighing.

> **HESI Hint** • People with anorexia gain pleasure from providing others with food and watching them eat. These behaviors reinforce their perception of self-control. Do not allow these clients to plan or prepare food for unit-based activities.

Bulimia Nervosa

Description: An eating disorder characterized by eating excessive amounts of food followed by self-induced vomiting. Bulimic clients usually report a loss of control over eating during the binging.

Nursing Assessment (Data Collection)

A. See Nursing Assessment (Data Collection) for Anorexia Nervosa.
B. Diarrhea or constipation, abdominal pain, and bloating.
C. Dental damage caused by excessive vomiting (gastric hydrochloric acid erodes dental enamel).
D. Sore throat and chronic inflammation of the esophageal lining with possible ulceration.
E. Financial stressors related to food budget.
F. Concerns with body shape and weight; bulimics usually are not underweight.

Analysis (Nursing Diagnoses)

A. Disturbed personal identity related to …
B. Interrupted family process related to …
C. Ineffective coping related to …
D. Risk for self-directed violence related to …

Nursing Plans and Interventions

A. Monitor weight, vital signs, and electrolytes (especially potassium).
B. Provide a structured supportive environment, especially around mealtime.
C. Monitor client after meals for possible vomiting.
D. Assist client to learn strategies, other than eating, to deal with feelings.
E. Encourage client to express feelings of anger and/or anxiety.
F. Discuss strategies to stop vomiting and laxative use.
G. Use positive reinforcement to build self-esteem and develop a realistic body image.
H. Administer antidepressant medications as indicated (see Table 7-6).
I. Promote family therapy.

> **HESI Hint** • Physical assessment and nutritional support are a priority; the physiologic implications are great. Nursing interventions should increase self-esteem and develop a positive body image. Behavior modification is useful and effective. Family therapy is most effective because issues of control are common in these disorders. Therapy is usually long term.

Review of Eating Disorders

1. Describe the clinical symptoms of anorexia nervosa.
2. State two psychodynamic differences between anorexia and bulimia.
3. A client with anorexia has her friend bring her several cookbooks so she can plan a party when she is discharged. What nursing intervention is appropriate in addressing this behavior?
4. Anorexia nervosa may be precipitated by what factors?
5. What might the initial treatment include for a client admitted to the hospital with a diagnosis of bulimia nervosa?

Answers to Review

1. Weight loss of at least 15% of ideal/original body weight; hair loss; dry skin; irregular heart rate; decreased pulse; decreased blood pressure; amenorrhea; dehydration; electrolyte imbalance.
2. Anorexia nervosa deals with issues of control and a struggle between dependence and independence. Bulimia deals with loss of control ("binge" eating) and guilt (purging).
3. Discuss activities that don't involve food, which may take place after discharge. Discuss the cookbooks with the treatment team and, if the treatment plan indicates, take books from client.
4. Mother-daughter conflicts, usually focusing on independence/dependence issues; discomfort with maturation; need for control; desire for perfection.
5. Blood work to evaluate electrolyte status; replenish electrolytes and fluids as indicated; carefully monitor for evidence of vomiting.

Mood Disorders

Definition: Disturbances in mood manifested by extreme sadness or extreme elation.

Depressive Disorders

Definition: Pathologic grief reactions ranging from mild to severe states.

Symptoms of Varying Degrees of Depression

A. Mild:
   1. Feelings of sadness
   2. Difficulty concentrating and performing usual activities
   3. Difficulty maintaining usual activity level
B. Moderate:
   1. Feelings of helplessness/powerlessness
   2. Decreased energy
   3. Sleep pattern disturbances
   4. Appetite/weight changes
   5. Slowed speech, thought, movement (may also be agitated and hyperactive)
   6. Rumination of negative feelings
C. Severe:
   1. Feelings of hopelessness, worthlessness, guilt, shame
   2. Despair

3. Flat affect
4. Indecisiveness
5. Lack of motivation
6. Change in physical appearance (slumped posture, unkempt)
7. Suicidal thoughts
8. Possible delusions and/or hallucinations
9. Sleep and appetite disturbances
10. Loss of interest in sexual activity
11. Constipation

HESI Hint • The most important signs and symptoms of depression are a sad mood with a loss of interest or pleasure in life. The client has sustained a loss. Other symptoms include:

- Significant change in appetite often accompanied by a change in weight—either weight loss or gain.
- Insomnia or hypersomnia (usually sleeping during the day—often because the client is not sleeping at night because of anxiety).
- Fatigue or a lack of energy.
- Feelings of hopelessness, worthlessness, guilt, or overresponsibility.
- Loss of ability to concentrate or think clearly.
- Preoccupation with death or suicide.

Nursing Assessment (Data Collection)

A. Determine type of depression:
   1. Exogenous: caused by a reaction to environmental or external factors.
   2. Endogenous: caused by an internal biologic deficiency (decreased biogenic amines at receptor sites in the brain).
B. Determine the degree of depression.
C. Determine current suicide risk (see Care of the Suicidal Client).
D. Lab tests and values:
   1. Dexamethasone-suppression test (DST):
      a. Indirect marker of depression.
      b. Considered positive/abnormal if post–dexamethasone cortisol level is greater than 5 mg/dL.
   2. Biogenic amines:
      a. Decreased serotonin indicative of depression.
      b. Decreased norepinephrine indicative of depression.

Analysis (Nursing Diagnoses)

A. Risk for self-directed violence related to …
B. Self-care deficit (specify) related to …
C. Disturbed sleep pattern related to …
D. Ineffective coping related to …

Nursing Plans and Interventions

A. Directly ask client about feelings/plans of harming self.
B. Implement suicide precautions if observation indicates risk (see Care of the Suicidal Client).

C. Monitor sleep, nutrition, and elimination patterns.
D. Initiate interaction with client (use nondemanding approach).
E. Direct client to participate in activities. Do not give the client a choice about participating in activities (e.g., "It's time to go to the gym for basketball").
F. Observe for sudden elevation in mood. May indicate increased potential for suicide risk.
G. Assist client in the identification of a support system.
H. Encourage discussion of feelings of helplessness, hopelessness, loneliness, or anger.
I. Administer antidepressant medication as indicated (Table 7-6, *Antidepressant Drugs*).
J. Sit in silence with client if client is nontalkative.
K. Spend time with client and return when promised.
L. Observe changes in client behavior and report to RN.

HESI Hint • Depressed clients have difficulty accepting compliments because of their lowered self-concept. Comment on signs of improvement by noting the behavior—for example, "I noticed you combed your hair today," *not* "You look nice today."

HESI Hint • The nurse knows depressed clients are improving when they begin to take an interest in their appearance or perform self-care activities that were previously of little or no interest.

Care of the Suicidal Client

Suicide Precautions

A. Review client record for history; a previous suicide attempt is a most significant risk factor. Other risk groups include those with biologic/organic causes of depression such as substance abuse, organic brain disorders, or other medical problems.
B. Be aware of the major warning signs of an impending suicide attempt:
   1. A client begins giving away his or her possessions.
   2. A previously depressed client becomes happy. He or she has made the decision to commit suicide, is no longer debating the possibility, and has figured out how to accomplish the suicide.
   3. A client may withdraw from friends or family.
C. Consider potential risk for suicide:
   1. Directly ask the client about his or her intent. Example: "Do you ever think about harming yourself?"
   2. If a client is currently contemplating suicide, ask about his or her plans for carrying out the attempt. Example: "Do you have a plan for harming yourself?"
   3. Identify the method chosen—the more lethal the method, the higher the probability that an attempt is imminent. Example: "What is your plan for harming yourself?" (A client mentions a shotgun and plans to put it to his head and pull the trigger.)

TABLE 7-6 **Antidepressant Drugs**

Drugs	Indications	Adverse Reactions	Nursing Implications
Tricyclics			
• Amitriptyline HCl (Elavil) • Desipramine HCl (Norpramin) • Imipramine HCl (Tofranil) • Nortriptyline HCl (Aventyl) • Protriptyline HCl (Vivactil) • Maprotiline (Ludiomil)	• Depression • Clients with morbid fantasies do not respond well to these drugs.	• Anticholinergic effects: dry mouth, blurred vision, constipation, and urinary retention • CNS effects: sedation, psychomotor slowing, and poor concentration • Cardiovascular effects: tachycardia, orthostatic, hypotension, quinidine-like effect on the heart (assess history of MI), prolongation of QTc interval • GI effects: nausea and vomiting • Narrow therapeutic index (can be lethal in overdose)	• Administer at bedtime to minimize sedative effect. • Takes 2 to 6 weeks to achieve therapeutic effects. • 1 to 3 weeks should elapse between discontinuing tricyclics and initiating MAO inhibitors. • Teach client to avoid alcohol. • Avoid concurrent use of antihypertensive drugs. • Carefully evaluate suicide risk. • Lethal in overdose
MAOIs (Monoamine Oxidase Inhibitors)			
• Isocarboxazid (Marplan) • Phenelzine sulfate (Nardil) • Tranylcypromine sulfate (Parnate) • Selegiline (Eldepryl)	• Depression • Phobias • Anxiety	• Tachycardia • Urinary hesitancy, constipation • Impotence • Dizziness • Insomnia • Muscle twitching • Drowsiness • Dry mouth • Fluid retention • *Hypertensive crisis:* severe hypertension, severe headache, chest pain, fever, sweating, nausea and vomiting • Confusion	• Must *not* be used with tricyclics (cause *hypertensive crisis*). • Major concern is need for dietary restrictions—*certain drug and food interactions can cause hypertensive crisis.* • Instruct client *not* to eat foods with high tyramine content: aged cheese, red wine, beer, beef and chicken, liver, yeast, yogurt, soy sauce, chocolate, bananas. • May not be used with SSRIs. • Teach client *not* to take over-the-counter drugs without physician approval. • Teach the warning signs of hypertensive crisis: headaches, palpitations, increased BP. • Teach client to use caution around machinery.
SSRIs (Selective Serotonin Reuptake Inhibitors)			
• Fluoxetine HCl (Prozac) • Paroxetine (Paxil) • Sertraline (Zoloft) • Fluvoxamine (Luvox) • Citalopram (Celexa)	• Depression • Anxiety • Panic disorder • Aggression • Anorexia nervosa • OCD	• Drowsiness • Dizziness, light-headedness • Headache • Insomnia • Depressed appetite	• Effective 2 to 4 weeks after treatment is initiated. • Should *not* be used with MAO inhibitors: cause hypertensive crisis (violent reaction). • Should wait at least 14 days between discontinuing MAO inhibitor and starting Prozac.

Continued

TABLE 7-6 **Antidepressant Drugs—cont'd**

Drugs	Indications	Adverse Reactions	Nursing Implications
• Escitalopram (Lexapro) • Vilazodone (Viibryd)	• Depression • Anxiety • Panic disorder • Aggression • Anorexia nervosa • OCD	• Serotonin syndrome • Sexual dysfunction • Allergic reaction or rash; withhold drug if occurs • Weight gain	• At least 5 weeks should lapse between discontinuing Prozac and initiating an MAO inhibitor. • May be given in evening if sedation occurs. • Monitor for serotonin syndrome (defined by at least 3 symptoms): →Rapid onset of altered mental states →Agitation →Myoclonus →Hyperreflexia →Fever →Shivering →Diaphoresis →Ataxia →Diarrhea • Caution client about OTC use of St. John's wort. • Must be tapered slowly if discontinuing or changing from one SSRI to another.
Atypical Antidepressants			
• Trazodone (Desyrel)	• Depression • With trazodone: insomnia, dementia with agitation	• Safer than tricyclics and MAO inhibitors in terms of side effects	• Effective 2 to 4 weeks after treatment is initiated.
S/NRIs (Serotonin/Norepinephrine Reuptake Inhibitors)			
• Duloxetine (Cymbalta) • Venlafaxine (Effexor) • Desvenlafaxine (Pristiq)	• Depression • Anxiety • Panic disorder • Aggression • Anorexia nervosa • OCD • Management of diabetic neuropathic pain	• Nausea • Dry mouth • Insomnia • Headache • Fatigue • Depressed appetite • Increased sweating • Sexual dysfunction • Withdrawal symptoms with abrupt cessation (agitation, tremors, headache, nightmares)	• Should not be used with MAO inhibitors: cause hypertensive crisis (violent reaction). • Should wait at least 14 days between discontinuing MAO inhibitor and starting S/NRIs. • Take baseline blood pressure and monitor periodically (can cause slight drop in BP). • Monitor for worsening of pretreatment symptoms and inform client of possibility. • (see Nursing Implications for SSRIs).
NDRIs (Norepinephrine Dopamine Reuptake Inhibitors)			
• Bupropion (Wellbutrin) • (Zyban) • Mirtazapine (Remeron)	• Second line of antidepressant when SSRI and SNRI are not effective for depression and smoking cessation • Anxiety and sleep disturbances	• Insomnia, tremor, anorexia and weight loss, dry mouth • Sleep disturbances, poor appetite, pain, sexual dysfunction, sedation	• Lowers seizure threshold; should not be used for patients with seizure disorders or eating disorders because of increased seizure incidence in this group. • Herbal considerations: Ephedra may cause hypertensive crisis. • Inform client of risk involved with alcohol use or other CNS depressants. Medication taken in evening due to sedative effects.

4. Determine the availability of the method chosen. If the method is readily available, the attempt is more likely. Example: The client has a loaded shotgun in his room so it is readily available.

Nursing Interventions

A. Express concern for the client. Example: "I am very concerned that you are feeling so bad that you want to harm yourself."
B. Tell the client that you will share this information with the staff. Example: "I need to share this with the staff so we can provide for your safety until you are feeling better."
C. Offer the client hope. Example: "You're feeling bad at this moment, but these feelings will pass. We have medications and treatments that can help you through the bad times."
D. Stay with the client—never leave a suicidal client alone. Maintain close observation and a safe environment. Legally, the PN should follow the policy of the institution regarding suicidal clients and should be able to demonstrate that these policies were carried out. Follow the agency policy regarding the removal of potentially hazardous objects such as razors, furniture, and so on.
E. Report to the RN immediately any changes in the client's behavior or expression of suicide ideation.

> **HESI Hint** • The nurse should suspect an imminent suicide attempt if a depressed client becomes "better" (e.g., happy or even elated). Be aware: a happy affect may signify that the client feels relieved that a plan has been made and that he or she is ready for the suicide attempt.

> **HESI Hint** • When dealing with a depressed client, the nurse should assist with personal hygiene tasks and encourage the client to initiate grooming activities even when the client does not feel like doing so. This helps promote self-esteem and a sense of control for the client.

> **HESI Hint** • An indication that a client's antidepressant medications are working is the client's ability to initiate and complete self-grooming activities.

> **HESI Hint** • An important nursing intervention for the depressed client is to sit quietly with the client. When answering NCLEX-PN questions, remember that you are working at Utopia General and there is plenty of time and staff to provide ideal nursing care. Do not let the realities of clinical situations deter you from choosing the best nursing intervention. The best intervention is to sit quietly with the client, offering support with your presence.

> **HESI Hint** • There are always drug questions on the NCLEX-PN. (see Table 7-9, Side Effects of Psychotropic Drugs and Nursing Interventions; Table 7-10, Antiparkinsonian Drugs)
> Here are some tips:
> 1. Know common side effects for drug groups—for example:
>   • Antianxiety drugs: sedation, drowsiness.
>   • Antidepressant drugs: anticholinergic effects, postural hypotension.
>   • MAOIs: hypertensive crisis.
> 2. Know specific problems or concerns for drug therapy—for example:
>   • Lithium requires renal function monitoring.
>   • Phenothiazines cause extrapyramidal effects (EPS); tardive dyskinesia can be permanent if client is not monitored regularly for signs of tardive dyskinesia!
> 3. Know specifics about drug therapy—for example:
>   • Phenothiazines: photosensitivity, need to wear protective clothing, sunglasses.
>   • MAOIs: dietary restrictions to prevent hypertensive crisis.

Bipolar Disorder or Manic-Depressive Illness

Description: Bipolar disorder is an affective disorder that is manifested by mood swings of euphoria, grandiosity, and an inflated sense of self-worth. This disorder may or may not include sudden swings to depression. To be diagnosed with a bipolar disorder, according to the DSM-IV-TR classification, a client must have at least one episode of major depression. Client may cycle, going from elation to depression with normal periods of activity in between.

Characteristics of Varying Degrees of Mania

A. Mild:
   1. Feeling of being on a high
   2. Feelings of well-being
   3. Minor alterations in habits
   4. Usually does not seek treatment because of pleasurable effect
B. Moderate:
   1. Grandiosity
   2. Talkative
   3. Pressured speech
   4. Impulsiveness
   5. Excessive spending
   6. Bizarre dress and grooming
C. Severe:
   1. Extreme hyperactivity
   2. Flight of ideas
   3. Nonstop activity—for example, running, pacing
   4. Sexual acting out; explicit language

5. Talkative
6. Overly responsive to external stimuli
7. Easily distracted
8. Agitated and possibly explosive
9. Severe sleep disturbance
10. Delusions of grandeur or persecution

Nursing Assessment (Data Collection)

A. Determine level of depression exhibited (see Symptoms of Varying Degrees of Depression).
B. Determine level of mania exhibited (see Characteristics of Varying Degrees of Mania, above).
C. Observe nutrition and hydration status.
D. Observe level of fatigue.
E. Observe danger to self and others in relation to level of impulse impairment present.

Analysis (Nursing Diagnoses)

A. Risk for self-directed/other-directed violence related to …
B. Interrupted family processes related to …
C. Self-care deficit (specify) related to …
D. Disturbed sleep patterns related to…

Nursing Plans and Interventions

A. Maintain client's physical health: provide nutrition, rest, and hygiene.
B. Provide safe environment (grandiose thinking and poor impulse control can result in accidents and/or altercations with other clients).
C. Decrease environmental stimulation (e.g., place in private room or seclusion room).

D. Implement suicide precautions if observation indicates risk; report immediately to RN.
E. Use consistent approach to minimize manipulative behavior.
F. Use frequent, brief contacts to decrease anxiety.
G. Implement constructive limit-setting.
H. Avoid giving attention to bizarre behavior (e.g., dress and language).
I. Try to meet needs as soon as possible to keep client from becoming aggressive.
J. Provide small, frequent feedings of food that can be carried—for example, small finger sandwiches.
K. Engage in simple, active, noncompetitive activities.
L. Avoid distracting or stimulating activities in the evening to help promote sleep/rest.
M. Praise self-control, acceptable behavior.
N. Promote family involvement in therapy, teaching, and medication compliance.
O. Administer lithium, sedatives, and antipsychotics as prescribed (Table 7-7, *Mood Stabilizing Drugs*).
P. Report significant changes in behavior and "acting out" episodes to the RN.
Q. Collaborate with the RN to establish realistic goals and limits/boundaries.

> **HESI Hint** • Monitor serum lithium levels carefully. The therapeutic and toxic levels are very close in readings. Signs of toxicity are evident when lithium levels are greater than 1.5 mEq/L.

TABLE 7-7 Mood Stabilizing Drugs

Drugs	Indications	Adverse Reactions	Nursing Implications
• Lithium carbonate (Carbolith)	• Bipolar disorders, especially the manic phase	• Nausea, fatigue, thirst, polyuria, and fine hand tremors • Weight gain • Hypothyroidism • Early signs of toxicity: diarrhea, vomiting, drowsiness, muscle weakness, lack of coordination • Possible renal impairment	• Lithium is excreted by the kidney. Maintain adequate serum levels. • Assess electrolytes, especially sodium. • Baseline studies of renal, cardiac, and thyroid status must be obtained before lithium therapy is begun. • Teach client *early* symptoms of lithium toxicity. If drug is continued, coma, convulsions, and death may occur. • Instruct client to keep salt usage consistent. • Use with diuretics is contraindicated. Diuretic-induced sodium depletion can increase lithium levels, causing toxicity.

TABLE 7-7 Mood Stabilizing Drugs—cont'd

Drugs	Indications	Adverse Reactions	Nursing Implications
Anticonvulsant Mood Stabilizers			
• Valproic acid (Depakene)	• Used in bipolar disorder alone or with lithium	• GI distress: nausea, anorexia, vomiting • Hepatotoxicity • Neurologic symptoms: tremor, sedation, headache, dizziness	• Administer with food. • Monitor and maintain target serum levels.
• Carbamazepine (Tegretol)	• Used in bipolar disorders • Used as alternative to lithium	• Dizziness • Ataxia • Blood dyscrasias	• Maintain serum levels at 8 to 12 g/mL. • Stop drug if WBC drops below 3000/mm^3 or neutrophil count goes below 1500/mm^3. • Monitor hepatic and renal function.
• Lamotrigine (Lamictal)	• Used in bipolar disorder alone or with other mood stabilizers	• Headache • Dizziness • Double vision • Rash (Steven-Johnson syndrome)	• To minimize risk of severe rash, give low dosage, 25 to 50 mg/day initially, then gradually increase to maintenance dose of 200 mg/day (used alone) or 100 mg/day (with Valproate) or 400 mg/day (with carbamazepine).

HESI Hint • Manic clients can be very caustic toward authority figures. Be prepared for personal "put-downs." Avoid arguing or becoming defensive.

HESI Hint • What activities are appropriate for a manic client? Noncompetitive physical activities that require the use of large muscle groups.

HESI Hint • Where should a manic client be placed on the unit? Make every attempt to reduce stimuli in the environment. Place the client in a quiet part of the unit.

HESI Hint • What interventions should the nurse use if a client becomes abusive?
• Redirect negative behavior or verbal abuse in a calm, firm, nonjudgmental, nondefensive manner.
• Suggest a walk or physical activity.
• Set limits on intrusive behavior. For example, "When you interrupt, I cannot explain the procedure to the others; please wait your turn."
• If necessary, seclude client or administer medication if client becomes totally out of control. Always remember to use compassion because nurses are "nice" people.

Review of Mood Disorders

1. Identify physiologic changes that often occur with depression.
2. A client who has been withdrawn and tearful comes to breakfast one morning smiling and interacting with her peers. Before breakfast she gave her roommate her favorite necklace. What actions should the nurse take and why?
3. Name the components of a suicide assessment.
4. A client on your unit refuses to go to group therapy. What is the most appropriate nursing intervention?
5. A client is standing on a table loudly singing "The Star Spangled Banner" encircled by sheets that have been set afire. In order of priority, describe appropriate nursing actions.

Answers to Review

1. Weight change (loss or gain), constipation, fatigue, lack of sexual interest, somatic complaints, and sleep disturbances.
2. Monitor for suicidal ideation, plan, and means to carry out plan. Place on precautions as indicated. A sudden change in mood and giving away possessions are two possible signs that a suicide plan has been developed.
3. Existence of a plan, method, availability of method chosen, lethality of method chosen, identified support system, and history of previous attempts.
4. Accompany client to the group; do not give client option. Client needs to be mobilized.
5. Remove client and other persons in the vicinity to a safe area and activate hospital fire plan. When area is safe, place client in quiet environment with low stimulation and medicate as indicated.

Thought Disorders

Schizophrenia

Definition: Schizophrenia is a psychiatric disorder characterized by thought disturbance, altered affect, withdrawal from reality, regressive behavior, difficulty with communication, and impaired interpersonal relationships.

> **HESI Hint** • There are five types of schizophrenia specified under the DSM-IV-TR (*Diagnostic and Statistical Manual [of Mental Disorders]*, 4th edition). The DSM-IV-TR is a diagnostic manual prepared by the American Psychiatric Association that provides diagnostic criteria for all psychiatric disorders.

Types of Schizophrenia

A. Catatonic:
  1. Stupor (decrease in reaction to the environment) or mutism
  2. Rigidity (maintenance of a posture against efforts to be moved)
  3. Posturing (waxy flexibility)
  4. Negativism (resistance to instructions)
  5. Excitement (severely agitated, out of control)
  6. Potential for violence to self or others during stupor or excitement
B. Disorganized:
  1. Incoherence
  2. Flat or inappropriate affect
  3. Disorganized, uninhibited behavior
  4. Unusual mannerisms
  5. Socially withdrawn
  6. Poor contact with reality
C. Paranoid:
  1. Systematized delusions and/or hallucinations related to a single theme
  2. Ideas of reference (misconstruing trivial events and remarks by giving them personal significance)
  3. Potential for violence if delusions are acted on

D. Residual:
  1. Socially withdrawn
  2. Inappropriate affect
  3. Eccentric or peculiar behavior
  4. Absence of prominent delusions and/or hallucinations
  5. No current psychotic behavior exhibited
E. Undifferentiated:
  1. Prominent delusions/hallucinations
  2. Incoherence and grossly disorganized behaviors
  3. Failure to meet any of the criteria for the other types

> **HESI Hint** • Use Bleuler's four As to help remember the important characteristics of schizophrenia:
> - Autism (preoccupied with self)
> - Affect (flat)
> - Association (loose)
> - Ambivalence (difficulty making decisions)

Nursing Assessment (Data Collection)

A. Observe for disturbance in thought process:
  1. Interpret content of internal and external stimuli:
    a. Symbolism: meaning given to words by client to screen thoughts and feelings that would be difficult to handle if stated directly.
    b. Delusions: fixed false beliefs that may be persecutory, grandiose, religious, or somatic in nature.
    c. Ideas of reference: belief that conversations or actions of others have reference to the client.
  2. Note form: construction of verbal communication:
    a. Looseness of association: lack of clear connection from one thought to the next.
    b. Tangential or circumstantial speech: fails to address the original point; gives many nonessential details.
    c. Echolalia: constantly repeats what is heard.
    d. Neologism: creates a new word.
    e. Preservation: repeats same word or phrase in response to different questions.
    f. Word salad: jumbled mixture of real and made up words.

3. Note process: flow of thoughts:
   a. Blocking: gap or interruption in speech caused by absent thoughts.
   b. Concrete thinking: thinking based on fact versus abstract and intellectual points.
B. Observe for disturbance in perception:
   1. Hallucinations: false sensory perception, usually auditory or visual in nature.
   2. Illusions: misinterpretation of external environment.
   3. Depersonalization: perceives self as alienated or detached from real body.
   4. Delusions: false, fixed beliefs that cannot be changed by reason.
C. Observe for disturbance in affect (feelings or mood):
   1. Blunted or flat
   2. Inappropriate
   3. Incongruent to context of situation or event
D. Observe for disturbance in behavior:
   1. Incoherent and disorganized
   2. Impulsive, uninhibited
   3. Posturing, unusual mannerisms
   4. Social withdrawal, neglects personal hygiene
   5. Exhibits echopraxia: repetition of another person's movements
E. Observe for disturbance in interpersonal relationships:
   1. Difficulty establishing trust
   2. Difficulty with intimacy
   3. Fear and ambivalence toward others

Analysis (Nursing Diagnoses)

A. Risk for caregiver role strain related to …
B. Disturbed sensory perception (auditory/visual) related to …
C. Disturbed personal identity related to…

Nursing Plans and Interventions

A. Establish trust.
B. Sit with mute clients.
C. Provide safe and secure environment.
D. Assist with physical hygiene and ADL.
E. Use matter-of-fact, nonjudgmental approach.
F. Use clear, simple, concrete terms when talking with client.
G. Accept and support client's feelings; use clarification.
H. Reinforce congruent thinking. Stress reality.
I. Avoid arguing or agreeing with inaccurate communication.
J. Set limits on behavior.
K. Avoid stressful situations.
L. Structure time for activities to limit time for withdrawal.
M. Encourage client to identify positive characteristics related to self.
N. Praise socially acceptable behavior.
O. Avoid fostering a dependent relationship.
P. Participate in the client plan of care.
Q. Promote family involvement in therapy; reinforce teaching and medication compliance.
R. Observe changes in client behavior and report to RN.

Delusional Disorders

Description: Characterized by suspicious, strange behavior that may be precipitated by a stressful event.

Nursing Assessment (Data Collection)

A. Determine degree of suspiciousness and mistrust of others and report to the RN.
B. Observe for degree of anxiety.
C. Determine if delusions are present:
   1. Reference or control
   2. Persecution
   3. Grandeur
   4. Somatic
   5. Jealousy
D. Observe for degree of insecurity.

Analysis (Nursing Diagnoses)

A. Risk for self-directed and/or other-directed violence related to …
B. Social isolation related to …

Nursing Plans and Interventions

(Box 7-1, *Nursing Interventions for the Delusional/Hallucinating Client*)
A. Establish trust.
B. Be truthful and honest; follow through on commitments.
C. Follow the established plan of care.
D. Assist client to identify situations that provoke anxiety and aggressive behaviors.
E. Avoid confrontation with the client over delusions.
F. Help client to focus on feelings that cause the delusions.
G. Assist in identifying thoughts, perceptions, and own conclusions of reality.
H. Observe changes in client behavior and report to RN.
I. Avoid talking and laughing where client can see but not hear you.
J. Engage in noncompetitive activities that require concentration.
K. Involve client in treatment plan.
L. Promote family involvement in therapy; reinforce teaching and medication compliance.
M. Avoid stepping into client's personal space or touching client!

> **HESI Hint** • Do not argue with a client about his delusions. Logic does not work; it only increases the client's anxiety. Be matter-of-fact and divert delusional thought to reality. Trust is the basis for all interactions with these clients. Be supportive and nonjudgmental. Stress increases anxiety and the need for delusions and hallucinations. Do not agree that you hear voices (you should be the client's contact with reality), but acknowledge your observation of the client—for example, "You look like you're listening to something."

BOX 7-1 *Nursing Interventions for the Delusional/Hallucinating Client*

Client Is Delusional	Client Is Hallucinating
A. Encourage recognition of distorted reality. B. Divert focus from delusional thought to reality; do not permit rumination of false ideas. C. Do not agree with or support delusions. D. Avoid arguing about the delusion. Be very matter-of-fact. E. Avoid physically touching client, especially if delusions are persecutory. F. Administer antipsychotic drugs (Table 7-8, *Antipsychotic Drugs*). G. Monitor and treat side effects of psychotropic drugs (Table 7-9, *Side Effects of Psychotropic Drugs and Nursing Interventions*). H. Administer anticholinergic drugs (Table 7-10, *Anticholinergic Drugs*).	A. Protect client from injury that might result from responding to commands of the voices; pay attention to the content. B. Avoid denying or arguing with client about the hallucination. C. Discuss your observations with client—for example, "You appear to be listening to something." D. Make frequent but brief remarks to interrupt the hallucinations. E. Administer antipsychotic drugs (see Table 7-8). F. Monitor and treat side effects of psychotropic drugs (see Table 7-9). G. Administer anticholinergic drugs (see Table 7-10).

HESI Hint • Observe for increased motor activity and/or erratic response to staff and other clients. The client may be experiencing an increase in command hallucinations. When this occurs, there is an increased potential for aggressive behavior.

HESI Hint • When monitoring client behaviors, consider the medications the client is receiving. Exhibited behaviors may be manifestations of schizophrenia or a drug reaction.

TABLE 7-8 Antipsychotic Drugs

Traditional Drugs	Indications	Adverse Reactions	Nursing Implications
Phenothiazines			

• Chlorpromazine HCl (Thorazine)
• Trifluoperazine HCl (Stelazine)
• Thioridazine HCl (Mellaril)
• Perphenazine (Trilafon)
• Triflupromazine (Vesprin)
• Loxapine (Loxitane)
	• To control psychotic behavior: hallucinations, delusions, and bizarre behavior	• Drowsiness
		• Orthostatic hypotension
		• Weight gain
		• Anticholinergic effects
		• Extrapyramidal effects
		  → Pseudo-parkinsonism
		  → Akathisia
		  → Dystonia
		  → Tardive dyskinesia
		• Photosensitivity
		• Blood dyscrasias: granulocytosis, leukopenia
		• Neuroleptic malignant syndrome
			• Extrapyramidal effects are *major* concern.
			• Monitor elderly clients closely.
			• Takes 2 to 3 weeks to achieve therapeutic effect.
			• Keep client supine for 1 hour after administration and advise to change positions slowly because of effects of orthostatic hypotension.
			• Teach client to avoid:
			  → Alcohol
			  → Sedatives (potentiate effect of CNS depressants)
			  → Antacids (reduce absorption of drug)

• Fluphenazine HCl (Prolixin)	• To control psychotic behavior • Useful in treatment of psychomotor agitation associated with thought disorders	• Same as other phenothiazines	• Absorbed slowly. • Used with noncompliant clients because it can be administered IM once every 14 days.

TABLE 7-8 Antipsychotic Drugs—cont'd

Traditional Drugs	Indications	Adverse Reactions	Nursing Implications
Nonphenothiazines			
• Haloperidol (Haldol) • Thiothixene HCl (Navane) • Pimozide (Orap)	• To control psychotic behavior • Less sedative than phenothiazines	• Severe extrapyramidal reactions • Leukocytosis • Blurred vision • Dry mouth • Urinary retention	• Teach client to avoid alcohol. • Orap is used only for Tourette's syndrome.
Long Acting			
• Fluphenazine decanoate (Prolixin Decanoate) • Haloperidol decanoate (Haldol Decanoate)	• Clients who require supervision with medication regimens	• Similar to Prolixin and Haldol	• Similar to Haldol and Prolixin. • Prolixin Decanoate can be given every 7 to 28 days. • Haldol Decanoate can be given every 4 weeks. • Requires several months to reach steady-state drug levels.
Atypical Antipsychotic Drugs			
• Risperidone (Risperdal) • Olanzapine (Zyprexa) • Quetiapine (Seroquel) • Aripiprazole (Abilify) • Ziprasidone (Geodon) • Clozapine (Clozaril)	• Treat positive and negative symptoms of schizophrenia without significant EPS • Clients who have not responded well to typical antipsychotics or who have side effects with typical antipsychotics • Fewer side effects • Clozapine has superior efficacy in clients who have been treatment resistant	• Risperdal: neuroleptic malignant syndrome (NMS), EPS, dizziness, GI symptoms (nausea, constipation), anxiety • Zyprexa: drowsiness, dizziness, EPS, agitation • Seroquel: drowsiness, dizziness, headache, EPS, weight gain, anticholinergic effects • Clozaril: agranulocytosis, drowsiness, dizziness, GI symptoms, neuroleptic malignant syndrome	• Monitor WBC weekly for first 6 months, then biweekly. • Baseline VS and ECG; report abnormal VS. • Monitor for symptoms of NMS and EPS. • Teach to change positions slowly. • Abilify is a new class of antipsychotic drugs, dopamine system stabilizers (DSSs) for schizophrenia and acute bipolar mania. • Seroquel: monitor lipids, especially for obese, diabetic, or hypertensive clients.

TABLE 7-9 Side Effects of Psychotropic Drugs and Nursing Interventions

Side Effect	Characteristics	Nursing Interventions
Blood Dyscrasias		
Agranulocytosis: occurs in first weeks of treatment	Sore throat, fever, chills	• Protect from infections. • Provide comfort measures: gargle for sore throat, use of lozenges and analgesics.
Thrombocytopenia: decreased platelets	Bruises easily, petechiae, tarry stools	Reinforce teaching about safety measures, monitor blood counts.
Extrapyramidal Effects		
Parkinsonism: occurs within 1 to 4 weeks after initiation of treatment	Rigidity, shuffling gait, pill rolling hand movements, tremors, dyskinesia, mask-like face	Administer anticholinergic drugs (e.g., Cogentin, Artane). Other drugs for extrapyramidal syndrome (EPS) include Benadryl, Symmetrel, Ativan, and Klonopin. Inderal for akathisia and vitamin E for tardive dyskinesia.
Akathisia: occurs within 1 to 6 weeks after initiation of treatment	Restlessness, agitation, and pacing; sudden difficulty sitting still (can be confused with tardive dyskinesia)	Rule out anxiety: Can ask client, "Are you feeling so restless that you can't sit still?"

Continued

TABLE 7-9 Side Effects of Psychotropic Drugs and Nursing Interventions—cont'd

Side Effect	Characteristics	Nursing Interventions
Dystonia: occurs within 1 to 2 days after initiation of treatment	Limb and neck spasms; uncoordinated, jerky movements; difficulty speaking and swallowing; rigidity and muscle spasms	• Emergency treatment is with IM anticholinergic drugs. • *Have respiratory emergency equipment available.*
Tardive dyskinesia: develops late in treatment	Involuntary tongue and lip movements, blinking, choreiform movements of limbs and trunk	• Permanent side effect; anticholinergic drugs are of no help in decreasing symptoms. • Reinforce teaching to client/family to report side effects EARLY.
Photosensitivity	Sunlight: exposed skin turns blue and color changes occur in eyes but does not cause vision impairment	• Reinforce teaching to client to stay out of sun, wear protective clothing and sunglasses. • Skin discoloration will disappear within 6 months after drug is discontinued.
Neuroleptic malignant syndrome	Life-threatening emergency; high fever, tachycardia, stupor, increased respirations, severe muscle rigidity	• Increased risk with phenothiazines. • Early recognition is important; transfer to medical facility for hydration, nutritional support, and treatment of possible respiratory failure and renal failure.
Serotonin syndrome	Confusion, disorientation, autonomic dysfunction	• Notify health care provider STAT. • Provide systems support.
Anticholinergic effects	Dry mouth, blurred vision, tachycardia, nasal congestion, constipation, urinary retention, orthostatic hypotension	• Encourage sips of water, chewing sugarless gum, or hard candy. • Increase fiber in diet. • Change positions slowly for dizziness. • Report urinary retention to health care provider. • Tolerance to these side effects will usually occur.

HESI Hint • Know the side effects of drugs commonly used to treat schizophrenia because client behavioral changes may be caused by drug reactions instead of schizophrenia.

TABLE 7-10 Anticholinergic Drugs

Drugs	Indications	Adverse Reactions	Nursing Implications
• Trihexyphenidyl HCl (Artane) • Benztropine mesylate (Cogentin) • Amantadine (Symmetrel)	• Acts on the extrapyramidal system to reduce disturbing symptoms	• Anticholinergic effects • Drowsiness • Headaches • Urinary hesitancy • Memory impairment	• Usually given in conjunction with antipsychotic drugs

Review of Thought Disorders

1. A client is sitting alone talking quietly. There is no one around. What nursing action should be taken?
2. A client dials 222-2222 and asks for his fiancé, naming a known movie star. This is an example of what type of thought disorder?
3. A client has been sitting in the same position for 2 hours. He is mute. What type of schizophrenia is this client experiencing? Describe appropriate nursing interventions for this client.
4. A client is very agitated. He believes that the CIA has tapped the phone and is sending messages through the television and that you are an agent who has been planted by the agency. In order of priority, list the appropriate nursing actions to intervene in this situation. What type of delusion is this client experiencing?
5. The nurse asks the client, "What brought you to the hospital?" The client's response is "The bus." What type of thinking is this client exhibiting?

Answers to Review

1. Quietly approach client and note the behavior. Assess content of the hallucinations (e.g., "I noticed you talking. Are you hearing voices? Can you tell me about the voices you are hearing?")
2. Delusion of grandeur.
3. Catatonic: spend time with client; assist with ADL; be alert to potential for violence toward self or others; be aware of fluid and nutrition needs.
4. Approach client and offer solitary activity to distract. Observe for behaviors that indicate a need for medication. Encourage verbalization of feelings and promote outlet for expression. Paranoid disorder with delusions of reference (CIA).
5. Concrete.

Substance Abuse

Description: Regular use of substances that affect the central nervous system, resulting in behavioral changes. Chemicals produce physiologic and/or psychologic dependence.

Alcoholism

Description: A drinking pattern that interferes with physical, social, familial, vocational, and emotional functioning.

Nursing Assessment (Data Collection)

A. Patterns indicative of alcoholism:
   1. Episodic drinking (binges)
   2. Continuous drinking
   3. Morning drinking
   4. Increase in family fighting about drinking
   5. Increase in absences from work or school, especially on Monday
   6. Blackouts
   7. Hiding drinking pattern
   8. Legal problems (DUIs)
   9. Health problems such as gastritis
   10. Defense mechanisms: denial, projection, and rationalization
B. Family history of alcoholism or substance abuse.
C. Dependent, yet resentful toward authority.
D. Impulsive, abusive behavior.
E. Impaired judgment, memory loss.
F. Incoordination, slurred speech.
G. Mood varies between euphoria and depression.
H. Intoxication as determined by blood alcohol level (BAL); BAL for intoxication varies by state.
I. Previous experience with treatment centers or Alcoholics Anonymous (AA).
J. Alcohol withdrawal symptoms:
   1. Begins shortly after drinking stops, as soon as 4 to 6 hours.
   2. Anxiety, nausea, insomnia, tremors, hyperalertness, and restlessness.
   3. Sudden or gradual increase in all vital signs.
   4. Delirium tremens (DTs) may appear 12 to 36 hours after last drink:
      a. Tachycardia, tachypnea, diaphoresis
      b. Marked tremors
      c. Hallucinations
      d. Paranoia
   5. Grand mal seizures possible
K. Chronic alcohol-related illnesses:
   1. Chronic gastritis
   2. Cirrhosis and hepatitis
   3. Korsakoff syndrome: organic syndrome that frequently follows delirium tremens, associated with chronic alcoholism; a major symptom is confabulation (making up answers to questions)
   4. Wernicke syndrome: a severe disorder (encephalopathy) occurring in chronic alcoholics, probably the result of a deficiency in vitamin B_1 (thiamin); may escalate Korsakoff syndrome; treat with thiamine chloride
   5. Malnutrition and dehydration
   6. Pancreatitis
   7. Peripheral neuropathy

Analysis (Nursing Diagnoses)

A. Risk for injury related to …
B. Ineffective family coping related to …
C. Imbalanced nutrition: less than body requirements related to …
D. Situational low self-esteem related to …

Nursing Plans and Interventions

A. Implement the previously established client plan of care.
B. Maintain safety, nutrition, hygiene, and rest.
C. Implement suicide precautions if indicated, and report observations to the RN.
D. Provide care during withdrawal:
   1. Monitor vital signs, I&O, electrolytes.
   2. Observe for impending delirium tremens.
   3. Prevent aspiration; implement seizure precautions.
   4. Reduce environmental stimuli.
   5. Medicate with antianxiety medication as prescribed, usually Librium or Ativan (see Table 7-4).

6. Provide high-protein diet and adequate fluid intake (limit caffeine).
7. Provide vitamin supplements, especially B_1 and B complex.
8. Provide emotional support.
E. Rehabilitation:
   1. Use direct, matter-of-fact, nonjudgmental attitude.
   2. Confront denial and rationalization (main coping styles used by alcoholics).
   3. Confront manipulations; set firm limits on behavior.
   4. Collaborate with the RN to set short-term, realistic goals.
   5. Help increase self-esteem.
   6. Explore ways to increase frustration tolerance without alcohol.
   7. Identify ways to decrease loneliness.
   8. Encourage client to accept responsibility for own behavior.
   9. Help client identify availability of support systems (family, friends, church, AA).
   10. Help client identify activities and friendships not related to drinking.
   11. Encourage group and family therapy; coordinate with support for family such as Al-Anon.
F. Reinforce client/family teaching regarding the side effects of disulfiram (Antabuse) if used as a deterrent to drinking (Table 7-11, *Alcohol Deterrents*).

Drug Abuse

Description: State of dependency produced by repeated use of a substance, which involves altered perception and/or mood.

Nursing Assessment (Data Collection)

A. Determine pattern of drug use:
   1. What drugs are used?
   2. What is the drug of choice?
   3. How much is used and how often?
   4. How long has the drug(s) been used?
B. Physical evidence of drug usage:
   1. Needle track marks
   2. Cellulitis at puncture site
   3. Poor nutritional status
   4. Inflammation of nasal passages
C. Possible causes of drug dependency:
   1. Desire to escape reality and problems
   2. Low self-esteem
   3. Peer or culture pressure
   4. Inherent susceptibility to drug dependence
D. Symptoms of withdrawal and overdose are particular for the drug used (Table 7-12, *Drug Withdrawal and Overdose Symptoms*).

Analysis (Nursing Diagnoses)

A. Risk for injury related to …
B. Situational low self-esteem related to …

TABLE 7-11 Alcohol Deterrents

Drugs	Indications	Adverse Reactions	Nursing Implications
• Disulfiram (Antabuse)	• Treatment of alcoholism; aversion therapy • Interferes with breakdown of alcohol causing an accumulation of acetaldehyde (a by-product of alcohol in the body)	Severe side effects occur if alcohol is consumed: • Nausea and vomiting • Hypotension, headaches • Rapid pulse and respirations • Flushed face and bloodshot eyes • Confusion • Chest pain • Weakness, dizziness	• Teach client what to expect if alcohol is consumed while taking the drug. • Be aware that some alcoholic clients use the side effects as a means of "punishing" themselves or as a form of masochism, and if a client repeatedly consumes alcohol while taking the drug, the health care provider should be notified. • Persons with serious heart disease, diabetes, epilepsy, liver impairment, or mental illness should not take Antabuse. • Use in motivated clients who have shown the ability to stay sober.
• Acamprosate (Campral)	• Treatment of alcohol dependence by reducing anxiety and unpleasant effects that trigger resuming drinking • Balances GABA and glutamate neurotransmitters	• Headache • Nausea and diarrhea	• Helps reduce cravings • Does not reduce or eliminate withdrawal symptoms

HESI Hint • What medications can the nurse expect to administer to chemically dependent clients?
   In treating alcohol withdrawal, Librium or Ativan are commonly used. Antabuse is often used as a deterrent to drinking alcohol. Client teaching should include the effects of consuming any alcohol while on Antabuse. Encourage client to read all labels of over-the-counter medications and food products because many may contain small amounts of alcohol.

TABLE 7-12 Drug Withdrawal and Overdose Symptoms

Drugs	Withdrawal	Overdose	Effect
Opiates			
• Heroin • Morphine • Codeine • Opium • Methadone	• Watery eyes, runny nose, dilated pupils • Anxiety • Diaphoresis, fever • Nausea, vomiting, and diarrhea • Achiness • Abdominal cramps • Insomnia • Tachycardia	• Respiratory depression leading to respiratory arrest • Circulatory depression leading to cardiac arrest • Unconsciousness leading to coma • Death	• General physical and mental deterioration • Rapid tolerance • Impaired judgment
• Cocaine	• Depression • Fatigue • Disturbed sleep • Anxiety • Psychomotor agitation	• Tachycardia • Pupillary dilation • Increased BP • Cardiac dysrhythmias • Perspiration, chills • Nausea, vomiting	• Psychologic dependence • Tolerance within hours or days
• Amphetamines	• Depression • Fatigue • Disturbed sleep	• Restlessness • Tremors • Rapid respiration • Confusion • Assaultive behavior • Hallucinations • Panic	• Paranoid delusions
• Hallucinogenics	• No withdrawal	• Panic • Psychosis	• Flashbacks • Impaired judgment
Antianxiety Drugs			
• Benzodiazepines: →diazepam (Valium) →oxazepam (Serax) →lorazepam (Ativan)	• Tremors • Agitation • Anxiety • Abdominal cramps • Grand mal seizures	• Drowsiness • Confusion • Hypotension • Coma: →Death	• Withdrawal occurs if there is abrupt cessation • Temporary psychosis

HESI Hint ● What type of therapy is used with chemically dependent clients? Group therapy is effective as well as support groups such as Alcoholics Anonymous, Narcotics Anonymous, and so on.

HESI Hint ● Harm reduction is a community health strategy designed to reduce the harm of substance abuse to families, individuals, community, and society.
Examples:
• More compassionate drug treatment options including abstinence and drug substitution models.
• HIV-related interventions such as needle exchanges.
• Directed drug use management should the client wish to continue use.
• Changes in laws concerning possession of paraphernalia and drug use.

C. Imbalanced nutrition: less than body requirements related to …
D. Ineffective family coping related to …

Nursing Plans and Interventions

A. Observe level of consciousness and obtain vital signs. (Rapid withdrawal can be fatal for persons addicted to barbiturates, antianxiety medications, and hypnotics.)
B. Monitor I&O and electrolytes.
C. Implement suicide precautions if observation indicates risk.
D. Provide adequate nutrition, hydration, and rest.
E. Administer medications according to detoxification protocol of medical unit.
F. Phenothiazines and benzodiazepines may be used to decrease the discomfort of withdrawal.
G. Confront denial (main coping style used by substance abusers):
   1. Focus on substance abuse problem.
   2. Confront placing blame on external problems.
H. Reinforce reality with simple, concrete terms.
I. Encourage verbal expression of anger and depression.
J. Assist with identification of stressors and areas of conflict.
K. Encourage exploration of alternate coping strategies.
L. Positively reinforce insight into behavior patterns.

M. Help identify an appropriate support system.
N. Provide support to significant others.
O. Reinforce the established teaching plan for danger of AIDS and other blood-borne diseases.

HESI Hint Know what defense mechanisms are used by chemically dependent clients. Denial and rationalization are the two most common coping styles used. Their use must be confronted so accountability for the client's own behavior can be developed.

HESI Hint What basic needs have priority when working with chemically dependent clients? Nutrition is a priority. Alcohol and drug intake has superseded the intake of food for these clients.

HESI Hint What behaviors are expected during withdrawal? In the alcoholic, delirium tremens (DTs) occur 12 to 36 hours after the last intake of alcohol. Know the symptoms. In drug abuse, withdrawal symptoms are specific to the type of drug.

Review of Substance Abuse

1. Three days ago, a client was admitted to the medical unit for a GI bleed. His BP and pulse rate gradually increased, and he developed a low-grade fever. What assessment data should the nurse obtain? What kind of anticipatory planning should the nurse develop?
2. What physical signs might indicate that a client is abusing intravenous medications?
3. What behaviors would indicate to the nurse-manager that an employee has a possible substance abuse problem?
4. A client becomes extremely agitated, abusive, and very suspicious. He is currently undergoing detoxification from alcohol with chlordiazepoxide (Librium) 25 mg every 6 hours. What nursing actions are indicated?
5. A client in the third week of a cocaine rehabilitation program returns from an unsupervised pass. The nurse notices that he is euphoric and is socializing with the other clients more than he has in the past. What nursing actions are indicated?

Answers to Review

1. Obtain a drug and alcohol consumption assessment, including type, frequency, and time of last dose/drink. Call the health care provider and report findings. Anticipate withdrawal/delirium tremens. Provide a quiet, safe environment. Place on seizure precautions. Anticipate giving a medication such as Librium.
2. Needle track marks; cellulitis at puncture site; poor nutritional status.
3. Change in work performance, withdrawal, increase in absences (especially Monday or Friday), increase in number of times tardy, long breaks, late returning from lunch.
4. Notify the health care provider immediately and anticipate an increase in dose or frequency of Librium. Provide a quiet, safe environment. Approach in a quiet, calm manner. Avoid touching client.
5. Notify health care provider of observed behavior change. Get a urine drug screen as prescribed. Confront client with observed behavior change.

Abuse

> **HESI Hint** • All victims of abuse have the potential to develop posttraumatic stress disorder (PTSD).

Child Abuse

Description: Includes physical and mental injury, sexual abuse, and neglect.

Nursing Assessment (Data Collection)

A. Most important indicators of child abuse:
   1. Injuries are not congruent with the child's developmental age or skills.
   2. Injuries do not correlate with the stated cause.
   3. Delay in seeking medical care.
B. Bruises in unusual places and in various stages of healing.
C. Bruises, welts from belts, cords, and so on.
D. Burns (cigarette, iron); immersion burns (symmetric in shape).
E. Whiplash injuries from being shaken.
F. Bald patches where hair has been pulled out.
G. Fractures in various stages of healing.
H. Failure to thrive, unattended physical problems.
I. Torn, stained, bloody underclothes.
J. Lacerations of external genitalia.
K. Bedwetting, soiling.
L. Sexually transmitted diseases.
M. Parent sees child as "different" from other children.
N. Parent uses child to meet own needs.
O. Parent seldom touches or responds to child; may be very critical of child.
P. Child appears frightened and withdrawn in the presence of parent or other adult.
Q. Family history of frequent moves, unstable employment, marital discord, and family violence.
R. One parent answers all the questions.

Analysis (Nursing Diagnoses)

A. Fear related to …
B. Impaired parenting related to …
C. Interrupted family process related to …

Nursing Plans and Interventions

A. PNs are legally required to report all cases of suspected child abuse to the appropriate local/state agency.
B. Follow the policy and procedure of the institution. Report observed data to RN.
C. Assist with collecting color photographs of injuries.
D. Document factual, objective statements of child's physical condition, child/family interaction, and interviews with family.
E. Establish trust, and care for the child's physical problems. These are the *primary* and *immediate* needs of these children.
F. Provide safe environment.
G. Recognize own feelings of disgust and contempt for the parents.
H. Use principles of crisis intervention.
I. Assist child/family to develop self-esteem.
J. Reinforce teaching of basic child development and parenting skills to family as established by the child's plan of care.
K. Support need for family therapy.

> **HESI Hint** • Select only one nurse to care for an abused child. Abused children have difficulty establishing trust. The child will be less anxious with one consistent caregiver.

Intimate Partner Violence

Description: A criminal act of physical, emotional, economic, or sexual abuse between an assailant and a victim who most commonly are, or were, in an intimate relationship (may be marital or dating).

A. Abuse is usually a tension-releasing action as well as a lack of impulse control.
B. Assailant may come from a family where battering and physical violence were present.
C. Persons act more violently when drinking or using drugs.
D. The relationship is usually characterized by extreme jealousy and issues of power and control.
E. Women in a battering relationship may lack self-confidence and feel trapped. They may be embarrassed about their situation, which results in isolation and dependency on the abuser.
F. Often begins during pregnancy and/or occurs more frequently during pregnancy.

Nursing Assessment (Data Collection)

A. Delay between time of injury and time of treatment
B. Anxious when answering questions about injury
C. Abdominal injuries during pregnancy
D. Looks to abuser for answers to questions related to injuries
E. Depression and/or suicidal ideation
F. Feeling of responsibility for "provoking" partner
G. Low self-esteem
H. Abrasions, cuts, lacerations, sprains, black eyes
I. Psychosomatic/somatoform complaints
J. Concurrent use of alcohol, drugs
K. Isolated from family and friends

Analysis (Nursing Diagnoses)

A. Risk for situational low self-esteem related to …
B. Fear related to …
C. Risk for injury related to …
D. Powerlessness related to …

Nursing Plans and Interventions

A. Establish trust; use nonjudgmental approach.
B. Treat physical wounds and injuries.
C. Document factual, objective statements of client's physical condition, injuries, and interaction with partner/family.
D. Interview clients without their partner present.
E. Determine potential for further violence.
F. Provide crisis intervention.
G. Assist with referral to shelter if necessary and/or desired with adult's consent.
H. Assist client with contacting authorities if charges are to be pressed.

> **HESI Hint** • A woman who is abused may rationalize the spouse's behavior and unnecessarily accept blame for his actions. The woman may or may not choose to press charges. Be sure to give her the number of a shelter or "help line" for future occurrences, as well as develop a safety plan.

Elder Abuse

Description: An act that causes physical, verbal, financial, or psychosocial injury or exploitation, as well as the physical neglect of an aged adult.

A. Abuse of the elderly is underreported; estimated number varies from 1% to 10% of the elderly population.
B. The majority of abuse is committed by spouses and children but also by other caregivers.

Nursing Assessment (Data Collection)

A. Bruises on the upper arms (bilaterally, from being shaken)
B. Broken bones from falls (resulting from being pushed)
C. Dehydration or malnourishment
D. Overmedication
E. Poor physical hygiene, improper medical care
F. Withdrawn behavior, feels hopeless, helpless
G. May be demanding, belligerent, and aggressive
H. Repeated visits to health care agency for injuries/falls
I. Injuries do not correlate with stated cause
J. Misuse of money by children or legal guardians

Analysis (Nursing Diagnoses)

A. Fear related to …
B. Interrupted family process related to …
C. Risk for injury related to …

Nursing Plans and Interventions

A. PNs are legally required to report all cases of suspected elder abuse to the appropriate local/state agency.
B. Follow the policy and procedure of the institution. Report observed data to RN.
C. Establish trust; use nonjudgmental approach.
D. Meet physical needs; treat wounds and injuries.
E. Document factual, objective statements of client's physical condition, injuries, and interaction with significant other/family.
F. Collaborate with the RN to arrange community resources to provide "respite care" for the caregiver.
G. Collaborate with the RN to arrange visiting nurses, nutrition services, or adult day care if possible.

> **HESI Hint** • It is difficult for an elderly person to admit abuse for fear of being placed in a nursing home or abandoned. Therefore, it is imperative to establish a trusting relationship with the elderly client.

Rape and Sexual Assault

Definition: A crime involving lack of consent, force, and sexual penetration; an act of aggression, not passion.

Nursing Assessment (Data Collection)

A. Careful documentation of observed injuries.
B. Emotional status: self-blame, anxious, fearful, humiliation, disbelief, and anger.
C. Coping behaviors.
D. Identify support system.
E. Obtain details of the assault; preserve evidence.

Analysis (Nursing Diagnoses)

A. Rape-trauma syndrome related to …
B. Powerlessness related to …
C. Fear related to …
D. Risk for injury related to …

Nursing Plans and Interventions

A. Communicate nonjudgmental acceptance.
B. Provide physical care to treat injuries.
C. Give clear, concise explanations of all procedures to be performed.
D. Document factual objective statements of physical assessment; record client's *exact* words in describing the assault.
E. Encourage victim to prosecute.
F. Assist with collection and labeling of evidence in the presence of a witness.
G. Notify Rape Crisis Team or counselor if available in the community.
H. Allow discussion of feelings about the assault.
I. Advise of potential for sexually transmitted disease, pregnancy, and HIV.
J. Provide information about medical care available.
K. Support client, family, and friends.
L. Report observed data to RN.

> **HESI Hint** • Rape victims are at high risk for posttraumatic stress disorder. Immediate intervention to diminish distress is vital. The nurse should monitor for and intervene with sequelae such as unwanted pregnancy, sexually transmitted diseases, and HIV risk.

HESI Hint • Questions on the NCLEX-PN exam regarding physical/sexual abuse usually focus on three aspects:
1. Physical manifestations of abuse
2. Client safety
3. Legal responsibilities of the nurse. In children, the nurse is legally responsible for reporting all suspected

Continued

cases of abuse. In intimate partner abuse, it is the adult's decision; the nurse should be supportive of his or her decision. Remember to document objective factual assessment data and the client's exact words in cases of sexual abuse/rape.

Review of Abuse

1. What family dynamics are often seen in child abuse cases?
2. What behavior might the nurse observe in a child who is abused?
3. Identify nursing interventions for dealing with an abused child.
4. When does battering of women often begin or escalate?
5. What dynamics prevent a battered spouse from leaving the battering situation?
6. Why is elder abuse so underreported?
7. What types of abuse are seen in the elderly?
8. Identify nursing interventions for working with a rape survivor.

Answers to Review

1. Parent sees child as "different" from other children. Parent uses child to meet his or her own needs. Parent seldom touches or responds to child. Parent may be very critical of child. Family history of frequent moves, unstable employment, marital discord, and family violence. One parent answers all the questions.
2. Child may appear frightened and withdrawn in the presence of parent or other adult.
3. Must report all cases of suspected abuse to appropriate local/state agency. Take color photographs of injuries. Document factual, objective statements of child's physical condition, child/family interactions, and interviews with family. Establish trust, and care for the child's physical problems. These are the *primary* and *immediate* needs of these children. Recognize own feelings of disgust and contempt for the parents. Teach basic child development and parenting skills to family.
4. During pregnancy.
5. A woman in a battering relationship may lack self-confidence and feel trapped. She is often embarrassed to tell friends and family, so she becomes isolated and dependent on the abuser.
6. It is difficult for an elderly person to admit abuse for fear of being placed in a nursing home or being abandoned.
7. Abuse can be physical, verbal, psychosocial, exploitive, or physical neglect.
8. Communicate nonjudgmental acceptance. Provide physical care to treat injuries. Give clear, concise explanations of all procedures to be performed. Notify police, encourage victim to prosecute. Collect and label evidence carefully in the presence of a witness. Document factual, objective statements of physical condition; record client's *exact words* in describing the assault. Notify Rape Crisis Team or counselor if available in the community. Allow discussion of feelings about the assault. Advise of potential for sexually transmitted disease, HIV, or pregnancy, and describe medical care available.

Organic Disorders

Description: Abnormal psychologic or behavioral signs and symptoms that occur as a result of cerebral disease, systemic dysfunction, or use/exposure to exogenous substances.
(Box 7-2, *Delirium and Dementia*)

Nursing Assessment (Data Collection)

A. Limited attention span; easily distracted
B. Confusion and disorientation; impaired judgment
C. Delusions, visual hallucinations, or sensory illusions
D. Labile affect; sudden anger
E. Anxiety and/or depression
F. Loss of recent and remote memory

BOX 7-2 *Delirium and Dementia*

Delirium	Dementia

Description: An acute process that, if treated, is usually reversible. It is recognized by its *sudden* onset.
A. Occurs in response to a specific stressor such as:
  1. Infection
  2. Drug reaction
  3. Substance intoxication or withdrawal
  4. Electrolyte imbalance
  5. Head trauma
  6. Sleep deprivation
B. Treatment of choice is the correction of the causative disorder.
	Description: Cognitive impairment characterized by gradual, progressive onset; it is irreversible. Judgment, memory, abstract thinking, and social behavior are affected.
	A. Most frequently seen in:
	  1. Alzheimer's disease (Table 7-13, *Alzheimer's Medications*)
	  2. Multi-infarctions (brain)
	B. Also occurs in:
	  1. Huntington chorea
	  2. Parkinson's disease
	  3. Multiple sclerosis and brain tumors
	  4. Wernicke-Korsakoff syndrome (chronic alcoholism)

HESI Hint • The basic difference between delirium and dementia is that delirium is acute and reversible, whereas dementia is gradual and permanent.

TABLE 7-13 **Alzheimer's Medications**

Drugs	Adverse Reactions	Nursing Implications
Acetyl Cholinesterase Inhibitors		
• Tacrine hydrochloride (Cognex) • Donepezil HCl (Aricept) • Rivastigmine (Exelon) • Galantamine (Razadyne)	• Overall: nausea and diarrhea • Cognex: considerable GI distress, elevated liver enzymes	• Reinforce teaching to clients that they should take *no* anticholinergic medication. • Medications should not be used in cases of severe liver impairment. • Take with meals to avoid GI upset. • Do not discontinue abruptly. • Implement the established plan of care. • Report significant changes to the RN.
N-Methyl D-Aspartate (NMDA) Antagonist		
• Memantine (Namenda)	• Headaches, dizziness, and constipation	• Add to acetyl cholinesterase inhibitors in moderate to severe Alzheimer's disease.

HESI Hint • May also use atypical antipsychotics such as risperidone and quetiapine. Clozaril is not a front-line agent because of side effects. May also give mood stabilizers and antianxiety medications as indicated.
See Dementia in Chapter 8, *Gerontologic Nursing*, p. 335, for additional interventions.

G. Confabulation (making up responses, stories to fill in lost memory)
H. Impaired coordination
I. Increased psychomotor activity
J. Slurring of speech
K. Decreased personal hygiene
L. Sleep deprivation, day/night reversal
M. Incontinence/constipation

Analysis (Nursing Diagnoses)

A. Risk for ineffective cerebral tissue perfusion related to …
B. Self-care deficit (dressing and grooming) related to …

Nursing Plans and Interventions

A. Provide safe, consistent environment.
B. Assist client with maintenance of health, nutrition, safety, hygiene, and rest.
C. Assist with ADL.
D. Provide support to client/family.
E. Provide routine in daily activities.
F. Clearly mark the bathroom.
G. Reorient the client as needed.
H. Use simple, direct statements.
I. Report client changes in mental status to the RN.

> **HESI Hint** Confusion in the elderly is often "accepted" as part of growing old. This confusion may be due to dehydration with resulting electrolyte imbalance. Think "sudden change" when reviewing a history. Such changes usually result from a specific stressor, and treatment for the causative stressor usually results in correcting the confusion.

> **HESI Hint** Nursing interventions for the confused elderly should focus on:
> - Maintaining the client's health and safety.
> - Encouraging self-care.
> - Reinforcing reality orientation (e.g., "Today is Monday," and call the client by name).
> - Providing a consistent, safe environment; engage client in simple tasks, activities to build self-esteem.

> **HESI Hint** Confabulation is not lying. It is a way in which confused clients may respond when they do not remember the answer to a question. Confabulation helps to decrease anxiety and protect the ego.

> **HESI Hint** Providing a consistent caregiver is a priority in planning nursing care for the confused older client. Change increases anxiety and confusion.

Review of Organic Disorders

1. List five causes of delirium.
2. Describe the nursing care for a client with Alzheimer's disease.
3. Identify three or more causes of dementia.

Answers to Review

1. Infection, alcohol withdrawal, electrolyte imbalance, sleep deprivation, and brain injury (i.e., subdural hematomas).
2. Provide a safe, consistent environment. (Do not make changes if possible. Change increases anxiety and confusion.) Stick to routines. If client wanders, make sure he or she has a name tag. Provide assistance as needed with ADL. Make sure bathroom is clearly labeled.
3. Alzheimer's disease, multi-infarcts (brain), Huntington chorea, multiple sclerosis, and Parkinson's disease.

Childhood and Adolescent Disorders

Attention Deficit (Hyperactivity) Disorder

Description: Attention deficit (hyperactivity) disorder (ADD/ADHD) is developmentally inappropriate attention, impulsiveness, and hyperactivity: may present without hyperactivity.

Nursing Assessment (Data Collection)
A. Review assessment data and report changes to the RN.
B. More prevalent in boys.
C. Failure to listen and follow instructions.
D. Difficulty playing quietly or sitting still.
E. Disruptive, impulsive behavior.
F. Distractibility to external stimuli.
G. Excessive talking.
H. Shifts from one unfinished task to another.
I. Underachievement in school performance.

Analysis (Nursing Diagnoses)
A. Risk for injury related to …
B. Social isolation related to …
C. Interrupted family process related to …

Nursing Plans and Interventions
A. Decrease environmental stimuli.
B. Set limits on behavior when indicated.
C. Provide a safe, comfortable environment.
D. Follow the behavior contract to help child manage own behavior.
E. Administer medications as prescribed (Table 7-14, *Stimulants*).

Conduct and Oppositional Defiant Disorders

Definition: Conduct disorder is an antisocial behavior characterized by violation of laws, societal norms, and the basic rights of others without feelings of remorse or guilt.

TABLE 7-14 Stimulants

Drugs	Indications	Adverse Reactions	Nursing Implications
• Dextroamphetamine sulfate (Dexedrine) • Methylphenidate HCL (Ritalin, Concerta) • Pemoline (Cylert) • Lisdexamfetamine (Vyvanse) • Amphetamine/dextroamphetamine (Adderal) • Dexmethylphenidate (Focalin)	• Treat ADD/ADHD • Methylphenidate is also used to treat narcolepsy	• May interact with MAO inhibitors, producing fever and hypertensive crisis • Nervousness and insomnia; dizziness • Tourette's syndrome • Tachycardia, palpitations, angina, dysrhythmias • Anorexia, weight loss, nausea, and abdominal pain	• Short-acting, 2 to 4 hours. • Teach to take last dose at least 6 hours before bedtime if insomnia occurs. • Administer 1 to 3 doses daily. • Administer with or after meals to avoid appetite suppression. • Monitor heart rate, rhythm, and BP. • Monitor height and weight to detect growth suppression.

Definition: Oppositional defiant disorder is characterized by behavior that fails to adhere to established norms but does not violate the rights of others.

Nursing Assessment (Data Collection)—Conduct Disorder

A. Physical fighting
B. Running away from home
C. Lying, stealing
D. Cruelty to animals
E. Frequent truancy
F. Vandalism, arson
G. Use of alcohol, drugs

Nursing Assessment (Data Collection)—Oppositional Defiant Disorder

A. Argumentative
B. Blaming others for problems
C. Defies rules and authority
D. Uses obscene language
E. Resentful, vindictive

Analysis (Nursing Diagnoses)—Conduct and Oppositional Defiant Disorders

A. Risk for other-directed violence related to …
B. Chronic low self-esteem related to …
C. Ineffective family coping related to …

Nursing Plans and Interventions—Conduct and Oppositional Defiant Disorders

A. Observe for verbal/nonverbal cues for escalating behavior to decrease outbursts.
B. Use a nonauthoritarian approach.
C. Avoid asking "why" questions.
D. Initiate a "show of force" for child who is out of control.
E. Use "quiet room" when external control is needed.
F. Clarify expressions or jargon if meaning is unclear.
G. Redirect angry feelings to "safe" alternative such as a pillow or punching bag.
H. Assist with implementation of behavior modification therapy if indicated.
I. Role-play new coping strategies with client.

HESI Hint • Children also experience depression, which often presents as headaches, stomachaches, and other somatic complaints. Be sure to assess suicidal risk, especially in adolescents.

HESI Hint • The client's lack of remorse or guilt about his or her antisocial behavior represents a malfunction of the superego or conscience. The id functions at the basic instinct level and strives to meet immediate needs. The ego is in touch with external reality and is the part of the personality that makes decisions.

HESI Hint • Important points to remember in answering NCLEX-PN exam questions: These children may be involved in self-fulfilling prophecy (e.g., "Mom says he or she is a troublemaker, so he or she must live up to Mom's expectations.").

Confront the client with his or her behavior—for example, lying. This gives the client a sense of security.

Provide consistent intervention—helps to prevent manipulation. Inconsistency does not help the client develop self-control.

Review of Childhood and Adolescent Disorders

1. A 7-year-old boy is disruptive in the classroom and is described by his parents as "hyperactive." What is the most probable psychiatric disorder? What are the signs and symptoms of this disorder? What drug is usually prescribed for this disorder?
2. A 15-year-old boy is threatening to drop out of school. His parents, both alcoholics, say they cannot stop him. He has just been arrested for stealing a car and breaking into a house. What is the most probable disorder?

Answers to Review

1. Attention deficit disorder (ADD/ADHD). More prevalent in boys; failure to listen or follow instructions; difficulty playing quietly; disruptive, impulsive behavior; difficulty sitting still; distractibility to external stimuli; excessive talking; shifts from one unfinished task to another; and underachievement in school performance. Methylphenidate (Ritalin).
2. Conduct disorder.

A. Aging is an individual process that affects each person differently.
B. The chronologic age of 65 is the standard in the United States for being considered an older adult (elderly).
C. By 2050, one in five Americans will be over the age of 65.
D. The concept of aging is further defined as young-old (65-74), middle-old (75-84), old-old (over 85), elite-old (over 90), and centenarian (100+).
E. Healthy aging is now an achievable goal for many.
F. Aging and disease are separate entities.
G. Eighty percent of people over the age of 70 have at least one chronic condition, and 50% have multiple health problems.

Theories of Aging

Psychosocial Theories

A. **Disengagement theory:** Progressive social disengagement occurs with aging.
B. **Activity theory:** Successful aging (as measured by the individual's satisfaction with life) depends on maintaining a high level of activity and involvement.

Biologic Theories

A. **Pacemaker theory:** A programmed decline or cessation of many components occurs in the nervous and endocrine systems.
B. **Immunity theory:** A programmed accumulation of damage and decline of the immune system's function (immunosenescence) takes place due to oxidative stress.
C. **Wear-and-tear theory:** After repeated use, damaged cells in the body structures wear out from the harmful effects of internal and external stressors, now known as free radicals.

Developmental Theories

A. **Erik Erikson's theory:** Theory identifies eight stages of developmental tasks throughout the life span; the eighth stage is integrity versus despair.
B. **Maslow's theory:** Maslow's hierarchy of needs ranks an individual's needs from the most basic to the most complex. Maslow uses the terms *physiologic, safety and security, belonging, self-esteem,* and *self-actualization* needs to describe the process that generally motivates individuals to move through life.

HESI Hint • Either a lack of stimulation or an overload of changes can result in stress. Provide as much consistency and routine as possible when caring for the older adult so as to reduce the possibility of creating stress and/or confusion.

Physiologic Changes

A. Aging affects every cell in every organ of the body but not at the same rate.
B. Three physiologic changes are clinically significant in making older adults vulnerable to injury and disease:
   1. Loss in compensatory reserve
   2. Progressive loss in efficiency of body to repair damaged tissue
   3. Decreased functioning of the immune system processes
C. Diseases in older adults do not always present with classic signs and symptoms.
D. Physiologic changes increase more rapidly with increasing age.
E. Aging changes are influenced by genetic makeup and environment.

HESI Hint • Changes in the heart and lungs result in less efficient use of O_2, which reduces an individual's capacity to maintain physical activity for long periods of time. Physical training for older persons can significantly reduce blood pressure and increase aerobic capacity. NCLEX-PN questions may ask about health maintenance factors for the older adult. Two important factors are physical activity and nutrition.

HESI Hint • Both systolic and diastolic blood pressure tend to increase with normal aging, but the elevation of the systolic is greater. REMEMBER: The physiology of blood pressure is expressed as a ratio of systolic to diastolic pressure. Systolic refers to the level of blood pressure during the contraction phase, whereas diastolic refers to the stage when the chambers of the heart are filling with blood. The healthy older heart is able to sustain adequate function for everyday life.

HESI Hint • Many older adults have problems with sleep; they cannot fall asleep at night and do not sleep soundly after they fall asleep. This is because they have shorter stages of sleep, particularly shorter cycles from stages 1 to 4, and REM sleep (stage 4 is deep sleep). They are easily awakened by environmental stimuli. They often compensate by napping during the day, which may lead to further disruptions of night sleep. The important point is that they get enough sleep to feel rested. A common response is the use of prescription sleeping pills, which can create even further problems. A healthier approach is to use nonpharmacologic methods to improve sleeping, such as developing a bedtime routine or using relaxation techniques.

Cardiovascular System

A. Age-related changes in the cardiovascular system predispose the older person to development of dysrhythmias and other cardiac problems.
B. Cardiac output decreases as a result of a decrease in heart rate and stroke volume (heart rate slows with age; resting heart rate remains unchanged).
C. Cardiac output decreases because vessels lose elasticity. The heart's contractility decreases in response to increased demands.
D. Diastolic murmurs are present in more than one half of older adults because the mitral and aortic valves become thick and rigid.
E. Dysrhythmias (bradycardia, tachycardia, atrial fibrillation, and heart block) become more common as one ages, in part because of higher systolic blood pressure (BP) and increased size of the atria.
F. Significant increases in systolic BP occur as a result of altered distribution of blood flow and increased peripheral resistance.
G. Arteriosclerosis increases with age and can cause cardiovascular problems:
   1. Peripheral vascular disease
   2. Edema
   3. Coronary artery disease: acute coronary insufficiency, myocardial infarction (MI), dysrhythmias, heart failure (HF)
H. Much heart disease is preventable.

Nursing Assessment (Data Collection)

A. Blood pressure and vital signs
B. History of dizziness or blackouts with sudden position change (orthostatic hypotension); may be related to medication(s)
C. Diuresis after lying down
D. Heart palpitations
E. Swelling in hands and feet (rings and shoes have become tight)
F. Weight gain without changes in eating pattern
G. Difficulty breathing at night (without elevation of the head of the bead)
H. Confusion or personality changes can result from O_2 deficit

Analysis (Nursing Diagnoses)

A. Activity intolerance related to . . .
B. Ineffective tissue perfusion (specify) related to . . .
C. Acute/chronic pain related to . . .
D. Decreased cardiac output related to . . .

Nursing Plans and Interventions

A. Monitor blood pressure in lying, sitting, and standing positions.
B. Encourage frequent rest periods to avoid fatigue.
C. Encourage regular, low-impact exercise.
D. Teach to change positions slowly to avoid falls and injuries.
E. Take apical and radial pulse; note deficits or rhythm abnormalities.
F. Teach to avoid extreme hot and cold because of decreased peripheral sensation.
G. Teach to avoid sitting with feet in a dependent position.
H. Monitor for edema: weigh daily if indicated.
I. Encourage strict adherence to medication regimen.
J. Teach not to stop medications without prior approval from health care provider.
K. Determine support system for follow-up.

HESI Hint • Dysrhythmias in older adults are particularly serious because they cannot tolerate decreased cardiac output, which can result in syncope, falls, and transient ischemic attacks (TIAs). Pulse may be rapid, slow, or irregular.

Respiratory System

A. Older adults have increased demands for oxygen. The life span of an older adult increases chances for exposure to toxic or infectious agents. Due to the aging process, multiple exposures over time can be damaging to the lungs and even life threatening.

B. Major age-related changes to the respiratory system:
1. Breathing mechanics: lungs lose elasticity; muscles become rigid and lose muscle mass and strength
2. Oxygenation: increased ventilation and perfusion are imbalanced; increased dead space in the lungs and a decrease of alveolar surface area
3. Ventilation control: decreased reaction of peripheral and central chemoreceptors to hypoxia and hypercapnia
4. Immune response: decrease of cilia; decreased ability to clear mucus secretions, decreased ability to cough and deep breathe, and a decreased immune response
5. Exercise capability: decrease of strength and muscle mass in the body
6. Breathing ability: decreased reaction to hypoxemia and hypercapnia

HESI Hint • With aging, the muscles that operate the lungs lose elasticity so that respiratory efficiency is reduced. Vital capacity (the amount of air brought into the lungs at one time) decreases. Breathing may become more difficult after strenuous exercise or after climbing up several flights of stairs. The rate of decline has been found to be slower in persons who are more active. The nurse should encourage older persons to remain physically active for as long as possible. Declining muscle strength may impair cough efficiency.

Nursing Assessment (Data Collection)

A. Confusion (may be the first sign of respiratory infection)
B. Vital signs for elevated temperature and blood pressure
C. Lungs for congestion or atelectasis
D. Vital capacity
E. Dyspnea and fatigue (COPD)
F. Cough reflex and sputum production

HESI Hint • COPD is the major cause of respiratory disability in the older adult.

Analysis (Nursing Diagnoses)

A. Ineffective breathing pattern related to . . .
B. Impaired gas exchange related to . . .
C. Ineffective airway clearance related to . . .
D. Activity intolerance related to . . .

Nursing Plans and Interventions

A. Encourage the client to receive the pneumonia vaccine every 5 years from initial dose until the age of 65. If the client receives the pneumonia vaccine after 65, a booster is not necessary.
B. Reinforce the importance of a yearly influenza vaccine.
C. Stress good hand washing and regular oral hygiene.
D. Remember that hypoxia can be manifested as confusion.
E. If the client is a smoker, encourage him or her to stop. (Regardless of age, both cardiovascular and respiratory statuses improve with smoking cessation and exercise.)
F. For the older postoperative clients, turning, deep breathing, and use of an incentive spirometer are imperative to help prevent complications.
G. Encourage deep breathing. Teaching breathing techniques, such as pursed lip breathing, can facilitate respirations.

Gastrointestinal System

A. Age-related changes are bothersome and can affect comfort, function, and quality of life but are rarely a direct cause of death.
B. Decreased saliva and dry mouth (xerostomia) are common.
C. Dental caries (tooth decay) and loss of teeth increase, resulting in decreased ability to chew food.
D. Hunger sensations decrease due to diminishing taste buds.
E. Relaxation of the lower esophageal sphincter or a sliding hiatal hernia increases the risk for GERD and aspiration.
F. The production of pepsin and hydrochloric acid decreases.
G. Delayed gastric emptying makes digestion of large amounts of food difficult.
H. Decreased peristalsis and decreased absorption in the small intestine of protein, fats, minerals (calcium), vitamins B_1 and B_2, and carbohydrates contribute to constipation problems.
I. Decreased enzyme production in the liver affects drug metabolism and detoxification processes.
J. Weight changes, especially weight loss, can be early indicators of health problems.

HESI Hint • The following are changes that occur with aging that contribute to chronic constipation:
• The number of enzymes in the small intestine is reduced, and simple sugars are absorbed more slowly, resulting in decreased efficiency of the digestive process.
• Smooth muscle content and muscle tone of the wall of the colon decrease. Anatomic changes in the large intestine result in decreased intestinal motility.

Continued

- Psychologic factors, as well as abuse of over-the-counter laxatives, can contribute to constipation.
- Decreases in fluid intake and mobility contribute to constipation.

illnesses that suppress appetite, hospitalization and surgery, difficulty chewing, alcohol use, cognitive changes, depression, grief, loneliness, social isolation, and problems with food procurement. An early sign of nutritional problems may be changes in weight.

Nursing Assessment (Data Collection)

A. Brittle teeth caused by thinning enamel
B. Receding gums resulting from periodontal disease (major cause of tooth loss after age of 30)
C. Decrease in taste and olfactory sensation as well as appetite
D. Dry mouth caused by a decrease in saliva production
E. Elimination pattern for evidence of constipation or diarrhea
F. Poor tolerance of high-fat meals and poor absorption of fat-soluble vitamins
G. Decreased glucose tolerance
H. Fluid intake

HESI Hint Tooth loss is *not* a normal aging process. Good dental hygiene, good nutrition, and dental care can prevent tooth loss.

Analysis (Nursing Diagnoses)

A. Constipation related to . . .
B. Excess or deficient fluid volume related to . . .
C. Impaired oral tissue mucous membrane related to . . .
D. Imbalanced nutrition: less than/more than body requirements related to . . .

Nursing Plans and Interventions

A. Encourage good oral hygiene (the use of a soft toothbrush, dental floss, and regular dental visits).
B. Monitor for proper fit of dentures.
C. Educate older clients about hidden sodium (canned soups, antacids, over-the-counter medications).
D. Promote adequate bowel functioning:
   1. Determine what is "normal" GI functioning for each individual.
   2. Increase fiber and bulk in the diet.
   3. Provide adequate hydration.
   4. Encourage regular exercise.
   5. Encourage eating small, frequent meals.
   6. Discourage the use of laxatives and enemas.
   7. Document bowel movements: frequency and consistency.
F. Encourage use of different spices to increase taste sensation.

HESI Hint Poor or inadequate nutrition and malnutrition are significant concerns in the older adult. Some reasons for poor nutrition include chronic

Genitourinary System

There are functional and structural changes as well as psychosocial changes in the older adult pertaining to the urinary system.

HESI Hint Older persons have a higher risk of developing renal failure because normal age-related changes result in compromised renal functioning. The nurse should pay careful attention to urinary output in older clients because it is the first sign of loss of renal integrity.

Physiologic Changes
Kidney

A. Size and weight of the kidney decrease due to reduced renal tissue growth.
B. Glomerular filtration rate decreases due to a decrease in renal blood flow resulting from lower cardiac output. Decreased renal clearance of drugs is the result.
C. Tubular function diminishes.
D. Increased risk for reflux of urine into the ureters.
E. Chronic diseases such as atherosclerosis and hypertension also decrease renal functioning in older adults.

Nursing Assessment

A. Signs of dehydration or electrolye imbalance:
   1. Skin turgor
   2. Intake/output
   3. Confusion
   4. Concentrated urine
B. Laboratory values:
   1. Proteinuria
   2. Increased BUN and creatinine
   3. Presence of blood in urine

Analysis (Nursing Diagnoses)

A. Risk for electrolyte imbalance related to . . .
B. Risk for imbalanced fluid volume related to . . .
C. Impaired urinary elimination related to . . .
D. Risk for ineffective renal perfusion related to . . .

Nursing Plans and Interventions

A. Encourage an intake of at least 2 to 3 liters of fluid daily, if not contraindicated.
B. Instruct client about signs and symptoms of dehydration and to contact health care provider immediately.

Continued

C. Instruct client about the importance of completing antibiotics until the entire prescription is gone, even if symptoms go away.
D. Write out antibiotic schedule, including any special instructions. Print in large letters.

Bladder

Nursing Assessment (Data Collection): Age-Related Changes

A. The capacity of the bladder decreases by one half, resulting in urinary frequency and nocturia.
B. Emptying the bladder may become difficult because of a weakening of the bladder and perineal muscles and a decrease in sensation or urge to void. (Consequently, UTIs become common because of residual urine in the bladder.)
C. Increased frequency and dribbling occur in men because of a weakened bladder and enlarged prostate.
D. Prostatic enlargement may cause urinary retention and bladder infection in males.
E. Women may experience stress incontinence.

Analysis (Nursing Diagnoses)

A. Disturbed personal identity related to . . .
B. Sexual dysfunction related to . . .
C. Risk for impaired skin integrity related to . . .
D. Disturbed sleep pattern related to . . .

Nursing Plans and Interventions

A. Initiate a bladder-training program if indicated.
B. Encourage older women to void at first urge when possible.
C. Initiate a skin care program if incontinence is present.
D. Provide methods of dealing with incontinence. Kegel exercises can help.
E. Teach to avoid sleeping pills and sedation, which may cause nocturnal incontinence.
F. Teach to avoid caffeine because it promotes diuresis.

HESI Hint • Kegel exercises consist of tightening and relaxing the vaginal and urinary meatus muscles. These exercises have been very successful in reducing the incidence of incontinence. They must be done consistently, but they can be done unobtrusively.

HESI Hint • Older adults with incontinence may seek isolation, thereby predisposing themselves to loneliness.

HESI Hint • Fifteen percent to 30% of community-based older adults and almost 50% of older adults living in nursing homes suffer from difficulties with bladder control. They may be more sensitive to alcohol and caffeine because these substances inhibit the production of antidiuretic hormone (ADH).

HESI Hint • MEDICATION ALERT! As one ages, the total number of functioning glomeruli decreases until renal function has been reduced by nearly 50%. This decrease in the filtration efficiency of the kidneys has grave implications for persons who are taking medication. Of particular importance are penicillin, tetracycline, and digoxin, which are primarily cleared from the bloodstream by the kidneys. These drugs remain active longer in an older person's system.

Reproductive System

A. Age-related changes are related to hormonal and nervous system control.
B. Age-related changes affect women more than men:
1. Women's ovarian function decreases; breast tissue involutes.
2. Ovaries and the uterus slowly atrophy, and neither may be palpable.
3. Perineal muscle weakness and atrophy of the vulva occur with age.
4. Vaginal mucous membrane becomes dry, elasticity of tissue decreases, surface becomes smooth, and secretions become reduced and more alkaline.
5. Libido may or may not decline.
C. Age-related changes in men include:
1. Testes atrophy, lose weight, and soften.
2. Erection changes are seen.
3. Prostate enlargement due to changes in testosterone levels.
4. Testosterone production decreases and libido can decline.

Nursing Assessment: Women

A. Vital signs (temperature), discharge, or labial or vulvar redness and pruritus for possible infections (vaginitis)
B. Complaints of hot flashes, mood swings, or night sweats
C. Dyspareunia (painful intercourse)

Nursing Assessment: Men

A. Monitor for complaints of urinary problems; prostate enlargement.
B. Monitor testosterone hormone levels.

Analysis (Nursing Diagnoses)

A. Disturbed body image related to . . .
B. Anxiety related to . . .
C. Sexual dysfunction related to . . .
D. Impaired urinary elimination related to . . .

Continued

Nursing Plans and Interventions: Women

A. Teach client signs of vaginitis; report and treat if present.
B. Promote perineal care as needed.
C. Prescription creams can help with vaginal dryness.
D. Encourage client to obtain mammogram per guidelines.

Nursing Plans and Interventions: Men

A. Encourage annual digital examination for early identification of prostate cancer.

Neurologic System

Neurologic disorders are the major cause of disability in older adults. Dementia, cerebrovascular disorders, and movement disorders (e.g., Parkinson's disease) are the major disorders in this category (see Medical-Surgical Nursing, p. 144).

A. The nervous system is the most complex of all systems and functions alone and in conjunction with many systems.
B. There is a decrease of neurons and neurotransmitters in the brain, which do not regenerate.
C. The neurologic system consists of two main components: the central nervous system (CNS) and the peripheral nervous system (PNS): decrease in both the CNS and PNS functioning.
D. Intelligence remains constant in a healthy older adult.
F. Central processing decreases; performance of tasks is slower.
G. Peripheral nervous system changes in aging people may include the following:
  1. Significantly lower or nonexistent vibratory senses in the lower extremities
  2. Decrease of tactile sensitivity
  3. Loss of connection in nerve endings in the skin
  4. Loss of proprioception, affecting balance

> **HESI Hint** • Alzheimer's disease is the most common irreversible dementia of old age. It is characterized by deficits in attention, learning, memory, and language skills. Discuss the problems family members have in dealing with Alzheimer's clients in relation to the following disease manifestations:
> • Depression
> • Night wandering
> • Aggressiveness or passiveness
> • Failure to recognize family members
> • Living in the past

Nursing Assessment (Data Collection)

A. Comprehensive functional assessment; weaknesses, tremors, and gait disturbances
B. History of falls
C. Pain, headaches, ROM, and neuropathies in extremities

D. Sudden changes in vision, cognition, and muscle weakness
E. Depression

Analysis (Nursing Diagnoses)

A. Risk for ineffective cerebral tissue perfusion related to . . .
B. Impaired verbal communication related to . . .
C. Risk for injury related to . . .
D. Risk for falls related to . . .

Nursing Plans and Interventions

A. Perform a complete mental status exam, including depression.
B. Screen for cognitive impairment.
C. Monitor blood pressure and hydration statuses.
D. Request physical and occupational service evaluations, if indicated.
E. Provide assistive devices as needed for ambulation.
F. Encourage walking, ROM, and balance exercises.
G. Teach individual relaxation techniques, stress management, and adaptive self-care management.
H. Minimize potential sources of injury in the environment.
I. Educate family and caregivers about support groups and other resources (agencies).
J. Allow as much autonomy as possible.

> **HESI Hint** • Strokes from cerebral thrombosis are more common in older persons than are strokes from cerebral hemorrhage.

> **HESI Hint** • Normal loss of brain cells is compounded by alcohol, smoking, and breathing polluted air. In relation to such losses, the nurse should teach older clients to shop at less crowded times in stores that are familiar to them, slow down well in advance of traffic signals, stay in the slower lane of the freeway, avoid freeways during rush hours, and leave for appointments well ahead of time.

Endocrine System

In the older adult, glands atrophy and decrease the rate of secretion. The impact is unclear, except it is more prevalent in women than in men due to the decline of estrogen, which causes menopause.

A. Endocrine system consists of the thyroid, parathyroid, pituitary, adrenal, and pineal glands; the thymus; and the pancreas.
B. Thyroid activity decreases (see Medical-Surgical Nursing, Hypothyroidism, p. 114). Symptoms are commonly undiagnosed in the older adult because they are attributed to being "normal for age."
C. Metabolic rate slows.

D. Estrogen production ceases with menopause; ovaries, uterus, and vaginal tissue atrophy.

E. Gonadal secretion of progesterone and testosterone decreases.

G. Insulin production decreases or insulin resistance increases.

H. T_4 (thyroxin) and T_3 (thyroid stimulating hormone; TSH) levels decrease and appear to be age related. Production of parathyroid hormone decreases, which is made evident by osteoporosis.

J. Adrenal changes may affect circadian patterns of adrenocorticotrophic hormone (ACTH).

Nursing Assessment

A. Signs and symptoms of diabetes in older adults; dehydration and confusion

B. History of recurrent infections, fatigue, nausea, delayed wound healing, and paresthesias

C. Weight loss or gain without change in eating pattern

D. Laboratory values; hemoglobin AIc, aldosterone, and cortisol levels

E. Bone density testing

F. Sleeping pattern

G. Depression

Analysis (Nursing Diagnoses)

A. Risk for imbalance in body temperature related to . . .

B. Risk for electrolyte imbalance related to . . .

C. Imbalanced nutrition related to . . .

D. Disturbed sleep pattern related to . . .

E. Risk for unstable glucose levels related to . . .

Nursing Plans and Interventions

A. Encourage thyroid testing for older clients who seem depressed. Hypothyroidism is often "dismissed" as depression.

B. Refer to Medical-Surgical Nursing, Hypothyroidism, p. 114.

C. Elderly clients may have difficulty with "lifelong" medication regimens. Develop memory cues for medications and caution against abrupt withdrawal.

D. See Medical-Surgical Nursing, Diabetes, p. 117.

E. Encourage annual physical examination with routine laboratory values.

F. Encourage annual eye examinations.

G. Teach daily foot care and monthly toenail care.

> **HESI Hint** • The most common endocrine disorders in the older adult are thyroid dysfunctions and diabetes.

Musculoskeletal System

Description: Age-related changes in the musculoskeletal system are gradual but have a significant impact on levels of mobility, which put older adults at risk for falls and fractures.

A. The musculoskeletal system is composed of bones, joints, tendons, ligaments, and muscles.

B. Age-related changes are not life threatening but can affect function and quality of life.

C. Bone loss begins around age 40 and is more common in women than in men; thus, osteoporosis occurs more often in women. (See Medical-Surgical Nursing, p. 61.)

D. There is a shortening of the trunk due to thinning of vertebral disks.

E. Loss of bone calcium, atrophic cartilage, and muscle occurs.

F. Bone mineral density (BMD) decreases, resulting in osteopenia and osteoporosis.

G. Range of motion (ROM) of joints decreases.

H. Progressive loss of cartilage occurs, resulting in osteoarthritis.

I. Muscle cells are lost and not replaced.

J. Lean body mass decreases with increased body fat.

Nursing Assessment

A. Dietary intake of calcium and vitamin D

B. Weight; underweight or overweight

C. Lifestyle habits; inappropriate nutrition, smoking, and inadequate exercise

D. History of fractures

E. ROM

F. Pain and chronic pain management strategies

Analysis (Nursing Diagnoses)

A. Acute/chronic pain related to . . .

B. Risk for disuse syndrome related to . . .

C. Risk for injury related to . . .

D. Impaired physical mobility related to . . .

Nursing Plans and Interventions

A. See Medical-Surgical Nursing, Osteoporosis, p. XXX.

B. Teach that adequate calcium intake may help lessen osteoporotic changes.

C. Establish muscle-strengthening program (small weights, aquatic therapy).

D. Prevent accidents by ensuring a clutter-free, safe environment.

E. Provide adequate lighting day and night to prevent falls.

F. Teach clients not to back up but to turn around to move in the direction they wish to go.

G. Teach clients to walk looking straight ahead instead of looking down at their feet to optimize balance.

H. Encourage regular exercise inclusive of balance, weight-bearing, and low-resistance training.

I. Teach to avoid excessive joint strain.

J. Teach that medications (diuretics and sedatives) may contribute to falls.

K. Discourage excessive alcohol intake and encourage smoking cessation.

L. Encourage older people to change positions slowly to prevent orthostatic hypotension.

> **HESI Hint** • Impaired mobility, impaired skin integrity, decreased peripheral circulation, and a lack of physical activity place older adults at risk for developing decubitus ulcers.

> **HESI Hint** • Ways to help prevent/decrease the occurrence of falls:
> - Ensure adequate lighting.
> - Paint the edges of stairs a bright color.
> - Place a bell on older person's pets (because small animals can move quickly and sometimes get underfoot).
> - Wear proper footwear that supports the foot and contributes to balance (made of nonslippery materials).
> - Remove throw rugs.

> **HESI Hint** • Fractured hips and hip replacements are common in older persons. Reinforce teaching about the proper way to sit and rise after hip replacement so that the hip is not adducted and not flexed more than 90 degrees. They should not lean forward while sitting (can cause dislocation of the prosthesis).

Integumentary System

Description: Skin, hair, and nail changes occur with aging and can cause problems concerning discomfort and self-esteem.

A. Thin skin provides a less effective barrier to trauma due to a loss of subcutaneous tissue:
1. Increased risk for dehydration due to decline in lean mass and loss of body water
2. Decreased ability of the skin to detect and regulate temperature
3. Dry skin resulting from a decrease in endocrine secretion
4. Loss of elastin and increased vascular fragility
B. Keratomocytes become smaller and regeneration slows; wound healing is slower.
C. Hair loss occurs; women have increased facial hair.
D. Vascular hyperplasia causes more varicosities (brown or blue discolorations).
E. There is an increased appearance of "age spots" and/or "liver spots" and raised lesions (seborrheic keratosis).
F. Nails become brittle and thick.

Nursing Assessment

A. Skin dryness and skin tears
B. Nails for changes in shape, color, and brittleness

C. Lesions to differentiate normal from abnormal
D. Bony prominences for signs of pressure points

Analysis (Nursing Diagnoses)

A. Impaired skin integrity related to . . .
B. Risk for injury related to . . .
C. Risk for infection related to . . .

Nursing Plans and Interventions

A. Encourage the use of oils or lubricants on the skin at least twice a day.
B. Discourage the use of powder, which can be drying.
C. Teach to avoid overexposure to sunlight.
D. Encourage balanced nutrition and increased fluid intake.
E. Teach to maintain adequate humidity in the environment.
F. Teach to avoid temperature extremes.
G. Teach good foot care.
H. Observe bony prominences for signs of pressure.
I. Teach that poor peripheral circulation may slow the healing of foot and hand lesions.

> **HESI Hint** • Older, immobile adults are at an increased risk for pressure sores (decubitus ulcers).

> **HESI Hint** • Peripheral circulation decreases as one ages. Regular assessment of the feet is very important because it increases the opportunity to discover and treat skin care problems early. These problems could become more serious because of decreased circulation.

> **HESI Hint** • Older persons have dry, wrinkled skin because they lose subcutaneous fat, and the second layer of skin, the dermis, becomes less elastic.

Sensory System

Description: The sensory system consists of vision, hearing, taste, touch, and smell. Changes in the sensory system, including balance, occur gradually and are often unnoticed.

A. A loss of cells in the olfactory bulb of the brain and a decrease in sensory cells in the nasal lining occur.
B. Sensitivity to smells declines.
C. Taste perception decreases due to loss of taste buds on the tongue.
D. Tear production decreases.
E. Abnormal, progressive clouding or opacity of the lens in the eyes occurs (cataracts).
F. A partial or complete white ring encircles the periphery of the cornea (Arcus senilis).

G. Increased intraocular pressure (IOP), usually bilaterally, leads to optic nerve damage (glaucoma).

H. Hearing of high pitches diminishes first; the ability to discriminate tones is lost (presbycusis).

Nursing Assessment

A. Monitor visual and hearing acuity, as well as glasses and/or hearing aids used.

B. Eyes for cloudiness or opacity

C. Ears for wax and hearing loss

D. Evaluate dietary intake for unplanned weight loss and salt and sugar intake.

Analysis (Nursing Diagnoses)

A. Risk for falls related to . . .

B. Risk for injury related to . . .

C. Social isolation related to . . .

D. Imbalanced nutrition: less than body requirements related to . . .

Nursing Plans and Interventions

A. Provide interventions to supplement loss of sensory input.

B. Encourage social interaction.

C. Make the client's environment as safe as possible to increase orientation and decrease confusion.

D. Maximize visual and nonvisual aids, such as bright colors, large print for written material, recorded books, lighted mirror, and glasses, if applicable.

E. Encourage the use of hearing aids with frequent battery changes if applicable.

F. Encourage the use of glasses and frequent cleaning if applicable.

G. Encourage the use of artificial tears; teach to avoid rubbing and touching of the eyes (increases risk for infection).

H. Encourage regular eye exams.

I. Directly face hearing-impaired clients so they may read lips and view facial expressions.

J. Adapt ethnic favorites to dietary and taste limitations.

K. Educate the client's support system about interventions to maintain a safe and comfortable environment.

> **HESI Hint** • Diminished eyesight results in:
> - A loss of independence (ADL and driving).
> - A lack of stimulation.
> - The inability to read.
> - A fear of blindness.

> **HESI Hint** • Lower the tone of your voice when talking to an older person who is hearing-impaired. High-pitched tones (i.e., women's voices) are the first hearing to go; therefore, lowering the pitch of your voice increases the likelihood that an older person with a hearing loss will be able to hear you speak.

> **HESI Hint** • Use frequent touch to decrease the sense of isolation and to compensate for visual and auditory sensory loss.

Psychosocial Changes

Loss

A. Loss includes loss of functional ability, decreased self-image, and death of significant others (family members, friends, or pets).

B. Loss is a universal, incontestable event of the human experience.

C. Regardless of the loss, each event has the potential to cause grief and the process called bereavement or mourning.

D. Grief is an individual response and is different depending on social and cultural norms.

E. Losses may be compounded (i.e., relocation, loss of support network, economic changes, and/or role changes), causing bereavement overload.

> **HESI Hint** • Older people undergo a great many changes, which are usually associated with loss (loss of spouse, friends, career, home, health, etc.). Therefore, older people are extremely vulnerable to emotional and mental stress, depression, and substance abuse.

Nursing Assessment

A. Any loss or losses

B. The older adult's day-to-day functioning—for example, eating and sleeping patterns

C. Level of depression and suicide risk

D. The support system in place to assist with loss

E. Ability to express emotions related to the loss or losses

F. Feelings of uselessness and nonparticipation in social events

G. Loss of income that affects health care needs and quality of life

H. Alcohol consumption on a daily or weekly basis

I. Past coping styles used with past losses

Analysis (Nursing Diagnoses)

A. Powerlessness related to . . .

B. Risk for social isolation related to . . .

C. Anxiety related to . . .

D. Grieving related to . . .

Nursing Plans and Interventions

A. Refer to grief counseling or a support group, if needed.

B. Encourage activities that allow the individual to use past coping strategies that will promote a feeling of self-worth and increased self-esteem.

C. Encourage the individual to share his or her feelings.
E. Encourage socialization with peers and reminiscing about significant life experiences.

> **HESI Hint** • Consider including review of medications (prescribed and OTC) and/or polypharmacy as possible cause for altered mental status (AMS).

> **HESI Hint** • *Integrity versus despair* is Erikson's final stage of growth and development. Reminiscing is a means of setting one's life in order (accepting life and self), which is the task of this stage of Erikson's development theory. The goal of this stage is to feel a sense of meaning in one's life rather than feel despair or bitterness that life was wasted. The major task of old age is to redefine self in relation to a "changed role." Those persons who had been in charge of situations most of their lives may now find themselves in dependent positions. Role adjustment is a major task of old age.

> **HESI Hint** • Think about the following situations and discuss the nursing care for each:
> - A nursing supervisor has a stroke and is sent to a long-term facility for rehabilitation.
> - An oil company executive retires after 42 years with the company to travel in his recreational vehicle with his wife and dog.
> - Shortly after their 53rd wedding anniversary, a woman who has never worked outside the home loses her husband to brain cancer.

Dementia

> **HESI Hint** • There are many conditions that can imitate dementia in the older adult. A key role for the nurse is to be observant to rule out other possible causes.

Description: The permanent, progressive impairment in cognitive functioning manifested by memory loss (both long-term and short-term) and accompanied by impairment in judgment, abstract thinking, and social behavior.
A. Characterized by the following:
1. Personality changes
2. Confusion
3. Disorientation
4. Deterioration of intellectual functioning, loss of memory

5. Decline of appropriate judgment and activities of daily living (ADLs)
B. The four As of cognitive impairment are agnosia, amnesia, apraxia, and aphasia.
C. Types of dementia:
1. **Alzheimer's disease:** The brains of individuals with Alzheimer's have an abundance of beta amyloid plaques, neurofibrillary tangles, and atrophic brain cells and tissue. Alzheimer's disease is the most common brain disorder and is one of the leading causes of death in the older adult.
2. **Vascular or multifocal dementia:** Ischemic brain lesions develop as a result of a history of hyperlipidemia, hypertension, smoking, or obesity.
3. **Dementia with Lewy bodies (DLB):** Microscopic deposits develop in the brain that damage nerve cells.
4. **Frontotemporal dementia (Pick's disease):** The frontal and temporal lobes of the brain degenerate.

Nursing Assessment
A. Memory complaints: short-term/long term; recognition of family, friends, or environment
B. Impaired physical functioning: shuffling, difficulty swallowing, and inability to perform ADLs
C. Conditions that mimic dementia
D. Unrecognized medical conditions
E. History of medications and changes

Analysis (Nursing Diagnoses)
A. Chronic confusion related to . . .
B. Self-neglect related to . . .
C. Readiness for enhanced family coping related to . . .
D. Impaired memory related to . . .

Nursing Plans and Interventions
A. Administer screening tools for depression and cognitive impairment.
B. Keep the client functioning and actively involved in social and family activities for as long as possible.
C. Maintain an orderly, almost ritualistic, schedule to promote a sense of security.
D. Maintain a regularly scheduled reality orientation on a daily basis.
1. Keep the client oriented as to time, place, and person (repeatedly).
2. Keep a calendar and clock within sight at all times.
   a. Display a calendar and clock that can be read by the older person (i.e., a clock with large numbers and a calendar that can be read by those with deteriorating vision).
   b. Be sure the date and time are accurate (i.e., keep the calendar current and the clock in working order).
E. Keep familiar objects, such as family pictures, in the older adult's environment to promote a sense of continuity and security.

F. Administer prescribed drugs to reduce emotional lability, agitation, and irritability or prescribed antidepressant, as indicated.

G. Speak in a slow, calm voice; avoid excitement.

H. Provide support and education to family and long-term caregivers.

I. Encourage end-of-life planning, including a will, DNR status, power of attorney, and funeral arrangements.

Health Maintenance and Preventive Care

Description: Diseases and conditions that affect older adults are the same as those that affect younger adults. However, in older adults, the signs and symptoms of pathology may be subtle, slow to develop, and very different from those seen in younger people (Table 8-1, *Diseases and Conditions in the Elderly (Older Adults)*).

Nursing Plans and Interventions

A. Encourage periodic health appraisal and counseling to prevent illness:
  1. ECG to detect subtle heart abnormalities
  2. Chest radiograph to detect tuberculosis or lung cancer
  3. Pulmonary function tests to detect chronic bronchitis and emphysema
  4. Tonometer test to measure intraocular pressure as a test for glaucoma
  5. Blood glucose to detect diabetes mellitus
  6. Pap smear to detect cancer of the cervix; digital rectal examination to detect cancer of the prostate
  7. Hearing and vision testing to detect sensory deprivation
  8. Breast self-examination and mammogram, if indicated
  9. Serum cholesterol as indicated by health status
  10. Screen at-risk older adults for bone density, thyroid functioning, and abdominal aneurysm
  11. Screen for depression and cognitive impairment
  12. Screen for BP as indicated by health status
  13. Screen for obesity
B. Promote accident prevention:
  1. Educate about safety measures to prevent falls.
  2. Encourage physical and mental activities to promote mobility and confidence.
  3. Encourage regular muscle-strengthening and balance-training exercises.
  4. Encourage the use of assistive devices when needed (e.g., cane, walker, glasses, hearing aids).
  5. Monitor driving skills.
C. Protect against infectious diseases:
  1. Encourage hand washing.
  2. Educate older adults to avoid individuals who are ill.
  3. Encourage immunization for influenza, pneumonia, and Td/Tdap.

  4. Recommend zoster; hepatitis A and B; and measles, mumps, rubella, and varicella immunizations if risk factors are present.
D. Avoid temperature extremes; prevent hypothermia.
E. Encourage the older person to stop smoking, and discourage excessive alcohol intake.
F. Educate clients about proper foot care.
G. Encourage proper nutrition and weight control.
H. Encourage social interaction and use of support services (e.g., Meals-on-Wheels) and support groups (e.g., church).
I. Discourage the use of over-the-counter medications.
J. Review all medications yearly, and encourage the client to throw away outdated drugs and prescriptions.

End-of-Life Care

Description: End-of-life care shifts care from invasive interventions aimed at prolonging life to supportive interventions that focus on control of symptoms. Insurance and hospice entities view the end-of-life stage as 6 months before death. However, a major problem with this definition is the difficulty in predicting the period of client survival. Health care providers may overestimate or underestimate survival time. End-of-life care includes the following:

A. Pain management is a priority in end-of-life care because untreated or undertreated pain consumes energy, interferes with function, affects quality of life and social interactions, and contributes to sleep disturbances, hopelessness, and loss of control.

B. Alleviating dyspnea can contribute to the client's comfort and decrease the family's anxiety. Dyspnea (distressing shortness of breath) may be related to pulmonary, cardiac, neuromuscular, or metabolic disorders; obesity; anxiety; and spiritual distress. Families need support, especially when the gurgling sound ("death rattle") occurs close to the end of life.

C. Listening, reassuring, and reinforcing nonpharmacologic interventions for helping to manage anxiety (a mild to severe subjective feeling of apprehension, tension, insecurity, and uneasiness) may need to be followed by pharmacologic agents.

D. Managing gastrointestinal symptoms of nausea, vomiting, gastritis, constipation, and diarrhea ensures comfort and quality of life.

E. Monitoring for psychiatric symptoms of depression and delirium common at the end of life and providing care as needed. If unrecognized, they can rob clients of quality of life and quality of care.

F. Recognizing the spiritual needs of the older adult can help them come to terms with their illness and the end of their life. *Spirituality* is a broad concept that encompasses the search for meaning in life experiences, relationships with others, and a sense of connectedness to a personal deity. Recognition of spiritual distress is important to help the dying client come to terms with the end of life.

TABLE 8-1 Diseases and Conditions in the Elderly (Older Adults)

Disease or Condition	Description in Terms of the Older Adult	Nursing Implications
Delirium	• Acute confused state with rapid onset, usually the result of systemic illness or medication. • Decreased level of consciousness.	• Establish a meaningful environment. • Help maintain body awareness. • Help client cope with confusion, delusions, and illusions. • See Nursing Interventions for Dementia.
Dementia	• Slow onset of symptoms. • Level of consciousness may be intact.	
Cardiac Dysrhythmias	• Incidence increases with age. • More serious in older adults because of lower tolerance of decreased cardiac output (can result in syncope, falls, TIAs, and confusion). • Symptoms result from compromised circulation and O_2 deficit.	• Monitor, prevent, and manage dysrhythmias. • Advise smoking cessation. • Encourage exercise and weight control.
Cataracts	• Often a result of normal aging changes. • Most common pathologic problem affecting the eyesight of older adults. • Treatment is surgical removal.	• Teach instillation of eye drops. • Reduce glare in environment. • Assistance is required postoperatively because affected eye is covered and disorientation may occur.
Glaucoma	• Risk of acquiring increases with age.	• Loss of sensory input can result in confusion. • Prevention: yearly pressure exams.
Macular Degeneration	• Principal cause of blindness.	• Loss of sensory input can result in confusion. • Prevention: yearly exams.
Cerebrovascular Accident (CVA) (Brain Attack)	• Interruption of cerebral circulation, caused by occlusion or hemorrhage in the brain. • Risk increases with age.	• Prevent deterioration of client's condition. • Maximize functional abilities (occupational therapy). • Assist client in accepting physical deficits. • Check gag reflex before client receives food or fluids. • Prevent injuries to paralyzed limbs.
Decubitus (Pressure) Ulcer	• Immobility puts older adults at risk for the development of decubitus ulcers.	• Reposition frequently. • Provide adequate nutrition.
Hypothyroidism	• Usually occurs after age 50. • Symptoms are often similar to normal aging changes and have an insidious onset, making it difficult to detect in older adults. • Elderly are at greater risk for development of myxedema coma, which is life threatening.	• Often diagnosed as depression; with treatment, signs of depression disappear. • Caution against abruptly discontinuing medication.
Thyrotoxicosis (Graves' Disease)	• Symptoms may be absent or attributed to other, more common diseases in older adults. • Weight loss and HF may be predominant symptoms.	• It is precipitated by stressful events such as trauma, surgery, or infection. Be alert for signs and symptoms. • Can be fatal if untreated.
COPD	• A major cause of respiratory disability in older adults. • Most older people exhibit both chronic bronchitis and chronic emphysema. • Fatigue is a common result because of the increased work required to breathe (dyspnea).	• Encourage client to stop smoking. • Keep in mind older person's state of confusion when teaching about treatment regimen. • Plan rest periods to allow client to maintain oxygen levels.
Urinary Tract Infections (UTIs)	• Their incidence increases with age. • Older people are often asymptomatic or exhibit vague, ill-defined symptoms. • With infections, older people often become confused.	• Suspect UTI when client's voiding habits change.

G. Supporting family caregivers is important because family caregivers may do everything for the client from assisting with ADLs to giving medications and managing medical equipment and treatments. Often they are the ones who serve as go-betweens for the client and health care providers. Although caregivers may find great satisfaction in their role, they often experience stress and diminished physical health.

H. Family bereavement support is essential because survivors are at an increased risk for illness or death. Normal responses to grief can be physical, psychologic, cognitive, and/or spiritual. Uncomplicated grief is a dynamic, pervasive, and highly individualized process. Individuals who are overwhelmed or remain interminably in the state of grief without progression through the mourning process to completion may be experiencing complicated grief. When the nurse identifies complicated grief, it should be reported so that a referral for help can be made to the correct provider, such as a bereavement counselor.

Review of Gerontologic Nursing

1. What are the normal memory changes that occur as one ages?
2. What three physiologic changes are clinically significant in older adults?
3. Why can the blood pressure of older adults be expected to increase?
4. What is the major cause of respiratory disability in older adults?
5. List five nursing interventions to promote adequate bowel functioning for older people.
6. What lifestyle factors negatively affect nearly every system in the older adult's body?
7. What visual problem most commonly occurs in older adults?
8. What are the three most common disorders that result from changes in the neurologic system?
9. What is the difference between delirium and dementia?
10. Falls are the result of what physiologic changes?
11. What are two factors that cause a decrease in the excretion of drugs by the kidneys?
12. What areas of care are important for end-of-life care?

Answers to Review

1. Short-term memory declines, whereas long-term memory stays the same.
2. Loss in compensatory reserve, progressive loss in efficiency of the body to repair damaged tissue, and decreased functioning of the immune system processes.
3. The heart's work increases in response to increased peripheral resistance.
4. Chronic obstructive pulmonary disease (COPD).
5. Determine what is "normal" GI functioning for each individual, increase fiber and bulk in the diet, provide adequate hydration, encourage regular exercise, and encourage eating small meals frequently.
6. Smoking, excessive alcohol intake, sedentary lifestyle (inactivity), and excessive dietary intake versus energy output.
7. Cataracts.
8. Dementia disorders, cerebrovascular disorders, and movement disorders (e.g., Parkinson's disease).
9. Delirium has a sudden onset and is reversible; dementia is a slowly progressive, irreversible disease.
10. Falls are the result of cardiovascular changes, musculoskeletal system changes, and neurologic system changes.
11. Decrease in glomerular filtration and slowed organ functioning.
12. Pain, dyspnea, anxiety, gastrointestinal symptoms, psychiatric symptoms, spirituality, support for family caregivers, and family support during bereavement period are important for end-of-life care.

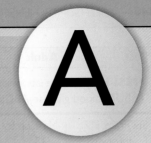

NORMAL VALUES

Test	Adult	Child	Infant/Newborn	Elder	Nursing Implications
Hematologic					
Hgb Hemoglobin: g/dL	Male: 14-18 Female: 12-16 Pregnant: >11	1-6 yr: 9.5-14 6-18 yr: 10-15.5	Newborn: 14-24 0-2 weeks: 12-20 2-6 months: 10-17 6 mo-1 yr: 9.5-14	Values slightly decreased	High-altitude living increases values Drug therapy can alter values Slight Hgb decreases normally occur during pregnancy
Hct Hematocrit: %	Male: 42-52 Female: 37-47 Pregnant: >33	1-6 yr: 30-40 6-18 yr: 32-44	Newborn: 44-64 2-8 weeks: 39-59 2-6 months: 35-50 6 mo-1 yr: 29-43	Values slightly decreased	Prolonged stasis from vasocon- striction secondary to the tourniquet can alter values Abnormalities in RBC size may alter Hct values
RBC Red blood cell count: million/mm^3	Male: 4.7-6.1 Female: 4.2-5.4	1-6 yr: 4.0-5.5 6-18 yr: 4.0-5.5	Newborn: 4.8-7.1 2-8 weeks: 4-6 2-6 months: 3.5-5.5 6 mo-1 yr: 3.5-5.2	Same as adult	Never draw specimen from an arm with an infusing IV Exercise and high altitudes can cause an increase in values Pregnancy values are usually lower Drug therapy can alter values
WBC White blood cell count: 1000/mm^3	Both sexes: 5-10	≤2yr: 6.2-17 ≥2 yr: 5-10	Newborn, term: 9-30	Same as adult	Anesthetics, stress, exercise, and convulsions can cause increased values Drug therapy can decrease values for 24 to 48 hours postpartum; it is normal to have a count as high as 25
Platelet count: 1000/mm^3	Both sexes: 150-400	150-400	Premature infant: 100-300 Newborn: 150-300 Infant: 200-475	Same as adult	Values may increase if living at high altitudes, exercising strenuously, or taking oral contraceptives Values may decrease because of hemorrhage, DIC, reduced production of platelets, infections, prosthetic heart valves, and drugs (acetamino- phen, aspirin, chemotherapy, H$_2$-blockers, INH, Levaquin, streptomycin, sulfonamides, thiazide diuretics)

Continued

Test	Adult	Child	Infant/Newborn	Elder	Nursing Implications
HESI Hint The laboratory values that are most important to know for the NCLEX-PN exam are Hgb, Hct, WBCs, Na, K, BUN, blood glucose, ABGs (blood gases), bilirubin for newborns, and therapeutic range for PT/INR and PTT.					
SED rate, ESR Erythrocyte sedimenta- tion rate: mm/hr	Male: up to 15 Female: up to 20 Pregnant: ↑ all trimesters	Up to 10	Newborn: 0-2	Same as adult	Rate is elevated during 2nd and 3rd pregnancy
PT Prothrom- bin time: seconds	Both sexes: 11-12.5 Pregnant: Slight ↓	Same as adult	Same as adult	Same as adult	Used in regulating Coumadin therapy Therapeutic range is 1.5 to 2 times normal or control
INR International Normalized Ratio	Both sexes: 0.8-1.1	Same as adult	Same as adult	Same as adult	Used to monitor anticoagula- tion therapy. INR must be individualized
PTT Partial thrombo- plastin time: seconds (see APTT)	Both sexes: 60-70 Pregnant: Slight ↓	Same as adult	Same as adult	Same as adult	It is used in regulating heparin therapy Therapeutic range is 1.5 to 2.5 times normal or control
APTT Activated partial thrombo- plastin time: seconds	Both sexes: 30-40	Same as adult	Same as adult	Same as adult	It is used in regulating heparin therapy Therapeutic range is 1.5 to 2.5 times normal or control
Blood Chemistry					
Alkaline phos- phatase: IU/l	Both sexes: 30-120	2-8 yr: 65-210 9-15 yr: 60-300 16-21 yr: 30-200	<2 yr: 85-235	Slightly higher than adults	Hemolysis of specimen can cause a false elevation in values
Albumin: g/dL	Both sexes: 3.5 to 5 Pregnant: slight ↑	4.5-9	Premature infant: 3-4.2 Newborn: 3.5-5.4 Infant 4.4-5.4	Same as adult	No special preparation is needed
Bilirubin total: mg/dL	Total: 0.3-1 Indirect: 0.2-0.8 Direct: 0.1-0.3	Same as adult	Newborn: 1-12	Same as adult	Client is to be NPO except for water for 8-12 hours before testing Prevent hemolysis of blood dur- ing venipuncture Do *not* shake tube; it can cause inaccurate values Protect blood sample from bright light

Test	Adult	Child	Infant/Newborn	Elder	Nursing Implications
Calcium total: mg/dL	Both sexes: 9-10.5	8.8-10.8	<10 days: 7.6-10.4 Umbilical: 9-11.5 10 days-2 yr: 9-10.6	Values tend to decrease	No special preparation is needed Use of thiazide diuretics can cause increased calcium values
Chloride: mEq/l	Both sexes: 98-106	90-110	Newborn: 96-106 Premature infant: 95-110	Same as adult	Do not collect from an arm with an infusing IV solution
Cholesterol: mg/dL	Both sexes: <200	120-200	Infant: 70-175 Newborn: 53-135	Same as adult	Do not collect from an arm with an infusing IV solution. Instruct client to fast 12-14 hours after eating a low-fat meal
High-density lipoprotein [HDL] (alpha lipoproteins)	Male: >45 mg/dL Female: >55 mg/dL	1 to 9 yr: 53-56 10 to 14 yr: 52-55 15 to 19 yr: 46-52	Newborn: 35	Same as adult	
Low-density lipoprotein [LDL] (beta lipoproteins)	Both sexes <130 mg/dL	1 to 9 yr: 93-100 10 to 14 yr: 97 15 to 19 yr: 94-96	Newborn: 29	Same as adult	Target LDL is <70 for client with high risk for CHD.
CPK Creatine phosphokinase: IU/l	Male: 55-170 Female: 30-135	Same as adult	Newborn: 65-580	Same as adult	Specimen must not be stored before running test
Creatinine: mg/dL	Male: 0.6-1.2 Female: 0.5-1.1	Child: 0.3-0.7 Adolescent: 0.5-1	Newborn: 0.2-0.4 Infant: 0.3-1.2	Decrease in muscle mass may cause decreased values	It is preferred but not necessary to be NPO 8 hours before testing A ratio of 20:1, BUN to creatine, indicates adequate kidney functioning
Glucose: mg/dL	Both sexes: 70-110	≤2 yr: 60-100 >2 yr: 70-110	Cord: 45-96 Premature infant: 20-60 Newborn: 30-60 Infant: 40-90	Increase in normal range after age 50	Client to be NPO except for water 8 hours before testing Caffeine can cause increased values Stress (i.e., MI, infection, general anesthesia) can cause iatrogenic hyperglycemia
Glycosylated hemoglobin (%)	Nondiabetic: 4-5.9 Diabetic Good control <7	Same	Same	Same	Used to monitor diabetic treatment Amount depends on glucose available over RBC's life span
HCO_3: mEq/l	Both sexes: 23-30	Same as adult	Infant: 20-28 Newborn: 13-22	Same as adult	None Included in assessments of electrolytes and acid base status

Continued

Test	Adult	Child	Infant/Newborn	Elder	Nursing Implications
Iron: mcg/dL	Male: 80-180 Female: 60-160	50-120	Newborn: 100-250	Same as adult	It is preferred but not necessary to be NPO 8 hours before testing
TIBC Total iron-binding capacity: mcg/dL	Both sexes: 250-460	Same as adult	Same as adult	Same as adult	None
LDH Lactic dehydrogenase: IU/l	Both sexes: 100-190	60-170	Infant: 100-250 Newborn: 160-450	Same as adult	No IM injections are to be given 8 to 12 hours before testing Hemolysis of blood will cause false positive
Potassium: mEq/l	Both sexes: 3.5-5	3.4-4.7	Infant: 4.1-5.3 Newborn: 3-5.9	Same as adult	Hemolysis of specimen can result in falsely elevated values Exercise of the forearm with tourniquet in place may cause increased potassium levels
Protein total: g/dL	Both sexes: 6.4-8.3	6.2-8	Premature infant: 4.2-7.6 Newborn: 4.6-7.4 Infant: 6-6.7	Same as adult	It is preferred but not necessary to be NPO 8 hours before testing
AST/SGOT Aspartate aminotransferase: IU/l	0-35 Female slightly lower than adult males	3-6 yr: 15-50 6-12 yr: 10-50 12-18 yr: 10-40	0-5 days: 35-140 <3 yr: 15-60	Slightly higher than adult	Hemolysis of specimen can result in falsely elevated values Exercise may cause an increased value
ALT/SGPT Alanine aminotransferase: IU/mL	Both sexes: 4-36	Same as adult	Infant may be twice as high as an adult	Slightly higher than adult	Hemolysis of specimen can result in falsely elevated values Exercise may cause an increased value
Sodium: mEq/l	Both sexes: 136-145	136-145	Infant: 134-150 Newborn: 134-144	Same as adult	Do not collect from an arm with an infusing IV solution
Triglycerides: mg/dL	Male: 40-160 Female: 35-135	Male 6-11 yr: 31-108 12-15 yr: 36-138 16-19 yr: 40-163 Female: 6-11 yr: 35-114 12-15 yr: 41-138 16-19 yr: 40-128	Male: 0-5 yr: 30-86 Female: 32-99	Same as adult	Client is to be NPO 12 hours before testing No alcohol for 24 hours before test
Urea nitrogen: mg/dL	Both sexes: 10-20	5-18	Infant: 5-18 Newborn: 3-12 Cord: 21-40	Slightly higher	None

Test	Adult	Child	Infant/Newborn	Elder	Nursing Implications
Thyroid-Stimulating Hormone (TSH, Thyrotropin) μ/mL	Both sexes: 2-10	Same as adult	Newborn: 3-18 Cord: 3-12	Same as adult	The TSH test is used to differentiate primary and secondary hypothyroidism
Triiodothyronine (T3) ng/dL	Both sexes: 70-205	1-5 yr: 105-270 6-10 yr: 95-240 ng/dL 11-15 yr: 80-215 ng/dL 16-20 yr: 80-210 ng/dL	Newborn: 100-740 Infant: 105-245	>50 yr: 40-180	Primarily to diagnose hyperthyroidism
Total thyroxine (T4) mcg/dL	Male: 4-12 Female: 5-12	1-5 yr: 7-15 5-10 yr: 6-13 10-15 yr: 5-12	Newborn: 1-3 days: 11-22 1-2 weeks: 10-16 Infant: 8-16	> 60 yr: 5-11	Newborns are screened to detect hypothyroidism so mental retardation can be prevented with early diagnosis. A heel stick is used to collect the blood
Arterial Blood Chemistry					
pH	Both sexes: 7.35-7.45	Same as adult	2 months-2 yrs: 7.34-7.46 Newborn: 7.32-7.49	Same as adult	Specimen must be heparinized Specimen must be iced for transport All air bubbles must be expelled from sample Direct pressure to puncture site must be maintained
P_{CO_2}: mmHg	Both sexes: 35-45	Same as adult	<2 yr: 26-41	Same as adult	Specimen must be heparinized Specimen must be iced for transport All air bubbles must be expelled from sample Direct pressure to puncture site must be maintained
P_{O_2}: mmHg	Both sexes: 80-100	Same as adult	Newborn: 60-70	Same as adult	Specimen must be heparinized Specimen must be iced for transport All air bubbles must be expelled from sample Direct pressure to puncture site must be maintained
HCO_3: mEq/l	Both sexes: 21-28	Same as adult	Infant/Newborn: 16-24	Same as adult	Specimen must be heparinized Specimen must be iced for transport All air bubbles must be expelled from sample Direct pressure to puncture site must be maintained

Continued

Test	Adult	Child	Infant/Newborn	Elder	Nursing Implications
O_2 saturation: %	Both sexes: 95-100	Same as adult	Newborn: 40-90	95	Specimen must be heparinized Specimen must be iced for transport All air bubbles must be expelled from sample Direct pressure to puncture site must be maintained

Urinalysis (UA)

Characteristic	Normal	Nursing Implications
Appearance	Clear	May be a midstream, clean-catch specimen Cloudy urine may be caused by the presence of pus (necrotic WBCs), RBCs, or bacteria, or ingestion of certain foods Urine that has been refrigerated for longer than 1 hour can become cloudy
Color	Yellow to amber	Pale yellow to amber color because of the pigment urochrome (product of bilirubin metabolism) The color indicates the concentration of the urine (dilute urine: straw colored; concentrated urine: deep amber and varies with specific gravity) Color can change with ingestion of certain foods or medications Urine darkens with prolonged standing
Odor	Aromatic	Diabetic ketoacidosis has the strong, sweet smell of acetone UTI, the urine may have a foul odor
pH	4.6-8.0 (average, 6.0)	Bacteria, UTI, or a diet high in citrus fruits or vegetables may cause increased urine pH
Protein	0-8 mg/dL 50-80 mg/24 hr (at rest) <250 mg/24 hr (during exercise)	Proteinuria is an indicator of renal disease Test urine of all pregnant women for proteinuria, an indicator of preeclampsia. If significant protein is noted at urinalysis, a 24-hour urine specimen should be collected so that the quantity of protein can be measured A first-voided specimen is best to test for protein
Specific gravity	Adult: 1.005-1.030 (usually, 1.010-1.025) Older adults: values decrease with age Newborn: 1.001-1.020	Renal disease tends to diminish concentrating capability Specific gravity is also a measurement of hydration status: overhydration of urine is more dilute, dehydration of urine is more concentrated
Ketones	None	Ketonuria is associated with poorly controlled diabetes Ketonuria may occur with acute febrile illnesses, especially in infants and children Special diets (carbohydrate-free, high-protein, high-fat) and some drugs may cause ketonuria
Red blood cells (RBCs)	≤2	Hematuria can be microscopic or gross Bladder, ureteral, and urethral diseases are the most common causes of RBCs in the urine
Volume		24-hour specimen is required If a 24-hour urine collection is needed, refrigerate urine during the collection period

Urinalysis (UA)—cont'd		
Characteristic	**Normal**	**Nursing Implications**
Glucose	In fresh specimen: none 24-hour specimen: 50-300 mg/24 hr	Glucose is not excreted by the kidney unless blood levels exceed approximately 180 mg/dL so can reflect the degree of glucose elevation in the blood Collect a fresh double-voided specimen In pregnancy glycosuria is common, but persistent and significantly high levels may indicate gestational diabetes or other obstetric illness
White blood cells (WBCs)	0-4 per low-power field	The presence of five or more WBCs in the urine indicates a UTI involving the bladder or kidneys, or both. A clean-catch urine culture should be done for further evaluation Vaginal discharge may contaminate the urine specimen and factitiously cause WBCs in the urine

Source: Pagana KD and Pagana TJ: *Mosby's diagnostic and laboratory test reference*, ed 10, St. Louis, 2011, Mosby.

RECOMMENDED DAILY REQUIREMENTS AND FOOD SOURCES

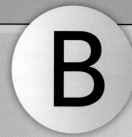

Food Sources for Fat-Soluble Vitamins	
Vitamin	**Food Source**
A	Liver, fish oils Whole milk, egg yolk, fortified margarine, and butter Dark green and deep orange fruits and vegetables—for example, apricots, broccoli, cantaloupe, carrots, pumpkin, winter squash, sweet potatoes, and spinach
D	Fortified and full-fat dairy products Egg yolks Can be synthesized in the skin when exposed to sunlight
E	Vegetable oil and their products such as salad oils, margarine, and peanuts Baby food such as peaches, apricots, and spinach
K	Green leafy vegetables such as lettuce, cabbage, spinach, peas, asparagus, and meat

Food Sources for Water-Soluble Vitamins	
Vitamin	**Food Sources**
C	Citrus fruits, cantaloupes, strawberries, tomatoes, potatoes, broccoli, green peppers, and spinach
B_1 (thiamine)	Pork, liver, whole grains, peas, eggs, milk, peanuts, oatmeal, and pasta
B_2 (riboflavin)	Milk and milk products, eggs, cheddar cheese, organ meats, and whole grains
B_3 (nicotinic acid)	Dairy products, beef, pork, fish, liver, whole grains, peanuts, and green vegetables
B_6 (pyridoxine)	Meat, liver, tuna, poultry, potatoes, wheat, and corn
Folic acid	Green leafy vegetables, broccoli, green beans, whole grains, and nuts
B_{12}	Glandular meats (such as liver), yeast, green leafy vegetables, milk, and cheese

Food Sources for Some Minerals	
Mineral	**Food Sources**
Calcium	Milk, cheese, dark green vegetables, and legumes
Phosphorus	Milk, cheese, poultry, and whole grains
Magnesium	Whole grains and green leafy vegetables
Iron	Meats, eggs, legumes, whole grains, green leafy vegetables, and dried fruit
Iodine	Marine fish, shellfish, dairy products, iodized salt, and some breads
Potassium	Citrus fruits and dried fruits, bananas, watermelon, potatoes, legumes, tea, and peanut butter
Zinc	Meats, seafood, and whole grains

Foods High in Sodium		
Vegetables	**Condiments**	**Miscellaneous**
Canned vegetables	Bouillon cubes	Bacon
Carrots, particularly canned	Mustard, prepared	Cheeses
Tomatoes, particularly canned	Olives, pickled; canned or bottled	Ready-to-eat breakfast cereals
Tomato catsup	Pickles, cucumber, dill	Peanut butters
Tomato juice	Salad dressings, commercially prepared	Soups, commercially prepared, canned
	Soy sauce	Corned beef

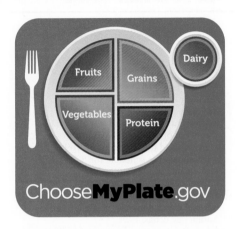

Information about healthy eating can be found at http://www.choosemyplate.gov/.

INDEX

A

AAA. *See* Abdominal aortic aneurysm (AAA)
ABC assessment, 163b
ABC rule, 70b
Abciximab (Reopro), 96t–97t
Abdomen, newborn, 252t–254t
Abdominal aortic aneurysm (AAA), 93–94
  nursing assessment (data collection) for, 93
  nursing plans and interventions for, 93
ABG. *See* Arterial blood gas (ABG)
Abortion, spontaneous, 259–260
Abruptio placentae, 261–262, 282b
Absence (petit mal) seizure, 191
Abuse, 319–321. *See also* Child abuse; Elder abuse; Intimate partner violence
Acamprosate (Campral), 316t
Acarbose (Precose), 119t–120t
Acceleration-deceleration injury, 139f
Accident
  child and adolescent deaths from, 169b
  prevention of, for elderly client, 336
Acetazolamide (Diamox), 133t
Acetyl cholinesterase inhibitor drugs, 322t
Acid-base balance, 40–42, 43t
Acid-base disorders, 41–42
Acidosis, 41, 175
Acquired immunodeficiency syndrome (AIDS)
  definition of, 49
  maternal/fetal effects of, 264t–265t
  stages of, 50t
Acrophobia, 293
ACTH. *See* Adrenocorticotropic hormone (ACTH)
Activated partial thromboplastin time, normal values for, 339
Acute glomerulonephritis (AGN), 195, 196t
Acute lymphocytic leukemia, 765, 205–206
Acute myelogenous leukemia, 150
Acute renal failure (ARF), 75–77
  nursing assessment (data collection) for, 76
  nursing plans and interventions for, 76–77
  types of, 76t
Acute respiratory distress syndrome (ARDS), 26
  nursing assessment (data collection) for, 26
  nursing plans and interventions for, 26
Acyanotic heart defect, 182–183, 185b
Acyclovir sodium (Zovirax), 52t–53t
Addison's crisis, 116b

Addison's disease, 115–116
Adenectomy, 114
Adenosine (Adenocard), 96t–97t
Adjuvant therapy, definition of, 152
Adolescent
  concept of bodily injury in, 169b
  growth and development of, 169
  immunization schedule for, 171f–172f
  pregnant, 263–266
  psychiatric disorders of, 323–325
  stages of development of, 9t
Adrenal gland, electrolyte balance and, 37
Adrenergic drugs, 179t
Adrenocorticotropic hormone (ACTH), 115, 143b
Adult
  normal values for, 339
  stages of development of, 9t
Aging
  biologic theories of, 326
  definition of, 326
  dementia associated with, 335–336
  developmental theories of, 326
  physiologic changes associated with, 326–334
  psychosocial changes associated with, 334–335
  psychosocial theories of, 326
  spine affected by, 126f
  theories of, 326
AGN. *See* Acute glomerulonephritis (AGN)
Agoraphobia, 293
Agranulocytosis, psychotropic drugs associated with, 313t–314t
Agraphia, 147b
AIDS. *See* Acquired immunodeficiency syndrome (AIDS)
Air embolism, 37
Airway obstruction, foreign body, 34–35
Akathisia, psychotropic drugs associated with, 313t–314t
Alanine aminotransferase, normal values for, 339
Albumin
  component therapy with, 31t–32t
  normal values for, 339
Albuterol (Proventil), 69t, 179t
Alcohol, newborn affected by maternal use of, 286–287
Alcohol deterrent drugs, 316t
Alcoholism, 315–316
  cirrhosis associated with, 108
  pancreatitis associated with, 110

Alexia, 147b
Alkaline phosphatase, normal values for, 339
Alkalosis, 41
Allopurinol, acute lymphocytic leukemia treated with, 206b
Alpha agonist drugs, 133t
Alpha-fetoprotein (AFP), 224
Alprazolam (Xanax), 294t
Altered state of consciousness, 136–138
  nursing assessment (data collection) for, 136
  nursing plans and interventions for, 137–138
Aluminum hydroxide/ magnesium hydroxide (Maalox, Mylanta, Riopan, Gelusil II), 103t
Alzheimer's disease
  dementia associated with, 331b, 335
  medications for, 322t
Amantadine (Symmetrel), 145t, 314t
Amikacin sulfate, 62t–65t
Amiloride (Midamor), 88t–89t
Aminoglycoside drugs, 62t–65t
Aminophylline, 69t
Amiodarone HCl (Cordarone), 96t–97t
Amitriptyline HCl (Elavil), 305t–306t
Amlodipine (Norvasc), 89t–90t
Ammonia, cirrhosis and, 108b
Ammonia detoxicant/stimulant laxative, 109t
Amnesia, psychogenic, 298
Amniocentesis, 224
Ampherotericin B (Fungizone), 52t–53t
Amphetamine/dextroamphetamine (Adderal), 324t
Ampicillin, 62t–65t
Ampicillin plus sulbactam (Unasyn), 62t–65t, 280t
Amprenavir (Agenerase), 52t–53t
Amputation, 130–132
Analgesic drugs, 56t, 240t
Analysis, disaster management and, 21
Anaphylactic shock, 28
Anemia, 149–150
  bone fracture and, 130b
  during pregnancy, 262–263
  nursing assessment (data collection) for, 149
  nursing plans and interventions for, 149–150
  pediatric, 203–204
  sickle cell, 204–205

---

b indicates boxes, *f* indicates figures, and *t* indicates tables.

Colic, 80b
Colitis, 51t
Colles fracture, 128t–129t
Colon cancer, 106–108
    nursing assessment (data collection) for, 107
    nursing plans and interventions for, 107
Colonoscopy, 107b
Colostomy, 201–202
Comminuted fracture, 127, 128t–129t, 209
Communication
    basic principles of, 289t
    effective leadership and, 16
    therapeutic, 288–292
Compartment syndrome, 209
Competency, determination of, 13
Competency hearing, 13
Complete abortion, 260
Complete fracture, 128t–129t, 209
Compound fracture, 209
Compression fracture, 128t–129t
Computer adaptive testing (CAT), 4, 6
Condom, 248t–249t
Conduct disorder, 323–325
Confabulation, 323b
Confusion, elderly client and, 323b
Congenital dislocated hip (developmental dysplasia of hip), 210–211
Congenital heart disorders, 182
    in newborn, 273
    nursing assessment (data collection) for, 184–185
    nursing plans and interventions for, 185
Congenital hypothyroidism, 206–207
Congenital/aganglionic megacolon, 201–202
Congestive heart failure (CHF), 185–186
    nursing assessment (data collection) for, 185
    nursing plans and interventions for, 186
Consciousness, altered state of, 136–138
Consent, description of, 12–13
Constipation
    in elderly client, 328b–329b
    postoperative, 48t
Continuous arteriovenous hemofiltration (CAVH), 78t
Continuous subcutaneous narcotic infusion (CSI), 56t
Contraception, 248t–249t
Conversion disorder, 296
Convulsions, preeclampsia and, 271
Coombs test, 2195
Coping styles (defense mechanisms), 288, 290t
Corticosteroid drugs, 69t, 115t
    Cushing's syndrome treated with, 116
    juvenile rheumatoid arthritis treated with, 212b
Cortisone, myasthenia gravis treated with, 143b
Courts, types of, 11t
Couvade syndrome, 219
Creatinine, 36t, 339
Creatinine phosphokinase, normal values for, 339
CRIES, pain assessment with, 170
Crime, description of, 10
Crisis intervention, 288–290
Critical pathways, 19
Critical thinking
    effective leadership and, 16
    management of care and, 18
Crohn disease, 104
Crutches, 127

Cryosurgery, 154b
Cryptococcal meningitis, 51t
CSF. See Cerebrospinal fluid (CSF)
Cushing's syndrome, 116–117
CVA. See Cerebrovascular accident (CVA)
CVS. See Chorionic villi sampling (CVS)
Cyanosis, Tetralogy of Fallot and, 184
Cyanotic heart disease, 183–184, 185b
Cyclophosphamide (Cytoxan), 196
Cycloserine, 72t–73t
Cystic fibrosis, 179–180
Cystitis, 79, 2195
Cystocele, 153–154
Cytomegalovirus (CMV), 51t
    colitis associated with, 51t
    maternal/fetal effects of, 264t–265t
    retinitis associated with, 51t
Cytoxan, myasthenia gravis treated with, 143b

D
Dalteparin (Fragmin), 92t
Damages, definition of, 11
Darifenacin (Enablex), 197t
Death rattle, 59
Death/dying, 58–60
    accidental, 169b
    nursing assessment (data collection) for, 58–59
    nursing plans and interventions for, 59–60
    signs and symptoms of, 59
Deceleration, fetal heart rate, 226f, 227
Decubitus (pressure) ulcer, 333b, 337t
Deep tendon reflex (DTR), preeclampsia and, 270–271, 272b
Defamation, definition of, 12
Degenerative joint disease (DJD), 125–126
Dehydration
    diarrhea as cause of, 175
    fluid volume deficit and, 36t
    in elderly client, 329
Delavirdine (Rescriptor), 52t–53t
Delegation
    do's and don'ts for, 18b
    effective leadership and, 16
    management of care and, 18
Delirium, 322b, 337t
Delirium tremens (DTs), 315, 318b
Delivery room, newborn care in, 238–239
Delusional disorders, 311–315
Delusional/hallucinating client, 312b
Delusions, 312b
Dementia, 322b
    aging associated with, 335–336
    description of, 337t
Dementia with Lewy bodies (DLB), 335
Denial, as defense mechanism, 290t
Dental hygiene, for older adult, 329, 329b
Dependent personality, 300
Depersonalization, 298
Depo-Provera, 248t–249t
Depression, 303–304
    nursing intervention for, 307
    pediatric, 324b
    symptoms of, 303–304, 304b
Dermis, burn injury to, 161f
Desensitization, phobia disorders treated with, 293b–294b
Desiccated thyroid (Armour thyroid), 115t
Desipramine HCl (Norpramin), 305t–306t
Desvenlafaxine (Pristiq), 305t–306t
Detached retina, 135
Detemir (Levemir), 120t–121t

Development. See Growth and development
Developmental theories of aging, 326
Dexamethasone, 115t
Dexamethasone (Decadron), 140
Dexlansoprazole (Kapidex), 103t
Dexmethylphenidate (Focalin), 324t
Dextroamphetamine sulfate (Dexedrine), 324t
Diabetes mellitus (DM), 117–124
    clinical characteristics of, 117–118
    in elderly client, 332
    maternal, nursing care for, 275
    nursing assessment of, 118
    nursing plans and interventions for, 118–124
    pregnancy and, 274–275
    treatment of, 117–118
    type 1, 117–118, 207–209
        nursing assessment (data collection) for, 207–208
        nursing plans and interventions for, 208–209
        pregnancy complications associated with, 274
        type 2 compared to, 117t
    type 2, 118, 208b
        pregnancy complications associated with, 274
        type 1 compared to, 117t
    type 3 (gestational), 274
Diabetic ketoacidosis (DKA), 118
Dialysis, types of, 78t
Diaphragm, contraception with, 248t–249t
Diarrhea, 174–176
    nursing assessment (data collection) for, 175–176
    nursing plans and interventions for, 176
Diazepam (Valium), 294t
DIC. See Disseminated intravascular coagulation (DIC)
Diclofenac potassium (Voltaren), 125t
Dicloxacillin sodium, 62t–65t, 280t
Diet. See also Nutrition
    colon cancer prevention and, 107b
    colostomy, 108
    during pregnancy, 221–222
    for Addison's disease, 116
    for anemia, 149
    hepatitis and, 110
    ileostomy, 108
    maternal diabetes mellitus managed with, 274
    recommended daily requirements for, 346t–347t
Differentiation, definition of, 152
Digitalis, 99t
Digitoxin (Crystodigin), 96t–97t, 99t
Digoxin (Lanoxin), 96t–97t, 99t, 186b
Diltiazem (Cardizem, Norvasc), 84t, 89t–90t, 96t–97t
Diphtheria, tetanus, pertussis vaccine, 171f–172f
Dipyridamole (Persantine), 92t
Disaster management
    levels of prevention in, 20
    triage in, 20
Disaster nursing, 20–25
Discoid lupus erythematosus (DLE), 125
Disopyramide phosphate (Norpace), 96t–97t
Displaced fracture, 128t–129t
Displacement, as defense mechanism, 290t
Disseminated cytomegalovirus, 49, 51t